"This *Manual of Clinical Phonetics* is an impressive collection of chapters authored by distinguished scholars from various fields of phonetic sciences. In addition to providing a comprehensive overview of the fundamentals of phonetics, capturing its inter- and multidisciplinary nature, it offers valuable insight into state-of-the-art instrumental techniques in clinical phonetics and gives phonetic transcription the attention it deserves, particularly in studying disordered speech."

— Professor Vesna Mildner, University of Zagreb, Croatia

"The *Manual of Clinical Phonetics* presents work by experts and influential researchers, communicating key concepts in clear language while drawing on cutting-edge research to convey the direction of travel for the next decade and more. The breadth of topics presented in four well-organized parts, is comprehensive. What's more, this manual pairs the core of the field (the foundations of clinical phonetics and phonetic transcription) with welcome explorations of variation. The manual also features a host of in-depth treatments of instrumentation, facilitating insightful quantitative and qualitative analyses."

— Professor James Scobbie, Queen Margaret University, Scotland

"This volume skillfully infuses a clinical perspective throughout comprehensive coverage of the science of phonetics. It is distinguished by extensive content in the area of instrumentation, including cutting-edge technologies like real-time MRI and automatic speech recognition. The choice to place multicultural and multilingual influences on phonetics at the forefront marks this volume as an essential collection for the modern scholar of clinical linguistics."

— Dr Tara McAllister, New York University Steinhardt, USA

MANUAL OF CLINICAL PHONETICS

This comprehensive collection equips readers with a state-of-the-art description of clinical phonetics and a practical guide on how to employ phonetic techniques in disordered speech analysis.

Divided into four sections, the manual covers the foundations of phonetics, sociophonetic variation and its clinical application, clinical phonetic transcription, and instrumental approaches to the description of disordered speech. The book offers in-depth analysis of the instrumentation used in articulatory, auditory, perceptual, and acoustic phonetics and provides clear instruction on how to use the equipment for each technique as well as a critical discussion of how these techniques have been used in studies of speech disorders.

With fascinating topics such as multilingual sources of phonetic variation, principles of phonetic transcription, speech recognition and synthesis, and statistical analysis of phonetic data, this is the essential companion for students and professionals of phonetics, phonology, language acquisition, clinical linguistics, and communication sciences and disorders.

Martin J. Ball is an honorary professor of linguistics at Bangor University, Wales, having previously held positions in Wales, Ireland, the US, and Sweden. He formerly co-edited *Clinical Linguistics and Phonetics* and co-edits the *Journal of Monolingual and Bilingual Speech,* as well as book series for Multilingual Matters and Equinox Publishers. He is an honorary fellow of the Royal College of Speech and Language Therapists, and a fellow of the Learned Society of Wales.

MANUAL OF CLINICAL PHONETICS

Edited by Martin J. Ball

Routledge
Taylor & Francis Group

LONDON AND NEW YORK

First published 2021
by Routledge
2 Park Square, Milton Park, Abingdon, Oxon OX14 4RN

and by Routledge
605 Third Avenue, New York, NY 10158

Routledge is an imprint of the Taylor & Francis Group, an informa business

© 2021 selection and editorial matter, Martin J. Ball

The right of Martin J. Ball to be identified as the author of the editorial material, and of the authors for their individual chapters, has been asserted in accordance with sections 77 and 78 of the Copyright, Designs and Patents Act 1988.

British Library Cataloguing-in-Publication Data
A catalogue record for this book is available from the British Library

Library of Congress Cataloging-in-Publication Data
A catalog record has been requested for this book

ISBN: 978-0-367-33629-5 (hbk)
ISBN: 978-0-367-33628-8 (pbk)
ISBN: 978-0-429-32090-3 (ebk)

Typeset in Times LT Std

Y tafawd, arawd eiriau,
Yw bwa'r gerdd heb air gau,
Arllwybr brig urddedig ddadl,
A'r llinyn yw'r holl anadl.
Guto'r Glyn 'Moliant i Rys ap Dafydd o Uwch Aeron' c.1435–1440

CONTENTS

Contents

CONTENTS

Contents

Contents

CONTRIBUTORS

Michael Ashby is an Honorary Senior Lecturer (Emeritus) in Phonetics at University College London (UCL) and President of the International Phonetic Association for 2019–2023. After graduating from Oxford, he trained in phonetics and linguistics at the School of Oriental and African Studies, London, and then at UCL, where he subsequently taught for 35 years. He was Director of UCL's Summer Course in English Phonetics, 2007–2014. Over the years, he has accepted numerous invitations to teach and lecture on phonetics across the world from Chile to Japan. His publications include a successful textbook, *Introducing phonetic science* (2005), written jointly with John Maidment. He was Phonetics Editor of five successive editions of the *Oxford Advanced Learner's Dictionary* from 1995 to 2015. His current main research field is in the history of phonetics. Michael is married to fellow phonetician Patricia Ashby.

Patricia Ashby is an Emeritus Fellow to the University of Westminster and a National Teaching Fellow of the Higher Education Academy. In addition to teaching at the University of Westminster for over 30 years, she taught phonetics and phonology all over the world, including Belgium, Germany, India, Poland, Spain, and Japan and in the UK at the universities of Reading, Oxford and UCL. She holds a PhD from UCL, and her main research interests now lie in the areas of phonetics pedagogy, English intonation and the history of phonetics. She is the author of two successful textbooks – *Speech Sounds (1995 and 2005)*, and *Understanding Phonetics (2011),* both published by Routledge. Patricia is the Examinations Secretary of the International Phonetic Association. She is married to Michael Ashby.

James Attard is an embedded Engineer and has been developing electrical commercial products since 2014. James received the Bachelor degree and MSc in Electrical Engineering from the University of Malta. His MSc studies focused on using automatic speech recognition algorithms to detect phoneme insertions, deletions and substitutions of speech impaired children. He obtained his engineering warrant in 2018 and his research interests consist of designing safety critical systems.

Harald Baayen studied general linguistics with Geert Booij in Amsterdam, and obtained his PhD degree in 1989 with a quantitative study on morphological productivity. From 1990 to 1998 he was a researcher at the Max Planck Institute for Psycholinguistics in Nijmegen,

The Netherlands. In 1998, upon receiving a career advancement award from the Dutch Science Foundation, he became associate professor at the Radboud University in Nijmegen, thanks to a Muller chair supported by the Dutch Academy of Sciences. In 2007 he took up a full professorship at the University of Alberta, Edmonton, Canada. In 2011, he received an Alexander von Humboldt research award from Germany, which brought him to the University of Tübingen. An ERC advanced grant is supporting his current research programme on discriminative learning. Harald Baayen has published widely in international journals, including *Psychological Review, Language, Journal of Memory and Language, Cognition, Complexity, Behavior Research Methods, PLoS ONE, Journal of Experimental Psychology, Journal of Phonetics* and the *Journal of the Acoustical Society of America*. He published a monograph on word frequency distributions with Kluwer, and an introductory textbook on statistical analysis (with R) for the language sciences with Cambridge University Press.

Elena Babatsouli is an Assistant Professor in the Department of Communicative Disorders at the University of Louisiana at Lafayette, the founding co-editor of the *Journal of Monolingual and Bilingual Speech*, President of the Association of Monolingual and Bilingual Speech, and founder of the International Symposium on Monolingual and Bilingual Speech. She received a BA in English from Royal Holloway, University of London, an MA in Languages and Business from London South Bank University, and a PhD in Linguistics from the University of Crete. Elena's research interests are on child/adult bilingual and monolingual (cross-linguistically) phonological acquisition and assessment, second language acquisition, speech sound disorders, culturally responsive practices in speech and language sciences, phonetics/phonology, morphology, psycholinguistics, clinical linguistics, and measures/quantitative methods. She has thirty publications, five edited books, three conference proceedings and two edited special issues in journals.

Ruth Huntley Bahr is Professor and Associate Dean for the Office of Graduate Studies at the University of South Florida. Her primary research interests include spelling and written language, phonological representations in dialect speakers and second language learners, between and within speaker variability in forensic situations, and voice production in individuals with vocal disorders. She has published numerous articles and book chapters in these areas and serves on several editorial boards. She is a Fellow in the American Speech-Language-Hearing Association (ASHA) and the International Society of Phonetic Sciences (ISPhS) and is a Board-Recognized Specialist in Child Language. She currently serves as the President and Treasurer of ISPhS and serves on the Boards of the International Association of Forensic Phonetics and Acoustics (IAFPA) and the American Board of Child Language and Language Disorders (ABCLLD).

Martin J. Ball is an honorary Professor of Linguistics at Bangor University, Wales, having previously held positions in Wales, Ireland, the US, and Sweden. He holds a PhD from the University of Wales, and a DLitt from Bangor University. He formerly co-edited the journal *Clinical Linguistics and Phonetics* and co-edits the *Journal of Monolingual and Bilingual Speech*, as well as book series for Multilingual Matters and Equinox Publishers. He has published widely in communication disorders, phonetics, sociolinguistics, bilingualism, and Welsh linguistics. Recently he completed co-editing the 4-volume *Encyclopedia of Human Communication Sciences and Disorders* for Sage publishers. He is an honorary fellow of the Royal College of Speech and Language Therapists, and a fellow of the Learned Society of Wales. He currently lives in Cork, Ireland.

Liam Barrett is working on a PhD in Experimental Psychology at University College London. He first worked on non-invasive brain stimulation in Sven Bestmann's Lab (also at University College London). Since graduating, he has worked extensively with a range of brain stimulation techniques (his current focus on work is with transcranial direct and alternating current stimulation). He has also conducted neuroimaging studies intended to understand the neural underpinnings of stuttering. The techniques include Electroencephalography and functional near infra-red spectroscopy. His current work employs machine learning to trigger forms of afferent stimulation during speech. He has presented his works at the British Psychological Society's Annual Conference and to a Special Interest Group of Speech and Language Pathologists who work on stuttering at Birmingham, UK.

Sally Bates qualified as a Speech and Language Therapist in 1998 following a PhD in Linguistics from the University of Edinburgh. Sally then gained experience in a range of pediatric settings including SureStart and a specialist provision for children with developmental language disorder before joining the SLT programme at Plymouth Marjon University as a Senior Lecturer. Sally's research focuses on speech sound disorder, the application of theory to practice and student education. She devised the online tool Webfon to support the development of phonetic transcription skills and is co-editor for the SLCN module within the Healthy Child Programme e-learning project. Sally has co-authored two speech assessment tools: PPSA (Phonetic and Phonological Systems Analysis) and CAV-ES (Clinical Assessment of Vowels – English Systems) and is a founder member of the Children's Speech Disorder Research Network (CSDRN). Sally is also author of the award winning Early Soundplay Series supporting development of phonological awareness.

Barbara M. Bernhardt, now Professor Emerita, was on faculty at the School of Audiology and Speech Sciences at the University of British Columbia, Vancouver, Canada, from 1990 to 2017. She has been a speech-language pathologist since 1972. Her primary focus is phonological development, assessment, and intervention across languages. In collaboration with co-investigator Joseph Paul Stemberger and colleagues in over 15 countries, she has been conducting an international crosslinguistic project in children's phonological acquisition (phonodevelopment.sites.olt.ubc.ca) since 2006. Other areas of expertise include the utilization of ultrasound in speech therapy, language development, assessment and intervention, and approaches to service delivery for Indigenous people in Canada.

Nicola Bessell is a lecturer in the Department of Speech and Hearing Sciences, University College Cork. After completing her PhD from the University of British Columbia, Canada, she taught and held a research position at the University of Pennsylvania, followed by a faculty position in the Linguistics Department at the University of Texas at Austin. She held a visiting teaching position at the University of California, Santa Barbara and now teaches at UCC in Ireland. She has collected data and published on several indigenous languages of the Pacific Northwest Coast, and now works on clinical data, database development and variation in Irish English.

Tim Bressmann is an Associate Professor in the Department of Speech-Language Pathology at the University of Toronto. He obtained a PhD in Phonetics from the University of Munich and an MA in Clinical Linguistics from the University of Bielefeld. Tim Bressmann's research focuses on speech production in individuals with craniofacial syndromes and head and neck cancer. He is a Section Editor of the *Cleft Palate-Craniofacial Journal* and an Associate Editor of *Clinical Linguistics and Phonetics*.

Loridana Buttigieg is a Speech and Language Pathologist (SLP) who graduated with a BSc (Hons.) degree in Communication Therapy in 2017. Loridana received the MSc degree in Communication Therapy from the University of Malta in 2019. Her special interest revolves around Speech Sound Disorders (SSD). In her postgraduate studies, Loridana evaluated the reliability and validity of an online version of an existing bilingual speech assessment, as well as the specificity and sensitivity of an automatic speech recognition system designed for Maltese children with SSD. Loridana is currently working as a SLP with the Primary Health Care and is part of the specialized division of SSD within the Speech and Language Centre.

Chiara Celata is Associate Professor of Linguistics at Urbino University, Italy, having previously held a position of post-doctoral researcher at Scuola Normale Superiore of Pisa. She has published in the sociophonetics and phonology of Tuscan Italian and Italo-Romance dialects, Italian dialect transmission in the context of long-term immigration, and phonotactic processing in Italian and German. Her recent research activity focuses on articulatory phonetics for the study and treatment of speech motor control disorders in Italian children. She is currently serving in the Executive Council of the Italian Association for the speech sciences (AISV).

Antonia Chacon works as a Speech Pathologist, Research Assistant and Clinical Educator within the Doctor Liang Voice Program. She graduated from The University of Sydney in 2016 with a Bachelor of Applied Science (Speech Pathology) Honours Class 1 and was awarded the University Medal for her academic and research achievements. Antonia is currently working upon a number of research studies within the program, which has involved the co-supervision of speech pathology honours research students. She coordinates The University of Sydney Voice Assessment Clinic to provide members of the community with comprehensive multidisciplinary voice assessment, diagnosis and recommendations, while simultaneously providing Speech Pathology students with clinical experience and insight into managing a voice disorder caseload through her role as a Clinical Educator. Beyond her role at the university, Antonia works as a Speech Pathologist within a private practice with a dominant caseload of voice disorder patients.

Yu-Ying Chuang studied phonetics with Janice Fon at the National Taiwan University in Taiwan. With a study on the perception of phonetic and dialectal variation in Taiwan Mandarin, she obtained her PhD degree in 2017. In the same year, she joined the Quantitative Linguistics group at the University of Tübingen, Germany. She is currently a postdoctoral researcher for the ERC advanced grant awarded to Harald Baayen. Her research focuses on the development of computational models for lexical processing with the framework of discriminative learning. Her published work can be found in journals such as *Behavior Research Methods* and *Lingua Sinica*.

Joanne Cleland, PhD, is a Speech and Language Therapist and a Senior Lecturer at the University of Strathclyde in Glasgow. Her main interests are in clinical phonetics and articulatory analysis, mostly using ultrasound tongue imaging. Her research focuses on visual biofeedback techniques for the assessment and treatment of motor speech disorders with a particular interest in speech disorders in children, particularly in children with developmental disabilities. Joanne is the chair of the Child Speech Disorder Research Network and the secretary of the International Clinical Phonetics and Linguistics Association. Recent publications include a systematic review of ultrasound biofeedback studies (https://pureportal.strath.ac.uk/en/publications/systematic-review-of-ultrasound-visual-biofeedback-in-interventio) and an investigation into whether using ultrasound tongue imaging can improve the reliability of transcription of cleft palate speech (https://pureportal. strath.ac.uk/en/publications/the-impact-of-real-time-articulatory-information-on-phonetic-tran).

John Costello, MA, CCC-SLP, has been a Speech Language Pathologist specializing in the area of Augmentative and Alternative Communication at Boston Children's Hospital (BCH) for 35 years. He is the Director of the Augmentative Communication Programs at BCH and an Adjunct Faculty member of Boston University. He has extensive experience in all aspects of augmentative and alternative communication (AAC), and has played many leadership roles in the International Society for AAC. Over the past two decades, he has led the field in innovations to support preservation of self and of dignity in the face of severe communication impairments. He has published in peer reviewed journals and has presented widely internationally on many different aspects of AAC.

Catia Cucchiarini holds a PhD from Radboud University, where she is now Principal Investigator in the research group Language and Speech, Learning and Therapy and the Centre for Language and Speech Technology. She worked at KU Leuven in Belgium and is now Senior Advisor at The Union for the Dutch Language in the Hague. She is a member of the editorial board of Computer Assisted Language Learning and advisor to the Dutch Organization for Language and Speech Technologies. She has conducted research on phonetic transcription, speech processing, language resources, language learning and speech technology applications in Computer Assisted Language Learning and e-health, for which she received several national and international grants.

Simon G. Fabri received the Bachelor degree in Electrical Engineering from the University of Malta, and the MSc and PhD degrees in Control Systems from the University of Sheffield, UK. He is currently Professor of Automatic Control Engineering at the University of Malta. His research interests include adaptive and intelligent control, artificial intelligence, nonlinear and stochastic control, systems modeling, signal processing and robotics. He has published numerous peer reviewed articles and co-authored a Springer textbook on Intelligent Control Systems. He is an Associate Editor of the *International Journal of Systems Science.*

Philip Farrugia received the B.Eng. (Hons) degree from the University of Malta (UM) in 2001 with First Class Honours and a PhD degree in product design from the same university. He is an Associate Professor at the Department of Industrial and Manufacturing Engineering (DIME) at UM. Philip has attracted over 1.3MEuros in research funding from various programmes, including Horizon2020, aimed at developing mostly medical devices, smart therapeutic and rehabilitation products. Prof. Ing. Philip Farrugia coordinated the taught Masters course in integrated product development managed by DIME for ten years. He has published over fifty peer reviewed research papers in fields related to product development. His current research interests revolve around the development of high-value added products and innovative product service systems for healthcare.

Janice Fon is currently an Associate Professor of Linguistics at the National Taiwan University. Trained as a phonetician and psycholinguist at The Ohio State University, she has always been mesmerized by the intricate nature of phonetic variation, and has focused on variants due to language contact at both production and perception levels. As variants are often more manifest in daily conversation, she also constructed a Taiwan Mandarin-Min bilingual spontaneous speech corpus, which holds more than 250 one-hour spontaneous language samples of Mandarin-Min bilinguals in Taiwan. She has received several national research awards and her publications include papers in *Language and Speech, Language and Linguistics, Journal of Chinese Linguistics* and *Lingua Sinica*, in addition to several book chapters.

Robert Allen Fox is a Professor and Chair in the Department of Speech and Hearing Science at The Ohio State University. He received a PhD in Linguistics from the University of Chicago and has held positions in Linguistics and Speech and Hearing Science at Ohio State. His research involves sociophonetics, speech perception, speech acoustics and second-language acquisition. He is the author or co-author of numerous publications and presentations in these areas. He was an associate editor for speech perception for the *Journal of the Acoustical Society of America*. He is a fellow of the Acoustical Society of America, and a fellow of the American Speech-Language-Hearing Association. He also served as a member of the Executive Board of Council of Academic Programs in Communication Science and Disorders, as a statistical consultant for several publishers, and as an expert witness in forensic phonetics.

Mária Gósy is Professor of Phonetics and Psycholinguistics at Eötvös Loránd University, and research consultant at the Linguistics Institute of the Eötvös Loránd Research Network. Her research areas cover various topics, with a main focus on speech processing, spontaneous speech production processes, and typical and atypical language acquisition. She teaches various courses at the university and is the Head of the Applied Linguistics Doctoral Program. She is a member of national and international committees, editorial boards, Secretary-General of the International Society of Phonetic Sciences (ISPhS) and works as Editor-in-Chief for the ISPhS journal, *The Phonetician*. She has published 12 books and more than 390 scientific papers in Hungarian and English. She has received various awards, including the Officer's Cross of the Order of Merit of the Hungarian Republic.

Professor **Helen Grech** is a registered audiologist and speech-language pathologist. She was awarded the PhD degree in 1998 by the University of Manchester, UK. Helen Grech has headed the Department of Communication Therapy within the Faculty of Health Sciences of the University of Malta, for 28 years. Her research interests are speech and language acquisition and disorders in multilingual populations. Helen Grech is involved in cross-linguistic research projects and Inter-Governmental COST Actions. She was awarded several research grants by the European Commission and is a regular reviewer of research proposals funded by the European Commission and other national agencies. She is a former President and an Honoured member of the International Association of Logopedics and Phoniatrics.

Christina Hagedorn is an Assistant Professor of Linguistics and director of the Motor Speech Laboratory at the City University of New York – College of Staten Island. She received her PhD in Linguistics from the University of Southern California, where she was a member of the Speech Production and Articulation Knowledge (SPAN) Group and the USC Phonetics and Phonology Group. She received her clinical training in Communicative Sciences and Disorders at New York University, and holds a certificate of clinical competency in Speech and Language Pathology (CCC-SLP). Her research aims to shed light on the precise nature of articulatory breakdowns in disordered speech and how this can inform theories of unimpaired speech production, as well as lead to the refinement of therapeutic techniques. Her current work focuses on both articulatory coordination patterns in apraxic speech and articulatory preservation and compensation mechanisms exhibited by oral and base of tongue cancer patients.

Gregory J. Hedlund is a Programmer at Memorial University (Newfoundland, Canada). His work focuses primarily on corpus creation and analysis software for research in linguistics, primarily in phonology and phonetics. As lead programmer, he has been an integral part of the design and development of the Phon open source software program and supporting utilities (https://www.phon.ca). He has also collaborated with members of the CHILDES project (https://childes.talkbank.org) on the TalkBank (https://talkbank.org) and PhonBank (https://phonbank.talkbank.org) database formats.

Peter Howell is Professor of Experimental Psychology at University College London where he has worked for most of his professional career. His main areas of interest are hearing and speech and he has published extensively in both of them. A particular interest throughout his career has been the relationship between speech perception and production. In early investigations he worked on explanations about why auditory perturbations whilst a person is speaking affect vocal control. This led to his discovery of the fluency-enhancing effects of frequency-shifted feedback on people who stutter that is incorporated in many contemporary prostheses. He has worked extensively on stuttering. Books he has authored include *Recovery from stuttering* and *Signals and Systems for Speech and Hearing Sciences*. His current interests include brain scanning and neurostimulation.

Ewa Jacewicz is a Research Associate Professor in the Department of Speech and Hearing Science at The Ohio State University. She holds a PhD from the University of Wisconsin-Madison, followed by a postdoctoral research fellowship from the National Institutes of Health. She has published on a wide range of topics in sociophonetics, speech perception and acoustics, speech development in late childhood and communication disorders. Her research interests are in phonetic variation and intelligibility of speech in the context of sociocultural dynamics and generational sound change. She was an associate editor for the *Journal of Speech, Language and Hearing Research* and served as an editorial board member for this journal. She is currently an associate editor for the *Journal of the Acoustical Society of America*.

Esther Janse is an Associate Professor in the Language and Communication department at Radboud University Nijmegen, the Netherlands. She holds a PhD from Utrecht University, also the Netherlands. She coordinates the language and speech pathology track within Linguistics at Radboud University, teaching courses on spoken language processing and experimental design in Radboud's Language and Communication Bachelor, Master and Research Master programmes. Esther Janse is chair of the Dutch Phonetics Association for the Netherlands and Flanders. Her research focuses on spoken language processing in healthy and pathological populations (including persons with aphasia or dysarthria and those with severe hearing impairment). She published multiple papers on the effects of ageing and hearing impairment on the perception and production of speech in multiple speaking styles.

Marie Klopfenstein, PhD, in an Associate Professor in the Speech-Language Pathology and Audiology program, which is part of the Department of Applied Health at Southern Illinois University Edwardsville. She teaches undergraduate and graduate classes in phonetics, speech science and voice. Dr. Klopfenstein has presented and published widely on acoustic and perceptual correlates of speech naturalness. Her other research includes voice services for transgender and gender non-conforming individuals, speech rate, sonority and phonetic transcription, with current focus on populations with unmet needs and issues with accessing speech and language services.

Christian Kroos is a Cognitive Scientist and Engineer with a focus on algorithm development. He received his MA and PhD in Phonetics and Speech Communication from Ludwigs-Maximilians-Universität, München, Germany. Over the last two decades, he has conducted research in Germany (Ludwig-Maximilian-Universität), Japan (ATR, Kyoto), USA (Haskins Laboratories, New Haven, CT), Australia (Western Sydney University, Sydney, & Curtin University, Perth) and the UK (University of Surrey, Guildford), spanning experimental phonetics, computer science, cognitive science, robotics, artificial intelligence and the arts. In his speech-related research he analyzed articulatory movements and investigated auditory-visual speech. He recently started a position at Fraunhofer Institute for Integrated Circuits (Erlangen, Germany) investigating novel machine learning algorithms for signal processing.

Alice Lee is a Speech and Language Therapist and Lecturer in Speech and Hearing Sciences at University College Cork, Ireland. Her research interest and expertise include perceptual and instrumental investigations of speech disorders associated with structural anomalies and neurological impairment; listener training for auditory-perceptual judgements of speech disorders; and Cochrane Systematic Review. In terms of teaching and learning, her primary interest is teaching and assessing auditory-perceptual judgements of speech disorders and using instrumental measures for speech assessment, with secondary interest in Visual Thinking Strategies. Alice is currently a steering group member of DELAD (website: http://delad.net/), a member of the United Kingdom Child Speech Disorder Research Network (CSDRN), a member of The Cochrane Collaboration (2018-2023), and a member on the Cleft Palate and Craniofacial Committee of the International Association of Communication Sciences and Disorders (known as IALP). She served as the Editor of *Journal of Clinical Speech and Language Studies* – the official journal of The Irish Association of Speech and Language Therapists (2010–2019) and currently, she is serving as a Section Editor of the Speech Section of *The Cleft Palate-Craniofacial Journal* – the office journal of the American Cleft Palate-Craniofacial Association.

Orla Lowry is currently a lecturer in English language and linguistics at Ulster University and tutor in phonetics at Queen's University Belfast, having previously had research and teaching positions at both universities. She holds a PhD in phonetics and linguistics from Ulster University. Her research has focused largely on the intonation of Northern Irish English, its communicative intent and the implications its structural diversity from "standard" varieties of English have for existing analytic frameworks for intonation. She has also co-authored articles and books on clinical phonetics, and for the last few years has regularly acted as reviewer for the journal *Clinical Linguistics and Phonetics*.

Catherine (Cate) Madill is an Associate Professor of Voice and Voice Disorders at the University of Sydney Australia, and a Certified Practising Speech Pathologist. She is co-director of the Dr Liang Voice Program at the University of Sydney. She holds a PhD and BAppSc (Speech Pathology) (Hons) and University Medal from the University of Sydney. She is an active researcher and educator, and has published widely in voice therapy and training, acoustic analysis, laryngeal physiology and voice disorders. She has developed an award winning online learning tool to support education and research in voice and communication disorders. She serves on the editorial board of numerous international peer reviewed journals across voice, speech pathology and performing arts medicine. She is also director and senior clinician in a large metropolitan private practice specializing in assessment and management of voice and upper airway disorders.

Robert Mayr is a Senior Lecturer in Linguistics at Cardiff Metropolitan University, Wales, and a research associate at the Centre for Research on Bilingualism, Bangor University. He previously held positions at the University of Vienna, Austria and at Sheffield University, England where he also completed his PhD. Dr. Mayr has published widely in the field of speech development of bilinguals and multilinguals across the lifespan, focussing particularly on the phonetic and phonological aspects of first and second language acquisition, first language attrition and atypical development. His research uses a number of behavioral measures, including acoustic methods of analysis and psycholinguistic experimentation.

Grant McGuire is an Associate Professor of Linguistics at the University of California, Santa Cruz. He received his PhD in Linguistics from The Ohio State University and spent time as a visiting scholar and post-doctoral researcher in the Phonology Lab at the University of California, Berkeley. His research is broadly within speech perception and production, specializing in perceptual learning, voice evaluation and recall, gender perception, and the articulation of palatalization and velarization contrasts. He is currently finishing a several year National Science Foundation grant using ultrasound to investigate palatalization in dialects of Irish.

Lisa McInnis, MS, CCC-SLP, is an ASHA certified pediatric speech-language pathologist with 19 years experience. She has provided early intervention services to the birth to three population in daycare centers, home based settings, school systems and through a U.S. military hospital. Mrs. McInnis has also worked as a clinical instructor, providing supervision to undergraduate and graduate students enrolled in clinical practicum. She has private practice experience and currently works for the Acadia Parish School Board in Crowley, Louisiana, USA. As an Army wife, she has traveled and proudly served communities of soldiers and their families.

Chiara Meluzzi has a PhD in Linguistics and is a Post Doc Fellow at University of Pavia. She has previously worked for the Free University of Bolzano/Bozen and Scuola Normale Superiore of Pisa, with different research projects on sociolinguistics both synchronically and diachronically. She has worked on experimental phonetics from both an acoustic and articulatory point of view. Her teaching activity at University of Pavia includes courses in Sociolinguistics, Phonetics and Phonology, and a course in Linguistics and Phonetics for speech therapists. From 2018 she is the Principal Investigator of a sociophonetic project on child speech in a mountain Italian area. Her main publications include a book on the Italian spoken in Bolzano as a result of a koineization process (Franco Angeli, 2020, Open Access), book chapters and articles on phonetics and sociophonetics (Equinox 2018, Loquens 2018).

Nicole Müller is Professor and Head of the Department of Speech and Hearing Sciences, University College Cork, Ireland. She has previously held professorships in the United States and Sweden. Her research interests include multilingualism and neurogenic and neurodegenerative conditions leading to cognitive-communicative impairments. She formerly co-edited the journal *Clinical Linguistics and Phonetics* (Taylor & Francis) and is co-editor of the book series *Communication Disorders Across Languages* (Multilingual Matters). She has published widely in journal and book form and was awarded a Fulbright scholarship in 2014 to study bilingual Irish-English communication in a retirement home in the west of Ireland. Among her recent publications are co-edited collections on sonority and on cross-linguistic language acquisition.

Daniel Novakovic is an Australian Otolaryngologist with postgraduate dual subspecialty fellowship training in the fields of Laryngology and Head and Neck oncology. He is a fellow of the Royal Australian College of Surgeons and is current Vice President of the Laryngology Society of Australasia. He is also a member of the Australian Voice Association, American Laryngological Association and American Broncho-Esophagology Associations. He is head of ENT department at Canterbury Hospital, and Associate Professor in the Department of Otolaryngology, Central Clinical School, as well as co-director of the Dr Liang Voice Program in the Faculty of Medicine and Health at University of Sydney. Dr Novakovic has active research interests in Laryngeal Papillomatosis, laser-tissue interactions and laryngeal surgery.

Duy Duong Nguyen has trained as Otolaryngologist at Hanoi Medical University (Vietnam) and has been practicing as a laryngologist and voice specialist at the National Hospital of Otorhinolaryngology in Hanoi. He is also a lecturer in otolaryngology at Thai Nguyen University of Medicine and Pharmacy (Vietnam). He completed masters by research (2003) and PhD (2009) in voice at The University of Sydney. Currently he is undertaking various voice research projects within The University of Sydney's Doctor Liang Voice Program. His research interests combine both otolaryngology and speech pathology methods and include control and physiology of phonation, acoustic and physiologic assessment of voice, strobolaryngoscopic assessment, voice outcome measures, effects of angiolytic laser on the larynx, early diagnosis and treatment of voice disorders, and effects of voice disorders on lexical tone phonation.

Ioannis Papakyritsis is an Assistant Professor in the Department of Speech and Language Therapy at University of Patras and a certified clinician. He has worked as an assistant professor in Western Illinois University. He holds a PhD from the University of Louisiana at Lafayette. His research interests include clinical acoustic phonetics and the analysis of suprasegmentals in neurogenic speech disorders. He is teaching classes on communication disorders at under-graduate and Master's levels and he has been working as a clinical supervisor of student clinicians and as speech & language therapist. He currently lives in Patras, Greece.

Joan Rahilly is Professor of Phonetics and Linguistics in the School of Arts, English and Languages in Queen's University, Belfast where she teaches phonetics, phonology and general linguistics. Her research focuses on atypical speech, and she is particularly interested in the role of prosody in communication. She also works on the phonetics of Irish English and is currently involved in a project (with Prof. Karen Corrigan from Newcastle University) which will create an open access resource for digitally mapping the linguistic structures of Northern Irish English. She is a Principal Fellow of the Higher Education Academy, a role which profiles her commitment to professionalism in learning and teaching in higher education, and specifically to phonetics and linguistics in Northern Ireland.

Vikram Ramanarayanan is a Senior Research Scientist in the Speech and NLP Group of Educational Testing Service R&D based out of the San Francisco office, where is he is also the Office Manager. He also holds an Assistant Adjunct Professor appointment in the Department of Otolaryngology - Head and Neck Surgery at the University of California, San Francisco. His work at ETS on dialog and multimodal systems with applications to language learning and behavioral assessment was recently awarded the prestigious ETS Presidential Award. Vikram's research interests lie in applying scientific knowledge to interdisciplinary engineering problems in speech, language and vision and in turn using engineering approaches to drive scientific understanding. He holds MS and PhD degrees in Electrical Engineering from the University of Southern California, Los Angeles, and is a Fellow of the USC Sidney Harman Academy for Polymathic Study. Vikram's work has won two Best Paper awards at top international conferences and has resulted in over 75 publications at refereed international journals and conferences. Webpage: http://www.vikramr.com/

Hannah Reece has training in Speech Pathology from The University of Queensland, Australia. She works in the Centre for Neuroscience of Speech at The University of Melbourne, Australia where she is Project Manager for SpeechATAX: a multi-national, multi-language randomised controlled trial for speech rehabilitation in people with progressive ataxia.

Irene Ricci is a Technician at the Experimental Linguistics Team (ELiTe) of Scuola Normale Superiore of Pisa. She has developed skills in carrying out experiments for linguistics studies in many fields such as psycholinguistics, sociophonetics, neurolinguistics, phonetics and phonology. Recently she focused on articulatory phonetics research, exploring the use of the ultrasound technique in the study of speech motor control disorders in children.

Toni Rietveld is an Emeritus Professor in the Department of Language and Communication at Radboud University Nijmegen, The Netherlands, where he has been lecturing for MA students in Language and Speech pathology. He was a research consultant for dysartrhria and aphasia at Sint Maartenskliniek, a hospital for rehabilitation. His main areas of research are phonetics, methodology of research in speech and language pathology and teletherapy for dysarthria. His most recent book is *Human Measurement Techniques in Speech and Language Pathology*, Routledge, 2020.

Yvan Rose is Professor of Linguistics at Memorial University (Newfoundland, Canada). His research focuses primarily on the integration of perceptual, acoustic and articulatory conditioning within formal models of phonology and phonological acquisition. Interested in the development of computer-assisted methods for corpus-based analysis of phonology, (acoustic) phonetics and language acquisition, Dr. Rose has been spearheading the development of Phon, a free (open-source) software program (https://www.phon.ca). Phon also provides the computational foundation for the PhonBank database project (https://phonbank.talkbank.org), co-directed by Drs. Brian MacWhinney and Rose. PhonBank provides researchers and students access to large datasets documenting phonological development and speech disorders across different languages and speaker populations as well as tools for analyzing these data.

Ben Rutter is a lecturer in Clinical Linguistics at the University of Sheffield. He has a degree in Linguistics and Phonetics from the University of York and did his PhD in the Department of Communicative Disorders at the University of Louisiana at Lafayette under the supervision of Martin J. Ball and Nicole Müller. His research focuses on the role of phonetics in Speech and Language Therapy and he has written extensively on interactional phonetics and dysarthria. More recently he has been working on topics related to the Medical Humanities. Ben is on the editorial board for the journal *Clinical Linguistics and Phonetics*.

Martine Smith, PhD, is Professor in Speech Language Pathology in Trinity College Dublin, Ireland. Her experience in the area of AAC stretches over three decades and is grounded in her clinical experience, research focus and teaching. A Past President of the International Society for Augmentative and Alternative Communication and former Editor-In-Chief of the flagship journal *Augmentative and Alternative Communication* (2015–2019), she has published extensively in the field and has an international reputation as a researcher. Her publications include one single-author text and one edited volume (co-edited with Prof Janice Murray, Manchester Metropolitan University), as well as over 70 peer reviewed journal publications, focusing on speech, language and interaction in AAC, as well as language learning and interaction in individuals with intellectual disability.

Joseph Paul Stemberger is an Emeritus Professor in the Department of Linguistics at the University of British Columbia. His research addresses language processing (especially for morphology, phonology, phonetics and interactions between them, for adult language production and first-language acquisition), and intersects linguistics, cognitive psychology and speech-language pathology. One goal is to compare across languages and explain what is similar and what is different. Current projects focus on typical and protracted phonological development in many languages: the Valley Zapotec project, and the Cross-Linguistic project. He also does traditional dancing (English and Slovenian), is in two choirs, and likes to go hiking and cycling.

Cara E. Stepp directs the STEPP LAB for Sensorimotor Rehabilitation Engineering and is an Associate Professor in the Departments of Speech, Language, and Hearing Sciences, Otolaryngology – Head and Neck Surgery, and Biomedical Engineering at Boston University. She received the S.B. in Engineering Science from Smith College, S.M. in Electrical Engineering and Computer Science from Massachusetts Institute of Technology, and PhD in Biomedical Engineering from the Harvard-MIT Division of Health Sciences & Technology. Prior to joining BU, she completed postdoctoral training in Computer Science & Engineering and Rehabilitation Medicine at the University of Washington. Dr. Stepp's research uses engineering tools to improve the assessment and rehabilitation of sensorimotor disorders of voice and speech.

Helmer Strik received his PhD in Physics from the Radboud University, where he is now Associate Professor in Speech Science and Technology. He is co-founder and Chief Scientific Officer (CSO) of the spin-off company NovoLearning, which develops advanced speech technology solutions for e-learning and e-health. He is Chair of the International Speech Communication Association (ISCA) "Special Interest Group" (SIG) on Speech and Language Technology in Education (SLaTE, http://hstrik.ruhosting.nl/slate/). He has obtained various national and international grants for research on speech processing, automatic speech recognition (ASR), pronunciation variation modeling, spoken dialogue systems and the use of ASR technology in real-life applications for language learning and speech diagnosis and therapy.

Jill Titterington has been a lecturer in Speech and Language Therapy at Ulster University (Northern Ireland) since 2006. She has over 20 years of clinical experience (mostly as a specialist for children with hearing impairment). Jill obtained her PhD from Ulster University in 2004. She has been responsible for design and delivery of the teaching, learning and assessment of clinical phonetic transcription for Ulster's pre-registration Speech and Language Therapy programme since 2012. Jill is a member of the UK and Ireland's Child Speech Disorder Research Network, Ireland's Clinical Phonetics Teaching Network and the UK's Clinical Phonetics Teaching Network. Jill's key clinical and research interests include speech sound disorder and supporting application of theoretically informed, evidence-based management for children with speech, language and communication needs within the complex context of everyday clinical work. To that end, Jill has co-authored an online resource co-produced with speech and language therapists supporting evidence-based practice for children with phonological impairment: Supporting and understanding speech sound disorder (SuSSD): https://www.ulster.ac.uk/research/topic/nursing-and-health/caring-for-people-with-complex-needs/research-themes/neurodevelopmental/ssd (Hegarty et al. 2018).

Pascal van Lieshout is a Professor and Chair in the Department of Speech-Language Pathology in the Faculty of Medicine at the University of Toronto. He is a former Canada Research Chair in Oral Motor Function and director of the Oral Dynamics Laboratory (ODL). He studies oral motor control mechanisms in a variety of populations, aiming to understand how people produce speech and what might cause problems performing this complex function. In his 30+ year career, he has published over 180 peer-reviewed publications (journal articles, book chapters, conference proceedings). His work is highly inter- and multi-disciplinary, working with colleagues in Psychology, Engineering, Linguistics and Rehabilitation Science to ensure an optimal learning environment for trainees. He is editor-in-chief of the *Journal of Fluency Disorders* and received the Richard H. Barrett Award 2011 for his research contributions to oral motor research from the International Association of Orofacial Myology.

Adam P. Vogel is Professor and Director of the Centre for Neuroscience of Speech at The University of Melbourne where his team work to improve speech, language and swallowing function in people with progressive and acquired neurological conditions. Adam holds a PhD in behavioral neuroscience from The University of Melbourne and degrees in psychology and speech science from the University of Queensland, Australia. He is a Humboldt Fellow at the Hertie Institute for Clinical Brain Research, Tübingen, Germany. He is also Founder and Chief Science Officer of Redenlab Inc, a neuroscience technology company that uses speech and language biometrics to enhance decision making in clinical trials.

Jennifer M. Vojtech is a Research Scientist at Delsys, Inc. She has a B.S. in Bioengineering from the University of Maryland, College Park and an MS and PhD in Biomedical Engineering from Boston University. Her doctoral work in the STEPP Lab for Sensorimotor Rehabilitation Engineering with Cara E. Stepp focused on developing computational methods to improve the clinical assessment of voice disorders and applying quantitative techniques to enhance augmentative and alternative communication device access. At Delsys, Inc., Jennifer collaborates with a multidisciplinary team of scientists and engineers to design technology for evaluating and augmenting communication in those with speech and voice disorders.

David J. Zajac is Professor in the Division of Craniofacial and Surgical Care at the Adams School of Dentistry, University of North Carolina at Chapel Hill and adjunct associate professor in the Division of Speech and Hearing Sciences. He is both a clinical speech-language pathologist and speech scientist at the UNC Craniofacial Center. He has authored two books, 10 book chapters, and over 50 peer-reviewed research articles. His research on cleft palate and other speech disorders has been regularly funded by NIH since 1993.

Fei Zhao is Reader in Hearing Science and Audiology, and Programme Director for the MSc Advanced Practice degree and audiology pathway lead, currently working at the Centre for Speech and Language Therapy and Hearing Science, Cardiff Metropolitan University. Dr Zhao qualified as an ENT surgeon at Tianjin Medical University (China) in 1992. He received his

PhD at the Welsh Hearing Institute, University of Wales College of Medicine in 1998. Between 1998 and 2002, he worked as a postdoctoral fellow and research associate in Japan, USA and the UK. He previously held lectureship positions in Swansea University and the University of Bristol. Dr Zhao has published regularly in key international journals in the fields of audiology, neuroscience, cognitive psychology and bioengineering. To date, Dr Zhao has published more than 80 scientific papers in peer-reviewed journals, two co-authored books and eight book chapters.

PREFACE

When I was first studying phonetics, longer ago than I intend to admit to, it was my wish (as with many of my colleagues) to get hold of a copy of the *Manual of Phonetics,* at that point as edited by Bertil Malmberg (Malmberg, 1968). The well-thumbed library copy was the go-to source for anything more advanced than our basic introductory textbooks. Unaffordable for most of us students, personal copies of the book were out of reach for us then. Years later I was able to buy a second-hand copy of the first printing of the 1968 edition. This copy of the book is on the desk beside me as I write this Preface and provided the motivation (as well as part of the title) for a brand-new collection on clinical aspects of phonetics. Malmberg's *Manual* is similar to this collection in some respects: it too has chapters on acoustic, articulatory and auditory phonetics, it has chapters devoted to prosody and to perceptual aspects of speech, it covers a range of phonetic instrumentation. However, it differs in several respects too. There is no special coverage of transcription or phonetic symbols, chapters are provided dealing with phonology, phonotactics, phonetic aesthetics and linguistic evolution (none of which are included in this collection), and sociophonetic variation is barely considered. Naturally, the instrumental phonetic techniques that are described are those common at the time. Thus, there is almost an entire chapter on x-radiography, but just a few pages on direct palatography (as publication predated by a few years the development of affordable electropalatography systems). Interestingly, there is a chapter on speech disorders, in this case a survey of different instrumental techniques and which disorders they can be best applied to.

In this new *Manual of Clinical Phonetics* many of the topics covered in Malmberg's collection are also covered but, naturally, as this book has a different focus, there are numerous differences as well. Scholars from 15 different countries on four different continents have been brought together to cover the range of topics that clinical phoneticians need to have a grounding in if they are to describe and analyze disordered speech.

The book is divided into four parts, each with its own dedicated introduction. Part 1 deals with the foundational aspects of phonetics needed by anyone interested in clinical aspects of speech. These cover articulatory, acoustic and auditory phonetics, perceptual aspects of phonetics, and suprasegmental phonetics. It is recognized that as well as readers who may need an introduction to one or more of these foundational aspects of phonetics, there will also be readers familiar with these basics but unfamiliar with the range of speech disorders that can occur; the final chapter of this Part, therefore, is just such a survey of disordered speech.

Part 2 is concerned with phonetic variation. This is discussed in four chapters. The first two examine phonetic variation between and within languages, with the second chapter mainly concerned with variation in English. The third chapter looks at stylistic variation in the case of a client with a speech disorder. The final chapter of the Part is an introduction to computer modeling of phonetic variation in both disordered and typical speech. In Part 3 the focus is on phonetic transcription. Chapters in this part examine the nature of phonetic transcription, the history of the International Phonetic Alphabet, and the history of the development of specialist symbols for atypical aspects of speech that may be encountered clinically. The use of phonetic transcription is described in two chapters: one on how to teach and learn transcription, the other on how to transcribe disordered speech. The final chapter of this part provides examples of a range of unusual articulations recorded from clients in the speech clinic and how these were transcribed phonetically using the symbol systems covered in the earlier chapters.

The final, and longest Part of the book—on phonetic instrumentation—can be considered as being divided into four sections. A *Preliminaries* section deals with the nature of phonetic instrumentation, recording speech for subsequent analysis, and how to use databases of disordered speech. The second section deals with instrumentation devoted to studying the articulation of speech: in particular, the muscles of speech, airflow, larynx activity, resonance and tongue-palate contact patterns. Also included are four chapters dealing with various imaging techniques although, due to its inherent dangers, this collection (unlike Malmberg's) does not cover x-radiography. In the third section, instrumentation used in the study of acoustic, auditory and perceptual phonetics is described. Thus, there are chapters on sound spectrography, audiometry, altered feedback in speech, dichotic listening and finally a range of perceptual phonetic techniques. The final section contains two chapters on speech recognition and speech synthesis (interestingly also covered in Malmberg's collection). Within the clinical context, reliable and detailed speech recognition would help considerably in the transcription of speech recorded in the clinic and speech synthesis can be a valuable resource for those working with alternative and augmentative communication.

The field of phonetics has grown considerably since Malmberg's *Manual of Phonetics*, and the area of clinical phonetics has come into existence as a separate aspect of phonetics since 1968. It is not surprising, therefore, that this Manual has twice as many chapters as the earlier collection. Of course, while Malmberg's *Manual of Phonetics* has served to some extent as an inspiration to this collection, the *Manual of Clinical Phonetics* is in no way connected to the earlier book in terms of authors, publishers, or aim. Nevertheless, just as the earlier book was the go-to collection for phonetics students when I was a student, the hope is that this collection will be the go-to book for students, researchers and practitioners in the field of clinical phonetics and the profession of speech-language pathology.

Reference

Malmberg, B. (Ed.) (1968). *Manual of Phonetics*. Amsterdam: North Holland.

ACKNOWLEDGEMENTS

I'd like to thank all those at Routledge who guided this collection from proposal to publication. Gratitude is especially due to Cloe Holland, Alex Howard, Lucy Kennedy, and Alison Macfarlane. Thanks also to the copy editors and typesetters.

PART I

Foundations of clinical phonetics
Introduction

A complete guide to clinical phonetics, which is the intention of this collection, needs to be able to provide an introduction to the basics of the field as well as to advanced theories and methods. This part of the *Manual of Clinical Phonetics* fulfils this role. Even for those who have received some training in phonetics or in communication disorders, there may well be some lacunae in their knowledge of these fields. For example, introductions to phonetics often concentrate on the segmental speech production area saying little about prosodic features or the transmission of speech, whereas speech science texts may be biased toward acoustics at the expense of speech production or speech reception. Even texts on auditory aspects of phonetics, or on audiology, may concentrate more on the mechanics of hearing and have little detail on how speech perception works. Finally, we need to bear in mind that this is a manual of *clinical* phonetics and thus that not all readers will be familiar with the range of communication disorders that can affect speech, even if they are well read in the study of typical speech. Part 1 of the *Manual*, therefore, provides a thorough foundation in both phonetics and speech disorders, allowing the reader to follow the content of later chapters which look in detail at specific aspects of phonetics and how these can be used to aid in the description and analysis of disordered speech.

This part of the book contains six chapters. The first of these, by Joan Rahilly and Orla Lowry, is a comprehensive account of articulatory phonetics. Clearly, in order to understand how the articulation of speech sounds can go wrong, one needs to understand how they are made. In this chapter, therefore, the production of vowels and of consonants is described. The chapter is not restricted to the sounds of any one language, however, and details of the whole range of sounds found in natural language are covered.

The second chapter, by Ioannis Papakyritsis, deals with acoustic phonetics. It introduces the main concepts in the study of acoustics and illustrates them by looking at both segmental and prosodic aspects of speech, covering both typical and disordered speakers. Elena Babatsouli describes the third main arm of phonetics—auditory phonetics—in the third chapter. This includes details of how hearing works, how it can be measured, and some of the ways in which it can go wrong.

The first three chapters, therefore, provide a grounding in what is traditionally thought of as the three arms of phonetics—articulatory, acoustic and auditory. However, there are two other areas which are important in phonetics and which are sometimes neglected: speech perception, and prosodic aspects of speech. In Chapter 4 Esther Janse and Toni Rietveld provide an introduction to the study of perceptual phonetics, including the important area of co-articulation, a topic sometimes neglected in clinical phonetic analyses. Orla Lowry, in Chapter 5, covers a range of suprasegmental features. These include those with potential for direct semantic impact (such as stress, tone, and intonation), and those with a more paralinguistic function (such as tempo, loudness, and voice quality), as both these types of suprasegmentals may be disturbed in various categories of disordered speech.

As noted above, this foundational part of the book is not restricted to the underpinnings of phonetics. To understand the contributions in the other three parts of this *Manual*, readers need to have a grounding in speech disorders as well as phonetics. The final chapter of this Part, by Martin Ball, provides just such a grounding. The chapter illustrates the wide range of communication disorders that impact speech, from child speech disorders, through acquired neurogenic disorders, to fluency disorders among several others. As each of these may impact speech production in different ways, the clinical phonetician needs knowledge of speech disorders as well as of phonetics.

1
ARTICULATORY PHONETICS FOR THE SPEECH CLINICIAN

Joan Rahilly and Orla Lowry

Introduction: What is articulatory phonetics?

It is no accident that the chapter on articulatory phonetics is the first one in the *Foundations* part of this book. Articulatory phonetics is indeed the foundational analytic, descriptive and therapeutic framework within which all speech clinicians must work to arrive at a clear picture of patients' abilities in speech production. Without a firm grounding in and understanding of articulatory phonetics, the task of speech analysis is impossible. The term *articulation* captures how the organs of speech function independently and collaboratively, in order to create speech sounds. Our articulatory descriptions of speech therefore allow us to identify aspects of sounds from the point at which the speaker begins to produce the sound, to the final product that is released; the latter being the material which listeners then use to decode meaning. This final product, then, is a composite of underlying and contributory factors, and when it does not conform to typical speech norms, it is usually possible to highlight which organs of speech are responsible and how specifically their behavior has affected the speech output. In general terms, we can state that speech provides listeners with a number of clues: some of these indicate regional and social background but, for our primary purpose of clinical assessment, they can provide important insights into patients' physical, physiological and even cognitive functioning. In the course of this chapter, we will introduce the key aspects of articulatory phonetics, beginning with a brief account of how and where speech sounds are initiated in the vocal apparatus, and moving on to a more detailed exploration of the standard framework for describing articulatory parameters.

A typical articulatory phonetic description requires us to identify what various organs of speech are doing during any given sound or stretch of sounds. Some of this activity is visible: we can usually see, for instance, when the upper and lower lips make contact with one another when we produce words beginning with *b* and *m* for instance, and when the upper teeth touch the lower lip in *f* or *v* (for the moment, we are using some orthographic letters which closely resemble phonetic symbols, and we will introduce a number of symbols as the chapter progresses, leading to a detailed account of transcription systems in Part 3). We may even see some tongue protrusion through the teeth when a speaker produces a *th* sound. Of course, many other speech sounds are produced inside the oral cavity (i.e. the mouth), and therefore cannot be seen or, at least, not easily seen. For *t*, *sh* or *g*, we cannot see the precise location of the sounds, but speakers can feel their tongue touch certain parts of their oral cavity in various ways. Furthermore, there are other sounds or aspects of sounds which cannot reliably be seen *or* felt and which need to be identified using the instrumental methods described in Part 4 of this book. Fortunately, the field of modern phonetics has developed convenient methods for describing the activity of speech sounds in considerable detail, drawing on the sort of visible, tactile and experimental knowledge we have outlined.

Overview of the stages of speech production

The first principle of articulatory phonetics is to recognize that there are four main stages in the production of any speech sound: *initiation*, *phonation*, *articulation* and, finally, the *coordination* which is required to make the relevant organs of speech work appropriately together. In practice, phonetic analysis tends to focus on the first three of these whilst acknow-ledging the importance of the coordination activities for creating fluent speech. To some extent, the terms initiation, phonation and articulation may seem self-explanatory (*initiation* for example, signals the beginning of the sound), but each has a specific, technical remit in articulatory phonetics. It is worth noting in passing that the term *articulation*, although used specifically to refer to the third stage of speech sound production, also invokes the broader sense of articulation in the entire production process. Each stage occurs in specific regions of the vocal tract (*vocal tract* is the term used to refer to the entire speech appar-atus, with the larynx as the central element which subdivides the apparatus into lower and upper regions): initiation occurs usually in the sublaryngeal portion, phonation in the laryn-geal area, and articulation in the supralaryngeal region. In each region, the sounds are formed and distinguished from one another by the actions of particular articulators and the location of this articulatory action, all of which will be discussed later in this chapter. Figure 1.1 provides an overview of the vocal tract, showing the location of the larynx and the key areas above and below it.

We now move on to explain how speech sounds are formed in the vocal tract, with ref-erence to the stages we have introduced above, i.e. initiation, phonation and articulation. To help readers combine the following descriptions with spoken examples of the sounds in question, we recommend reading this chapter whilst cross-referring to the online IPA charts provided by York University (http://www.yorku.ca/earmstro/ipa/index.html). With regard to atypical speech, we should note that the frameworks introduced in this chapter still serve as the descriptive basis for those working with all clinical speech types, with two caveats. First, what is regarded as a usual means for producing any given sound may not apply in various disorders. In the case of initiation, for example, Ball and Müller (2007) show the prevalence of non-pulmonic-egressive systems in clinical data, even though such systems are relatively rare in non-clinical speech. Second, there are instances where clin-ical speech cannot be described solely according to standard IPA criteria and, for this reason, the Extensions to the IPA for the Disordered Speech (known as *extIPA*) are used to capture atypical articulations such as consistent interdental protrusion of the tongue. For a detailed account of developments in phonetic notation, we urge readers to consult Esling (2010), particularly for his own elaborations of consonantal elements of both the IPA and extIPA, (both alphabets are discussed in Chapters 12 and 13 of this book), all in pursuit of providing as comprehensive a resource as possible for transcribing articulation in all speech types.

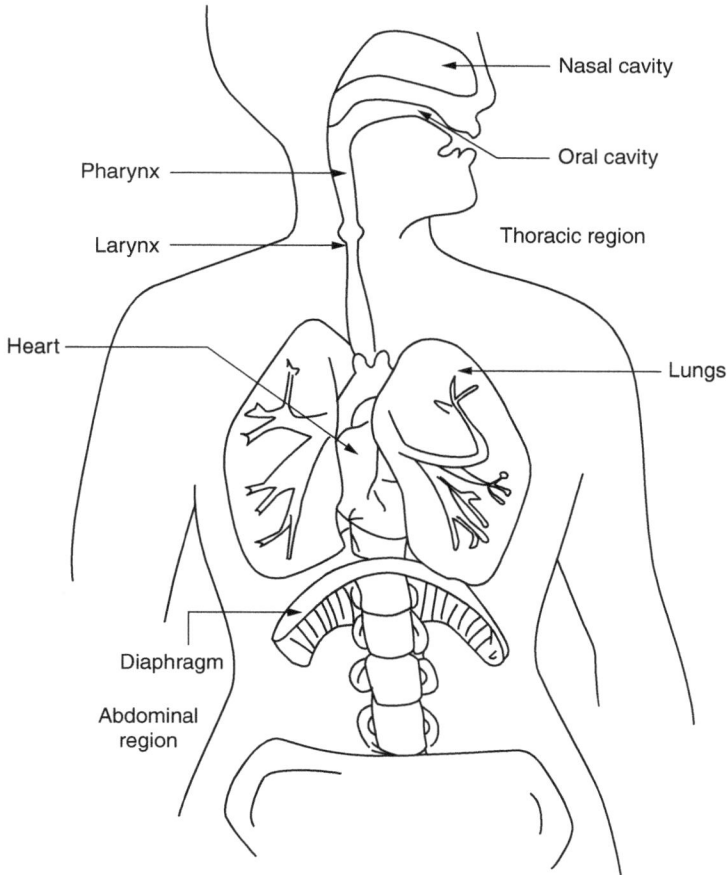

Figure 1.1 Overview of the vocal tract.

Source: Courtesy of S. Qiouyi Lu.

Initiation

Any sound, whether speech or not, must obviously begin somewhere, even though speakers and listeners rarely focus on the beginning point of sounds. The core component of sound is a moving body of air which is acted upon in various ways by the channels through which it travels. In musical instruments, for example, bodies of air are pushed through cavities of differing sizes and shapes, with varying force applied to the air at a range of points within the cavity in question. When we produce speech sounds, we are usually aware of what comes out of our mouths, i.e. the end point, without thinking of what precedes it, but the complete trajectory of a sound from start to finish is crucial in articulatory phonetics and it is a key element of the diagnostic process in therapy. The initiation of speech sounds requires speakers to set in motion the body of air somewhere within the vocal tract, usually by pushing air upward and outward through the system, although movement of air inward is also possible. These bodies of air, in whichever direction they travel, are known as *airstream mechanisms*. There are three such airstream mechanisms in speech, defined according to the particular point of initiation in question: the lungs, the velum and the glottis.

Lungs as initiators: Pulmonic airstreams

Airstream mechanisms which begin in the lungs, with the latter contained within the ribcage and controlled by the diaphragm, are known as *pulmonic* systems, while those which are initiated by other organs of speech are called *non-pulmonic* (*pulmo* is the Latin term for *lung*). In order to bring useable air into the pulmonic system (we use the term *useable* to refer to air that is used for both normal respiration and for speech), the ribcage contracts and in doing so increases the volume of air within the lungs. To release air from the system, the ribcage expands thereby exerting pressure on the lungs and forcing the air upward and out of the lungs. The *pulmonic egressive airstream* mechanism (*egressive* means *exiting*) is the most common one in speech. While the pulmonic *ingressive* airstream does exist, formed by air being sucked into the system more rapidly than during standard inhalation, it is used only rarely in non-clinical speech (in gasps, for instance).

The distinction between pulmonic and non-pulmonic sounds is signaled in the two consonants grids in the IPA chart. The non-pulmonic category consists of sounds which do not involve lung activity, and it subdivides into the three main groupings known as *clicks*, *implosives* and *ejectives*: the first are produced on a *velaric airstream* mechanism, and the remaining two on a *glottalic airstream*. Figure 1.2 shows a stylized cross-sectional area of the speech organs which create non-pulmonic airstreams, i.e. the velum and the glottis. This representation is also referred to as a *midsagittal* diagram, drawing on information from speech imaging techniques

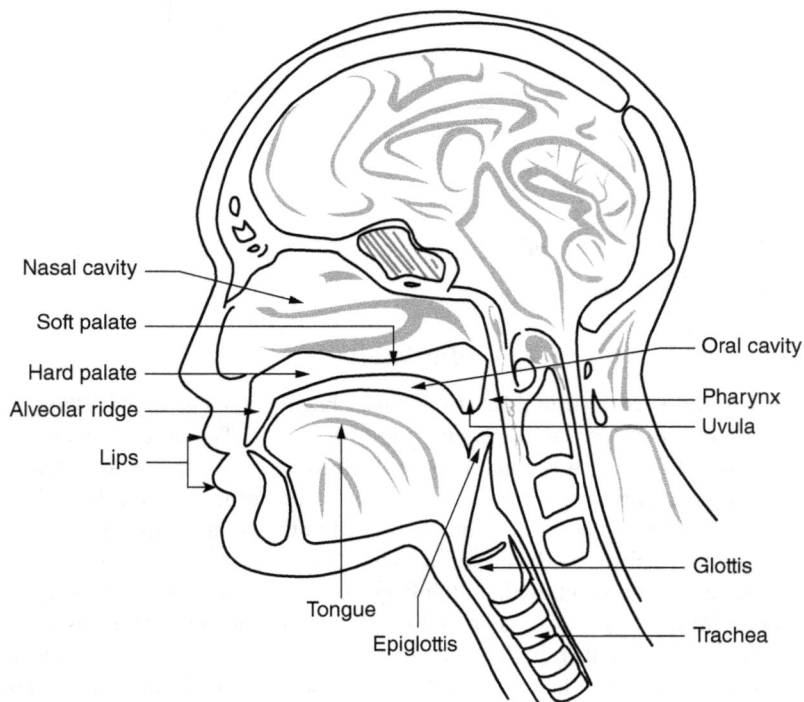

Figure 1.2   Midsagittal section, showing regions responsible for non-pulmonic initiation, oral and nasal cavities.

Source: Courtesy of S. Qiouyi Lu.

to present the medial plane of this portion of the vocal tract. Figure 1.2 also identifies areas of the oral and nasal cavities which are referred to in the following sections of this chapter.

Velum as initiator: Velaric airstreams

The velum, also known as the *soft palate*, is located at the back of the oral cavity and its main role during speech production is to direct the flow of air from the lungs into either the oral or nasal cavity: for most of the time, the velum is raised thereby closing off access to the nasal cavity resulting in oral sounds. Otherwise, it is lowered, allowing air to pass into the nasal cavity for either normal breathing or production of nasal sounds. However, the velum also plays an independent role as an initiator. In this case, the body of the tongue (see the section below on articulation, for information on individual parts of the tongue) makes a closure with the velum, and this closure blocks off the passage of air rising from the lungs. A second closure is also made, at the lips for instance, or between the tongue and some portion of the roof of the mouth. The pressurized build-up of air between the two closures, and its subsequent inward release, results in sounds known formally as *clicks*, which we often recognize as kissing and tutting sounds.

Glottis as initiator: Glottalic airstreams

In glottalic airstream mechanisms, the body of air used to produce speech sounds begins in the larynx area, specifically with a closure made at the glottis. This glottal closure blocks the passage of air from the lungs as the air travels upward and, in addition to the glottal closure, a second point of articulation must be made further forward in the oral cavity. The air thereby contained within the two closures becomes pressurized and the release of front-most closure is sometimes heard as a popping sound, particularly when the front closure involves the lips. The majority of glottalic sounds are produced on an egressive airstream and they are also referred to as *ejectives*, but *ingressive glottalic* airstreams do exist. Sounds made on ingressive glottalic airstreams are known as *implosives*: these are formed similarly to their egressive counterparts up to the point at which the front closure is released. At that point, the glottis closure loosens slightly and permits vocal fold vibration to take place, thereby involving air from the lungs in the articulation: for this reason, implosive consonants are not fully glottalic but, rather, they combine aspects of glottalic and pulmonic ingressive initiation.

Having established the three airstream mechanisms on which speech sounds are formed, we now move on to focus on the next stage of the production process, i.e. phonation.

Phonation

The second stage in the production of pulmonic egressive speech sounds, which is by far the most common type of sound in typical speech, is phonation; though, as mentioned above, pulmonic ingressive, velaric and glottalic initiation often occur in clinical data (Ball and Müller, 2007). This process refers to the actions of the two vocal folds, also known as the vocal cords, which are strings of tissue located in the larynx. Sometimes termed the *voice box*, the larynx is a structure composed of muscle and cartilage, and is positioned at the top of the trachea. Modifications to the position of the vocal folds are of great importance in differentiating speech sounds, as we will see in the following sections.

The main cartilages are the *cricoid* cartilage, which is ring-shaped and situated at the base of the larynx where it joins the trachea, and the *thyroid* cartilage, which can be felt as a protuberance at the front of the neck. This is often visible in many speakers and referred to informally as the *Adam's Apple*. At the back of the larynx and above the cricoid are the two *arytenoid* cartilages, one of which attaches to each vocal fold. These cartilages move during the process of speech production and, in doing so, open a triangular space between the vocal folds, known as the *glottis*. For normal breathing, the glottis is open, allowing air from the lungs to pass through. The *epiglottis* is a flap of tissue which closes the entrance to the larynx, primarily to prevent food from entering the trachea during swallowing. The *hyoid* bone does not constitute part of the laryngeal structure itself, but has muscular attachments which assist in the movements of the larynx. Figure 1.3 shows the front, back and top views of the larynx and its surroundings.

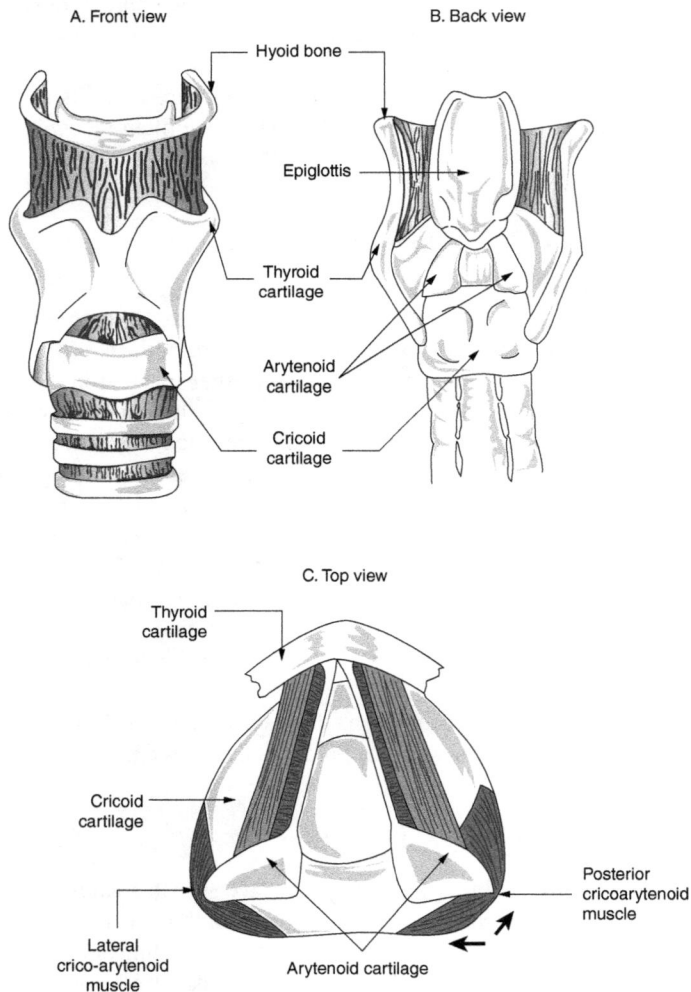

Figure 1.3 Front, back and top views of the larynx and its surroundings.

Source: Courtesy of S. Qiouyi Lu.

Voiced and voiceless

Consonant sounds in natural speech are distinguished by two main configurations of the vocal folds: at a fairly basic level of description, if they are held loosely together and vibrating, the sound produced is *voiced*; if held apart in the open position, the sound is *voiceless*. The action of holding the vocal folds apart is *abduction*, and is achieved by movements of the *posterior crico-arytenoid* muscle, which connects the arytenoids and cricoid at the back of the larynx. The bringing together of the vocal folds is *adduction*, and this is brought about by movements of the *lateral crico-arytenoid* muscles and the *interarytenoid* muscles (the latter connect the posterior surfaces of the arytenoid cartilages and are not shown in Figure 1.3). For a voiced sound to be produced, the adducted vocal folds are held taut, which first obstructs the air flowing upward from the lungs; a pressurized airflow then builds up and pushes between the folds, forcing them apart and allowing air through. As the air passes through the narrowed glottis, the speed of flow accelerates and pressure decreases—a principle known as the Bernoulli Effect—which has the effect of sucking the vocal folds back together again (see, for example, Story (2015), for a comprehensive account of the aerodynamics of speech). The elastic nature of the vocal folds facilitates the procedure since the folds, once pushed apart, begin to pull back toward one another. The cycle begins again after the folds come together completely, repeats itself, and thus, continuous vibration occurs, for as long as there is suffi-cient air supply.

Examples of voiced sounds are those at the beginning and end of the word *zoom*. If a finger is placed on the front of the neck while the sounds in question are being uttered (i.e. those which correspond to the emboldened letters), vibration will be felt. Examples of voiceless sounds are those at the beginning and end of the word *pat*. No vibration will be felt at the larynx during the production of these sounds, since the vocal folds are held apart.

In English, the voiced-voiceless distinction is contrastive, in that this single sound diffe-rence semantically differentiates words. Examples of such distinctions are: *fan, van; sat, sad; bitter, bidder*. There are other laryngeal settings, which are often used paralinguistically (i.e. to convey communicative aspects, such as attitude or emotion), and these will be considered in Chapter 5 on suprasegmental phonetics.

Closed and close glottal settings

Two English consonants which entail glottal settings other than the open and vibrating vocal folds described above are the glottal stop and the glottal fricative (fricatives are particular manners of consonant articulation, discussed below). The latter is the sound at the beginning of *head*, and requires the vocal folds to be closer than they are for voicelessness, but not in contact with each other: this increased closeness between the vocal folds causes turbulence in the air flow. A glottal stop is produced when the vocal folds are tightly shut, and depending on the regional accent, or the style of speech (e.g. whether careful, as in a public address, or more informal, as in a conversation between friends) can be a variant of *t* sounds between vowels, or at the end of words. For example, *matter* may be pronounced with the middle consonant as a glottal stop by many speakers. Glottal stops may also be used as a compensatory sound for target oral stops in speech disorders; e.g. in the case of speakers with cleft palate, deformity of the palate renders the usual articulation impossible, so a glottal stop may be used in place of the target sound (Bressmann et al., 2011).

Articulation

Place

The third main stage of speech production is *articulation.* The term refers to the shaping of the airstream into recognizable sounds which takes place in the supralaryngeal area. We use the term *place of articulation* to denote the articulators which affect the maximum degree of constriction to the body of air. These are placed along the top of the IPA consonant chart and move from the front of the oral cavity (the lips) to the back (the larynx). Articulators may be described as *passive* or *active:* the active articulator is the more mobile, while there is relatively less movement in the passive articulator during the production of the sound. For example, to produce the first sound in *pin*, the lower lip moves upward, and is thus active, to make contact with the upper lip which moves comparatively little.

Lips and teeth

We begin by considering the lips and teeth as places of articulation, before making our way backward in the vocal tract. Sounds made with both lips, such as those at the beginning and end of the word *palm* (the IPA symbols are [p] and [m], respectively) are *bilabial.* The consonant [p] is voiceless, since the vocal folds are not vibrating, and [m] is voiced, since vibration is present. When the lower lip makes contact with the upper teeth to produce a sound, the sound is *labiodental.* The consonant at the beginning of *far*, [f], and that in the middle of *never*, [v], are labiodental, the former being voiceless since there is no vibration of the vocal folds and the latter, voiced. *Dental* consonants are pronounced with the tongue making contact with the upper teeth; for some speakers, it is placed at the back of the upper teeth, and for others it protrudes between the teeth. An example of a voiceless dental sound is that at the end of *tooth* and symbolized in the IPA as [θ]; its voiced counterpart is the middle consonant in *weather* and the symbol is [ð].

Alveolar ridge, hard palate and velum

Directly behind the upper teeth is a bony structure known as the *alveolar ridge* and consonants made at this location are classified as *alveolar.* Examples of alveolar sounds are [t] and [s], as in *cat* and *sit*, which are both voiceless. Voiced alveolar sounds are [d] and [z] as in *shudder* and *zeal.* Other English consonants made at the alveolar place of articulation are [ɹ], as in *red*, [l], as in *letter*, and [n], as in *den.* At the back edge of the alveolar ridge is the *postalveolar* place of articulation. An example of a voiceless sound made at this location is [ʃ] in *wash,* and a voiced postalveolar sound is the middle consonant in *measure*, transcribed as [ʒ]. The *retroflex* place of articulation entails a curling back of the tip (the frontmost part) of the tongue. Some speakers of English may use the retroflex [ɻ] for *r* sounds, as in *red*, but this is generally accepted as idiosyncratic, and is more usually the alveolar consonant described above. Behind the alveolar ridge is the hard palate, which is the passive articulator in the production of the first sound in *young* and *university* (note the different spellings of the same sound). This is transcribed as [j], described as *palatal*, and is a voiced consonant. Most varieties of English have this as their only palatal sound in typical speech, although Esling's elaborations to the IPA chart include an extensive range of possible palatal consonants, incorporating those also found in atypical speech. At the back of the oral cavity, behind the hard palate is the *velum*, also known as the *soft palate* as mentioned earlier. Sounds made at this point are *velar*, and examples are the

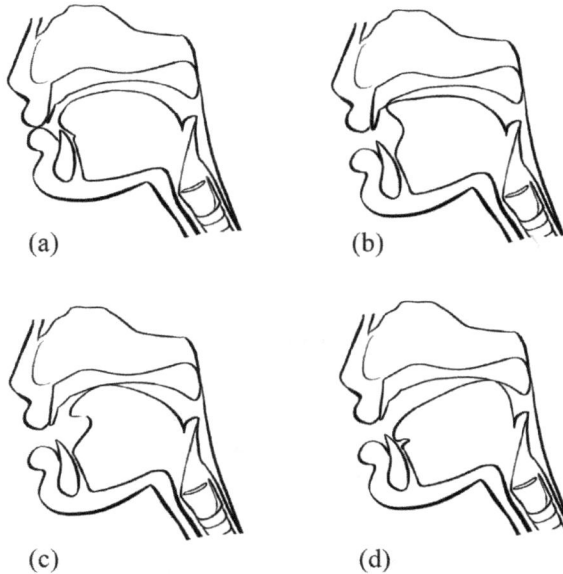

Figure 1.4　Four different places of articulation: (a) bilabial, (b) alveolar, (c) palatal, (d) velar.

Source:　Courtesy of S. Qiouyi Lu.

voiceless [k] at the beginning of *king*, the voiced [g] at the end of *dog*, and the voiced [ŋ] at the end of *song*; the latter is considered a single sound phonetically, despite the two orthographic symbols. The *uvula* is the back part of the velum, and is the appendage which is visible at the back of the oral cavity when the mouth is wide open. Sounds made here are described as *uvular*, and do not typically occur in English. Most French *r* sounds, as in *rouge* (*red*) are made at this place of articulation, and transcribed as [ʁ]. Figure 1.4 shows constrictions at four places of articulation: lips, alveolar ridge, palate and velum.

Pharynx and glottis

The *pharynx* is a chamber located above the larynx. Sounds made at this location are *pharyngeal*, and do not occur in English, but are found in Hebrew and Arabic. The glottalic place of articulation was discussed above: the glottal stop, which is often a variant of the *t* sound, is transcribed as [ʔ], and the glottal fricative at the beginning of *head* is [h].

The tongue

When the tongue is involved in the production of a sound, it is the active articulator, and is divided into sections for the purposes of precision of classification. The front extremity is the *tip*, behind which is located the *blade*. The blade is the part which lies under the alveolar ridge when the tongue is at rest, and either the tip or blade is used in the production of alveolar consonants. The *front* of the tongue lies under the hard palate, and is active in the pronunciation of palatal sounds. The *back* of the tongue articulates with the velum in velar sounds and uvular sounds, and the *root* of the tongue forms a constriction with the pharynx rear wall in pharyngeal consonants.

11

Double articulation

Several sounds have two places of articulation, and are situated in the *Other Symbols* section of the IPA chart. Only one of these occurs in typical speech and is classified as *labial-velar*. The *double articulation* description is due to the fact that the sound's production entails a constriction at the velar place of articulation and a rounding of the lips. The sound begins the word *wind* and its IPA symbol is [w]. Some varieties of Irish and Scottish English also have a voiceless labial-velar sound, with a fricative manner of articulation, at the beginning of *wh* words, such as *which, why* and *when*. This is transcribed as [ʍ].

Manner

Throughout this chapter, we have referred to the airstream as the raw material for speech sounds, and we have seen that the airstream can be altered at various stages (the places of articulation) from initiation to exit points. We now need to consider *how* the airstream is modified, by asking three main questions about it: Is the air stopped entirely? Is it constricted to some degree? Does it flow freely or relatively freely? We use the term *manner of articulation* to refer to the ways in which the airflow is modified during the production of speech sounds, and it is typically one of the three labels that is used (along with phonation mode and place of articulation) to describe consonants rather than vowels. On the IPA consonant chart, for instance, descriptions of manner are clearly visible in the leftmost column where eight manners are listed: plosive, nasal, trill and so on. Vowels, on the other hand, are sounds which are made on an open, or mostly open, vocal tract; so the manner labels used for consonants are not entirely relevant. We say that they are not *entirely* relevant because there is occasional overlap in the manner terminology used for vowels and consonants.

Plosive consonants, also frequently known as *stops* or *stop consonants* are those in which the relevant articulators come together and stop the air from exiting the system. For example, to make the [b] sound in *big*, we must bring the two lips tightly together to stop the airflow which has left the lungs and travelled up past the larynx area into the oral cavity. We refer to [b] as a voiced, bilabial, plosive (*voiced* captures the phonation mode, *bilabial* the place of articulation, and *plosive* the manner). Because the air is effectively trapped in the oral cavity during plosive sounds, there is usually some build-up of air pressure behind the closure in question and, when the articulators come apart and release the pressure, a small puff or pop of air can be heard. The plosive sounds listed in the top row of the IPA chart ([p, b, t, d], for example) are known as *oral stops* because the airflow on which they are based exits the oral cavity (i.e. the mouth). In the second row, several *nasal stops* are listed: these are sounds (such as [m and n]) which also contain an oral closure but one that is released via the nasal cavity.

Fricative sounds are those in which the articulators approach one another but do not make a complete closure. Their proximity to one another has the effect of narrowing the airflow so that it is forced through a relatively narrow aperture, thereby causing friction. This friction is usually heard as a hissing or sibilant sound, as in [s] (in *see*), the voiceless, alveolar fricative, and [f] (*fee*), the voiceless labiodental fricative.

Affricate is the term used to capture sounds which contain both a plosive and a fricative element, produced in such quick succession that they are considered effectively to count as a single sound. Examples of affricates are [tʃ] (the last sound in *itch*), the voiceless, postalveolar affricate, and [dʒ] (the first sound in *John*), the voiced, postalveolar affricate. In these examples, the plosive sound is released immediately into the fricative airflow, rather than out through the oral or nasal cavity. Because affricates are not single sounds like other consonants, they do not occur on the IPA consonant chart. They can be found, though, in the *Other Symbols* section of the IPA.

Plosive, fricative and affricate manners of articulation tend to be the main options for classifying manner in consonants, but there are many others which are used commonly in speech. For instance, *approximant* is a manner in which the articulators come close together but neither touch nor create a narrowed airflow. The passage of air through the articulators is, therefore, unhindered but not as unhindered as it would be for vowel sounds. Examples of approximant sounds are [ɹ] as in *rail*, the voiced, alveolar approximant, and [j] as in *yes*, the voiced, palatal approximant. Trills are sounds in which there are rapid successive closures between an active and passive articulator, as in [r] (in the Spanish *perro*), the voiced, alveolar trill. Taps and flaps (the terms tend to be used synonymously) involve a rapid closure between the relevant articulators, and these are often illustrated using examples from General American English (where the *tt* in *butter* might be realized as the [ɾ] flap). Laterals are sounds in which the tongue makes contact with some portion of the roof of the mouth and allows the airflow to pass over the sides of the tongue ([l, ɭ, ʎ, ʟ]). Depending of the degree of constriction caused by the tongue, lateral sounds may also contain friction, leading therefore to the category of lateral fricatives ([ɬ, ɮ]).

Any sound which is produced on a plosive, fricative or affricate manner of articulation is known as an *obstruent* sound whilst those produced on unobstructed airflows are known as *sonorants* (the latter allows sounds to resonate within the oral or nasal cavities.) Whilst the terms *obstruent* and *sonorant* are not strictly manners of articulation (they refer to classes of sounds, rather than the airflow), they are helpful in identifying some commonalities between vowels and consonants. For example, all vowels are sonorant sounds but so, too, are approximants, the nasal stops and lateral sounds.

As indicated earlier in this chapter, extIPA and Esling's (2010) elaborations of the IPA provide means for symbolizing articulations which fall outside those indicated by standard IPA descriptions. To take one illustration, extIPA reframes the traditional *fricative* and *lateral fricative* into three sections: *median*, *lateral+median* and *nareal*. The lateral+median fricatives are those in which there is a central and a lateral gap from which air escapes, usually at the alveolar place of articulation, and nareal indicates the presence of nasal friction. ExtIPA also includes a *percussive* manner of articulation to refer to sounds made by continuous striking together of two articulators. In the *others* section of extIPA, we also see resources for indicating *indeterminate* aspects of airflow, and *silent articulation*. Esling's elaborated phonetic chart foregoes many of the separate IPA categorizations (pulmonic and non-pulmonic consonants are provided in the same chart, for example), and provides a rich and arguably more comprehensive coverage of both typical and atypical sounds.

Vowels

As stated above, vowel sounds are produced with an open configuration of the vocal tract, in that there is no, or very little, constriction to the airflow. They are also usually voiced, although certain contexts, such as occurring between two voiceless obstruents, may cause them to be devoiced. Contrastive voiced and voiceless vowels have been reported for some languages, including Ik, spoken in North-Eastern Uganda, and Dafla, a Himalayan mountain language (Ladefoged and Maddieson, 1996). Articulatory descriptions of vowel production depend mainly on three parameters: the height of the highest part of the tongue during the articulation in relation to the palate, the degree of frontness or backness of the highest part of the tongue within the oral cavity, and the lip position. The vowel section on the IPA chart is known as either a *trapezium* or *quadrilateral* and is a schematized representation of the speaker's *vowel space*, postulating four positions for tongue height and three for tongue frontness-backness. In addition, lips can be rounded, spread or neutral, and where vowel symbols occur in pairs on the trapezium, the one on the right is rounded. Tongue height labels are: *close* when the highest part of the tongue is close to the palate, *open* when the jaws are open and the tongue far from the palate, and in between are two mid degrees of height, which are *close-mid* and *open-mid*. Tongue frontness-backness labels are: *front* when the front of the tongue is highest, approximately aligning with the hard palate, *back* when the back of the tongue is highest, approximately aligning with the velum, and *central*, when aligning with a point intermediate between back and front.

Illustrations of some English vowels are the vowel in *see*, which is a close, front, unrounded vowel, and symbolized as [i], the vowel in *luck*, which is an open-mid, back, unrounded vowel and transcribed as [ʌ], and the vowel in *bird*, which is an open-mid, central, unrounded vowel and transcribed as [ɜ]. It must, of course, be noted that vowel realizations will vary according to regional accent.

Diphthongs and monophthongs

The quality of a vowel sound, i.e. the sum of its articulatory parts which differentiate one vowel from another, may remain unchanged, or may vary during its production. Those exemplified above have a stable quality for their duration, and are *monophthongs*. If the quality changes, due to a movement of the tongue from one position to another, the vowel is a *diphthong*. Examples of English diphthongs are contained in the words *eye* and in *toy*, transcribed as [aɪ] and [ɔɪ], respectively.

Cardinal Vowels

Cardinal Vowels are a system of fixed reference points devised by phonetician Daniel Jones in the early 20th century. Jones's intention was that vowels of any language or language variety could be described by linguists using a commonly-understood framework. There are eight primary cardinals and eight secondary cardinal vowels, all of which are given numerical references and arranged around the periphery of the vowel space. Cardinal Vowel 1 is produced with the front part of the tongue as far forward and raised as is possible without creating friction and with unrounded lips, Cardinal Vowel 5 is produced with the tongue as far back and as lowered as possible and with unrounded lips, and Cardinal Vowel 8 is produced with the tongue as high and back as possible and with rounded lips. The remaining points are arranged in terms of the perceived auditory distance between Cardinal Vowels 1, 5 and 8. For example, Cardinal Vowels 6 and 7 are perceived to be equidistant between 5 and 8, and vowels 5, 6, 7 and 8 are defined as having an equal auditory distance between them (see International Phonetic Association, 1999) for further explanation of how the Cardinal Vowels are defined and arranged in the vowel quadrilateral). The secondary Cardinal Vowels have identical tongue positions to the primary Cardinals, but reverse the lip position.

Conclusion

This chapter has discussed the systems involved in speech articulation by way of explaining and exemplifying the key stages of (1) initiation, which takes place usually in the lungs, but may also occur at the glottis or velum; (2) phonation, which takes place in the larynx; and

(3) articulation, which occurs above the larynx. Consonant sounds are produced with constriction in the vocal tract, and the specification of individual consonants depends on the degree of constriction and its location, as well as on the presence or absence of vocal fold vibration. Vowel sounds are produced with little constriction in the vocal tract, and the main parameters for their description are tongue height, tongue frontness-backness and lip rounding. Monophthongs are vowels which maintain a stable quality throughout their duration and diphthongs involve a change in quality due to tongue movement. Cardinal Vowels are a set of articulatory- and auditory-based reference points to which any vowel can be related. Obstruents and sonorants are broader classes of sounds which distinguish those entailing obstruction to the airflow (obstruents) and those which do not (sonorants), and which cut across the consonant-vowel distinction. The information presented in this chapter provides a number of tools to enable speech clinicians to deconstruct patients' productive abilities by way of accessible and agreed frameworks. As will be shown in the course of this book, certain tools and analytic procedures will be more relevant than others for particular varieties of atypical speech, and many of the following chapters explain how existing frameworks have been expanded and developed to deal comprehensively with atypical speech.

References

Ball, M.J. and Müller, N. (2007). Non-pulmonic-egressive speech in clinical data: A brief review. *Clinical Linguistics & Phonetics*, 21 (11–12), 869–874. DOI: 10.1080/02699200701602433.

Bressmann, T., Radovanovic, B. Kulkarni, G.V., Klaiman, P. and Fisher, D. (2011). An ultrasonographic investigation of cleft-type compensatory articulations of voiceless velar stops. *Clinical Linguistics & Phonetics*, 25 (11–12), 1028–1033. DOI: 10.3109/02699206.2011.599472

Esling, J. (2010). Phonetic Notation. In W.J. Hardcastle, J. Laver and Gibbon, F.E. (Eds.), *The Handbook of Phonetic Sciences* (pp. 678–702), Hoboken: John Wiley.

International Phonetic Association. (1999). *Handbook of the International Phonetic Association: A Guide to the Use of the International Phonetic Alphabet*. Cambridge: Cambridge University Press.

Ladefoged, P. and Maddieson, I. (1996). *The Sounds of the World's Languages*. Oxford: Blackwell.

Story, B.H. (2015). Mechanisms of Voice Production. In M.A. Redford (Ed.), *The Handbook of Voice Production* (pp. 34–58), Malden MA: Wiley-Blackwell.

2

ACOUSTIC PHONETICS FOR THE SPEECH CLINICIAN

Ioannis Papakyritsis

Introduction

Acoustic phonetics is the study of physical properties of speech. When we talk to each other, speech sound waves travel from the mouth of the speaker to the ear of the listener. This acoustic signal can be easily captured, analyzed and displayed. The study of the acoustic characteristics of speech has provided researchers with a window into the less observable aspects of speaker/ listener interaction, including the processes of language formulation and processing in the brain.

In the field of communication disorders, the careful description and analysis of the client's speech is a central part of the clinical appraisal and intervention practices employed by speech and language pathologists (SLPs). Perceptual assessment of speech is justifiably regarded as the gold standard in clinical practice, given that speaking is a perceptual phenomenon and the effects of treatment are determined by changes in global measures such as intelligibility and naturalness that are largely based on perceptual judgments. However, human perception has certain limitations and the reliability and validity of perceptual measures has often been questioned (see for example Kent, 1996; Kreiman, Gerratt, and Ito, 2007). Acoustic analysis can be a valuable complement to perceptual evaluation. Given the decreased costs and increased convenience of acoustic analysis, joint perceptual-acoustic analysis is becoming increasingly common even in routine clinical settings.

The essence of acoustic phonetics is the conversion of sound waves to visual representations that can be measured and related to phonetic features and physiological components of speech production. By recording the client and analyzing speech samples offline, the clinician can carefully inspect the acoustic display, accurately document the rapid alternations of the speech signal and focus on any detail relevant to the assessment. Additionally, acoustic analysis can generate quantitative and qualitative measures that can inform treatment practices. Collection of pre- and post-treatment samples allows for ongoing longitudinal tracking of the effects of intervention by monitoring changes that might be missed if relying only on perceptual methods. Clinicians can also collect multiple samples to provide feedback to clients during therapy; there are free or low-cost software programs that provide real-time acoustic information of pitch, volume or even segmental production.

Despite their documented clinical value, acoustic analysis has its own limitations. Clinicians should be cautious when they infer information from acoustic measurements, since the relationship between perceptual and acoustic data is not always straightforward. Additionally, the speech output of clients with a communication disorder typically generates a diminished acoustic signal often characterized by poor accuracy and reduced contrast compared to normal speech, making acoustic analysis and subsequent interpretation more challenging (Kent, Weismer, Kent, Vorperian, & Duffy, 1999).

Speech recordings

Overall, the goal of recording is to capture a speech signal that is clear, and has minimal distortion and background noise. In a clinical setting, SLPs seldom have the luxury to record in a high-quality sound isolation booth, however, they should try to record in a quiet recording environment, free of extraneous sounds. A common setup involves recording speech samples directly into a computer using an external unidirectional microphone placed in a fixed position from the mouth of the client. A unidirectional head-mounted microphone, which is more sensitive to the sound originating from the client, would be particularly helpful when recording in a noisy clinic room. The audio files are usually analyzed using one of the several readily available, open access, downloadable acoustic software (e.g. Praat, Paul Boersma and David Weenick; Institute of Phonetic Sciences, University of Amsterdam, The Netherlands, http://praat.org). Apart from computer-driven recordings, there are also portable digital devices that can be used to capture and analyze speech signals. These have typically involved digital recorders, such as solid-state compact flash recorders, with an external microphone. Recently, however, the advancements in cellphone technology have made recording and analyzing speech even more convenient and user friendly (Carson & Ryalls, 2018). Smartphones have been found comparable to external microphones in terms of recording quality for voice analysis (Lin, Hornibrook, & Ormond, 2012). Smartphones, equipped with a variety of apps for acoustic analysis, can be used not only by clinicians, but also by clients, either independently or with minimal guidance, for self-assessment. In that way, clinicians and clients can obtain a more accurate representation of real-life speech performance, and they can monitor treatment generalization.

Types of acoustic analysis

Generally, the acoustic signal can be analyzed as (1) an amplitude-by-time display (e.g. a waveform), (2) an amplitude-by-frequency display (e.g. a power spectrum) or (3) an amplitude-by-time-by-frequency display (e.g. a spectrogram). Amplitude indicates the power or intensity of the sound. Waveforms represent the changes in air pressure and/or the displacement of air particles over time. Power spectra display the amplitudes of the frequency components of the speech signal at a specific point in time. Finally, spectrograms are three-dimensional displays of acoustic information that can be considered as combinations of spectra and waveforms. Spectrograms can accurately capture the rapid alternations of the speech signal. They provide an analysis of the frequency component of the speech signal in terms of either the harmonic structure of the glottal source (in a narrowband spectrogram) or the formants, i.e. the peaks of resonance in the vocal tract (in a wideband spectrogram). The portions of the spectrographic signal with a high concentration of acoustic energy, such as harmonics and formants, are rendered darker compared to other, less intense, parts of the signal. Although spectrograms can be used to infer information regarding the overall intensity and fundamental frequency (F_0)

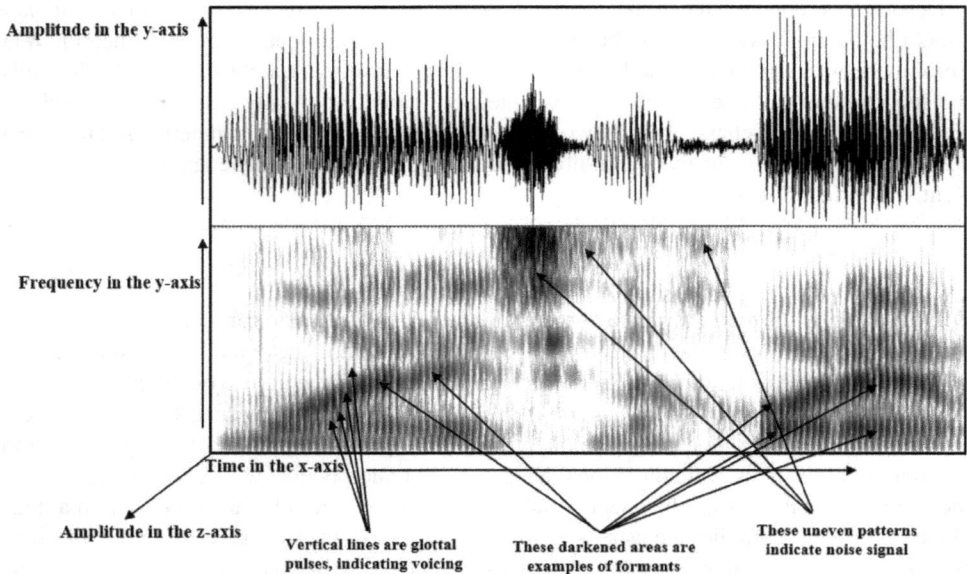

Figure 2.1 Example of a waveform paired with a wideband spectrogram of the Greek utterance [mu aˈresi na xoˈrevo] ("I love to dance").

variation of the speech signal, most acoustic software have analysis routines that isolate and depict changes of F_0 and amplitude either superimposed or below a time-linked spectrogram. Some of the features depicted in a spectrographic display can be seen in Figure 2.1.

The acoustic description of atypical speech output can be a valuable tool for the assessment and remediation of a number of different speech disorders across the lifespan, including, but not limited to, neurogenic speech disorders (dysarthria and apraxia of speech), voice disorders, craniofacial anomalies, speech sound disorders, stuttering, hearing disorders in children and adults, etc. Given that acoustic phonetics offer a wide variety of tools for the display and description of the speech signal, SLPs should carefully consider the purpose and interpretation of the acoustic measurements they apply. Most of the acoustic measures reported in the literature (see Kent et al, 1999; Kent & Kim, 2003, for neurogenic speech disorders), refer to spectral-temporal features of individual events in the acoustic record that usually correspond to specific phonetic aspects or to physiological components of speech production. For example, the voice onset time (VOT) measure signals the phonetic contrast of voicing in oral stops. Similarly, measurements of the formant frequencies of vowel segments, indicate vowel type and can be used as indices of tongue position and trajectory during vowel articulation. Acoustic metrics can also be developed for suprasegmental characteristics of speech, for instance a combination of vowel duration, intensity and F_0 measures, can be used to index the prominence relations between stress and unstressed syllables.

Other acoustic measures are statistical features or indices emerging from long spans of speech and can represent the overall use of a variable during a speaking event. For instance, there have been several attempts to quantify speech rhythm between and within languages and in neurogenic speech disorders by quantifying timing patterns in connected speech using a variety of duration-based metrics such as speaking rate and the standard deviation of vowel and/or consonant duration over an utterance or longer stretches of speech (Liss et al., 2009).

The selection and interpretation of acoustic measures is directly related to the speaking tasks used. Relevant tasks include, but are not limited to, vowel prolongation, syllable repetition, word and sentence production, reading and conversation. To illustrate, the vowel prolongation task, the simplest task for isolating the respiratory-phonatory speech systems (Kent, Vorperian, Kent, & Duffy, 2003) is used for the acoustic assessment of laryngeal function via a series of measures, taken from the steady middle potion of the vowel. Most of these measures, however, will generally not be considered valid if they are obtained from connected speech samples. Connected speech, especially conversation and free play, are the most meaningful areas for speech assessment, including acoustic analysis. However, spontaneous speech is difficult to control, highly variable and requires extensive samples to obtain stable measurements. Thus, making quantifications and between subject comparisons based on acoustic analysis of conversational data is often problematic and should be made cautiously (Rosen, Kent, Delaney, & Duffy, 2006). Clinicians should be aware that performance in a task does not predict patterns in conversational speech and ideally clinical decisions should be based on data, including acoustic metrics, from a variety of different speech events.

In the remaining part of this chapter we will present examples of acoustic indices that have been discussed in the literature of speech disorders and have been proven useful in clinical settings. These include both segmental and suprasegmental acoustic measures.

Segmental characteristics

Vowel articulation

Speech production involves the generation of a complex periodic sound source in the larynx, which is then filtered via changes in the size and shape of the vocal tract. Some frequencies resonate and have high amplitudes, and the remaining frequencies are attenuated. Each vocal tract configuration results in different resonance patterns; the resulting resonant frequencies are the formants which are important acoustic cues for speech perception. The first three resonant frequencies (formants F_1, F_2 and F_3) are the most widely used acoustic indices for the description of vowel articulation. Generally, the first two formants (F_1 and F_2) correlate with the articulatory dimensions of tongue height and tongue advancement (Ladefoged, 2005). As the tongue moves forward, the first formant decreases and the second formant increases. As the degree of constriction becomes smaller, F_1 decreases and F_2 increases. Finally, as the degree of lip rounding increases, F_1 and F_2 decrease. A high front vowel such as [i], is realized with a wide formant spread (low F_1, high F_2), [æ] that requires a lower and somewhat anterior tongue position is produced with a higher F_1 and a lower F_2, i.e. a more narrow formant spread, while [u], a back, rounded vowel has a low F_1 and low F_2, i.e. a minimal formant separation. The values of the first two formant frequencies are also affected by the presence of nasality and this should be taken into account when analyzing data from hypernasal speech. Diphthongs in contrast to monophthongs, consist of a movement from one vowel to another, they are produced with a continually moving tongue shape and changing sound quality, and thus they are acoustically characterized by patterns of formant transitions rather than stable formant frequencies.

Vowel formants for monophthongs and formant trajectories for diphthongs can be readily measured by identifying the darker bands in a wideband spectrogram. Most acoustic software have built-in linear predictive coding (LPC) algorithms that automatically generate formant tracks from spectrogaphic data and allow the computation of formant values at any point of the given vowel segments. Additionally, the acoustic vowel space, calculated by plotting the values of the first two vowel formants, can be used as an index of the vowel working space (Kent et al, 1999).

Although formant information is used to differentiate vowels from one another acoustically, given the individual differences in terms of fundamental frequency and vocal tract size, absolute formant frequencies will differ for different speakers. It is safer to rely on the degree of the formant separation, expressed as the ratio relationships among the first two formant frequencies, to differentiate vowels spoken by different speakers. In clinical populations, a variety of different patterns of atypical vowel production has been reported. For instance, in neurogenic speech disorders these patterns are usually associated with restricted tongue movement and include aberrant formant frequency values for high and for front vowels or the centralization of formant frequencies and the compression of the acoustic vowel space. The latter appears to be a general characteristic of many different types of speech disorders that is related to intelligibility (Weismer, 1997).

Consonant articulation

Consonants are diverse in terms of their perceptual and acoustic characteristics and it is difficult to describe them using a single set of acoustic indices (Kent & Read, 2002). Sonorant consonants, i.e. glides, liquids and nasals, have vowel-like properties and can be acoustically analyzed by describing patterns of formants (frequency regions that resonate), as well as antiformants (frequency regions in which the amplitudes of the source components are substantially attenuated). For instance, the articulatory placements and thus the formant patterns associated with the glides [j] and [w] are very similar to those of the vowels [i] and [u]. Similarly, nasal stops, such as [m], [n] and [ŋ], display two distinct resonance patterns; a severe amplitude attenuation in the high frequency range as the velum lowers and acoustic energy is absorbed by the nasal cavity tissues, and a concentration of the energy (formant or nasal murmur) in the lower frequency regions which are rendered darker in a wideband spectrogram display. Quantitative data on formant and antiformant patterns can be automatically generated using LPC algorithms as in the case of vowel formants. In the following section we will focus on nonsonorant consonants and specifically oral stops that have been emphasized in the acoustic literature.

Oral stops

Oral stops, [p, t, k] and [b, d, g] in English, are produced in three stages: (i) articulators are brought together, (ii) articulators are held together and pressure builds up behind the constriction and (iii) the constriction is released abruptly leading to a burst of noise. Voice onset time (VOT) is a simple and widely researched durational measure for syllable initial stops (Kent & Kim, 2003). It is defined as the acoustic interval between the burst and the onset of periodic energy in the speech signal that corresponds to the physiological interval between the release of the constriction of the stop consonant and the onset of vocal fold vibration of the following vowel. VOT is the most reliable acoustic cue for the distinction between voiced and voiceless stops (Auzou et al., 2000). VOT patterns have been used to describe oral stops both cross-linguistically and in the field of speech disorders. In English voiceless stops, voicing ceases during the closure interval and resumes after the release phase with a delay, i.e. positive VOT values ranging from 60 ms to 100 ms, whereas in most voiced stops release of closure and voicing happen almost at the same time, i.e. positive VOT values up to about 25 ms. On the other hand, in French, Greek and other languages, voiceless stops are normally produced with a brief voicing lag, as most English voiced stops, and voiced stops are realized with a voicing lead, i.e. vocal folds are vibrating during the time of closure. In some types of neurogenic speech disorders, including ataxic dysarthria and apraxia of speech, it is often assumed

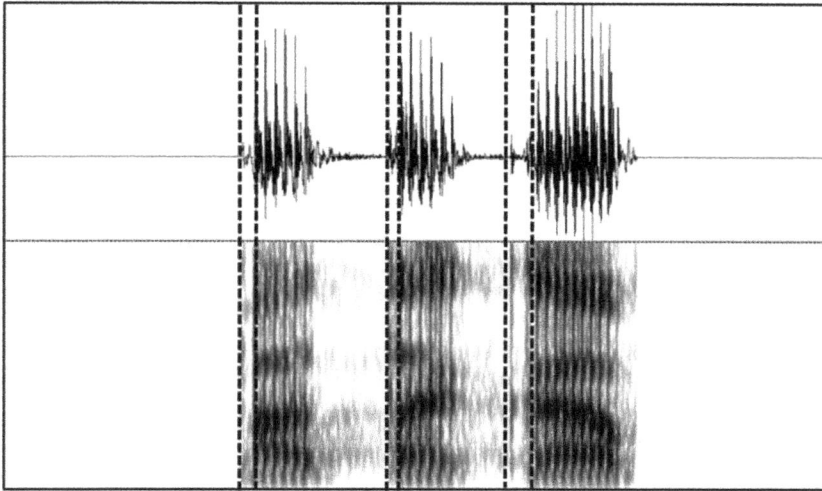

Figure 2.2 A waveform and a wideband spectrogram display of the sequence [pataka], produced by a typical Greek speaker. VOT values, the intervals between the dashed lines, are very brief since in Greek voiceless stops the release of closure and the commencement of voicing happen almost at the same time.

that atypical VOT values reflect problems with the timing and coordination of laryngeal and supralaryngeal activity (Morris, 1989; Ackermann & Hertrich, 1993). Clinicians can readily analyze the acoustic characteristics of their client's oral stop productions by inspecting the spectrographic data, and they can carry out VOT measurements using the wideband spectrogram and the waveform display to determine the onset of the burst and the voicing of the vowel. Figures 2.2 and 2.3 provide examples of VOT boundary identification from acoustic data of typical and atypical speakers.

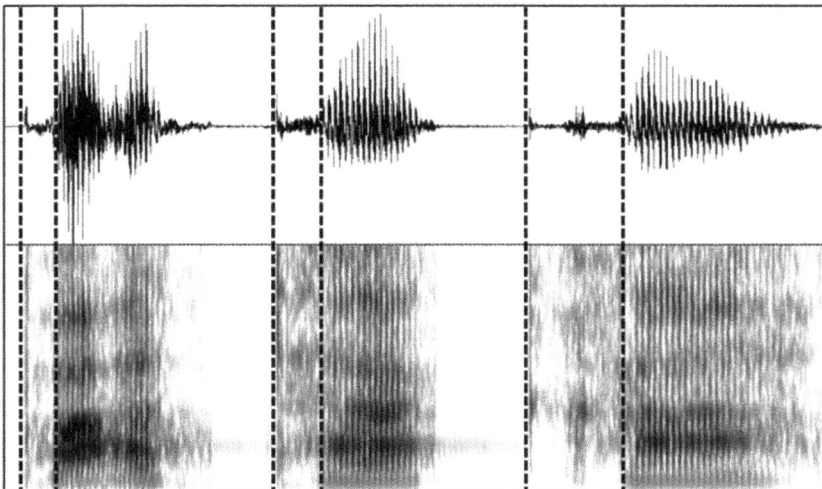

Figure 2.3 A waveform and a wideband spectrogram display of the sequence [pataka], produced by a Greek speaker with dysarthria. Note that VOT values are much longer indicating a difficulty to alternate between voiceless and voiced states.

Suprasegmental characteristics

Suprasegmental characteristics refer to aspects of speech that are not restricted to individual segments, but extend over larger units, i.e. syllables, words, phrases or sentences. In this review we will focus on voice quality, intonation and speaking rate.

Voice quality

Voice quality is a speech characteristic that has been notoriously difficult to describe and transcribe phonetically (Ball, Esling, & Dickson, 1995). Most of the clinical labels used for the assessment of dysphonic patients do not clearly correlate with specific vocal fold configurations, they are strictly perceptual and have been criticized as subjective (Duffy, 2019). Acoustic analysis of voice can involve several tasks (sustained phonation, phonation with loudness and pitch changes, voice-voiceless alternations, etc.) but sustained vowel prolongation, typically using the low back vowel [a], is the main task used to obtain measures of voice quality. Given that pathologic voice quality is commonly characterized by changes in the regularity of the vibratory cycle, most work on acoustic analysis has focused on the measurement of the periodicity of the voice signal. Pitch and amplitude perturbation measures (jitter and shimmer, respectively) are the most commonly used estimates of signal periodicity. They refer to the cycle-to-cycle fluctuations in the period duration (jitter) and the amplitude (shimmer) of adjacent pitch pulses. Another periodicity measure, harmonic-to-noise ratio (HNR) is the ratio of the energy present in the fundamental frequency and harmonics to the energy in the aperiodic component of speech, averaged over several cycles. These metrics are easily obtained, selecting the middle steady portion of the vowel prolongation to avoid unusual phenomena associated with the onset and offset of phonation, and applying automatic analysis routines that are readily available in most acoustic software. Although increased jitter has been associated with the perception of roughness (Hillenbrand, 1988), and HNR was found to correlate with perceptual ratings of breathiness (de Krom, 1995), there is no consistent research evidence that jitter, shimmer and HNR measures can classify patients by diagnostic category with the precision required in clinical settings, or that there is a straightforward relationship between them and the perceptual dimensions of voice quality. Accurate perturbation and HNR measures presuppose the precise determination of cycle-to-cycle boundaries, a task that requires high-quality recordings with no background noise and distortion, and signals without significant aperiodicity (Hillenbrand, 2011). Jitter, shimmer and HNR are recommended for patients with a mild voice disorder that generate nearly periodic voice signals in the vowel prolongation task, with harmonics that are clearly identifiable in a narrowband spectrogram (Bielamowicz, Kreiman, Gerratt, Dauer, & Berke, 1995). For patients with moderate and severe dysphonia and in cases when high quality recordings are not realistically feasible, it is suggested that it is more beneficial to carefully and consistently inspect the signal for disordered features than to run quantitative voice metrics.

Considering the methodological issues related to time-based voice measures, alternative metrics that use an amplitude-by-frequency analysis of speech, i.e. the spectrum, to calculate the distribution of signal energy, have been proposed (Hillenbrand, 2011). These include measures of the distribution of signal energy in the harmonic and the non-harmonic frequencies that are based on the idea that in a perfectly periodic signal all spectral energy will be found in the harmonic regions of the spectrum and the ratio of harmonic to non-harmonic energy is expected to decrease in dysphonic voices. Similar metrics quantify the distribution of high and low frequency energy in the voice signal, based on the premise that a voice produced with incomplete glottal closure would show an increased ratio of high to low frequency energy.

Both types of spectral metrics appear to correlate well with listener ratings of breathiness (e.g. Hillenbrand & Houde, 1996). An additional advantage of such metrics is that they can be calculated not only for sustained vowels but also for connected speech samples using long-term average spectra (LTAS), that are essentially power spectra calculated for regular intervals (e.g. every 5 ms) averaged over a given stretch of speech, a full utterance or a longer text. It is clinically useful having measures that can be applied across a number of different speaking tasks, given that some voice dysfunctions are only manifested, or become more evident, in connected speech. For example, the vocal disturbances in spasmodic dysphonia often become much more noticeable in connected speech than in vowel prolongation (Kent et al, 2003).

Another acoustic measure that can be obtained from both vowels and connected speech signals and it is recommended for use with voices in the moderate to severe range is a metric called Cepstral Peak Prominence (CPP) (Hillenbrand, Cleveland, & Erickson, 1994). It is obtained by performing a Fourier transformation of the spectrum, creating a cepstrum. In the cepstrum, periodic voices should display prominent harmonics that emerge as elevated peaks. CPP is an amplitude-normalized measure of the amplitude of the cepstral peak corresponding to the harmonic regularity. Several acoustic software, including Praat, offer automatic analysis routine for computing CPP. This cepstral estimate is considered a robust clinical index that correlates well with listener ratings of severity of dysphonia (Awan, Roy, & Dromey, 2009) and can differentiate distinct types of voice pathology (Awan & Roy, 2005).

Intonation

Intonation refers to patterns of pitch variation over an utterance, rather than a syllable or a word. Pitch perception depends mainly on changes in the frequency of vocal fold vibration, i.e. the fundamental frequency (F_0), that can be readily extracted from the acoustic signal, visualized and measured. Intonation is used to signal the function of an utterance. A very common use of intonation in several languages, including English, is a rising F_0 at the end of a question and falling F_0 at the end of a statement. In English, questions are marked either via intonation or syntactically, i.e. "You ate my ice-cream?" or "Did you eat my ice-cream?" while in other languages, including Greek, intonation is the only means to signal a polar question. Changes in intonation in a sentence can also change meaning or emphasize what is important, i.e. "Who ate my ice-cream? "Kate ate your ice-cream." In clinical populations, it possible to witness issues related to the linguistic use of pitch, such as difficulty signaling questions vs. statements. However, the most frequent pattern of disordered intonation, common in neurogenic speech disorders, results from problems with sustaining the normal variations of F_0 in connected speech which bring about the perceptual impressions of flat, monotonous intonation, also described with the labels "monopitch" and "reduced stress" (Duffy, 2019). In these cases, even if acceptable levels of intelligibility can be achieved, speech lacks naturalness, which can be detrimental to the patient's overall communicative effectiveness. The acoustic analysis of intonation in clinical settings typically involves the extraction of the pitch track from a connected speech signal and the calculation of measures that express the level, shape and variation of the F_0 contour (e.g. mean F_0, F_0 range and standard deviation, etc.), which are readily available in most acoustic software. Figure 2.4 shows an example of the use of the pitch track display to document spontaneous recovery of speech in the early stages following traumatic brain injury. As evident in the F_0 contours in 4A and 4B, initially the patient had flat intonation with minimal F_0 variation, but within a period of two months she could produce the same wh-question with the typical melody for Greek, i.e. an initial high pitch gesture on the wh- element, followed by a gradual fall and an utterance final rise.

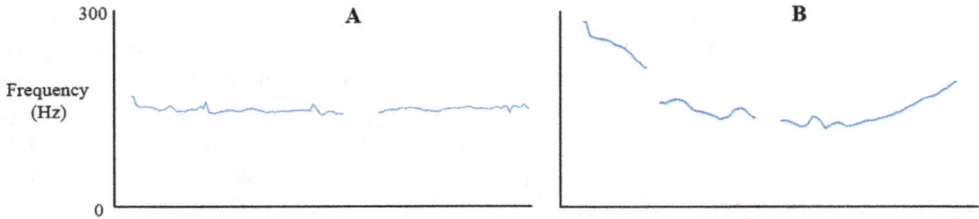

Figure 2.4   Pitch track of the wh-question [ti ˈefaɣes to proˈi] ("What did you eat in the morning?") generated from a Greek patient with traumatic brain injury: (A) one week post onset and (B) two months post onset.

Speaking rate

Speaking rate is very straightforward in terms of its measurement and physiologic interpretation. It is usually measured in terms of syllables per minute and reflects the speed of articulatory movement. It is important to keep in mind that speaking time involves both articulation time and pause duration. Speaking rate is clinically relevant, given its assumed correlation with articulatory precision and thus, intelligibility. Clinicians often aim to reduce their clients' rate of speech to work on intelligibility, monitoring at the same time their naturalness which can be significantly affected at very slow speaking rates (Yorkston, Beukelman, Strand, & Hakel, 2010). The duration of segments, words and utterances as well as pause time can be easily measured from a waveform and a spectrographic display. Additionally, it is often useful to divide the speech signal into breath groups based on the presence of inter-word pauses, and measure their length and duration. Apart from segment durations, articulatory gestures can be acoustically analyzed by monitoring the trajectory change in formant patterns. As a matter of fact, the slope of the transition of the second formant (F_2) has been used as an index of intelligibility (Kent et al, 1999). Figure 2.5 shows an example of articulatory slowness in a patient with cerebral palsy. Her utterance was about five times longer in duration compared to that of

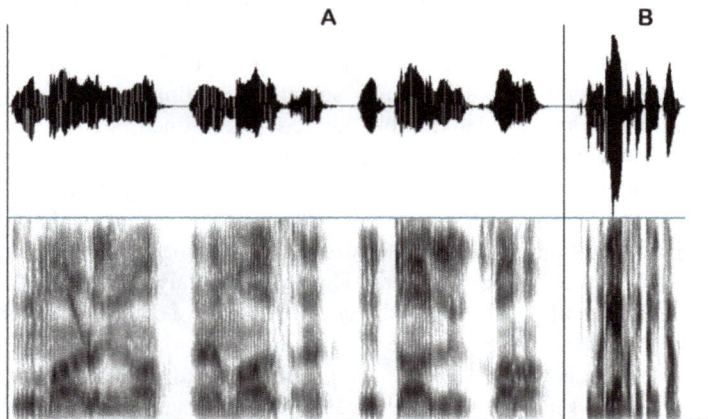

Figure 2.5   A waveform and a wideband spectrogram of the Greek phrase [i maˈria ˈemaθe italiˈka] ("Maria learned Italian") produced by (A) a Greek speaker with cerebral palsy and (B) a typical Greek speaker. The patient produces the sentence in about 7.5 seconds, while the control speaker takes only 1.5 seconds. You can see the patient's phrasal pauses, and her slow articulatory gestures evident in the very gradual formant transitions and the long segments.

the control speaker. This slowness was evident by the long segment durations, the slow formant transitions and the extensive inter-word pauses.

In this chapter, we have outlined many of the main aspects of speech acoustics and how these can be measured and displayed. In Chapter 30 of this book, more details on spectrographic analysis are provided together with examples of analyses of a range of different speech disorders.

References

Ackermann, H. & Hertrich, I. (1993). Dysarthria in Friedreich's ataxia: Timing of speech segments. *Clinical Linguistics and Phonetics*, 7, 75–91.

Auzou, P., Ozsancak, C., Morris, R. J., Jan, M., Eustache, F., & Hannequin, D. (2000). Voice onset time in aphasia, apraxia of speech and dysarthria: A review. *Clinical Linguistics and Phonetics*, 14(2), 131–150.

Awan, S. & Roy, N. (2005). Acoustic prediction of voice type in women with functional dysphonia. *Journal of Voice*, 19, 268–282.

Awan, S., Roy, N., & Dromey, C. (2009). Estimating dysphonia severity in continuous speech: Application of a multi-parameter spectral/cepstral model. *Clinical Linguistics and Phonetics*, 23, 825–841.

Ball, M.J., Esling, J., & Dickson, C. (1995). The VoQS system for the transcription of voice quality *Journal of the International Phonetic Association*. 25(2), 71–80.

Bielamowicz, S., Kreiman, J., Gerratt, B., Dauer, M., & Berke, G. (1996). Comparison of voice analysis systems for perturbation measurement. *Journal of Speech, Language and Hearing Research*, 9, 126–134.

Carson, C.K. & Ryalls, J. (2018). A new era in acoustic analysis: Use of smartphones and readily accessible software/applications for voice assessment. *JSM Communication Disorders*, 2(1), 1006.

de Krom, G. (1995). Some spectral correlates of pathological breathy and rough voice quality for different types of vowel fragments. *Journal of Speech and Hearing Research*, 38(4), 794–811.

Duffy, J.R. (2019). *Motor Speech Disorders: Substrates, Differential Diagnosis, and Management*. St. Louis: Mosby.

Hillenbrand, J.M. (1988). Perception of aperiodicities in synthetically generated voices. *Journal of the Acoustical Society of America*, 83, 2361–2371.

Hillenbrand, J.M., Cleveland, R. A., & Erickson, R. L. (1994). Acoustic correlates of breathy vocal quality. *Journal of Speech and Hearing Research*, 37, 769–778.

Hillenbrand, J.M. & Houde, R. A. (1996). Acoustic correlates of breathy vocal quality: Dysphonic voices and continuous speech. *Journal of Speech and Hearing Research*, 39, 311–321.

Hillenbrand, J.M. (2011). Acoustic analysis of voice: A tutorial. *Perspectives on Speech Science and Orofacial Disorders*, 21(2), 31–43.

Kent, R.D. (1996). Hearing and believing: Some limits to the auditory-perceptual assessment of speech and voice disorders. *American Journal of Speech-Language Pathology*, 7, 7–23.

Kent, R.D. & Kim, Y.J. (2003). Towards an acoustic typology of motor speech disorders. *Clinical Linguistics and Phonetics*, 17(6), 427–445.

Kent, R.D. & Read, W.C. (2002). *The Acoustic Analysis of Speech*. San Diego: Singular Publishing Group.

Kent, R.D., Vorperian, H.K., Kent, J.F. & Duffy, J.R. (2003). Voice dysfunction in dysarthria: Application of the multi-dimensional voice program. *Journal of Communication Disorders*, 36, 281–306.

Kent, R.D., Weismer, G., Kent, J.F., Vorperian, J.K. & Duffy, J.R. (1999). Acoustic studies of dysarthric speech. Methods, progress and potential. *Journal of Communication Disorders*, 32, 141–186.

Kreiman, J., Gerratt, B.R., & Ito, M. (2007). When and why listeners disagree in voice quality assessment tasks. *Journal of the Acoustical Society of America*, 122, 2354–2364.

Morris, R.J. (1989). VOT and dysarthria: A descriptive study. *Journal of Communication Disorders*, 22, 23–33.

Ladefoged, P. (2005). *Vowels and Consonants*. Oxford: Blackwell.

Lin, E., Hornibrook, J., & Ormond, T. (2012). Evaluating iPhone recordings for acoustic voice assessment. *Folia Phoniatrica et Logopaedica*, 64, 122–130.

Liss, J.M., White, L., Mattys, S.L., Lansford, K., Lotto, A.J., Spitzer, S.M., & Canivess, J.N. (2009). Quantifying speech rhythm abnormalities in the dysarthrias. *Journal of Speech, Language, and Hearing Research*, 52, 1334–1352.

Rosen, K., Kent, R., Delaney, A., & Duffy, J. (2006). Parametric quantitative acoustic analysis of conversation produced by speakers with dysarthria and healthy speakers. *Journal of Speech, Language and Hearing Research*, 49, 395–411.

Weismer, G. (1997). Motor speech disorders. In W.J. Hardcastle & J. Laver (Eds.), *The Handbook of Phonetic Sciences* (pp.191–219). Cambridge: Blackwell.

Yorkston, K.M., Beukelman, D.R., Strand, E.A., & Hakel, M. (2010). *Management of Motor Speech Disorders*. Austin: Pro-Ed.

3

AUDITORY PHONETICS FOR THE SPEECH CLINICIAN

Elena Babatsouli

Introduction

Phonetics is a branch of linguistics (the study of language) that is concerned with human speech sounds. The *<phone>* part of the word *phonetics* originates in the Greek φωνή [foˈni] which means "voice." Voice is an attribute that may be simultaneously associated with different entities: the speaker, the sound itself, the listener. Because of this, the study of phonetics is distinguished into three main categories: *articulatory* (planning and execution of movements for speech production), *acoustic* (the physical properties of speech sounds) and *auditory* (the conversion of speech sounds into linguistic information), as also represented in the thematic contents of this volume. Expertise in phonetics is a vital asset in the speech clinician's repertoire of skills.

The present chapter focuses on the latter of the three categories, *auditory phonetics*, in lay terms referring to "hearing," as derived from the Latin term *audire* "to hear." Thus, what follows is a succinct discussion of the fundamental themes and notions involved in the systematic study of normal and impaired hearing within the scientific field of *audiology*. Audiology came about in the mid-1900s as a result of the fields of speech pathology (*<pathos>* Greek "suffering," *<logy>* Greek "speaking of") and otology (*<oto>* Greek "ear") coming together to represent, respectively, nonmedical and medical perspectives in our understanding of human hearing, the identification of hearing impairment, the assessment of hearing capacity/loss and subsequent rehabilitation procedures (Newby, 1979).

As with most scientific fields, audiology is wide-spectral in that it may be tackled from different perspectives while also informing and being informed by experts from diverse fields of investigation, three of which are medical: pediatrics (*<pedia>* Greek "children"), gerontology (*<gero>* Greek "elderly") and neurology (*<neuron>* Greek "nerve"); and three are nonmedical: physics (*<physi>* Greek "nature"), psychology (*<phycho>* Greek "soul") and education (*educare*, Latin "bring up, rear"). Pediatrics and gerontology are closely related to audiology because they are concerned with patients at two extreme age-groups that mostly evidence hearing impairment/loss. Similarly, neurology is germane to audiology because of the involvement of human nerves in transmitting the speech signal/sound to the brain for processing during communicative acts.

Among the nonmedical fields just mentioned, the physics of the speech signal refer, first, to *acoustics* (waves, the physical propagation of sound) and, second, to *electronics* (technological applications dealing with the emission, flow and control of electrons in matter) as used in diagnostic and rehabilitation procedures of hearing impairment (e.g. audiometers, hearing aids). Consultation with a psychology expert may also be required when hearing impairment adversely affects the psychological wellbeing of the person suffering it. Finally, hearing impairment/loss in children may have detrimental effects to the development of language and communicative skills, and the way these affect several aspects of children's educational development.

The clinical emphasis of the present volume necessitates the inclusion of information on what is involved in hearing, both normal and in the presence of impairment/disorder—a dichotomy that will be also reflected in the thematic undercurrent of this chapter. Within the study of speech science, normal speaker/listener interaction is represented by a diagram referred to as *The Speech Chain* (e.g. Denes & Pinson, 1993), pictorially depicting interrelationships between a *Speaker's* mouth, brain and nerves, the speech *Sound* waves, and a *Listener's* outer ear, brain and nerves. Illustrations of the speech chain diagram are freely available online. Thus, the "fundamentals of hearing" involve: (i) the *ear* ("peripheral auditory anatomy and physiology"); (ii) the *sound* itself ("auditory stimulus"); (iii) the listener's *sensitivity* to the sound ("auditory sensation") in relation to *pitch, loudness, sound localization*, i.e. the ability to identify the location/origin of the sound, and *sound masking*, i.e. the ambient sound, specifically engineered to match human speech and used to minimize the extent of conversational distractions, (iv) *how the speech sound is processed* and the intermediary role of nerves transmitting signals to the brain ("auditory perception and the central nervous system") (Yost, 2013).

Figure 3.1 is an illustration of the speech chain notion that is specifically adapted here to have a focus on hearing for the requirements of this chapter.

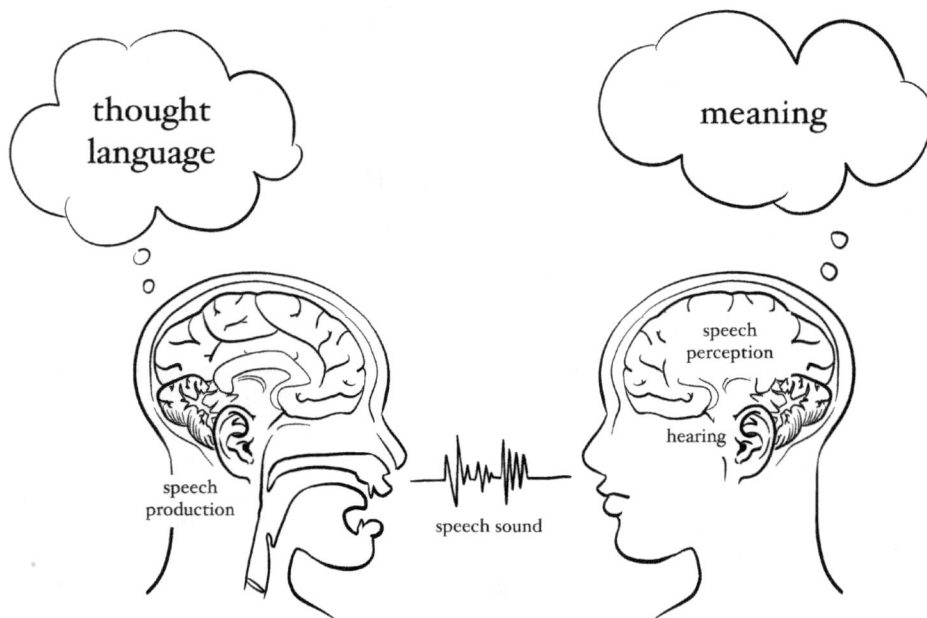

Figure 3.1 Hearing in the speech chain.
Source: S. Qiouyi Lu.

Because terminological clarity is not *de facto*, disambiguation of terms is also addressed where necessary. Both hearing "impairment" and "disorder" are in use in medical and non-medical academic articles and books to refer to a range of hearing problems, including hearing loss (Bagai et al., 2006; Crandell & Smaldino, 2000; Hudson & DeRuiter, 2019; Katz, 2014; Kennedy et al., 2005; Libb et al., 1985; Miceli et al., 2008). "Hearing impairment" will be the generic term preferred here. Definitions of "impairment" and "disability" allude to divergent but associated concepts: *impairment* is the loss of a body part or a significant deviation of a body function or structure, whereas *disability* is a person's inability to be functional in personal, social or professional settings as a result of the presence of impairment (e.g. Dobbie & Van Hemel, 2005).

The remaining of this chapter consists of the following sections: the hearing mechanism, anatomy and physiology of the auditory system, routes of hearing, the measurement of hearing, causes and types of hearing impairment, and conclusion.

The hearing mechanism

Oral language in a speaker's voice (speech signal or sound stimulus) takes the form of sound waves that enter the ear; the speech signal is then transmitted through the ear, and onward via the nerves to the brain where the meaning associated with the original linguistic signal is processed. In other words, the ear behaves like a biotransducer that changes the form of energy from sound wave, to mechanical vibration, to electrical impulse.

Anatomy and physiology of the auditory system

The human ear may be described in terms of its peripheral (*peripheral auditory system*) and internal (*internal auditory system*) constituents. The peripheral component is an exterior section, or a prefatory stage, leading to internal or more central organs and functions of the hearing mechanism.

The peripheral auditory system (PAS)

This section will describe the anatomy (or physical apparatus) of the ear. Figure 3.2 is an abstract representation of the right ear's PAS (assuming it is facing the reader); see also Clark et al. (2007). Anatomical illustrations are freely available online.

There are three parts in the PAS: the *external* ear, the *middle* ear and the *inner* ear. The external ear consists of the *auricle* or *pinna* (the only visible part of the human ear) and the *external auditory canal* (or *meatus*). The auricle functions like a funnel capturing the sound signal in the environment (cf. similarly, the hand cups behind the ear in noisy contexts); then, the sound wave passes through the auditory canal and briefly stumbles on the *eardrum* penetrating it to enter the middle ear. The eardrum, *tympanic membrane* (Greek "thin tissue shaped like a drum") has a semitransparent, quasi-circular shape coning inwards. It is the physical boundary of the middle ear between the auditory canal and the first of the three *auditory ossicles* (tiny bones) that form a chain (*ossicular chain*) in the middle ear. In order of appearance and decreasing size, these bones are: the *malleus* (Latin "hammer"), the *incus* (Latin "anvil") and the *stapes* (Latin "stirrups")—the last one being the smallest in the human body (3 mm long).

The ossicular chain has two functions: (i) it is a mechanical lever system that increases the force of the transmitted signal and ii) it behaves like an acoustic reflex mechanism that contracts to regulate the sound level when the noise reaching the middle ear is extremely loud.

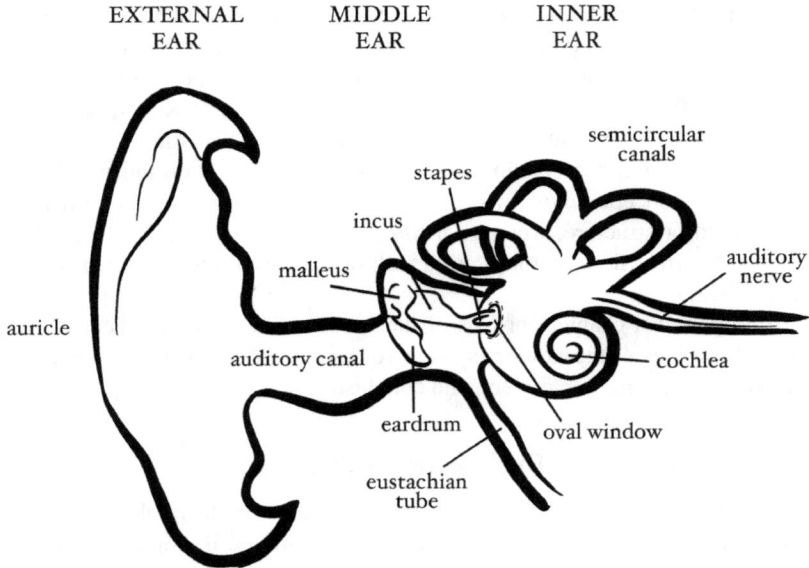

Figure 3.2   The peripheral auditory system.

Source: Courtesy S. Qiouyi Lu.

It is the *stapedius* muscle that actually stabilizes the stapes, attenuating intense sounds in the area. The degree of movement of the ossicular chain resulting from the stapedius' contraction is called *amplitude*. The time between the onset of sound and the contraction is called *latency*. The entire middle ear section is called the *tympanum* "drum," because it transforms the sound pressure vibrations coming from the auditory canal into actual mechanical movements of the ossicular chain, as the ossicles vibrate consecutively, much like a chain reaction.

The stapes are attached to the *oval window*, a breach in the skull's bone structure which actually has a smaller surface than the eardrum. Given that pressure is great on a smaller surface than on a larger one, the resulting acoustic energy on the oval window is 35 times greater than on the eardrum. Pressure differences between the external and the middle ear are balanced by the *Eustachian tube* (*pharyngotympanic tube*) that connects the middle ear with the nasal and oral cavities releasing the pressure (cf. the function of swallowing to equalize pressure in the ear in airplane flights). The purpose of the middle ear, thus, is to transmit, regulate and amplify the incoming signal, as the signal is further thrust toward the inner ear.

The inner section of the ear, also referred to as the *labyrinth*, is very complex in structure, and it includes *fluid*, the *cochlea*, a snail-like organ that coordinates hearing, and the *vestibular apparatus* that is responsible for balance. Balance is achieved because of the position of the organs of the vestibular apparatus that stays the same irrespective of the position of the head in space. The *semicircular canals* form part of the vestibular apparatus. The cochlea and semicircular canals are connected in a shared area, the *vestibule*. One side of the cochlea, the *base*, connects to the oval window leading to the stapes and the other side, the *apex*, is the innermost section of the cochlea. The cochlea itself consists of three tubes rolled up like the shell of a snail—each tube divided by the next by a membrane: the *vestibular* and the *basilar*. Inside the basilar membrane, the *organ of Corti* has tiny inner and outer hair cells that link to the auditory nerve. Fluid in the cochlea is of two types: *perilymph* and *endolymph* that stimulate the sensorineural hair cells of the organ of Corti. The function of the organ of Corti is pivotal for our perception of the speech signal.

The inner ear has a similar function to that of the middle ear transmitting, altering and evaluating incoming sounds. First, the inner ear converts the vibrations coming from the middle ear into neural signals, as follows: middle ear vibrations are transported by the cochlear fluid into the basilar membrane, which sets in motion the hair on the organ of Corti, and the hairs convert vibrations into electrical impulses that are sent, in turn, to the brain via neurotransmitters. It is, thus, apparent that proper functioning of the hair on the organ of Corti is critical for normal hearing. Another function of the inner ear is that of sound analysis. This is done by the vibration of the hair of the organ of Corti that amplifies sounds. The basilar membrane sorts out the incoming sounds based on their frequency: sounds with higher frequency (max. 32,000 Hz for humans) activate the cochlea at the base, while sounds with lower frequency (min. ca. 20 Hz for humans) activate the cochlea at the apex; intermediate frequencies are activated accordingly around the cochlea curl. Due to higher frequencies processed there, the cochlea base is more vulnerable to damage from intense vibration, especially around the 3,000–6,000 Hz range. In fact, the point of most hearing loss is localized around the 4,000 Hz dip. Figure 3.3 shows the *tonotopy,* i.e. the spatial arrangement (Greek <*topos*> "place") of *tones* (sounds of different frequency) in the cochlea; see also Lahav and Skoe (2014).

Finally, the basilar membrane has a bidirectional function in that neural vibrations coming from the brain can also affect its resting status due to cellular or mechanical causes, thus, causing it to move; this vibration forms a brain-prompted sound, known as *otoacoustic emission* (OAE) (e.g. Kemp, 2002). OAEs can be measured with sensitive microphones and are routinely used as a simple, noninvasive hearing test; complete lack of OAEs is evidence of hearing impairment of the inner ear.

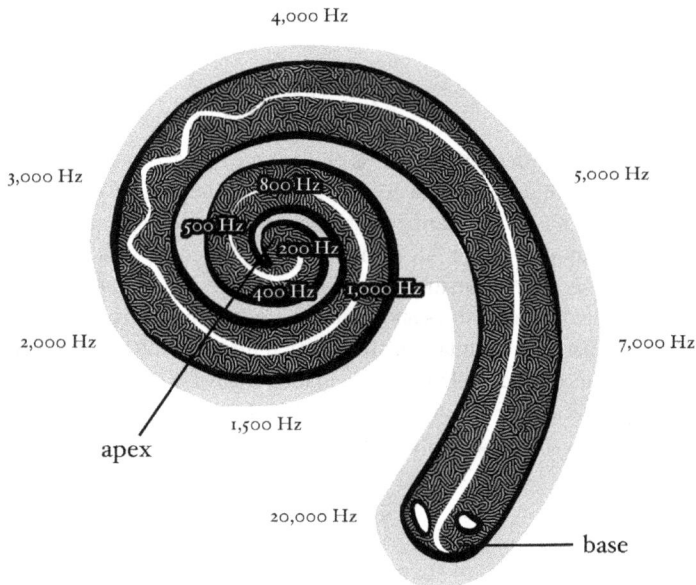

Figure 3.3 Cochlea and its tonotopy across the frequency spectrum.

Source: S. Qiouyi Lu.

The internal auditory system (IAS)

The IAS is responsible for transmitting sound information to the brain for processing (*high executive function*). The IAS consists of the *auditory nerve* and the *central auditory system (CAS)*. The auditory nerve utilizes electrical impulses to transfer the speech signal information that was coded in the cochlea to the brain. In particular, the inner hairs act as transducers converting vibration into neural discharge. The bending of the hairs on the inner hair cells causes a neuroelectrical response, while the size of the outer hairs changes leading to mechanical alteration of the cochlea. This coupling activates a response from the nerves which is transferred through the auditory nerve to different parts of the brain for further analysis. Different nerve cells (and their fibers) are linked to different parts of the organ of Corti, each specializing in a specific sound frequency. Under normal hearing, the nerve fibers go past the auditory nerve, enter the *brainstem* (posterior part of the brain) at the cochlea nucleus, gradually proceeding to the *superior olivary complex* (SOC) and the *inferior culliculi* in order to eventually reach the *cerebral cortex* (or *auditory cortex*). The areas of auditory reception are mainly in the *temporal lobes* on both sides of the cortex, but other parts of the cortex are also involved in the representation of hearing. Each ear's representation in the cortex is bilateral; as a result, disruption of the auditory track on one side of the brain does not impede hearing in either ear. The interested reader is directed to Musiek and Baran (2007), Rouse (2019) and Seikel et al. (2020) for more detailed anatomical descriptions of IAS, and Delgutte (1997) for a discussion on auditory neural processing of speech sounds.

The function of the auditory nerve is often investigated in disorders caused by a tumor (*acoustic neuroma*) and in rehabilitation procedures using *cochlear implants*. Similarly, if the capacity of nerve fibers to process different sound frequencies is compromised, our hearing capacity is also compromised. An unexpected loud sound, or long-term exposure to high and intense noise, may permanently impair hair cells that lose their biotransducer capacity and are incapacitated. Hearing impairment due to aging also results from nerve failure to process sound frequencies and transmit the processed information to the auditory cortex.

The acoustic reflex

The *acoustic reflex (AR)* is often utilized as a clinical tool to assess the healthy status of the hearing mechanism in the middle ear, the cochlea, cochlea nucleus, as well as the low auditory brainstem in the function of SOC. Nevertheless, conductive hearing loss (discussed below) limits ability to observe a patient's AR. The AR primarily functions to prevent damage to the cochlea from high intensity sounds (see above the function of stapedius). The stapedius contracts more at high intensities and less at low intensities and in silence. When the AR is activated in one ear, both stapedius muscles (one per ear) simultaneously contract, informed by facial nerves on either side of the head. Typical AR thresholds in humans are in the range of 80–90 dB, with frequencies over 250–4,000 Hz having little effect. The amplitude of the AR is proportional to the sound's intensity level, while its latency is disproportional to the sound's high intensity and frequency.

Tinnitus

The normal perception (sensation) of sound in the ear with a lack of external acoustic stimulus is called *tinnitus* and is described as a buzzing, hissing, humming, ringing or whistling sound. Common experiences of tinnitus include the aftermath of having been close to loud speakers playing in concerts, or sensing a pulse beat. Tinnitus can be either *objective* (rare occurrence with an internal acoustic stimulus, e.g. turbulent blood flow near the ear) in that the audiologist can hear it, or *subjective* (occurring with no acoustic stimulus at all) in that it is only heard by the person experiencing it.

Tinnitus is common in people with hearing loss, but not all people with hearing loss experience it. It may be the result of broken/damaged auditory hair cells, turbulence in a carotid artery or jugular vein, temporomandibular joint (TMJ) issues and problems in the auditory processing pathways of the brain. Tinnitus *tones* (sound frequencies) are close to the frequencies people have difficulty hearing. The intensity of an external tone matched in loudness to a person's tinnitus is usually less than 10 dB above that person's threshold for the tone. Tinnitus does not customarily cause suffering, though trouble concentrating and understanding speech, emotional issues (anxiety, depression, etc.), and sleep disturbance have been reported in extreme cases (e.g. Tyler & Baker, 1983).

Routes of hearing

While anatomists are interested in the physiology of the hearing mechanism, audiologists and physicians focus on measuring hearing for the assessment and diagnosis of hearing impairment. In this point of view, the function of the ear can be seen as either *conductive* or *sensorineural*. Conduction refers to the process by which sound waves travel through a medium and is distinguished into *air conduction* and *bone conduction*. The two fork-like symbols in Figure 3.4 point out the two different conduction paths, but they also represent a tuning-fork, which is an

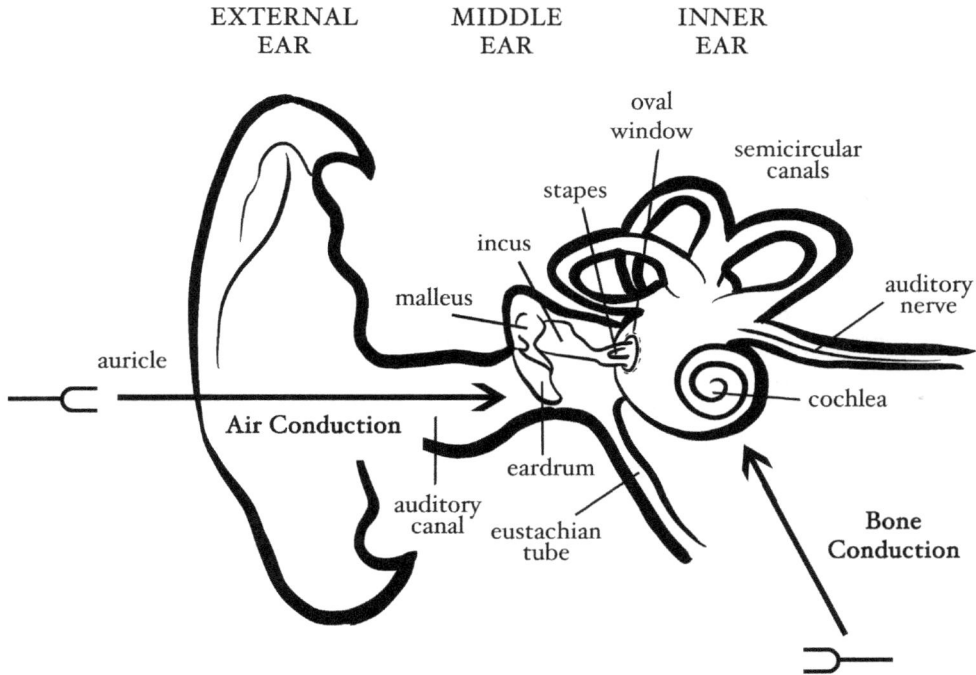

Figure 3.4   Conductive versus sensorineural hearing.

Source: Courtesy S. Qiouyi Lu.

instrument producing tones at different pitch values and traditionally used by audiologists to test *hearing sensitivity* (i.e. how well the ear hears).

Most of the sounds we hear are airborne; air conduction takes place in the external ear, middle ear and beyond, as sound pressure is channeled via the eardrum (external ear) and ossicles (middle ear) to the inner ear composed of fluid and tissue. This phenomenon whereby a medium carries ("admits") sound inward is called *admittance*. As the medium admitting the sound stimulus changes from less to more dense (i.e. from air to fluid and tissue), the process of admitting pressure is impeded, with a pressure loss of up to 35 dB, a phenomenon called *impedance*. This conduction of pressure inside the ear is known as *acoustic immitance* (from *im*[pedance]+[ad]*mitance*). In spite of this, the entire hearing apparatus functions in a way that tries to counteract the 35 dB impedance.

Conduction by bone involves vibrations reaching the ear through the movement of the bone section of the skull in which the inner ear is nested. Thus, bone conduction can only happen in the inner ear and beyond. Hearing by bone conduction is admittedly less effective than by air conduction. This is because: (i) the sound stimulus must be very intense to cause vibrations in the skull, and (ii) no matter how intense the sound is, its progress through the outer layers of human body (skin, flesh) to reach the bone, dissipates the vibration eventually reaching the bone. For this reason, bone conduction generally results in sound distortion. Also, hearing by bone conduction is less conscious to us than by air, as when we rest our head on the floor and feel the vibration of footsteps. The reason that our voice sounds different in recordings is because this is how *others* hear our voice by air conduction. The way we hear *our own* voice is (i) while we talk: by a combination of air and bone conduction, as the sound is first air-conducted via the cavities of the head and neck and, subsequently, bone-conducted through the skull's bones and (ii) after we talked, that is, via external air conduction that sends the sound wave of our voice to our ears. This multi-plane process leads to our "distorted" acuity regarding our voice.

Last, *sensorineural* hearing refers to the part of the auditory track where no conduction takes place; on the other hand, there is transmission of the sound stimulus within and beyond the inner ear via mechanical and electrical impulses to the auditory nerve ultimately reaching the cerebral cortex.

The measurement of hearing

The normal *threshold of hearing* for humans is between 20 and 30 Hz (hertz, cycles per second) and 0 and 20 dB (decibel, sound level). The normal hearing range is between 20 and 30 Hz and 32,000 Hz and at intensities between 10–90 dB (<30 dB: whisper, leaves rustling, birds chirping; 30–60 dB: conversation; 60–90 dB: car passing, dog barking, baby crying, telephone ringing, loud music; 90–110 dB, discomfort: motorcycle, airplane, train; >110, pain: thunder, explosion; 140 dB: ear damage). The hearing range for speech and language is 500–8,000 Hz. In frequencies above 1,000 Hz, our capacity to hear small changes in frequency decreases, while our capacity to hear high-frequency sounds deteriorates with age. Voiced speech sounds (phones: z, v, j, m, l, o, i) have high frequencies, while voiceless speech sounds have low frequencies (phones: t, s, ʃ, f, θ). A combination of sounds is called "white noise" when all frequency components have the same average sound level. Hearing sensitivity in normal, impaired hearing or *hearing loss* is measured by *audiometry*. Specifically, to test hearing sensitivity, *pure tones* (simple sinusoidal waves) with different frequencies spanning from low to high, are successively played to a listener's ear and the listener is expected to indicate when the tone was heard. The average threshold for different frequencies is used to give an estimate of auditory sensitivity or hearing loss. This is referred to as the pure-tone average (PTA) threshold, where the frequencies used for threshold averaging are listed in abbreviated form, e.g. a PTA threshold obtained at 300 Hz (.3 kHz), 1,000 Hz (1 kHz) and 2,000 Hz (2 kHz) is noted as PTA 512. An audiogram shows the hearing threshold for each frequency established. Based on such PTAs, loss of hearing, indicated by dB, is classified as follows:

	Hearing loss
16–25 dB	*slight*
26–40 dB	*mild*
41–55 dB	*moderate*
56–70 dB	*moderately severe*
71–90 dB	*severe*
>90 dB	*profound*

The criteria that determine hearing disability require that the ear functioning better shows one of the two following: (1) a PTA air conduction threshold, for 500, 1,000 and 2,000 Hz, (PTA 512) of 90 dB hearing level or greater, with corresponding bone conduction thresholds, or, (2) a speech discrimination score of ≤40%, at a sufficient level to decide maximum discrimination skill.

Types and causes of hearing impairment

Normal hearing refers to the hypothetical average hearing of a young adult (aged 18–22) with no known hearing pathology (infection, disorder). Any considerable deviation from normal ear behavior is considered a disorder, classified under hearing impairment (HI). In lay terms, differentiation in the seriousness of HI has led to two characterizations: *hard-of-hearing* and *deaf*, the first denoting variable degrees of loss of hearing sensitivity, and the second denoting complete lack of hearing. HI may be *organic* or *nonorganic*. Nonorganic HI has *psychogenic* (i.e. psychological disorder) origins. On the other hand, impairments resulting from malfunction or damage in the operation of any intercepting link within the hearing apparatus are organic and form four categories: *conductive HI* (hindrance in the auditory track involving conduction), *sensorineural HI* (setbacks within the inner ear and auditory nerve), *mixed HI* (instances of both conductive and sensorineural HI) and finally, *central auditory processing disorder* (where hearing loss is caused by damage in the neural pathway of sound inside the brain). These impairments are called *organic*.

HI involves *hearing loss* (HL), i.e. *attenuation* of a sound's strength at variable degrees from slight to profound, as seen before. Further subcategories specify whether one or both ears are affected (*unilateral* vs. *bilateral*), whether both ears are equally affected (*symmetrical* vs. *assymetrical*), and the onset of HI compared to language development (*prelingual* vs. *postlingual*). Hearing loss may also be described as *progressive* or *sudden, fluctuating* or *stable*, and *congenital* (present at birth) or *acquired* (developed later in life).

Conductive hearing impairment

Conductive HI (CHI) results from impaired air conduction, though bone conduction is normal. The symptoms include: speaking with a low voice (the patient hears himself well but not environmental noise), hearing speech better in noise contexts because noise has a masking effect (*paracusis willisiana*), better tolerance of sounds at discomfort level, loss of sensitivity to all sound frequencies (*flat loss*), and tinnitus. Likely settings of conductive HI include: blockage of the external meautus by, e.g. *cerumen* (wax) accumulation, or by tiny objects children play with; in infants born with missing auricle(s) (*agenesis*) or occluded canals (*atresia*). Atresia is curable if the inner ear is functioning well. Medical conditions leading to CHI include upper respiratory infections (*otitis media*) that cause the eardrum to be either distended or retracted, in the second case affecting the patency (opening) of the Eustachian tubes. Another medical condition causing CHI is *otosclerosis* (the inner ear bone capsule becomes spongy). CHI can in most cases be treated via medication or surgery. CHI is less common than sensorineural HI and rarely leads to deafness; hearing aids and surgical rectification, as necessary, prove beneficial.

Sensorineural hearing impairment

Sensorineural hearing impairment (SHI) refers to hearing loss due to pathology either in the inner ear or the neural track linking the inner ear to the brainstem. Other terms to refer to SHI are *perceptive impairment* and *nerve loss*. For SHI to be diagnosed, all conductive hearing is normal, i.e. the sound is conducted by the ear but not processed or perceived. SHI symptoms include: speaking excessively loud (since the patient cannot hear either himself or others) unless the patient has learned to regulate his voice level, better hearing for low frequencies (e.g. for high frequency phones: [f, s, k] in *fake*, *shook*, *kick*, the patient only hears the vowel), difficulty in speech discrimination (even at loudness levels above the hearing threshold), discomfort at loud noise (due to a disproportionate increase of sensation of loudness in the inner ear, when an actual loud sound is heard), and tinnitus that is much higher pitched than in normal or CHI tinnitus (e.g. like a doorbell or phone ringing). SHI is the predominant disorder in infants born with HI, with the exception of congenital atresia mentioned above.

Generally, the causes of SHI may be grouped into *congenital* and *acquired*. Congenital causes include *heredity* (defective genes) and *damage to the embryo in utero* (due to mother's diseases, e.g. rubella, in the first three months of pregnancy). Acquired SHI may occur any time in the lifetime as a result of aging, disease, exposure to drugs, or injury, while susceptibility to hearing loss varies across people. Normal loss of hearing, as a result of aging (*presbycusis*) starts at about 30 years of age, and worsens every following decade. *Ménières syndrome* (or *endolymphatic hydrops*) is a disease specific to the inner ear, caused by increased fluid pressure, and it exhibits dizziness (*vertigo*), hearing loss and tinnitus. The clinician plays an important role in diagnosing *Ménières syndrome* and referring the patient to an otologist. Diseases causing SHI due to toxicity are influenza, diphtheria, mumps, measles and virus infections.

Exposure to chemicals and drugs may also lead to SHI; in the past, a drug commonly causing hearing loss was quinine, but nowadays dangerous drugs for hearing health are *neomyscin*, *kanamycin* and *dyhydrostreptomysin* that are usually reserved for use in life-threatening circumstances only. Other SHI causes, though less common, are abrupt hearing loss, even overnight (as in autoimmune system attacks), and mechanical injury like bone fracture. Trauma, or *noise-induced hearing loss* (NIHL) is another common cause of SHI. All HI that is not noise-induced is commonly referred to as *non-noise-induced hearing loss* (NNIHL). NIHL mostly results from sustained exposure to high-frequency/high-intensity sounds, and it is a result of cumulative exposure over several years. Temporary hearing loss (*threshold shift*) may also occur following short-lived exposure to intense noise though, in this case, normal hearing sensitivity returns. By and large, however, SHI does not on the whole respond well to treatment. When hearing aids are used, they amplify sounds but do little to increase the clarity of speech. In such cases, *cochlear implants* (surgically implanted devices) are used to stimulate the hearing nerve which increases the ability to hear sounds and, thus, comprehend speech. Sensorineural abnormality leads to hearing sensitivity loss that is greater by air conduction than by bone conduction. This is because the sound travelling by air conduction is attenuated by the processes taking place in both the middle and the inner ear, while the sound travelling by bone conduction is attenuated only by impairment of the inner ear.

Mixed hearing impairment

Mixed hearing loss (MHI) refers to hearing problems demonstrating characteristics from both conductive and sensorineural HI. MHI is not uncommon. A typical example would be an elderly person with presbycusis that also demonstrates conductive hearing loss caused by otitis media. Figure 3.5 is a diagram (see also Martin, 1975, 5) showing all three types of organic hearing impairment discussed above.

Central auditory processing disorder

Central auditory processing disorder (CAPD) (or *auditory processing disorder, central loss*) is caused by interferences in the neural pathways from the brainstem to, and including, the temporal lobes of the cerebral cortex. Patients with CAPD exhibit difficulties *comprehending* what is heard (*auditory imperception*) rather than actually hearing the sound stimulus. Loss

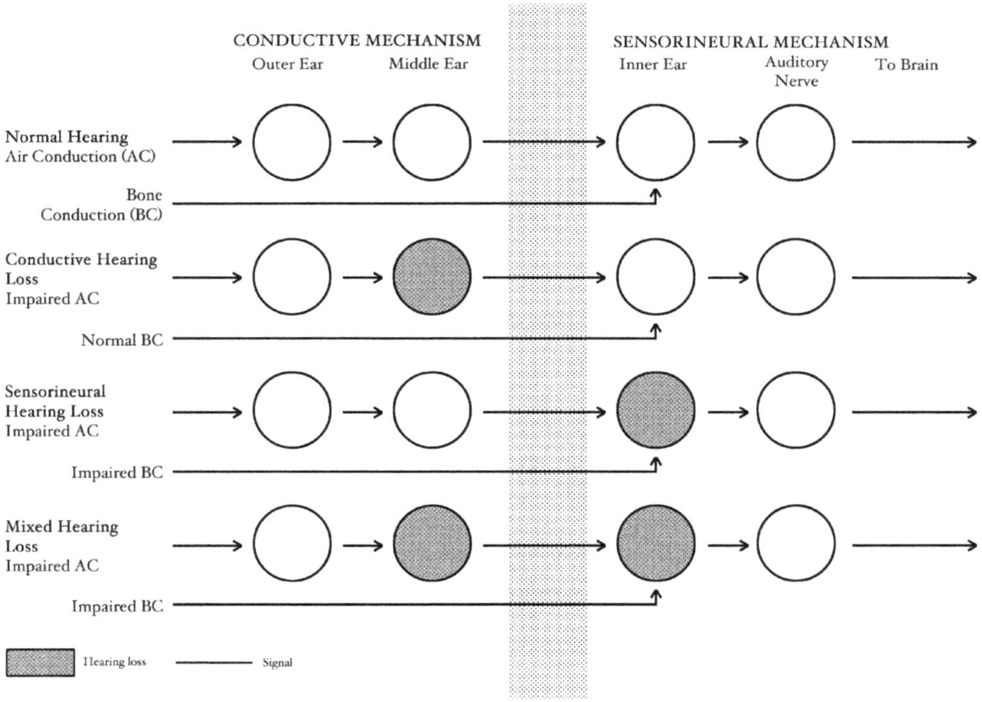

Figure 3.5   Normal and impaired hearing.

Source: Courtesy S. Qiouyi Lu.

of hearing sensitivity is less easily diagnosed in CAPD than in conductive and sensorineural HI. Central loss may also result from lesions in the brain. If CAPD occurs after language has been developed, lesions are not identifiable through routine audiometry, because the ears will respond normally to the demands of these tests, although the patient cannot recognize what he hears. The causes of CAPD may also be brain tumor(s), an abscess, brain damage from trauma, vascular (vein) changes in the brain (e.g. *arteriosclyrosis*), infections (e.g. *meningitis, encephalitis*), degenerative diseases (e.g. *Parkinson's, multiple sclerosis*), *erythroblastosis fetalis* (a hemolytic disease resulting from blood-group compatibility between mother and fetus), etc. It should be emphasized, further, that the hearing loss discussed in CAPD is not the same as the one discussed for peripheral and internal HI, in the sense that CAPD is a neurological disorder rather than a disorder of the hearing mechanism *per se*. As a neurological disorder, it has similar symptoms to those of *auditory agnosia* (ability to hear but not recognize sounds) and *auditory verbal agnosia* (hearing but not recognizing speech sounds). Auditory agnosia is a type of *receptive aphasia* (affecting language comprehension), associated with injury of the dominant cerebral hemisphere. *Congenital aphasia* in children is characterized by auditory imperception, visual imperception, or both; in such cases, children have typical intelligence and hearing sensitivity, but cannot develop language. Although the treatment of CAPD falls within the field of neuropsychology, a speech clinician needs to be able to differentiate between peripheral hearing and central hearing disorders for diagnosis purposes.

Nonorganic hearing impairment

Nonorganic (or *functional*) hearing impairment (NHI) is instigated by psychological factors, like emotional stress, as a defense against the painful situation. Other terms for NHI are *conversion deafness* and *hysterical deafness*. In such cases, the patient is truly convinced that he has suffered hearing loss despite the fact that his hearing apparatus is intact. Similarly to CAPD, hearing loss in functional hearing impairment is not a loss that relates to breakdown of the hearing mechanism, and it requires referral to a psychologist.

Conclusion

A person with normal hearing is always in the midst of a noisy milieu. To a large extent, we are all unaware or less conscious of the constant array of sounds that surround us. Thus, while reading something or having a conversation, we may not pay attention to other noises in the environment like a car going by, the sound of the refrigerator, a TV playing in another room, or the sound of keys being struck when typing. This type of unconscious primitive hearing is taken for granted, but once we are removed from this setting of familiar noise, uneasiness is immediately felt. It is plainly understood, then, how hearing impairment or loss can place patients at a distinct disadvantage. By elaborating on what constitutes normal and impaired hearing, the present chapter has served to highlight the significance of the ability to hear for general quality of living. The chapter is presented to the speech clinician reading this volume as a comprehensive preface to the substantive study of auditory phonetics (part of audiology), a field that verges on speech language pathology, medicine, psychology, physics and linguistics.

References

Bagai, A., Thavendiranathan, P., & Detsky, A.S. (2006). Does this patient have hearing impairment? *JAMA*, *295*(4), 416–428. doi:https://doi.org/10.1001/jama.295.4.416

Crandell, C.C., & Smaldino, J.J. (2000). Classroom acoustics for children with normal hearing and with hearing impairment. *Language, Speech, and Hearing Services in Schools*, *31*(4), 362–370. https://doi.org/10.1044/0161-1461.3104.362

Clark, J., Yallop, C., & Fletcher, J. (2007). *An Introduction to Phonetics and Phonology* (3rd ed.). Malden, MA: Blackwell Publishing.

Delgutte, B. (1997). Auditory neural processing of speech. In W.J. Hardcastle & J. Laver (Eds.), *The Handbook of Phonetic Sciences* (pp. 507–538). Oxford, UK: Blackwell.

Denes, P.B., & Pinson, E.N. (1993). *The Speech Chain: The Physics and Biology of Spoken Language* (2nd ed.). Oxford, UK: Freeman.

Dobbie, R.A., & Van Hemel, S. (2005). *Hearing loss: Determining eligibility for social security benefits*. National Research Council (US) Committee on Disability Determination for Individuals with Hearing Impairments. Washington (DC): National Academies Press.

Hudson, M.W., & DeRuiter, M. (2019). *Professional Issues in Speech-Language Pathology and Audiology* (5th ed.). San Diego, CA: Plural Publishing.

Katz, J. (2014). *Handbook of Clinical Audiology*. Philadelphia, PA: Wolters Kluwer.

Kemp, D.T. (2002). Otoacoustic emissions, their origin in cochlear function, and use. *British Medical Bulletin*, *63*, 223–241.

Kennedy, C., McCann, D., Campbell, M.J., Kimm, K., & Thornton, R., (2005). Universal newborn screening for permanent childhood hearing impairment: An 8-year follow-up of a controlled trial. *Lancet*, *366*(9486), 660–662. https://doi.org/10.1016/S01406736(05)67138-3

Lahav, A., & Skoe, E. (2014). An acoustic gap between the NICU and womb: A potential risk for compromised neuroplasticity of the auditory system in preterm infants. *Frontiers in Neuroscience*, *8*, 381.

Libb, J.W., Dahle, A., Smith, K., McCollister, F.P., McLain, C. (1985). Hearing disorder and cognitive function of individuals with Down syndrome. *American Journal of Mental Deficiency*, *90*(3), 353–356.

Martin, F.N. (1975). *Introduction to Audiology*. Englewood Cliffs, NJ: Prentice-Hall.

Miceli, G., Conti, G., Cianfoni, A., et al. (2008). Acute auditory agnosia as the presenting hearing disorder in MELAS. *Neurological Science*, *29*, 459. https://doi.org/10.1007/s10072-008-1028-9

Musiek, F., & Baran, J.A. (2007). *The Auditory System: Anatomy, Pshysiology, and Clinical Correlates*. Boston, MA: Pearson Education.

Newby, H.A. (1979). *Audiology*. Englewood Cliffs, NJ: Prentice Hall. Publications.

Rouse, M.H. (2019). *Neuroanatomy for Speech-Language Pathology and Audiology*. Burlington, MA: Johns & Bartlett Learning.

Seikel, J.A., King, D.W., & Drumright, D.G. (2020). *Anatomy and Physiology for Speech, Language, and Hearing* (4th ed.). Clifton Park, NY: Delmar Cengage Learning.

Tyler, R.S., & Baker, L.J. (1983). Difficulties experienced by tinnitus sufferers. *Journal of Speech and Hearing Disorders*, *48*(2), 150–154.

Yost, W.A. (2013). *Fundamentals of Hearing: An Introduction*. Leiden: Brill Academic Publishers.

4

PERCEPTUAL PHONETICS FOR THE SPEECH CLINICIAN

Esther Janse and Toni Rietveld

Ease of articulation vs. perceptual clarity

Speech articulation has been modeled to be a kind of compromise between ease of articulation for the speaker and speech signal clarity that is needed by the listener. This compromise is most clearly reflected in Lindblom's Hyper- and Hypoarticulation theory of speech (1990), in which speech realization is the result of speaker- and listener-oriented constraints. Hypo-speech, or sloppy speech, is modeled to be convenient for the speaker who can speak with minimal effort if the communicative situation allows it. However, speakers may need to resort to hyper-speech, or clear speech, if communication occurs against a noisy background or if there are listener-related constraints (e.g. the listener being hearing-impaired or being a non-native speaker of the language at hand).

Phonetic realization (clear or more reduced realization of words and sounds) has been linked to contextual predictability, such that highly predictable items tend to be realized with shorter durations and with more articulatory "undershoot" (e.g. Aylett & Turk, 2006). This observation of predictability-related reduction has been accounted for by referring to the listener (in listener-oriented accounts of phonetic reduction) or to the speaker (in speaker-driven accounts of phonetic reduction). Listener-oriented or intelligibility accounts emphasize that listeners can do with less signal clarity for words that are contextually predictable, where speaker-driven accounts of reduction argue that speakers are slower to retrieve less predictable words from memory, and that this lexical-retrieval delay spills over in the slower (and hence, clearer) way they pronounce less probable words. Tearing these two accounts apart is complicated because the two accounts often make similar predictions. Nevertheless, there may be some more evidence in favor of the speaker-driven account of phonetic reduction (Gahl, Yao, & Johnson, 2012).

Coarticulation

*Co*articulation means the articulation of different sounds at the same time; another term being *co*production. At first sight, this process may seem quite counter-intuitive as we tend to think that speech consists of sequences of distinct speech sounds. Speech sounds are the result of movements of the articulators and consequently a comparison with limb movements is obvious, see Grimme, Fuchs, Perrier, and Schöner (2011). When different successive body postures are required, like kneeling and standing, transition movements can be observed between the two target postures. These movements are naturally influenced by the distance the articulators need to travel from the starting position to the new target position, for instance when reaching different heights is required. In Figure 4.1 we show the movement of the tongue dorsum for two utterances which only differ noticeably in the last phoneme: /a/ vs. /i/.

When we focus on the positions of the dorsum during the articulation of the schwas, we see a clear difference in "tongue height" in /kəməma/ and /kəməmi/, with the position of the tongue dorsum being clearly lower in the latter than in the former. It is obvious what the influencing factor is: vowel height in utterance-final /a/ ("low") and in utterance-final /i/ ("high"). In "normal" speech coarticulation always occurs (inevitably) as is the case with transition phases between body postures. In that respect, coarticulation is a process that fundamentally differs from that of *assimilation*. Assimilation is a process that is directed by the linguistic system of the language in question and that can be avoided. For instance, in the contact of – voiced stops and + voiced fricatives, anticipatory assimilation (effect from right to left) does occur in Russian but not in English. Russian "from" [at] is pronounced as [ad] in the context [ad_zɑlə] "from the hall," whereas in English /kz/ is preserved in that context of voiceless plosive preceding voiced fricative: [plæstɪk_zɪps].

Coarticulation occurs, like assimilation, in two directions: from left to right (*carry-over* or *perseverative coarticulation*) and from right to left (*anticipatory* or *regressive coarticulation*). Coarticulation going both ways, i.e. from left to right and from right to left, also exists, and is called *reciprocal coarticulation*. The example shown in Figure 4.1 is a case of anticipatory coarticulation and can be seen as the result of motor planning. Preservative coarticulation is often considered to be the result of inertia of the articulators, a somewhat less interesting phenomenon than articulatory planning. Coarticulation is not limited to lingual movements

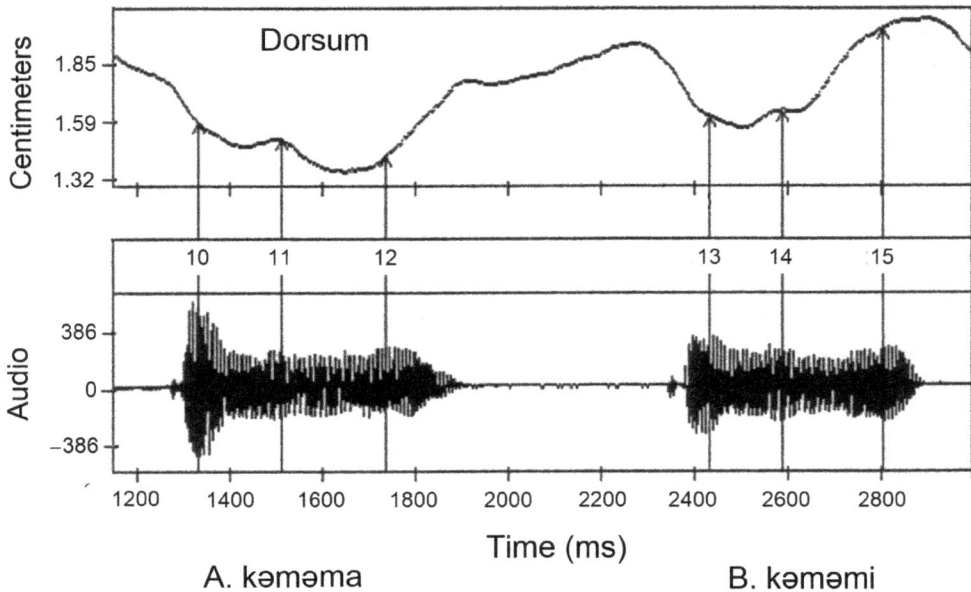

Figure 4.1 Movement of tongue dorsum—recorded with EMA (see Van Lieshout, Chapter 26)—and associated waveforms in two Dutch non-word utterances: /kəməma/ and /kəməmi/.

Source: Adapted version of Figure 9.9 in Rietveld and Van Heuven (2016), with permission.

(although they are frequently discussed in research), but can also be observed in laryngeal (Voice Onset Time), velar (nasality) and labial (rounding) activity.

Factors which play a role in coarticulation

Coarticulation is an inevitable and universal phenomenon in articulation. However, the extent, or better, magnitude of coarticulation depends on multiple factors, which are as follows:

- *Prosodic weight*: Speech segments differ in prosodic weight (see section 5). It seems obvious that stronger segments—for instance vowels in stressed syllables—are less vulnerable to influences of lighter segments (this is called *coarticulation resistance*) than the other way round. At the same time, stronger segments have a relatively stronger effect on surrounding segments than weaker segments. This prosodic-weight effect is illustrated in Figure 4.1 discussed earlier: the last (strong) syllable affects tongue dorsum height in the preceding schwas. However, the effects of prosodic weight are not the same for all languages and all speech dimensions. In an extensive study on vowel-to-vowel coarticulation in English (Cho, 2004), the prosodic-weight effect was not found, at least not for English. For nasality, Cho, Kim and Kim (2017) showed that "prominence" (for instance stress, accentuation) enhances the nasalization of consonants due to coarticulation but makes vowels less vulnerable to nasality.
- *Boundary strength*: The extent of coarticulation between two speech segments will clearly depend on boundary strength as hardly any coarticulation can be expected to be observed between two utterances with a relatively long pause between the two. However, there are gradations in boundary strength, with strength ranging from boundaries between segments, syllable onset and rhyme, syllables, morae, words, intonational phrases to boundaries between utterances. Cho (2004) found clear effects of boundary strength in English on coarticulation of tongue position: the stronger the boundary is (i.e. the higher the prosodic boundary is), the more resistant vowels are to coarticulation. Boundary strength induces different types of enhancement patterns as a function of prosodic position (Cho, 2004).
- *Segment specificity*: Not all segments are prone to coarticulation to the same extent as they differ in articulatory precision requirements. Apart from the density in articulatory space of vowels, there is less freedom in the movement of the tongue in the realization of a high vowel like /i/ than in a low vowel such as /a/, which makes /i/ more resistant to coarticulation (Cho, 2004).
- *Intersegmental distance and segmental composition*: In fact, the distance and segmental composition of that distance can be considered as aspects of boundary strength. It is quite obvious that the longer the distance between two segments is, the less the segments will be affected by coarticulatory processes. Apart from distance, the type of intervening segments also matters, both for the direction of coarticulation as well as for its magnitude. For Catalan, for instance, Recasens (2015) found that in [Vłi] sequences anticipatory coarticulation was favored (both dark /l/ and /i/ require tongue dorsum retraction), whereas in [Vli] (clear /l/) this anticipation effect during the first vowel (V) was not consistently present.
- *Speech rate*: Faster speech rate is associated with increased coarticulation (Agwuele, Sussman, & Lindblom, 2008; Tjaden, 2000). The effect of speech rate on coarticulation is also modulated by segmental characteristics. In faster speech, Li and Kong (2010) found a linear increase of temporal coarticulation in consonant clusters embedded in V1C1C2V2 clusters. The gestural overlap, however, was—not surprisingly—constrained by the consonant production manner and the lingual specification for flanking vowels. For instance, /s/ is more resistant than /t/ to

overlap with a preceding nasal consonant. This greater resistance apparently follows the aerodynamic requirements for high-pressure buildup for an intelligible fricative.

- *Language dependency*: The last factor mentioned here is language dependency. This means that the extent and magnitude of coarticulation often vary as a function of language. Classical examples of language dependency are given by Manuel (1990) who showed that coarticulation from vowel to vowel is stronger in languages with a small vowel inventory, like Greek or Spanish with only five vowels, than in languages with larger vowel inventories, such as Dutch, English and German. These language differences may arise because confusion is less likely to occur in languages with a small number of vowels than in languages with a crowded vowel inventory. Language-specificity does not just concern V-to-V coarticulation but also coarticulation in consonant clusters (e.g. Bombien & Hoole, 2013).

Modeling coarticulation

Coarticulation is part of speech planning and not only the result of mechanical inertia. Thus, it calls for a planning model which can predict the observed coarticulatory phenomena. Several coarticulation models have been developed since the sixties of the 20th century. One model which is still influential is Keating's *window model* (1988). We illustrate this model on the basis of Figure 4.2. A fundamental element of the model is the distinction between three types of speech segments depending on the specification of a segment for a specific feature (+, 0, or −).

A segment can be specified positive (+) for a given feature, for instance [+round] for the vowel /y/ in Figure 4.2, negative (−), for instance [-round] for /ɑ/ and neutral (0) for consonants like /l/, /s/ and /t/. The specification in (−), (0) and (+) determines the freedom of movement of the associated articulators, in our example of the lips. The extent of freedom is indicated by the breadth of the windows linked to the segments. In our example the lips can move freely after a [-round] specification for /ɑ/ to a [+round] specification for /y/, as the intermediate consonants are (0) specified (i.e. they are unspecified) for the feature [round]. The window model allows flexibility in window length, which makes it possible to account for a number of observations. In our example, coarticulation takes quite a long time as the interval between the two vowels in

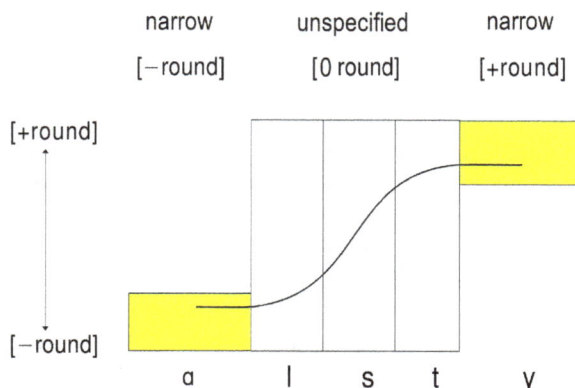

Figure 4.2 Coarticulation windows for the feature [round] in part of the Dutch word *alstublieft* ("please"). The colored boxes represent the critically specified windows.

Source: Adapted illustration from Rietveld and Van Heuven (2016), with permission.

question is rather long; in a short VCV-sequence like /ɑly/, the curve representing the transition of the lips from [-round] to [+round] will be steeper.

Coarticulation and speech perception

At first sight, one might think that coarticulation impedes speech perception. Coarticulation affects the "pure" characteristics of segments, and confusion might be the result. The opposite appears to be the case. In a classic article, Strange, Verbrugge, Shankweiler, and Edman (1976) compared identification of vowels presented in noise for isolated vowels (#V#) and vowels presented in a consonantal environment (CVC). Vowel identification for vowels with flanking consonants was better than identification of isolated vowels. This consonantal-context benefit illustrates that the acoustic information distributed over the speech segments (due to coarticulation) is used by listeners to identify vowels. Warner, McQueen and Cutler (2014) confirmed the availability of acoustic information beyond the boundaries of isolated speech segments in an experiment in which fragments of increasing length ("gates") of diphones were presented to listeners. This availability was not identical for all (classes of) speech segments. For obvious reasons, information was "highly localized" (i.e. present in the speech sound itself, and not so much outside of it) in affricates and diphthongs, whereas information on stops and sonorants already becomes available in the preceding segment.

Listeners are also known to perceptually compensate for coarticulation. When presented with an ambiguous sound that is acoustically halfway between a synthetic "da" to "ga" continuum, listeners will report hearing "ga" when the ambiguous sound was preceded by the VC syllable [ɑl], but will report hearing "da" when preceded by [ɑr] (Mann, 1980). This is because tongue retraction in [r] (as evident from F3 movement) will make listeners expect (coarticulatory) tongue retraction in the following segment too, and hence a stop more like "g" than "d" (Johnson, 2012). This compensation for coarticulation has also been observed with a non-phonetic precursor tone (a simple sine wave matching the ending frequency of the F3 of [ɑr]), making compensation for coarticulation similar to other auditory contrast effects (Lotto & Kluender, 1998).

Coarticulation in clinical research

The sections on coarticulation above provide general information on coarticulation, and hence provide a starting point for studies comparing motor behavior of patient groups with speech disorders to those of typical speakers. Obviously, in those comparisons, between-group speech rate differences will always need to be accounted for given their effect on coarticulation, as well as any between-group differences in prosodic and boundary composition of the spoken utterances. Coarticulation behavior has already been studied in multiple groups with speech impairment, such as persons with aphasia (Katz, 2000) and persons with multiple sclerosis or Parkinson's disease (PD), see Tjaden, 2003. For patients with PD, studies have also investigated effects of Lee Silverman Voice Treatment on coarticulation patterns (Sauvageau, Roy, Langlois, & Macoir 2015). Developmental research has shown that children differ from adults in the temporal organization of (overlapping) speech gestures, but evidence is mixed as to whether young children are reported to display more or less coarticulation than adults (cf. Rubertus & Noiray, 2018, for a review). Evidence of decreasing or increasing coarticulation with age is relevant to theoretical debates about age-related change in organizational units for speech planning. Studies on developmental speech disorders have used coarticulation to probe motor programming behavior in children with developmental apraxia of speech, providing evidence of a motor programming deficit (e.g. Nijland, Maassen, & van der Meulen, 2003).

Categorical perception

Categorical perception has been a widely discussed phenomenon since its introduction by Liberman, Harris, Hoffman and Griffith (1957) and its official labeling as such by Eimas (1963). The basis was the interesting "relation" between classification (identification or labeling of a single sound) and discrimination of speech sounds (deciding whether two speech sounds are the same or different) on a continuum of stimuli. In Figure 4.3 we show the spectrograms of a series of seven [Ca:]-stimuli to illustrate this relationship between classification and discrimination of speech sounds. All characteristics of the stimuli are equal, but for the so-called locus of the F2. F2 on the left side of the continuum starts quite low (typical for /p/) and is moved upward in the synthesis until it reaches a relatively high value, typical for /t/ (visible on the right side of the continuum).

Listeners are presented with sounds 1-7 from the continuum, and are asked to report whether they classify the speech sound as "pa" or "ta." The classification results are depicted in Figure 4.4. The first three stimuli are predominantly classified as "pa," but the fourth and following stimuli are mainly classified as "ta." The change from "pa" to "ta" identifications (also called classifications, see Figure 4.4A) is quite abrupt, or "categorical." In a discrimination task, all pairs of the stimuli are presented: (1, 2), (1,3) …. (6,7). Participants are asked to say whether they members of the pair sound the same or different. The discrimination results are summarized in Figure 4.4B: the listeners only discriminated above chance those stimulus pairs straddling the phonetic boundary: pairs could only be discriminated well if one member was originally classified as "pa," and the other as "ta." Such a relation between discrimination and classification implies that the phonetic labels direct the discrimination. This combined effect of identification and discrimination is called *categorical perception*.

Several claims have been made regarding categorical perception. One of those claims is that categorical perception is limited to human speech. Another claim is that, as far as speech is concerned, categorical perception is limited to consonants. The first claim, based on the idea that labels of speech sounds were either innate or learned, was not confirmed. The phenomenon of categorical perception has been observed in a large number of domains, such as perception of colors, facial expressions and robot non-linguistic sounds (Read & Belpaeme, 2016), and perception of objects with artificial categories (see Feldman, Griffiths, & Morgan, 2009). The second claim can

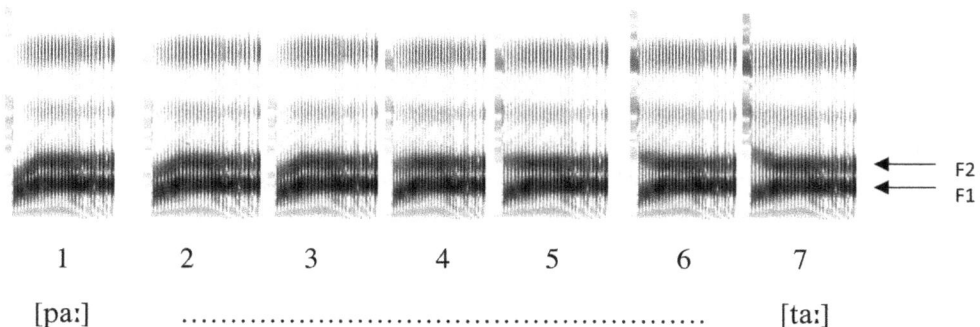

Figure 4.3   Spectrograms of {p….t}a: stimuli.

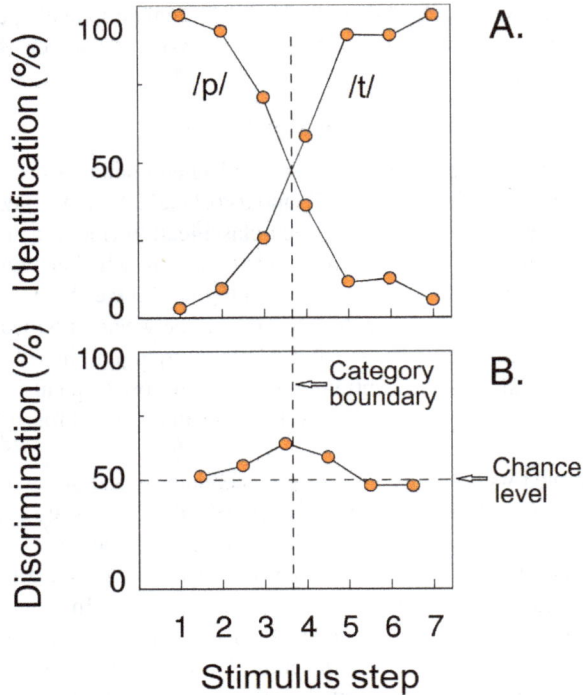

Figure 4.4   Results of identification and discrimination tasks with the seven stimuli displayed in Figure 4.3.

Source: Adapted version of Figure 10.17 in Rietveld and van Heuven (2016), with permission.

be regarded as partially confirmed (Chao, Ochoa, & Daliri, 2019; Gerrits & Schouten, 2004). Many consonants have faster transitions of acoustic characteristics than vowels, which may relate to the more categorical nature of their perception.

Categorical perception in clinical research

Differences in the way categorical perception manifests itself have been used for quite a long time in order to establish speech perception differences between patient groups and (age-matched) controls, or, in developmental research, between adults and children or between age groups in children. Many studies report phonetic identification behavior that is less categorical in nature, and hence is characterized by shallower identification slopes and worse or better discrimination, for pathological groups compared to control groups. The fact that deviant categorical perception behavior can be found across multiple different speech or language impairments may relate to evidence that categorical perception relies on "intact functioning of a large network of neural regions" (Ravizza, 2005). Deviant identification behavior has been reported for persons with aphasia (Blumstein, Tartter, Nigro, & Statlender, 1984) and for diverse child patient populations, including children with specific language impairment (e.g. Ziegler, Pech-Georgel, George, Alario, & Lorenzi, 2005), reading impairment or dyslexia (Bertucci, Hook, Haynes, Macaruso, & Bickley, 2003) and cleft palate and persistent posterior placement of /t/ (Whitehill, Francis, & Ching, 2003). It is important to note, however, that results on categorical perception in clinical populations have been very mixed and inconsistent for identification as well as discrimination behavior (e.g. Messaoud-Galusi, Hazan, & Rosen, 2011 for children with reading impairment; Coady, Evans, Mainela-Arnold, & Kluender, 2007 for language-impaired groups). These inconsistent results have led some researchers to suggest that differences in reported categorical perception results across studies should be attributed to task (Rietveld, 2021) and stimulus differences rather than to true underlying speech perception differences between groups. Group or individual differences in categorical perception could thus be task-artefact, and due to the memory load of the tasks, or the way listeners approach the tasks, rather than revealing much about the (spoken) language impairment under study itself. Following this line of reasoning, several studies have used psycholinguistic methods to measure the dynamics of spoken word recognition to investigate the nature of the impairment at hand (Milberg, Blumstein, & Dzworetzky, 1988). Spoken-word recognition is generally assumed to involve activation of a number of word candidates, and competition and selection among them (e.g. in the Shortlist B model; see Norris & McQueen, 2008). Rather than differences in phonological or auditory abilities, subtle deficits in these word activation, competition and selection processes may characterize speech perception deficits in aphasia (Janse, 2006; Mirman, Yee, Blumstein, & Magnuson, 2011) and language impairment (McMurray, Munson, & Tomblin, 2014).

Perceptual units

The previous section on categorical perception implies that segments can be considered perceptual units. The syllable (σ) is another well-known (perceptual or organizational) unit in linguistics, used in psycholinguistics, phonetics and phonology. Although clear and universal phonetic features for establishing the boundaries of this unit—in most cases consisting of more than one speech segment—are still lacking, its functional presence has been observed in many domains: speech errors, effects of stress, accentuation on its constituents, etc. This almost universal presence of syllables in language description and analysis might suggest that it is the only possible unit above the constituents of a syllable: onset, nucleus and coda. That is not true, however. There is another unit, the mora (symbolized as μ), a Latin word which means "short interval"; plural: morae. It is known as a unit for the description of Japanese and Telugu (the latter is a Dravidian language spoken by 70 million people in India). Figure 4.5 shows the structure of syllables in languages without the mora (A) and with the mora (B) as constituents of the syllable.

An example of a familiar word illustrating the structure of the mora is the Japanese pronunciation of the place name "Washington" as "wasinton" (Kubozono, 1989), as illustrated in Figure 4.6.

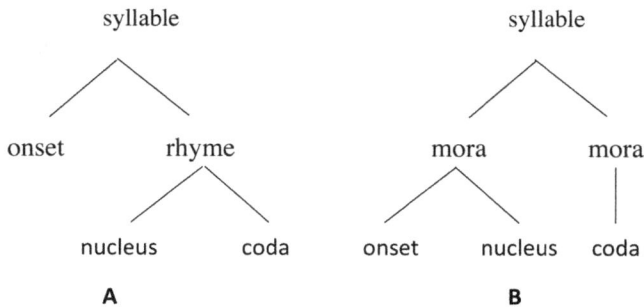

Figure 4.5 Structure of the syllable in languages without the mora (A), such as English, Spanish, Chinese etc. and with the mora (B): Japanese, Telugu.

σ   σ   σ

μ   μ μ μ μ

/wɑsɪnton/   was si n to n

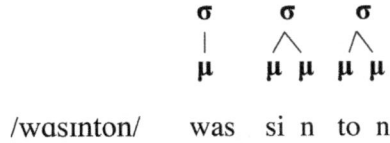

Figure 4.6 Syllabic/moraic structure of the loan-word "Washington" in Japanese, with each μ sign representing a mora.

When a syllable consists of one mora (as in "was" in our Japanese example), the mora is called a syllabic mora. When syllables consist of multiple morae, all composite morae are called non-syllabic morae. In the example depicted in Figure 4.6 "si," "n," "to," "n" are non-syllabic morae. There are multiple sources of evidence for the existence of the mora as constituent of the syllable. We will give some examples in the following domains: syllable counting by Japanese and English listeners, patterns of speech errors in Japanese and other languages, and the mora as an aid in segmentation of continuous speech.

When English speakers are asked to report the number of syllables in a word, they will seldom make an error. The performance of a Dutch or Spanish speaker—when asked to count syllables in English words—will not be very different. However, when Japanese participants are asked to carry out the same task, their performance will deviate to a great extent from that of the English participants. Erickson (1999), for instance, reported accuracy rates of 98% for English listeners and 51% for Japanese listeners (overall) in an experiment with this task. These results do not prove the existence of the mora, but at least show that Japanese speakers' awareness of the syllable is not present. However, Japanese listeners can be taught to develop an awareness of the syllable, as research with Japanese L1-children has shown (Murakami, Miyatani, & Cheang, 2017).

Speech errors have been an important source of information on the structure of continuous speech and on the structure of the syllable in particular. One of the frequently reported patterns in speech errors is the transposition of syllables and onsets of syllables. An example of syllable transposition is "Moran and Fader"→ "Morer and Fadan" (example taken from Nooteboom, 1969). An example of syllable onset transposition is "smart + clever" being pronounced as "smever." In Japanese, different patterns of speech errors are observed, often involving a split of long vowels and "long" consonants, such as /s/. We illustrate this pattern with a loan word: "motorbike," normally pronounced by Japanese as "mo-ta ba-i-ku."

A possible speech error is the split of the long vowel "o," and the transposition (or anticipation) of the "i" toward a position after the "o," as illustrated in Figure 4.7 (after Kubozono, 1989). The result is mo. i – ta. a ba. i – ku (with a dot symbolizing a mora boundary and a dash for a syllable boundary), see Figure 4.7. This example makes it clear that in speech errors long

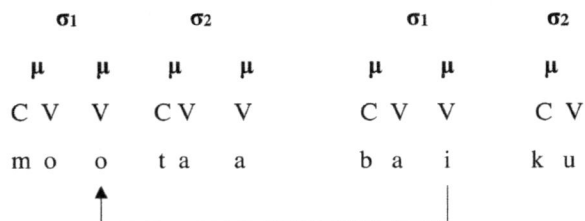

σ_1 σ_2 σ_1 σ_2

μ   μ   μ   μ   μ   μ   μ

C V   V   C V   V   C V V   C V

m o   o   t a   a   b a i   k u

Figure 4.7 Speech error in the loan-word "motorbike" in Japanese, resulting in *mo . i – ta . a ba . i – ku.*

vowels can be split. This splitting process can only be understood when there is another unit in the structure of a syllable, not being the rhyme or the onset, but a unit called the mora.

The syllable appears to play a role in many languages when participants are presented with tasks involving speech segmentation, for instance if the task involves the detection of specific speech sounds. Although Japanese contains both syllables and morae as structural units, the mora overrules the syllable for Japanese listeners when engaged in speech segmentation tasks. Cutler and Otake (1994) carried out an experiment in which listeners were asked to indicate whether a specific speech sound was present in a stimulus. The performance of Japanese listeners was better, both in accuracy and reaction times, for moraic (= the target is the only constituent of a mora) than for "nonmoraic" targets (i.e. targets which do not constitute a mora on their own; for an illustration, see Figure 4.7).

The examples given above (which can easily be extended, see for instance Verdonschot & Kinoshita, 2018) illustrate that the mora is not only a theoretical concept but also a unit that plays a role in accounting for speech and language processing behavior of speakers with Japanese (and Telugu) as their L1.

Sonority

The concept of sonority has always been controversial (see *The Sonority Controversy*, by Parker, 2012). This controversy is unparalleled for other phonetic concepts, such as coarticulation, formants, locus, fundamental frequency, etc. For the latter (more concrete) concepts, any controversy is limited to measurement techniques, application domain, (theoretical) modeling, etc. One of the reasons for the "sonority controversy" is that the name of the phenomenon suggests physical reality, and thus general applicability. Obvious associations of the word sonority are "loudness," "salience," "audibility" and "intensity." The first three associations refer to the perceptual domain, the latter to the physical domain. One of the first authors who used a sonority-like term was Sievers (1883) when he introduced the (German) term "Schallfülle" ("sound fullness"). This term, however, could also refer to both acoustic and perceptual phenomena. At first sight, the term "sonority" seems to be useful in determining the boundaries of syllables. This is because in most languages a syllable always contains a vowel—intuitively to be considered as the loudest part of the syllable—which is surrounded by zero consonants, by single consonants, or by consonant clusters that differ in loudness in a specific way. For instance, in a word like "plank," sonority is assumed to increase from /p/ to /l/ and then from /l/ to the vowel, and to decrease again from the vowel to the nasal /n/, and from /n/ to the final stop /k/. That is why the structure of a syllable is often written as indicated in Figure 4.8.

Thus, sonority increases from the left syllable boundary into the vowel, and decreases from the vowel onward to the right boundary. An often reproduced rank order of sonority is that proposed by Ladefoged and Johnson (2010), of which we show below only the rank order of the consonants:

(1) [l] > [n] > [m] > [z] > [v] > [s] > [ʃ] > [d] > [t] > [k]

$$C_1 \ldots C_n \ [+syl] \ C_{n+1} \ldots C_k$$

$$- \quad \longrightarrow \quad + \quad \longleftarrow \quad -$$

sonority

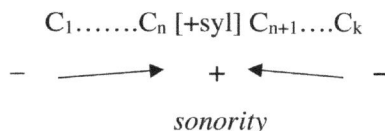

Figure 4.8 Sonority and syllable structure.

In many languages, sequences of segments making up syllables seem to conform to the sonority principle. In English, sequences like /slV.../ and /....Vls/ are allowed (*slice*, *kills*), but not */ lsV.../ and */ ...Vsl/. However, in Russian the words "*rtut*" (English: "mercury") and "*mlga*" (English: "fog") are one-syllabic words; in most accounts of sonority rankings, however, /t/ is considered to be less sonorous than /r/, and /l/ less loud than /m/. A Persian example violating the sonority principle is the word [satl] for "bucket." Thus, the conventionally operationalized definition of sonority (with each syllable having sonority increasing from its left edge into the vowel and decreasing from to its right edge) is not universally applicable. Although loudness (perceptual correlate, measured in sones) or intensity (physical correlate, expressed in dB) may seem good correlates of sonority, in fact they are not. Perceived loudness is a function of a number of physical units: intensity, duration and spectral composition. The latter is often not taken into consideration. Glave and Rietveld (1975) showed that vowels realized in a normal speech-like condition and shouted, will differ in loudness when equalized in intensity. The difference is the result of spectral widening which occurs when the voice pulses become more abrupt, as happens, for instance, in shouting. There are also reasons why intensity should be questioned as a reliable correlate of sonority. Segments like /s/, which conventionally have a lower position on the sonority scale than vowels like /i/, often have a larger intensity than the vowel. See the waveform presented in Figure 4.9, of the Dutch word "schip" (English: ship): [sχɪp]. Both the fricatives [s] and [χ] have a higher intensity than [ɪ]: The maximum intensity of [s] is around 75 dB, whereas that of [ɪ] is only 70 dB.

Most proposed scales of sonority are used and have been used to predict or explain phonological and/or phonetic phenomena, both in typical speech (development) and in disordered speech. An important concept in speech research on language development and disorders is the Sonority Sequence Principle (SSP). This principle states that speech in which the sonority scale (be it a "universal" scale or a language-specific scale) is violated, should be seen as marked speech. Violation of SSP may thus be reason for further clinical speech examination (see Ball, Müller, & Rutter, 2010).

In order to relate audibility of speech segments in everyday listening settings to the concept of sonority, Meyer, Dentel, and Meunier (2013) set up an experiment to test the intelligibility of (French) speech segments. Segments were presented in natural background noise of fluctuating

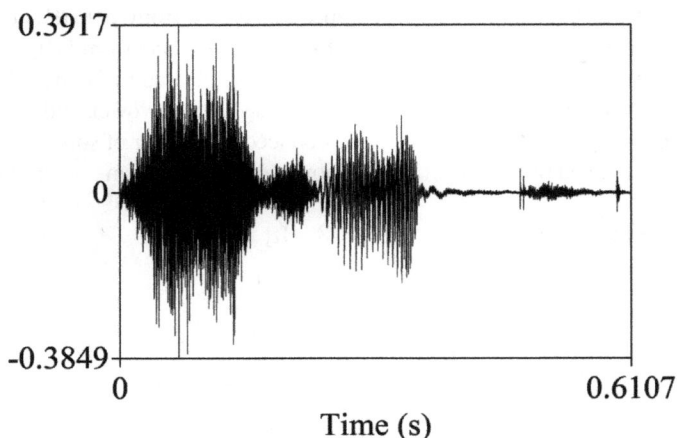

Figure 4.9   Waveform of Dutch word "schip" [sχɪp]; (English: "ship").

intensity so as to simulate varying distance between speaker and listener. Below we reproduce the rank order of the consonants as a function of the robustness of intelligibility (or audibility):

(2a) [ʃ, s] > [ʒ] > [j] > [l] > [ʁ] > [m,n] > [k] > [t] > [g] > [z] > [b] > [d] > [p] > [v] > [f]

Meyer and colleagues summarized the results of their intelligibility-in-noise study as follows (HE = High Energy, LE = Low Energy):

(2b) HE Sibilants > Semivowel > Liquids > Nasals > HE Obstruents > LE (Obstruents, Fricatives)

Obviously, there are some similarities in rank ordering between (1) and (2a,b), but also clear discrepancies: in (1) [l] is seen as more sonorous than [s], whereas in (2) it is the other way round. The surprising "high" positions of [ʃ] and [s], compared to those on conventional sonority rankings, are explained by the narrow frequency band and the location within the range of best perceived frequencies in human hearing of these consonants (Meyer et al., 2013). Even though the results of segment intelligibility in noise are, to some extent, dependent on the spectral composition and possible amplitude variation of the chosen noise masker, results like those of Meyer and colleagues can be used in the design of investigations in the audibility of speech segments after therapy, for instance of speakers with Parkinson's Disease.

References

Agwuele, A., Sussman, H., & Lindblom, B. (2008). The effect of speaking rate on consonant vowel coarticulation. *Phonetica, 65*, 194–209.

Aylett, M., & Turk, A. (2006). Language redundancy predicts syllabic duration and the spectral characteristics of vocalic syllable nuclei. *Journal of the Acoustical Society of America, 119*, 3048–3058.

Ball, M.J., Müller, N., & Rutter, B. (2010). *Phonology for Communication Disorders*. New York, NY: Psychology Press.

Bertucci, C., Hook, P., Haynes, C., Macaruso, P., & Bickley, C. (2003). Vowel perception and production in adolescents with reading disabilities. *Annals of Dyslexia, 53*, 174–200.

Blumstein, S.E., Tartter, V.C., Nigro, G., & Statlender, S. (1984). Acoustic cues for the perception of place of articulation in aphasia. *Brain and Language, 22*(1), 128–149.

Bombien, L., & Hoole, P. (2013). Articulatory overlap as a function of voicing in French and German consonant clusters. *Journal of the Acoustical Society of America, 134*, 539–550.

Chao S-C., Ochoa, D., & Daliri, A. (2019). Production variability and categorical perception of vowels are strongly linked. *Frontiers in Human Neuroscience, 13*, 96.

Cho, T. (2004). Prosodically conditioned strengthening and vowel-to-vowel coarticulation in English. *Journal of Phonetics, 32*, 141–176.

Cho, T., Kim, D., & Kim, S. (2017). Prosodically-conditioned fine-tuning of coarticulatory vowel nasalization in English. *Journal of Phonetics, 64*, 71–89.

Coady, J. A., Evans, J. L., Mainela-Arnold, E., & Kluender, K. R. (2007). Children with specific language impairments perceive speech most categorically when tokens are natural and meaningful. *Journal of Speech, Language, and Hearing Research, 50*(1), 41–57.

Cutler, A., & Otake, T. (1994). Mora or Phoneme? Further evidence for language-specific listening. *Journal of Memory and Language, 33*, 824–844.

Eimas, P. D. (1963). The relation between identification and discrimination along speech and nonspeech continua. *Language and Speech, 6*, 206–217.

Erickson, D., Akahane-Yamada, R., Tajima, K., & Matsumoto, K.F. (1999). Syllable counting and mora units in speech perception. In J.J. Ohala (Ed.), *Proceedings of the XIVth International Congress of Phonetic Sciences* (pp. 1479–1482). Berkeley, CA: Department of Linguistics.

Feldman, N.H., Griffiths, T.L., & Morgan, J.L. (2009) The influence of categories on perception: Explaining the perceptual magnet effect as optimal statistical inference. *Psychological Review*, *116*(4), 752–782.

Gahl, S., Yao, Y., & Johnson, K. (2012). Why reduce? Phonological neighborhood density and phonetic reduction in spontaneous speech. *Journal of Memory and Language, 66*, 789–806.

Gerrits, E., & Schouten, M.E.H. (2004). Categorical perception depends on the discrimination task. *Perception & Psychophysics, 66*(3), 363–376.

Glave, R.D., & Rietveld, A.C.M. (1975). Is the effort dependence of speech loudness explicable on the basis of acoustical cues? *Journal of the Acoustical Society of America, 58*, 1418–1424.

Grimme, B., Fuchs, S., Perrier, P., & Schöner, G. (2011). Limb versus speech motor control: A conceptual review. *Motor Control, 15*, 5–33.

Janse, E. (2006). Lexical competition effects in aphasia: Deactivation of lexical candidates in spoken word processing. *Brain and Language, 97*, 1–11.

Johnson, K. (2012). *Acoustic and Auditory Phonetics* (3rd ed.). Malden, MA: Blackwell.

Katz, W.F. (2000). Anticipatory coarticulation and aphasia: Implications for phonetic theories. *Journal of Phonetics, 28*(3), 313–334.

Keating, P.A. (1988). Coarticulation and timing. *UCLA Working Papers in Phonetics, 69*, 1–29.

Kubozono, H. (1989). The mora and syllable structure in Japanese: Evidence from speech errors. *Language and Speech, 32*(3), 249–278.

Ladefoged, P., & Johnson, K. (2010). *A Course in Phonetics*. Boston, MA: Wadsworth.

Li, Y-H, & Kong, J. (2010). Effect of speech rate on inter-segmental coarticulation in standard Chinese. In *Proceedings of 7th International Symposium on Chinese Spoken Language Processing* (pp. 44–49).

Liberman, A.M., Harris, K.S., Hoffman, H.S., & Griffith, B.C. (1957). The discrimination of speech sounds within and across phoneme boundaries. *Journal of Experimental Psychology, 54*, 358–368.

Lindblom, B. (1990). Explaining phonetic variation: A sketch of the H&H theory. In W.J. Hardcastle and A. Marchal (Eds.), *Speech Production and Speech Modeling*(pp.403–439), Dordrecht, The Netherlands: Kluwer.

Lotto, A.J., & Kluender, K.R. (1998). General contrast effects in speech perception: Effect of preceding liquid on stop consonant identification. *Perception & Psychophysics, 60*, 602–619.

Mann, V.A. (1980). Influence of preceding liquid on stop-consonant perception. *Perception & Psychophysics, 28*, 407–412.

Manuel, S. (1990). The role of contrast in limiting vowel-to-vowel coarticulation in different languages. *Journal of the Acoustical Society of America, 88*, 1286–1298.

McMurray, B., Munson, C., & Tomblin, J.B. (2014). Individual differences in language ability are related to variation in word recognition, not speech perception: Evidence from eye-movements. *Journal of Speech, Language, and Hearing Research, 57*(4), 1344–1362.

Messaoud-Galusi, S., Hazan, V., & Rosen, S. (2011). Investigating speech perception in children with dyslexia: Is there evidence of a consistent deficit in individuals? *Journal of Speech, Language, and Hearing Research, 54*(6), 1682–1701.

Meyer, J., Dentel, L., & Meunier, F. (2013). Speech recognition in natural background noise, *PLOS ONE, 8*(11), 1–14.

Milberg, W., Blumstein, S.E., & Dzworetzky, B. (1988). Phonological processing and lexical access in aphasia. *Brain and Language, 34*, 279–293.

Mirman, D., Yee, E., Blumstein, S.E., & Magnuson, J.S. (2011). Theories of spoken word recognition deficits in aphasia: Evidence from eye-tracking and computational modeling. *Brain and Language, 117*(2), 53–68.

Murakami, K., Miyatani, M., & Cheang, A. (2017). Developing English phonological awareness in elementary school: Focusing on rhyme and syllable. *JASTEC Journal, 36*, 1–14.

Nijland, L., Maassen, B., & van der Meulen, S. (2003). Evidence of motor programming deficits in children diagnosed with DAS. *Journal of Speech, Language, and Hearing Research, 46*(2), 437–450.

Nooteboom, S.G. (1969) The tongue slips into patterns. In A.G. Sciarone, A.J. van Essen, & A.A. van Raad (Eds.), *Nomen, Leyden Studies in Linguistics and Phonetics* (pp. 114–132). The Hague, The Netherlands: Mouton.

Norris, D., & McQueen, J.M. (2008). Shortlist B: A Bayesian model of continuous speech recognition. *Psychological Review, 115*(2), 357–395.

Parker, S. (2012). *The Sonority Controversy*. Berlin/Boston, MA: De Gruyter Mouton.

Ravizza, S.M. (2005). Neural regions associated with categorical speech perception and production. In H. Cohen & C. Lefebvre (Eds.), *Handbook of Categorization in Cognitive Science* (pp. 601–615). Amsterdam, The Netherlands; Oxford, UK: Elsevier Press.

Read, R., & Belpaeme, T. (2016). People interpret robotic non-linguistic utterances categorically. *International Journal of Social Robotics*, *8*, 31–50.

Recasens, D. (2015). The effect of stress and speech rate on vowel coarticulation in Catalan vowel-consonant-vowel sequences. *Journal of Speech, Language and Hearing Research*, *58*, 1407–1424.

Rietveld, A.C.M., & Van Heuven, V.J. (2016). *Algemene Fonetiek* (4th ed.). Bussum, The Netherlands: Coutinho.

Rietveld, T. (2021). *Human Measurement Techniques in Speech and Language Pathology.* London/New York: Routledge (*in press*).

Rubertus, E., & Noiray, A. (2018). On the development of gestural organization: A cross-sectional study of vowel-to-vowel anticipatory coarticulation. *PLos ONE*, *13*(9), e0203562.

Sauvageau, V.M., Roy, J-P., Langlois, M., & Macoir, J. (2015). Impact of the *LSVT* on vowel articulation and coarticulation in Parkinson's disease, *Clinical Linguistics & Phonetics*, *29*(6), 424–440.

Sievers, E. (1883). *Grundzüge der Phonetik.* Leipzig, Germany: Bretitkopf & Hartel.

Strange, W., Verbrugge, R.R., Shankweiler, D.P., & Edman, T.R. (1976). Consonant environment specifies vowel identity. *Journal of the Acoustical Society of America*, *60*, 198–212.

Tjaden, K. (2003). Anticipatory coarticulation in multiple sclerosis and Parkinson's disease. *Journal of Speech, Language, and Hearing Research*, *46*(4), 990–1008.

Tjaden, K. (2000). An acoustic study of coarticulation in dysarthric speakers with Parkinson disease. *Journal of Speech, Language, and Hearing Research*, *43*(6), 1466–1480.

Verdonschot R. G., & Kinoshita, S. (2018). Mora or more? The phonological unit of Japanese word production in the Stroop color naming task. *Memory & Cognition*, *46*, 410–425.

Warner, N.L., McQueen, J.M., & Cutler, A. (2014). Tracking perception of the sounds of English. *Journal of the Acoustical Society of America*, *135*, 2995–3006.

Whitehill, T.L., Francis, A.L., & Ching, C.K-Y. (2003). Perception of place of articulation by children with cleft palate and posterior placement. *Journal of Speech, Language, and Hearing Research*, *46*, 451–461.

Ziegler, J.C., Pech-Georgel, C., George, F., Alario, F.X., & Lorenzi, C. (2005). Deficits in speech perception predict language learning impairment. *Proceedings of the National Academy of Science USA*, *102*, 14110–14115.

5

SUPRASEGMENTAL PHONETICS

Orla Lowry

In previous chapters, we have encountered the vowel and consonant sounds, which are termed as the *segments* which make up speech. These two combine to form syllables, which in turn make up words, phrases and longer utterances. Phonetic characteristics, such as stress and pitch, which spread over units longer than the segment are known as *suprasegmentals*. This chapter will explore the main suprasegmental features which extend over syllables and longer domains, and will consider: stress, length, pitch, voice quality, tempo and loudness. Before dealing with these, it is necessary to discuss the concept of the syllable, this being the smallest unit of speech above the level of the segment.

The syllable

Structure

Most people can agree on the quantification of the number of syllables in the majority of words, but there is no single definitive means of phonetically characterizing and determining the location of boundaries of a syllable where uncertainty arises. It is, however, generally accepted that syllables have a particular structure, consisting minimally of a *nucleus*. The nucleus is usually a vowel, but may also be a sonorant consonant (see explanation of *sonorant* in Chapter 1). One syllable, made up only of a nucleus, can constitute a single word; for example, *awe* and *I*. Syllables can also have an *onset*, which is a consonant or consonant cluster (two or more contiguous consonants) preceding the nucleus, and/or a *coda*, which is a consonant or consonant cluster succeeding the nucleus. *Tea* has an onset and a nucleus ([ti]); *it* has a nucleus and a coda ([ɪt]); *strike* has an onset, nucleus and coda ([stɹaɪk]). The nucleus and coda combine to make up the *rime* or *rhyme* of the syllable. The number and order of consonants which are permissible in the onset and coda of syllables is language-specific: English, for instance, cannot have [ts] in an onset, nor [h] in a coda, and a small number of languages, such as Hawaiian and Mba (Ubangian language spoken in the northern Democratic Republic of the Congo) are reported never to allow a coda (Maddieson, 2013a). Syllables with no coda are referred to as *open*, while those with a coda are *closed*. Figure 5.1 shows the structure of the word sleep; σ is the conventional symbol for the representation of the syllable.

σ

onset   rhyme

nucleus   coda

[s   l   i   p]

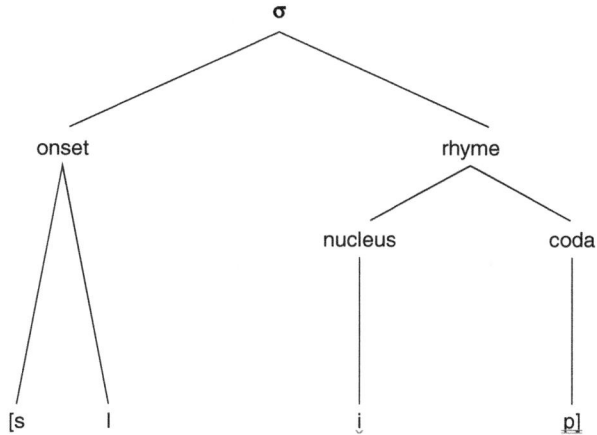

Figure 5.1   Syllable structure of the word *sleep* [slip].

Examples of consonants which may constitute a syllable nucleus are the [l] at the end of *little* and the [n] at the end of *fasten*, and occur in the absence of the schwa vowel. In IPA terms, these are signaled by a diacritic below the symbol; respectively, [lɪtl̩] and [fasn̩].

Sonority

In attempting to define a syllable nucleus, the most sonorous segment of those in question is often proposed. *Sonority* is the relative loudness of a sound, and correlates with the degree of openness of the vocal tract: the more open it is, the more sonorous the sound. Low vowels, then, which are produced with the most open configuration of the vocal tract are the most sonorous of the speech sounds. Increased sonority also entails increased acoustic intensity, oral air pressure, air flow volume and sound duration. Mid vowels have the next highest degree of sonority, followed by high vowels. These can all constitute the nucleus of a syllable. Sounds with the lowest degree of sonority are voiceless plosives, which only ever occupy onset or coda position. The sonority scale below depicts the order of sonority of the sounds in between.

Sonority scale of sounds, from most to least sonorous:

1. Low vowels
2. Mid vowels
3. High vowels and glides ([j] and [w])
4. Taps, flaps and [ɹ]
5. Laterals
6. Nasals
7. Voiced fricatives
8. Voiceless fricatives
9. Voiced affricates
10. Voiceless affricates
11. Voiced plosives
12. Voiceless plosives

The concept of sonority has been used to explain many types of consonant deletion in child speech disorders, but there is an ongoing debate as to whether sonority is an innate aspect of language, or simply a pattern that emerges from commonly occurring combinations of consonants and vowels in natural language.

Maximal onset principle

In the case of multisyllabic words, one way of deciding on syllable boundaries, in cases of doubt, is according to the *Maximal Onset Principle*. In the word *describe* ([dəskɹaɪb]), for example, there will be agreement that there are two syllables, but there may be debate over where the first syllable ends and the second begins. According to the principle, if the consonant or consonant cluster is permissible as an onset in English, or the language in question, it is assigned to the second syllable. In this case, then, the word will be syllabified as [də.skɹaɪb], where the full stop marks the division between syllables, since the cluster [skɹ] can make up the onset of a number of English words, such as *scream, scrap* and *scribble*. In the case of the word hanger, the division would be [haŋ.ə], since the velar nasal, [ŋ] cannot form an onset in English. It must therefore be affiliated with the first syllable, as its coda.

Stress

Stress is the relative prominence of a particular syllable, either in the context of a single word or a longer utterance, such as a phrase or sentence. This perceived prominence is due to a combination of such physical properties as increased duration, greater intensity and changes in the rate of vocal fold vibration, this latter of which is perceived as pitch change and will be discussed in more detail later. In the case of English words pronounced in isolation, known as their *citation form*, the location of the stressed syllable, known as *lexical* or *word-level* stress, is at times unpredictable, and indeed, often variable, both between and within varieties of English. The words *controversy*, for example, can be pronounced with either the first *or* the second of the four syllables as salient. In American English, the word *inquiry* is usually pronounced with the stress on the first syllable, while in Standard Southern British English, it is normally on the second. Stress can sometimes be contrastive in English, usually with the effect of differentiating a noun from a verb. For example, *record* is a noun when the stress is on the first syllable, and a verb when on the second; the same pattern applies for *insult* and *conduct*. The IPA marks stress with ['] preceding the relevant syllable; thus, the noun is 'record and the verb is re'cord. Longer words, usually of more than three syllables, can have a *secondary* stress as well as the main stress, or *primary* stress. Syllables with secondary stress are not as prominent as those with primary stress, but neither are they unstressed; i.e. they have lesser degrees of length, loudness and pitch level or movement. They are marked by the IPA's secondary stress mark, [ˌ], and examples of words with primary, secondary and unstressed syllables are: ˌsupraseg'mental, ˌdiagno'stician and aˌcade'mician.

In atypical speech, the typical or expected stress patterning can be impaired, which is often related to syllable duration or to excessive stress on typically unstressed syllables, resulting in stress contrast being reduced. See, for example, Haley and Jacks (2019) on the effects of apraxia of speech—a motoric speech disorder which is caused by left-hemisphere lesions, which adversely affects planning and programming of speech production—on lexical stress.

Stress location, in the context of longer utterances than single words, contributes to the rhythm of the utterance. This type of stress is *rhythmic* or *sentence-level* stress, and it can supersede the lexical stress. In English, apart from some Asian and African varieties, stress in phrases typically occurs at regular time intervals, which means that some of the lexical stresses are omitted. English is thus known as a *stress-timed* language. In the utterance *Quick big brown foxes jump over lazy dogs*, each word would have a stress when pronounced in isolation (in the two-syllable words, *foxes, over* and *lazy*, the stress is on the first syllable). However, in the context of the full utterance, the stresses may occur as 'Quick big brown 'foxes jump 'over lazy 'dogs as a likely production in conversational speech. Other languages, such as French, Italian and Spanish, are said to be *syllable-timed*, which means that syllables have more or less equal timing, whether or not they are stressed. As is the case for lexical stress, expected rhythmic stress patterns can be disrupted in atypical speech.

Length

The physical duration of a syllable is not often contrastive (i.e. the cause of a meaning difference between words) in English, although varieties of Australian English have been reported to distinguish some pairs of words purely by length. For example, Harrington, Cox, and Evans (1997) claim that the pairs *bed-bared* and *bard-bud* are differentiated only by their vowel lengths in some varieties of Australian English. Finnish and Maltese have contrastive vowel length (Laver, 1994), while Japanese and Italian have contrastive consonant length; Italian, for example, contrasts the words *sete* (thirst) and *sette* (seven) by means of the lengthened medial consonant [t] in the second word. Increased duration of consonant sounds is known as gemination and lengthening of both consonant and vowel sounds are indicated by the diacritic [:].

A syllable's duration can also be conditioned by surrounding sounds. The main manifestation of this in English is the lengthening of a vowel preceding a voiced consonant. The word *sat*, for example, is perceived as containing a shorter vowel sound than that in the word *sad*. Similarly, *bus* has a shorter vowel than *buzz*, and *leaf* is shorter than *leave*.

A variety of speech disorders can affect length. For example, in dysfluent speech segments and syllables may be lengthened excessively or sometimes reduced. Motor speech disorders (see Chapter 6) may also affect the ability to control length.

Pitch

Pitch is the auditory perception which correlates with the rate of vibration, known as the *fundamental frequency* of the vocal folds during speech. An increase in the rate of vibration of the vocal folds, which is affected by such aspects as degree of tension of the vocal folds and amount of lung air, is perceived as higher pitch; decrease in rate is perceived as lower pitch. The pattern of pitch changes for communicative purposes over the course of an utterance is termed *intonation*.

Tone languages

Many of the world's languages, and in particular, those of Africa (for example, Somali and Luganda) and Southeast Asia (for example, Vietnamese and Mandarin Chinese), use pitch height and pitch shape in syllables to distinguish meaning; thus, the segmental material of a syllable can remain the same, but the word's meaning will be determined by the pitch level or shape. Languages that use pitch contrastively like this are *tone languages*. In Thai, for example, the syllable [kʰaa] corresponds to five different words and the meaning of the word depends on the tone type. If pronounced with a high tone, it means *to trade*, with a mid-tone, it means *to get stuck*, and with a rising tone, means *leg* (Maddieson, 2013b). Certain types of aphasia (see Chapter 6) have been shown to disrupt correct tone production in various tone languages.

Intonation languages

Pitch is not used in English, nor in the majority of European languages, to determine lexical meaning (that is, the dictionary definition of a word). However, intonation patterns do have important communicative functions in these languages, which are various and often context-dependent. Languages which utilize pitch in this way are *intonation languages*. Perhaps the most often-reported function of intonation in the majority of commonly-described varieties of English (Standard Southern British English, General American English and Standard Australian English) is to indicate whether the utterance type is a statement or a question: statements are pronounced with falling intonation, while questions have a rising pattern. (This is, however, something of an oversimplification; *wh*-questions in Standard Southern British English, at least, are often produced with falling pitch.) Figure 5.2 shows a schematized diagram depicting two different pitch contours associated with the phrase *I'm late*.

Several analytic frameworks for the formal description of intonation have been put forward (see below), and although these may differ in specific details and notation conventions, they all share two premises: that speech can be divided into manageable sections by using particular intonation features, and that within these sections, there is at least one relatively prominent syllable. The sections are termed *intonation phrases* (older analyses have used the terms *tone group, breath group* and *sense group*) and the beginnings and end of these intonation phrases are characterized by one or both of pause and pitch resetting. More often than not, these boundaries coincide with syntactic boundaries, such as those in a phrase or sentence. In most frameworks, the particularly prominent syllable in the intonation phrase is termed the *nucleus*, and as well as being longer and louder than the others (as is the case with stressed syllables discussed above), its particular perceived salience is due to a pitch movement during the syllable, or due to a step-up or step-down in pitch from a preceding syllable. This is known as an *accent* or a *pitch accent*. Changes to the location of intonation phrase boundaries and to the

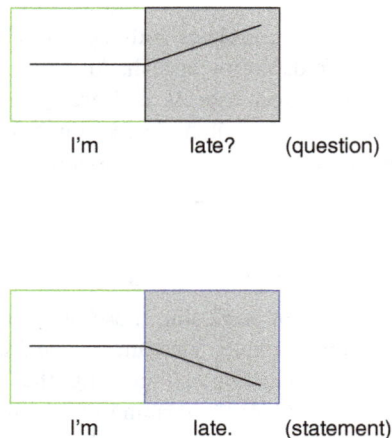

I'm   late?   (question)

I'm   late.   (statement)

Figure 5.2 Typical intonation patterns for statements and questions. The black line represents the pitch contour and the shaded area is the accented syllable (the nucleus).

location or shape of the nucleus can change the function of the utterance. Examples of these follow, but it must be remembered that the functions of particular intonational features are usually dependent on the specific situation, as opposed to being constant, one-to-one mappings between form and function.

If we consider the utterance, *A woman without her man is nothing*, which is often given as part of a light-hearted exercise or Internet meme, with the aim of showing the importance of punctuation, very different interpretations can be gleaned by different placements of intonation phrase boundaries. These boundaries can be considered the oral equivalent of written punctuation. The insertion of three intonation phrase boundaries, marked here by the symbol ‖ (the IPA symbol for a pause) could result in the utterance,

A woman ‖ without her ‖ man is nothing ‖

which presents the woman in favorable terms and the man in a very much less commendatory light. This would correspond to the written version, *A woman: without her, man is nothing*. If, however, the boundary number and locations were changed, a resulting, plausible utterance could be,

A woman without her man ‖ is nothing ‖

and would correspond to the written, *A woman without her man, is nothing.* and has quite the opposite interpretation. This type of signaling of grammatical structure, then, is an important function of intonation.

Varying the position of the nucleus can also have a significant effect on the meaning of the utterance, particularly in relation to its focus. The utterance *John is twenty* could be pronounced with the nucleus on *John* or *is*, or on the first syllable of *twenty*. If *John is TWENty* is produced (where the capital letters mark the accented syllable), the interpretation is likely to be that the phrase in its entirety is new information; the intonation phrase is thus said to have *broad focus*. In English, broad focus utterances usually have the nucleus on the stressed syllable of the final content word as the default position. Shifting the position of the nucleus to the first word, as in, *JOHN is twenty* causes the focus to move to John, and the focus thus becomes *narrow*. A possible context is that the speaker is contradicting something that has just been said erroneously (for example, *Jane is twenty*) and is emphasizing *John* for a particular effect (for example, to make sure that the interlocutor has understood correctly that it is John, and not Jane, who is twenty). In this case, the remainder of the information in the utterance (i.e. that someone is twenty) has already been stated and is therefore *given*. Given information is in the shared background of knowledge of the speaker and hearer, because it has been stated, or is inferred from the context, and is usually deaccented. Finally, a possible context of the narrow-focus utterance, *John IS twenty* may be that a previous debate entailed uncertainty as to whether or not John is twenty. This rendition of the utterance may be interpreted as confirmatory of the fact, following some new discovery or revelation.

Modifying the shape of the nucleus is another main way of altering the meaning of the intonation phrase. Most analytic frameworks recognize at least five types of nuclear pitch pattern in English: falling, rising, level, falling-rising and rising-falling. The statement-question example, illustrated in Figure 5.2, shows how the change from a rising nucleus to the falling nucleus changes the utterance from a question to a statement. Falling versus rising or falling-rising nuclei can also have the function of signaling completeness versus continuation. This can often be seen in lists. The shopping list, *eggs, beans, oranges, apples* could have the following intonation pattern, where the iconic/preceding a syllable signals a rising nucleus, and \ a falling nucleus:

/eggs ‖ / beans ‖ / oranges ‖ \ apples ‖

The rising nucleus on the first three items signals that more is to come and that the list is not complete, while the falling nucleus on the final items indicates that it is complete.

Intonation patterns can contribute to conveying the attitude or emotional state of the speaker. A very high-pitched utterance, for instance, could indicate that the speaker is excited or frightened, while low-pitched, monotonous speech may indicate tiredness or boredom. Context is particularly important here and other physical factors may be involved, such as facial expression or hand gesticulation; as stated above, definitive form-function relationships do not exist.

Conventional intonation patterns can be disrupted for several reasons in atypical speech. Children with autism, for example, have been reported to display monotonous speech, where there is very little variability in pitch movement and type (see, for example, Shriberg et al., 2001). Motor disorders, such as dysarthria and Parkinson's disease, can also cause unexpected intonation patterns (see, for example, Lowit & Kuschmann, 2012) as can the speech of people with hearing impairment (Rahilly, 1991, 2013).

Transcribing intonation

A large number of intonation transcription systems have been proposed over the years, and we do not have space to consider all of them. Some of these have been iconic, using lines to denote the movement up and down of Bolinger, D. (1986, 1989); others have used diacritics or numerals to denote different parts of an intonation pattern; and others again have used a set number of alphabetic abbreviations to represent major tone movements.

A variety of the iconic approach (often termed "tadpole" notation) can be seen in Chapter 13 (Figure 13.4), where the dots stand for syllables (large dots represent stressed syllables) and the tail of the tadpole shows the direction and extent of pitch movement over time. O'Connor and Arnold (1973) used a system of diacritics, whereas Halliday (1970) employed numbers to denote major pitch types, and Pike (1945) and Trager and Smith (e.g. Trager, 1964) used numerals to denote different pitch levels. We can compare the O'Connor and Arnold approach with that of Trager in the example below[1]. The transcriptions show an utterance with the first few syllables said with a low pitch (a "low pre-head"), the syllables from the word "typically" pronounced at a high level pitch ("high head"), and the main pitch movement on the word "day" said with a fall in pitch from a medium to a low level ("low fall").

a. it was a 'typically sunny˳ day
b. ¹it was a ⁴typically sunny ²⁻¹day

In (a) the low pre-head is deemed the default value so is unmarked, the head is marked with a vertical dash placed high, and the low-fall with a grave accent placed low. In the Trager example, the numerals denote one of four pitch levels, where (1) is the lowest and (4) the highest.

More recently, work by Beckman and colleagues (e.g. Beckman, Hirschberg, & Shattuck-Hufnagel, 2005) outlined an analysis system for intonation that can also be used as a form of transcription: the ToBI system (Tones and Breaks Indices). There are various tiers involved in a full ToBI analysis, but we can look very briefly at the tones tier and how it links to the orthographic level (the word tier). In this system, the pitch on important stressed words is marked as H* or L* (high or low), phrase accents (those between the final accented syllable and the phrase edge) are marked H- and L-. Boundary tones display the pitch movement at the end of a phrase and can be H% or L%. Applying these to the phrase used earlier, we get:

c. it was a typically sunny day

    H*   H-   H* L-L%

It can be noted that the syllables of the pre-head are unmarked in ToBI, but a derivative of ToBI (the IViE system, Grabe, Post, & Nolan, 2000) does allow a fuller marking of the pre-head and simplifies some other aspects of the ToBI formalism.

Many of these systems, being based on normal patterns of intonation for the language concerned, are not readily adaptable to disordered prosody. Iconic systems such as the tadpole approach illustrated in Chapter 13 may well be the most useful, therefore, as specific intonation units are not presupposed in such a transcription.

Voice quality

In Chapter 1, we encountered the glottal settings which apply to individual segments and determine their status as *voiced* or *voiceless*. The term, *voice quality*, however, refers to articulatory settings which spread over longer stretches of speech, imbuing it with particular longer-term characteristics, such as nasality or breathiness. These settings affect either the glottalic (at the larynx) or the supraglottalic area (above the larynx), and are not contrastive in English, but may be in other languages. Some of the main muscular adjustments which occur in order to produce these different qualities are described below.

Glottalic/Laryngeal settings (phonation types)

The laryngeal *falsetto* setting entails a very high-frequency vibration of the vocal folds, which are stiff and thin, due to the movements of the muscles of the larynx (see Chapter 1 for illustrations of the larynx). The result is unusually high-pitched speech in relation to the speaker's default voice. *Creaky voice* is produced when subglottal air pressure is low, meaning that the anterior parts of the vocal folds vibrate very slowly. The arytenoid cartilages are close together and laryngeal muscles are tensed. This type of phonation is informally known as *glottal fry* or *vocal fry,* and is sometimes produced by English speakers toward the end of the utterance. It has also been relatively recently described as a social or stylistic phenomenon of the speech of young American female speakers (see, for example Yuasa, 2010). Languages such as Somali and some Austro-Asiatic languages are reported to have contrastive creaky voice in plosives (Ladefoged & Maddieson, 1996). In *breathy voice*, there is low muscular tension, which leads to incomplete closure of the glottis during vibration, allowing more air to escape. This voice quality is often associated with English-speaking female actors to signal seductiveness. Plosives in Indo-Aryan languages, of which Hindi is an example, use breathy voice contrastively (Ladefoged & Maddieson, 1996). *Whisper* involves a constriction in the vocal folds, which is greater than that involved in voiceless sounds, and is often used in English when the speaker is obliged to speak very quietly. *Modal voice* is the neutral setting for the larynx. Combinations of these settings are also possible; for example, whispery falsetto or nasal whispery may occur.

Glottalic voice quality settings can be affected and impaired by a number of speech disorders. For instance, laryngeal cancer, even after treatment and rehabilitation, can cause such qualities as increased breathiness or creak (Millgård & Tuomi, 2020).

Supraglottalic/Supralaryngeal settings

These settings involve muscular modifications in the area above the larynx. *Nasality* refers to the escape of air through the nasal, as well as the oral, cavity which entails the velum lowering. English has nasalized vowels when followed by or preceded by a nasal consonant; French, on the other hand, contrasts nasalized and oral vowels. The words *bon* (*good*) and *beau* (*beautiful*), for example, are distinguished by having a nasalized vowel in the former and an oral vowel in the latter. Some speakers may idiosyncratically keep the velum lowered over longer stretches of speech, giving the speech a characteristic nasal quality. In cases of clinical speech, excessive nasality or *hypernasality* may occur in cases where a speaker is not able to raise the velum to close off the nasal cavity and direct air exclusively through the oral cavity. This means that the speech will have a consistent nasal quality. The speech of persons with cleft palate is often characterized by hypernasality. Conversely, speakers may be unable to lower the velum, which means that air cannot enter the nasal cavity, so all sounds will be oral. This *hyponasality* can be a temporary condition, caused by rhinitis, colds and swelling in adenoids and/or tonsils.

The area above the larynx can be modified width-wise and length-wise, which has an effect on the voice quality characteristics. In terms of the width-wise or latitudinal settings, the tongue may move in particular ways in relation to the palate. If it is consistently directed upward and forward toward the hard palate, *palatalized* voiced is produced, which is characterized by raised pitch. This voice quality may be observed in speakers with Down's syndrome, due to the often-underdeveloped palate in relation to the large size of the tongue. If the tongue is drawn backward, toward the velum, the voice quality is *velarized,* and the overall pitch of the voice is lowered.

The length-wise or longitudinal adjustments may include lowering or raising of the larynx, which has the effect of lengthening and shortening the vocal tract, respectively. Speech produced with a raised larynx will have high pitch and with a lowered larynx will have lower pitch. Labial protrusion (pushing the lips outward) and labial retraction also vary the length of the supralaryngeal area, and as is the case for any of these modifications, has an effect on the voice quality.

Tempo and loudness

The final two suprasegmental features that we will consider are tempo and loudness. In the study of phonology (i.e. the linguistic use of phonetics in specific languages or dialects), these two features are often ignored as they rarely contribute to differences in meaning. However, clinical phoneticians are interested in them as they are disturbed in a variety of speech disorders. While it is possible to measure both tempo and loudness instrumentally and produce measurements in syllable per second, or in decibels, it is usually enough for clinical purposes to state whether the tempo or loudness is within normal limits, is too much or too little. For example, the extIPA chart of symbols to transcribe disordered speech (see Chapter 13) uses terms derived from musical notation to denote loudness (*p,* or *pp* to denote soft and very soft, *f* or *ff* for loud and very loud; *allegro* or *lento* to denote fast and slow). Hearing-impaired speakers are one client type that may display disorders to their control of loudness (speaking either too loudly or not loudly enough); clients with dysarthria may display problems with tempo and loudness.

We can also note here that tempo can be measured in terms of speech rate (for example, syllables per second) or articulation rate. Speech rate includes all the normal pauses, hesitations and false starts that speakers may use; thus, the rate does not reflect how fast a speaker articulates an utterance without these interruptions. Articulation rate, on the other hand, is a measurement of tempo with all these features excluded. This difference may also be important for clinical phoneticians, for example in calculating how much the speech of a person who stutters has been slowed down due to their dysfluencies.

Conclusion

In this chapter, we have considered some of the main aspects of speech which affect units larger than the segment. The smallest of these units is the syllable, although the effects discussed may spread over longer units, such as words, phrases, sentences and longer utterances. The structure of the syllable and syllable sonority were explained, although there is no conclusive phonetic definition. The suprasegmental feature of lexical stress, both primary and secondary, was examined, and we saw how lexical stress, which applies to words pronounced in isolation, can be overridden (in English) by rhythmic stress when the words are in the context of connected speech. Syllable length and how it may be conditioned by its surrounding sounds was then discussed. Intonation can be considered to be the melody of speech, or the tone of voice, and has a variety of functions in English, depending principally on the location of intonation phrase boundaries, nucleus location and nucleus type. Tone languages, unlike English, use different pitch patterns to distinguish words lexically. Then we looked at some different types of voice quality, which are particular characteristics of speech caused by muscular adjustments made at the glottis and the area above the glottis. Finally, we looked at the speed and volume of speech and ways of denoting them. All of these suprasegmental features can be affected and impaired by a number of speech disorders, and these will be considered in detail in later chapters.

Note

1 Trager also used some diacritics but these are omitted for the sake of simplicity.

References

Beckman, M.E., Hirschberg, J., & Shattuck-Hufnagel, S. (2005). The original ToBI system and the evolution of the ToBI framework. In S.-A. Jun (Ed.), *Prosodic Typology – The Phonology of Intonation and Phrasing*(pp. 9–54). Oxford, UK: Oxford University Press.

Bolinger, D. (1986). *Intonation and its Parts. Melody in Spoken English*. Stanford, CA: Stanford University Press.

Bolinger, D. (1989). *Intonation and its Uses. Melody in Grammar and Discourse*. Stanford, CA: Stanford University Press.

Grabe, E., Post, B., & Nolan, F. (2000). Modelling intonational variation in English: The IViE system. In *Proceedings of Prosody 2000* (Vol. 5, pp. 1–57).

Haley, K.L. & Jacks, A. (2019). Word-level prosodic measures and the differential diagnosis of apraxia of speech. *Clinical Linguistics and Phonetics*. 33(5), 479–495. doi:10.1080/02699206.2018.155 0813

Halliday, M.A.K. (1970). *A Course in Spoken English: Intonation*. London, UK: Oxford University Press.`

Harrington, J., Cox, F., & Evans, Z. (1997). An acoustic phonetic study of broad, general, and cultivated Australian English vowels. *Australian Journal of Linguistics*, 17(2), 155–184. doi: 10.1080/07268609708599550

Laver, J. (1994). *Principles of Phonetics*. Cambridge, UK: Cambridge University Press.

Lowit, A. & Kuschmann, A. (2012) Characterizing intonation deficit in motor speech disorders: An autosegmental-metrical analysis of spontaneous speech in hypokinetic dysarthria, ataxic dysarthria, and foreign accent syndrome. *Journal of Speech, Language and Hearing Research*, 55(5), 1472–84. doi: 10.1044/1092-4388(2012/11-0263)

Ladefoged, P. & Maddieson, I. (1996). *The Sounds of the World's Languages*. Cambridge, UK: Cambridge University Press.

Maddieson, I. (2013a). Syllable structure. In: M.S. Dryer & M. Haspelmath (Eds.) *The World Atlas of Language Structures Online*. Leipzig, Germany: Max Planck Institute for Evolutionary Anthropology. (Available online at http://wals.info/chapter/12.)

Maddieson, I. (2013b). Tone. In: M.S. Dryer & M. Haspelmath (Eds.) *The World Atlas of Language Structures Online*. Leipzig, Germany: Max Planck Institute for Evolutionary Anthropology. (Available online at http://wals.info/chapter/13.)

Millgård, M. & Tuomi, L. (2020). Voice quality in laryngeal cancer patients: A randomized controlled study of the effect of voice rehabilitation. *Journal of Voice*, 34(3), :486.e13–486.e22. https://doi.org/10.1016/j.jvoice.2018.09.011

O'Connor, J.D. & Arnold, G. (1973). *The Intonation of Colloquial English*. London, UK: Longman.

Pike, K. (1945). *The Intonation of American English*. Ann Arbor, MI: University of Michigan Press.

Rahilly, J. (1991). *Intonation patterns in normal hearing and postlingually deafened adults in Belfast*. Unpublished PhD thesis, Queen's University of Belfast.

Rahilly, J. (2013). Vowel disorders in hearing impairment. In M.J. Ball & F.E. Gibbon (Eds.), *Handbook of Vowels and Vowel Disorders*(pp. 364–383). New York, NY: Psychology Press.

Shriberg, L.D., Paul, R., McSweeny, J.L., Klin, A.M., Cohen, D.J., & Volkmar, F.R. (2001). Speech and prosody characteristics of adolescents and adults with high-functioning autism and Asperger syndrome. *Journal of Speech, Language and Hearing Research*. 44, 1097–1115.

Trager, G.L. (1964). The intonation system of American English. In D. Abercrombie, D. Fry, P. MacCarthy, N. Scott, & J. Trim (Eds.), In *Honour of Daniel Jones: Papers Contributed on the Occasion of His Eightieth Birthday, September 12, 1961* (pp. 266–270). London, UK: Longmans, Green.

Yuasa, I.P. (2010). Creaky voice: A new feminine voice quality for young urban-oriented upwardly mobile American women? *American Speech*, 85, 315–337.

6

AN INTRODUCTION TO SPEECH DISORDERS

Martin J. Ball

Clinical Phonetics is the interaction between phonetics and disordered speech. That is, the contribution of phonetics to the description of speech disorders, and the contribution of the study of speech disorders to phonetic theory and phonetic analysis. The chapters of this collection deal with this interaction but, to set the scene, we need first to consider the range of communication problems that fall under the heading of "speech disorders."

There are several different ways we could divide up this topic. We could classify speech disorders according to characteristics of the speakers concerned, for example, in terms of their age. We could classify them in terms of the phonetic/linguistic aspects affected, for example, segmental versus suprasegmental, or in terms of levels of organization of speech (phonetic versus phonological). We could classify them in terms of the cause, for example, genetic causes as opposed to a stroke, or surgical intervention, or even more basically, known versus unknown causes. Finally, we should note that disorders can usually be classified by several of these types. In the following descriptions, we use the headings suggested in Ball (2016).[1]

Genetic etiology

The first category is disorders with a genetic etiology. This category includes disordered speech due to cleft lip and/or palate, and due to a variety of genetic syndromes. Cleft lip and/or palate disorders are often grouped under the heading craniofacial or orofacial anomalies. These may derive from a large number of different genetic syndromes (see Russell, 2010) and may affect any combinations of the lip, prepalate/alveolar ridge, hard palate and soft palate.

Hypernasality in the speech of speakers with cleft palates is often described as being part of a grouping of velopharyngeal inadequacy (or insufficiency), or VPI. However, VPI can be due to a range of problems, some genetic, some acquired.

The speech consequences of cleft palate, as Russell (2010) notes, include obligatory and compensatory patterns. Obligatory patterns are those that are a direct result of the organic abnormality. In the case of cleft palate, the absence of a barrier between the oral and the nasal cavities means that intraoral air pressure cannot be built up: pressure that is needed in the production of target oral stops, for example. Thus, these target sounds are replaced by nasal stops, as they lack the requirement of intraoral air pressure and involve airflow through the nasal cavity. Compensatory patterns are those adopted by speakers to get around the difficulties they encounter in producing certain sounds or sound classes. For example, the production of many fricatives of a target language may prove difficult if first there is a cleft in the area where the target fricatives are normally produced (depending on the language this could include any-where from the lips back to the soft palate); and second, due again to the need for a certain amount of intraoral air pressure to produce the turbulence necessary for frication in speech. In these cases, therefore, speakers may compensate by producing fricatives behind the location of the cleft, resulting in dorsal, pharyngeal and glottal fricatives for targets normally produced anterior to these locations. There may also be pervasive glottal usage for a variety of conson-antal targets. Other unusual places of articulation have been reported; Russell (2010) notes both linguolabial and dentolabial articulations compensating for bilabial and labiodental, respect-ively. Such compensatory patterns can be thought of as active articulatory processes devised by the speaker, as opposed to passive processes where as much as possible of the target sound remains (e.g. place of articulation), but affected by the loss of the oral-nasal distinction. In this latter case, target fricatives, for example, may be realized as nasalized, or accompanied by velopharyngeal friction, or by audible nasal turbulence (sometime called nareal fricatives, see Ball & Müller, 2005).

In western countries, cleft palates are generally repaired in early childhood (but after the onset of speech), but as Russell (2010) notes there is considerable variation in the precise age of such repairs. Some of the speech characteristics used presurgically may resolve rela-tively easily post-surgery, but some may not, and if therapy is delayed these patterns become phonologized (that is, the learnt speech behavior of the child) and thus resistant to therapy.

In one way, separating genetic syndromes from craniofacial anomalies (especially cleft lip and palate) is artificial, as these anomalies are consequent to a variety of such syndromes. Nevertheless, a large number of genetic syndromes (over 300 according to Stojanovik, 2010) have implications for both speech and language, and it is therefore not unusual to treat them separately from cleft lip and palate.

Stojanovik (2010) describes three syndromes in detail: Williams, Down and Fragile-X. However, others have also been the subject of clinical phonetic research: Prader–Willi (for example, Kleppe, Katayama, Shipley, & Foushee, 1990), Noonan syndrome (Pierpont et al., 2010; Wilson & Dyson, 1982) and Cri-du-chat (Kristoffersen, 2008) among others. While many of these syndromes have consequences for language ability, most also have some effect on speech. Briefly, Williams children exhibit delay in speech development coupled with articu-latory problems caused by muscle tone problems. As Stojanovik (2010) points out, Down children also suffer speech and language delay, and have been described as having both pros-odic disruptions (e.g. Heselwood, Bray, & Crookston, 1995) and unusual misarticulations (Heselwood, 1997).

Stojanovik (2010, p.123) describes the speech characteristics of people with fragile-X syndrome as follows: "Similarly to children with DS, children with FXS also have speech dif-ficulties which can often make their speech unintelligible … due to hypotonia that involves the orofacial musculature." Kleppe et al. (1990) reported a range of misarticulations, disfluencies and resonance problems in children with Prader–Willi syndrome. The misarticulations affected singleton consonants and clusters, with problems especially noted with fricatives, affricates and glides, and with tongue tip and blade consonants. At least part of the explanation could be connected to an excessively high palatal arch that Kleppe et al. (1990) note as commonly encountered with this syndrome. Noonan syndrome too has associated craniofacial anomalies, including high palatal arch, dental malocclusion, intellectual impairment and delayed motor development (Wilson & Dyson, 1982). Kristoffersen (2008) reviews a range of studies on cri-du-chat and a range of linguistic levels. In terms of speech (for those who can use the spoken medium), he notes the generally high-pitched voice of these speakers, the restricted consonant and vowel inventories, and simplified syllable structures. He also notes frequent and variable misarticulations.

Disorders with a surgical origin

The two main surgical procedures that affect speech are laryngectomy and glossectomy. Laryngectomies may be total or partial (Bressmann, 2010). The removal of the larynx has a devastating effect on speech. In normal spoken communication, the larynx has a variety of functions: airstream initiation, phonation and pitch control. The airstream initiation function of the larynx is restricted to those languages that use implosives and ejectives (see Chapters 1 and 16). Neither of these consonant types is possible following a total laryngectomy.

More widely applicable is the role of the larynx in phonation, in that all languages have at least a binary distinction between voiced and voiceless consonants, and some have further phonatory distinctions (Laver, 1994); all these being controlled by vocal fold activity. Finally, pitch (as used linguistically in intonation and tone) is also controlled laryngeally. In this case, the relative frequency of vocal fold vibration corresponds to changes in pitch; clearly; after total laryngectomy pitch changes can no longer be made in this way.

Total laryngectomy, therefore, removes the ability to signal via speech phonation differences and pitch movement. In order to compensate for this loss, speakers may receive therapy to use esophageal speech. Esophageal speech involves the use of a moving column of air from the esophagus, which causes vibration at the sphincteric pharyngoesophageal junction which acts as a pseudoglottis. The speaker then modifies the resultant airflow with the supraglottal articulators in the same way as for pulmonic egressive speech (Ball, Esling, & Dickson, 2000). Lung air is not available for speech as, following the removal of the larynx, the trachea ends in a stoma in the throat. A variety of air intake techniques exists for esophageal speech and is described in Bressmann (2010). Voice quality in esophageal speech clearly differs from that in pulmonic speech; one major difference being the smaller amount of air available for each "exhalation." Apart from the shorter breath units, the use of a pseudoglottis rather than the real glottis results in an unnatural voice quality: low pitched and rough. Little control is available for pitch or volume or for the voiced-voiceless distinction.

Tracheoesophageal speech is possible for those clients where the laryngectomy operation has resulted in a tracheoesophageal junction controlled by a valve in the throat (see Bressmann, 2010). In this case, although the trachea still terminates with a stoma in the throat, a puncture is made between the trachea and the esophagus just at the level of the tracheal opening. Therefore, lung air can still be used for speech by directing it (via the valve) to the esophagus and then through the upper esophageal sphincter as for esophageal speech. This form of speech allows longer breath groups, but still suffers from reduced pitch range and a rough voice quality. Nevertheless, it is generally deemed more acceptable than simple esophageal speech (Bressmann, 2010; Ball et al., 2000).

A final method of voice production we can briefly consider is the use of an electrolarynx. Bressmann (2010) describes the range of these devices in some detail. These devices produce an artificial buzz to compensate for the loss of vocal fold vibration. Even competent users of an electrolarynx, however, will have speech that sounds highly unnatural.

Partial laryngectomies can result in a wide range of different structural changes to the larynx, as described fully in Bressmann (2010). Thus, partial laryngectomy clients may have almost unchanged speech and voice quality at one end of a continuum, or may have to utilize ventricular or partial ventricular partial glottal phonation at the other end. In these latter instances, the voice quality is again going to sound rough and unnatural, but less so than for esophageal or tracheoesophageal speech.

Although glossectomy is the second major type disruption to speech caused by surgery, it is difficult to give details of typical speech problems due to the diverse nature of the procedure. Glossectomies today are usually partial (though total glossectomy can occur) and thus can range from removals of small amounts of tissue to quite extensive resections (Bressmann, 2010). Further, the surgeon may compensate for the missing part of the tongue using flap reconstruction. Thus, clients having undergone glossectomies may be left with differing tongue mass and motility. Bressmann (2010) describes research showing how clients can compensate for the results of the glossectomy with greater speech and articulatory effort, and many clients may well re-achieve acceptable and intelligible speech.

Neurogenic speech disorders

Neurogenic disorders are those acquired through damage caused to the brain, for example through a cerebrovascular accident, brain tumors, or traumatic brain injury. Not all acquired disorders of communication affect speech production, but we will concern ourselves here with the commonest disorders that do cause speech problems.

Aphasia

We follow Code (2010) here in positing a basic distinction between fluent and nonfluent aphasia. Interestingly, both types may affect speech production. Nonfluent aphasia may manifest itself in slow, hesitant speech and disruptions to both prosody and articulatory precision. However, because this type of aphasia is often found with concomitant apraxia of speech, we will deal with the characteristics of nonfluent aphasia under that heading.

Fluent aphasia may show speech impairments. In particular, phonemic paraphasias may occur. These take the form of incorrect phoneme use or incorrect phoneme placement. Code (2010) gives the example of /pæt/ for target "cat"; there may also be transpositions of phonemes: *tevilision* for target "television" (Brookshire, 1997) and additions (e.g. *fafter* for target "after," Buckingham, 1989), among others.

If a speaker produces mostly, or only, paraphasic substitutions, their speech may be unintelligible, and classed as *jargonaphasia*. The speech of clients with jargonaphasia sounds fluent (as noted, it is an aspect of fluent aphasia), with preserved prosody and phonotactic constraints. It is rarely intelligible; however, it sounds as if it is the target language. (Some words may be preserved, but it is not always clear whether these correct words are the intended words of the speaker or just accidental.) Indeed, bilingual clients with jargonaphasia may sound as if they are switching from one language to another, even when the entire communicative event is unintelligible; examples can be found in a study by Müller and Mok (2012) of a premorbidly French–English bilingual.

Apraxia of speech

This disorder is usually characterized as being an impairment of phonetic planning (rather than abstract phonological assembly, or of phonetic execution) (see Jacks & Robin, 2010; Code 1998). That is to say, the construction of motor plans for novel utterances is compromised, but formulaic utterances (that do not need planning *ab initio* and are assumed to be stored as wholes) may be unaffected. This gives apraxic speech the character of having islands of clear speech among the impaired sections. The impairments can consist of a range of disruptions to fluent speech. These include: slow speech rate, distortions to consonants and vowels, prosodic impairments, and inconsistency in errors (Jacks & Robin, 2010). Other features often noted are: articulatory groping, perseverative errors, increasing errors with increasing word length and increasing articulatory complexity, and difficulties initiating speech.

A disorder most often called *progressive apraxia of speech, aphemia* or *anarthria* involves speech deterioration over time without a localized lesion site, though usually accompanying general cortical atrophy (often due to a degenerative condition) (Code, Ball, Tree, & Dawe, 2013). A number of cases of progressive speech deterioration have been described in recent research that occur either in combination with some progressive language or other cognitive impairment or are reported as relatively pure speech production impairments (see references in Code et al., 2013), but nonetheless are not primarily dysarthric nor (par) aphasic conditions.

Dysarthria

Dysarthria is the term applied to speech impairments resulting from "disturbances in muscular control over the speech mechanisms due to damage of the central or peripheral nervous system" (Duffy, 2005, p. 5). Underlying causes of dysarthria are many. Ackermann, Hertrich, and Ziegler (2010) give, among others, Parkinson's disease, Huntington's chorea, focal damage to the basal ganglia, and pseudobulbar palsy. This range of underlying causes also manifests itself in a range of dysarthria types, described, for example, in Ackermann et al. (2010) and in Darley, Aronson, and Brown (1975). The speech sequelae of these different types are listed below, where the consequences for respiration (and thus pulmonic initiation), phonation, resonance, articulation and prosody are shown (derived primarily from Darley et al., 1975). The dysarthria types are flaccid, spastic, hypokinetic, hyperkinetic and ataxic. It should also be noted that mixed dysarthria types are also known where, naturally, the effects on speech depend on which types of dysarthria combine in the particular client.

In terms of respiration, flaccid, spastic and hypokinetic dysarthria are characterized by short expiratory cycles (unlike typical speech where expiration is slowed), hyperkinetic dysarthria is usually described as demonstrating lack of respiratory control and the use of frequent breaths, while ataxic is described as having audible inspiration and inadequate breath control.

For phonation, flaccid and hypokinetic dysarthria are noted as having breathy phonation, flaccid and spastic as having harsh voice quality, spastic and hyperkinetic as having strained voice quality, hypokinetic as having high pitch, and ataxic as having fluctuating pitch, loudness and voice quality.

With resonance, flaccid and spastic have hypernasality, with hyperkinetic having alternating hypernasality. Hypokinetic and ataxic have normal resonance. Articulation for all dysarthria types is noted as imprecise but this is variable for hyperkinetic and ataxic. Finally, prosody is characterized as showing a slow tempo in flaccid and spastic dysarthria, normal or accelerated in hypokinetic, disrupted by pausing in hyperkinetic, and showing a scanning rhythm in ataxic dysarthria (i.e. breaking the utterance into separate syllables, often with pauses between them).

Childhood speech sound disorders

The term "childhood speech sound disorders" is used here for all speech disorders occurring in children. There has been considerable debate in recent years over both what to call this category of disordered speech and how to subdivide it, and these points are discussed in detail in Ball (2016) and Bowen (2009); in this sketch of disordered speech, we adopt the categories used in the former.

Therefore, we posit a first division into "phonetic" and "phonological" disorders or, more precisely, disorders affecting the ability to produce articulations, and disorders affecting the ability to organize speech. Under the first heading, we include articulation disorders and childhood motor speech disorders. Under the second we include phonological delay and various nontypical phonological error patterns. Because this book is concerned mostly with phonetics, we will not go into much detail on these phonological types.

Articulation disorders

One of the diagnostic factors distinguishing an articulation disorder from a phonological disorder is whether the client is stimulable for a sound or group of sounds (i.e. can repeat a sound correctly when prompted by a therapist); if they cannot, then it is likely a problem of articulation (Bowen, 2009). Other considerations include whether the errors affect a large category of sounds or just one or two (the former more likely to be a phonological error), and whether the error falls within the small group of articulatory difficult sounds (such as, for English, sibilants and rhotics). Further, articulation disorders tend to be fairly consistent in terms of the errors produced, whereas phonological disorders may not be. Articulation disorders, then, do seem to have a motoric basis for their difficulty, but this is deemed to differ from motor speech disorders such as dysarthria, as the latter have overt damage to the motor system whereas the former do not. There are numerous illustrations in the literature of sibilant and rhotic problems (for example, Bacsfalvi, 2010; Ball, Manuel, & Müller, 2004; Gibbon & Hardcastle, 1987).

Motor Speech Disorders in children

Cerebral palsy, a nonprogressive motor control disorder caused by damage to the developing brain before, during or just after birth (Bauman-Waengler, 2008), is one of the commonest causes of dysarthria in children. It produces speech disruptions similar to those in adult dysarthria described above, but mainly of the spastic type (ataxic dysarthria and a third type, termed "dyskinesia" may also be encountered).

As the name suggests, "childhood apraxia of speech" (CAS) has many similarities in its effect on speech production as acquired apraxia of speech. While this diagnostic category has in the past been controversial (Shriberg & McSweeny, 2002), it is now generally accepted that CAS is a developmental condition (i.e. no neurological injury can be identified) causing disruption to speech (among other possible effects). There are several checklists that illustrate typical speech disruptions in CAS, and Bauman–Waengler (2008) includes the following speech behaviors: errors greater in sounds requiring more complex oral movements; unusual errors (e.g. repetitions, prolongations, additions); large number of omissions; difficulty producing and maintaining voicing; vowel and diphthong errors; difficulty sequencing sounds and syllables; difficulty with nasality and nasal emission; groping behavior; prosodic impairment. Other checklists exist and are described in Ball (2016).

Phonological disorders in children

"Phonological delay" is perhaps both the easiest to describe and the easiest to treat. A child that exhibits only delay (without the chronological mismatch that Grunwell, 1981, described) has a phonology that resembles the normal phonology of a younger child; it is as if phonological development has simply stopped. Dodd and Bradford (2000) and Grunwell (1987) both discuss and illustrate this category of phonological disorder.

"Phonological deviancy, consistent" and "phonological deviancy, inconsistent" are the two remaining categories of phonological disorders proposed by Dodd (e.g. Dodd, 1995; Dodd, Holm, Hua, Crosbie, & Broomfield, 2006). These disorder types involve phonological patterns not typically encountered in phonological development; in the first grouping the patterns are realized consistently, in the second a range of realizations of certain target sounds are used with no observable pattern.

Others

In this category, we include three disorder types that directly or indirectly affect speech: voice disorders, fluency disorders and hearing impairment. The term *voice disorders* applies to impairments to voice quality which, in turn, refers to aspects of both phonation and long-term supralaryngeal settings (Morris & Harmon, 2010). Voice disorders may arise from a variety of causes, some physical (such as growths on the vocal folds), some acquired (such as neurogenic: see the description of dysarthria above), some from surgical intervention (see discussion earlier on partial and complete laryngectomy) and some functional (in that there is no known cause). While the majority of voice disorders seen clinically involve phonatory problems, problems related to supralaryngeal settings may also be encountered. Common among these are hyper- and hypo-nasality, but favorite articulation in child speech may also manifest itself in settings such as pervasive palatalization, and children exhibiting tongue thrust will have pervasive interdentalization as a voice quality.

Fluency disorders usually have an effect on speech prosody for, as the term suggests, the speech is not fluent due to a variety of possible disruptions. In stuttering, these include repetitions of various kinds (part and whole word), excessive pauses and prolongations of sounds. In cluttering, the speech is characterized by fast and slurred speech. (Tetnowski & Scaler Scott, 2010). However, apart from these prosodic aspects, people who stutter may use a variety of unusual segmental features, possibly as mechanisms to move beyond either repetitions or "blocks" (that is points in the utterance where the speaker is unable to continue usually accompanied by articulatory tension and sometimes other physical manifestations such as grimaces or head and neck movements). Developments in phonetic transcription such as the extIPA and VoQS systems allow the transcription of many of these features (see Chapter 13).

The effect of hearing impairment on speech depends partly on the severity of the impairment and partly upon whether the hearing loss occurred before or after the development of spoken language (i.e. prelingual or postlingual hearing impairment) (see Ball, 1993; Cowie and Douglas-Cowie, 1983; Rahilly, 2013). Prelingually hearing impaired persons are likely to have difficulties producing both segmental and prosodic aspects of speech (see details on consonant and vowel errors in Cowie and Douglas–Cowie, 1992) and so may opt to use sign as well as or instead of spoken communication. With postlingually deafened speakers, prosodic aspects of speech may first be noted as disordered (including loudness and intonation), but eventually segmental aspects may also be affected. Non-normal voice quality of both pre- and postlingually hearing impaired speakers has been noted as a particular characteristic of "deaf speech," and Abberton (2000) describes this in some detail. Non-pulmonic consonants may be found in the speech of the hearing impaired and those with cochlear implants (see Chapter 16, and Ball & Müller, 2007).

This sketch of the range of disorders of speech production has demonstrated the variety of both the underlying causes and the resultant articulatory realizations. To describe these adequately, clinical phoneticians need to be able to use a full range of both transcriptional and instrumental approaches. In the following chapters we provide introductions to the main branches of phonetics, detailed accounts of phonetic transcription for both normal and disordered speech, and practical introductions to over 20 instrumental techniques used in experimental investigations of speech.

Note

1 The following descriptions of types of speech disorder derive closely from those given in Chapter 2 of Ball (2016). This publication also provides copious illustrations of the disorders listed in this introduction.

References

Abberton, E. (2000). Voice quality of deaf speakers. In R.D. Kent & M.J. Ball (Eds.). *Voice quality measurement* (pp. 449–459). San Diego, CA: Singular.

Ackermann, H., Hertrich, I., & Ziegler, W. (2010). Dysarthria. In J. Damico, N. Müller & M.J. Ball (Eds.), *The handbook of language and speech disorders* (pp. 362–390). Chichester, UK: Wiley-Blackwell.

Bacsfalvi, P. (2010). Attaining the lingual components of /r/ with ultrasound for three adolescents with cochlear implants. *Canadian Journal of Speech-Language Pathology and Audiology, 34*, 206–217.

Ball, M.J. (1993). *Phonetics for speech pathology* (2nd ed.). London, UK: Whurr.

Ball, M.J. (2016). *Principles of clinical phonology. Theoretical Approaches*. New York, NY: Psychology Press.

Ball, M.J., Esling, J., & Dickson, C. (2000). The transcription of voice quality. In R.D. Kent & M.J. Ball (Eds.), *Voice quality measurement* (pp. 49–58). San Diego, CA: Singular.

Ball, M.J., Manuel, R., & Müller, N. (2004). Deapicalization and velodorsal articulation as learned behaviors: A videofluorographic study. *Child Language Teaching and Therapy, 20*, 153–162.

Ball, M. J. & Müller, N. (2005). *Phonetics for communication disorders*. Mahwah, NJ: Erlbaum.

Ball, **M.J.** & Müller, **N.** (2007). Non-pulmonic egressive speech sounds in disordered speech: A brief review. *Clinical Linguistics and Phonetics, 21*, 869–874.

Bauman–Waengler, J. (2008). *Articulatory and phonological impairments: A clinical focus* (3rd ed.). Boston, MA: Allyn and Bacon.

Bowen, C. (2009). *Children's speech sounds disorders*. Chichester, UK: Wiley-Blackwell.

Bressmann, T. (2010). Speech disorders related to head and neck cancer. In J. Damico, N. Müller & M.J. Ball (Eds.). *The handbook of language and speech disorders* (pp. 497–526). Chichester, UK: Wiley-Blackwell.

Brookshire, R.H. (1997). *Introduction to neurogenic communication disorders* (5th ed.). St. Louis, MO: Mosby.

Buckingham, H.W. (1989). Phonological paraphasia. In C.F. Code (Ed.), *The characteristics of aphasia* (pp. 81–110). London, UK: Taylor and Francis.

Code, C.F. (1998). Models, theories and heuristics in apraxia of speech. *Clinical Linguistics and Phonetics, 12*, 47–65.

Code, C.F. (2010). Aphasia. In J. Damico, N. Müller & M.J. Ball (Eds.). *The handbook of language and speech disorders* (pp. 317–336). Chichester, UK: Wiley-Blackwell.

Code, C.F., Ball, M.J., Tree, J., & Dawe, K. (2013). The effects of initiation, termination and inhibition impairments on speech rate in a case of progressive nonfluent aphasia with progressive apraxia of speech with frontotemporal degeneration. *Journal of Neurolinguistics, 26*, 602–618.

Cowie, R. & Douglas-Cowie, E. (1983). Speech production in profound postlingual deafness. In M. Lutman & M. Haggard (Eds.), *Hearing science and hearing disorders* (pp. 183–230). London, UK: Academic Press.

Darley, F.L., Aronson, A.E., & Brown, J.R. (1975). *Motor speech disorders*. Philadelphia, PA: W.B. Saunders.

Dodd, B. (1995). *Differential diagnosis and treatment of children with speech disorder*. London, UK: Whurr.

Dodd, B. & Bradford, A. (2000). A comparison of three therapy methods for children with different types of developmental phonological disorder. *International Journal of Language and Communication Disorders*, *35*, 189–209.

Dodd, B., Holm, A., Hua, Z., Crosbie, S., & Broomfield, J. (2006). English phonology: acquisition and disorder. In Z. Hua & B. Dodd (Eds.), *Phonological development and disorders in children. A multilingual perspective* (pp. 25–55). Clevedon, UK: Multilingual Matters.

Duffy, J.R. (2005). *Motor speech disorders: Substrates, differential diagnosis and management* (2nd ed.). St. Louis, MO: Elsevier Mosby.

Gibbon, F. & Hardcastle, W. (1987). Articulatory description and treatment of "lateral /s/" using electropalatography: A case study. *British Journal of Disorders of Communication*, *22*, 203–217.

Grunwell, P. (1981). *The nature of phonological disability in children*. London, UK: Academic Press.

Grunwell, P. (1987). *Clinical phonology* (2nd ed.). London, UK: Chapman and Hall.

Heselwood, B. (1997). A case of nasal clicks for target sonorants: A feature geometry account. *Clinical Linguistics and Phonetics*, *11*, 43–61.

Heselwood, B., Bray, M., & Crookston, I. (1995). Juncture, rhythm and planning in the speech of an adult with Down's syndrome. *Clinical Linguistics and Phonetics*, *9*, 121–137.

Jacks, A. & Robin, D. (2010). Apraxia of speech. In J. Damico, N. Müller & M.J. Ball (Eds.). *The handbook of language and speech disorders* (pp. 391–409). Chichester, UK: Wiley-Blackwell.

Kleppe, S.A., Katayama, K.M., Shipley, K.G., & Foushee, D.R. (1990). The speech and language characteristics of children with Prader–Willi Syndrome. *Journal of Speech and Hearing Disorders*, *55*, 300–309.

Kristoffersen, K. (2008). Speech and language development in cri du chat syndrome: A critical review. *Clinical Linguistics and Phonetics*, *22*, 443–457.

Laver, J. (1994). *Principles of phonetics*. Cambridge, UK: Cambridge University Press.

Morris, R. & Harmon, A.B. (2010). Describing voice disorders. In J. Damico, N. Müller & M.J. Ball (Eds.). *The handbook of language and speech disorders* (pp. 455–473). Chichester, UK: Wiley-Blackwell.

Müller, N. & Mok, Z. (2012). Nonword jargon produced by a French-English bilingual. In M. Gitterman, M. Goral & L. Obler (Eds.), *Aspects of multilingual aphasia* (pp. 224–241). Bristol, UK: Multilingual Matters.

Pierpont, E.I., Weismer, S.E., Roberts, A.E., Tworog-Dube, E., Pierpont, M.E., Mendelsohn, N.J., & Seidenberg, M.S. (2010). The language phenotype of children and adolescents with Noonan Syndrome. *Journal of Speech, Language, and Hearing Research*, *53*, 917–932.

Rahilly, J. (2013). Vowel disorders in hearing impairment. In M.J. Ball & F. Gibbon (Eds.). *Handbook of vowels and vowel disorders* (pp. 364–383). New York, NY: Psychology Press.

Russell, J. (2010). Orofacial anomalies. In J. Damico, N. Müller & M.J. Ball (Eds.). *The handbook of language and speech disorders* (pp. 474–496). Chichester, UK: Wiley-Blackwell.

Shriberg, L. & McSweeny, J. (2002). Classification and misclassification of childhood apraxia of speech. *Phonology Project Technical Report #11*. Madison, Wis: University of Wisconsin-Madison.

Stojanovik, V. (2010). Genetic syndromes and communication disorders. In J. Damico, N. Müller & M.J. Ball (Eds.), *The handbook of language and speech disorders* (pp. 115–130). Chichester, UK: Wiley-Blackwell.

Tetnowski, J. & Scaler Scott, K. (2010). Fluency and fluency disorders. In J. Damico, N. Müller & M.J. Ball (Eds.). *The handbook of language and speech disorders* (pp. 431–454). Chichester, UK: Wiley-Blackwell.

Wilson, M. & Dyson, A. (1982). Noonan syndrome: Speech and language characteristics. *Journal of Communication Disorders*, *15*, 347–352.

PART II

Variationist clinical phonetics
Introduction

Looking at the history of linguistics during the second half of the twentieth century, a disinterested observer might wonder why one major part of the linguistics community were searching for ever more economical, but psycholinguistically unconvincing, ways to model a non-varying form of language that no-one speaks, while another major part was spending its time collecting as much variation in spoken language as it could and correlating this with non-linguistics factors. While this dichotomy is evident in phonology as well as syntax, it is less obvious in our field of phonetics, and specialism of clinical phonetics. Nevertheless, phonetic descriptions of typical speech often seem to suggest that variant realizations of phonological units are almost always constrained by phonological context and all other variation is "free," i.e. at the whim of the speaker. Within disordered speech research too, there has been a tendency to search for neat "phonological processes" whereby target sounds, when in error, are realized by a set of invariant substitutions.

Recently, the insights of variationist linguistics have been adapted and applied to phonetics as well. Some of the findings are at the level of fine phonetic details—for example, subtle changes in prosodic features to signal the approach to the end of a turn in conversation. Other findings are at the level of dialect or language differences—for example, differences in articulation that still produce auditorily identical sounds (as in English apical and bunched-r). These sociophonetic approaches have also been applied to disordered speech. Thus, the examination of fine phonetic detail uncovered the phenomenon of covert contrasts—that is, subtle articulatory differences when a client attempts two different, but similar, target sounds even though the auditory percepts of their realizations are the same (Gibbon & Lee, 2017). At a broader level, an understanding of the phonetic resources available to a language or dialect can help explain patterns of errored realizations (as, for example, Welsh-English bilingual children who have been noted to use [w] for target English /ɹ/, but [v] for target Welsh /r/; Ball, Müller & Munro, 2001). The study of fine phonetic detail, coupled with the ability to use narrow phonetic transcription, has illustrated quite how much variation there may be in some clients with inconsistent phonological disorders; for example, Müller, Ball and Rutter (2006) recorded 12 different realizations of target /t/ in the client being investigated.

The first three chapters in this part of the book explore clinical aspects of sociophonetics at these different levels, while the fourth illustrates computational approaches to analyzing phonetic data (both clinical and non-clinical). Barbara May Bernhardt and Joseph Stemberger's chapter covers, among other topics, the phonetic aspects of an international crosslinguistic project on children's speech development that the authors led. Thus, aspects of language, multilingualism, and dialect are central to this chapter. Robert Fox and Ewa Jacewicz's chapter on the other hand is more concerned with variation within the context of American English (though not solely so), and they explore phonetic variation as linked to regional, ethnic, and social factors, as well as to features of second language English. In the third chapter, Martin Ball, Orla Lowry and Lisa McInnis look in detail at the speech of a single client who displayed multiple realizations of target English /ɹ/. Their analysis showed that a variety of factors correlated with these realizations—primarily the formality of the speech event, but also position within the syllable and whether a singleton or in a cluster. Interestingly, the authors also include the point that therapy may have introduced a new, errored sound to the client's repertoire rather than resolving the problem.

The final chapter in this part, by Yu-Ying Chuang, Janice Fon, Ioannis Papakyritsis and Harald Baayen introduces generalized additive mixed models (GAMS) that is, computerized approaches to modelling phonetic data. The chapter starts with an illustration of how GAMS can analyze data from a study of syllable stress errors in the speech of Greek clients with dysarthria. The chapter also looks at other types of phonetic data (such as regional variation, response time testing, and prosodic characteristics over time) and, although these are not clinical data sets, the authors describe the clinical applications of the program in these areas.

Phonetic variation is central to the description and analysis of typical and disordered speech. The insights from the chapters in this part of the book can and should be applied to the various approaches to transcription and instrumentation described in the remaining chapters.

References

Ball, M. J., Müller, N. & Munro, S. (2001). The acquisition of the rhotic consonants by Welsh-English bilingual children. *International Journal of Bilingualism, 5,* 71–86.

Gibbon, F. & Lee, A. (2017). Preface to the special issue on covert contrasts. *Clinical Linguistics and Phonetics, 31,* 1–3.

Müller, N, Ball, M.J. & Rutter, B. (2006). A profiling approach to intelligibility problems. *Advances in Speech-Language Pathology, 8,* 176–189.

7

CLINICAL PHONETICS ACROSS LANGUAGES AND DIALECTS

Barbara M. Bernhardt and Joseph Paul Stemberger

This chapter addresses clinical phonetics in crosslinguistic, multilingual and dialectal contexts. The perspectives and data in the chapter are drawn primarily from an international crosslinguistic project on children's monolingual speech development (Bernhardt & Stemberger, 2017), but the observations pertain more broadly to other populations and multilingual/multidialectal environments. In clinical multilingual/multidialectal contexts, speech-language therapists (SLTs) often aim to determine whether a client's difficulties in speech production/perception stem from the complex language learning context (simultaneously learning two or more languages or dialectal variants) or from an underlying difficulty in the phonological/phonetic domain (Goldstein & Gildersleeve-Neumann, 2015). Until recently, SLTs often used only their own language(s) or dialect(s) in assessment and treatment, due to lack of knowledge and resources for addressing other languages or dialects. However, use of only one language or dialect makes it difficult to differentiate accent or dialect from developmental speech issues, because there is no direct evidence to confirm that the client's first language or dialect is relatively intact, or (in the developmental case) at age level (Hack, Marinova-Todd, & Bernhardt, 2012). The SLT might erroneously assume that the client has a general difficulty and initiate treatment that is neither needed (wasting resources and potentially leading to stigmatization; Ball & Bernhardt, 2008) nor specifically addresses accent or dialect, if such is the client's wish. Further, in the case of true difficulty, the SLT might assume that patterns observed in the SLT's language extend across all the client's languages. However, even if the same restrictions underlie both of a bilingual's phonological systems, differences between the languages and a client's relative proficiency in each can result in different outputs or complex interactions between the languages that are not observable in monolinguals (Stow & Dodd, 2003). The more the SLT can learn about a client's languages and general level of proficiency in each, the more informed the assessment and treatment approaches can be (Verdon, McLeod, & Wong, 2015).

Definitions, assumptions, and topics

By "clinical," we refer to characteristics of speech production and perception that are different enough from what is locally considered typical that assessment and, potentially, remediation may be required. By phonetics, we refer to articulatory and acoustic aspects of speech production and perception, noting that these aspects cannot easily be separated from what is called "phonology," which focuses on the long-term storage and (re)construction of pronunciation-related information during language processing. In adopting a non-modular perspective, we presuppose that motor, perceptual and cognitive systems are in constant interaction when a speaker or listener is actually "doing" language and speech, so that every level is influenced by every other level. We note too that language and speech are not fixed in childhood, but are in a continuous state of change across the lifespan of every individual as well as across generations, and that one source of change is contact with other dialects and other languages (including where the other language is a colonizer/settler language).

In light of those assumptions, the following chapter first addresses issues in variability that affect methodological considerations in data collection and evaluation. These considerations are a foundation for the subsequent overview of key developmental patterns concerning segments and word structure, where differences among languages or dialects can result in variable developmental profiles. The final section provides a brief perspective on treatment in bilingual/multilingual contexts.

Variability

For humans to understand each other, there must be some degree of consistency in speech production and perception. However, all human activities are subject to variability, including languages, which evolve over time. Further, variability is a prerequisite for development: systems must allow for variability so that change can happen. The SLT may be able to exploit variability in accelerating development, and in fact, some studies suggest that clients with a high degree of inconsistency may require a specific treatment approach to reduce variability (e.g. Dodd, Holm, Crosbie, & McIntosh, 2006). Thus, documentation of variability goes hand in hand with documentation of commonalities across observations. Although there are many sources of variability in speech production, we focus on three that are especially relevant for clinical phonetics: description of speech, context of speech production and acceptability.

Variability: Speech description

The primary system for describing speech sounds is the International Phonetic Alphabet (IPA, 1999), with its extension, the Extended IPA (Duckworth, Allen, Hardcastle, & Ball, 1990) (see Chapters 11–13 of this volume). Several websites (e.g. Esling, 2010; Isotalo, 2003) provide detailed audio/video examples to help users become conversant with speech sounds outside their own language(s). There are three cautionary notes for the crosslinguistic context. First, the IPA intentionally does not provide symbols for all the speech sounds that exist. Some speech sounds that are relatively uncommon across languages must be approximated by extending the use of a symbol or diacritic slightly beyond its usual interpretation. For example, there are no symbols for a uvular tap or approximant, and no diacritics that denote that something is a tap or approximant. However, using the shortening diacritic, a uvular tap can, by convention, be transcribed as a short uvular trill [ʀ̆]; similarly, using the diacritic for widening, a uvular approximant can be indicated as a uvular fricative with a widened constriction [ʁ̞]. Second, researchers may employ a particular symbol even if a more phonetically accurate alternative exists in the IPA. For example, for English dialects without trilled [r], the Latin letter "r" may be used to denote the English approximant [ɹ]. Similarly, the Spanish "ch" (as in the word *chili*) is transcribed as if it were a palatoalveolar [t͡ʃ] (to make it look comfortably like the "ch" affricate in English and many other languages), even though it is in fact an alveolopalatal [t͡ɕ] (Kochetov & Colantoni, 2011). Third, the IPA symbols and diacritics define "standard" consonants and vowels with the recognition that boundaries between particular vowels or consonants may differ across languages. For example, in a given language the tongue position for the vowel [i] might be slightly lower and more central than in another language, or the consonant [k] might be slightly more fronted or backed than in another language. A consonant or vowel that lies somewhere between the "perfect" IPA categories might be perceived as, e.g. [i] in one language but [e] in another. Different location of boundaries can lead to non-native perception that two IPA categories are involved with a particular speech sound whereas native-speaker perception might treat it as one. For example, Slovenian /v/ is described as the fricative [v] in the onset of a syllable (especially in word-initial syllables) but as the approximant [ʋ] before consonants in words such as *vlak* "train" (e.g. Toporišič, 2004). Srebot-Rejec (1973), however, suggests that the [v] in syllable onsets is a weakly articulated fricative that is just one end of a continuum from (weak) fricative to approximant, and that all tokens should be considered to be instances of the approximant /ʋ/. This also illustrates the fact that the cues for a particular speech sound may not be identical across all languages.

Instrumental analysis may be used to supplement phonetic transcription (e.g. acoustic or articulatory such as ultrasound, electropalatography) and can show further variation across speakers, languages and dialects for what appear to be the same IPA segments. For example, vowels with the same IPA symbol have different formant regions in different languages and speakers. Within a language, perceptual "normalization" allows the listener to identify varying formant patterns as the same vowel across speakers (Miller, Engebretson, & Vemula, 1980). Across languages, perception tends to be biased early on by the first language(s) (Werker, Gilbert, Humphrey, & Tees, 1981) with the consequence that certain contrasts between very similar speech sounds may either be missed for another language or ascribed to a single category within one's own language (Bohn & Flege, 1990). For consonants, one divergence between IPA use and acoustics concerns stop voicing. In postpausal position, prevoiced word-initial stops [b, d, g] in French and Spanish contrast with short-lag unaspirated stops [p, t, k], whereas in English, short-lag "voiced" stops [b̥, d̥, g̊] contrast with long-lag aspirated stops [pʰ, tʰ, kʰ]; however, these differences between languages are often not reflected in phonetic transcriptions, where the English and French "voiced" stops are both broadly transcribed with the symbols [b, d, g], and the French unaspirated and English aspirated voiceless stops are transcribed broadly with plain [p, t, k]. (Further, in English, /b, d, g/ additionally vary in VOT across phonological/ phonetic contexts; they are usually short-lag [b̥, d̥, g̊] postpausally but prevoiced [b, d, g] between vowels, e.g. in *Dogs!* vs. *The dog!*) Within a monolingual context, the details of VOT may be relevant or not, depending on the goal of analysis. However, in crosslinguistic or multilingual comparisons, adjusting the IPA conventions to take such acoustic details into account will enhance the validity of the comparisons.

Beyond the segment

Description of characteristics such as stress, tone and segment length can be particularly challenging. They are inherently more relative than consonants and vowels, leading to considerable crosslinguistic variation in their production and description. In many languages, such as English (e.g. Ladefoged & Johnson, 2014), a stressed syllable is louder, longer and of higher pitch than an equivalent unstressed syllable (though not every token shows a contrast along all three dimensions). However, in Valley Zapotec (Chávez-Peón, 2010), where stressed syllables also contrast for high versus low tone, stressed syllables differ from unstressed only by being louder and longer. In French, stressed syllables are longer than unstressed but do not differ in pitch or loudness (e.g. Frost, 2011). A transcriber whose native language uses a set of cues for stress which differs from that of the language being transcribed will not necessarily perceive stress in the same way as native speakers of that language.

Tonal systems can range from a simple system of level high versus low tone, or can additionally have level mid tones and contour tones of various sorts (IPA, 1999). Although the IPA describes tones as involving differences only in pitch, there can be other differences (such as in duration, intensity or glottalization) across languages. Native speakers are sensitive to these additional differences (e.g. Whalen & Levitt, 1995) and can use them as cues to tones when pitch is artificially neutralized; a non-native speaker may not be aware of these subsidiary cues and consequently transcribe the tones only based on pitch. Stress and tone make use of general properties (since all vowels have a pitch and some degree of loudness and duration) that differ in their exact definition across people and contexts. For example, the raw pitch of tones shifts relative to the inherent pitch of the speaker's voice, something that is particularly evident comparing children's and most adult women's tonal pitches versus those of adult men. Even within the same voice, pitch for stress and tone may vary by context, i.e. when speaking quietly vs. loudly, or when superimposing sentential prosody that raises sentence-final pitch in questions but lowers it in statements. There are no universal values for what constitutes "high" versus "low" tone. In addition, boundaries can shift for a number of reasons, such as whether both possible values of a contrast make a real word (e.g. as in *big* vs. *dig*, but **bish* vs. *dish* or *built* vs. **dilt*); when only one value makes a possible word, listeners shift their boundaries to be accepting of tokens that would otherwise be intermediate between two sounds (so that the same acoustics that lead to perception of /b/ in *big* may be perceived as /d/ in *dish*). Similarly, an intermediate pitch value may potentially be perceived as high tone if low tone would create a non-word, or as low tone if high tone would create a non-word; such information is generally only available to a native speaker as an automatic characteristic of perception. By extension to child language, it also means that less-than-perfect child tokens may (legitimately) be perceived differently by adult speakers both within and across languages.

In terms of segment length, some languages contrast long versus short consonants, or long versus short vowels, while other languages have no such contrasts. In the latter case, consonants and vowels are usually described only as short. However, "short" consonants or vowels in a language without a length contrast are not necessarily as short as short consonants or vowels in a language with such a contrast. Further, the boundary between "long" versus "short" is not consistent across languages, leading to possible inconsistency of transcription by transcribers with different native languages. The situation is not helped by the fact that differences in the length of consonants or vowels can be confounded with other features or with different contexts. In English, for example, the vowel in the word *bit* is short [ɪ], while the vowel in *beat* is long [iː]; there is a difference in length that co-occurs with a difference in vowel quality. This confounding of vowel quality and length has led to a commonly used convention of transcribing only the vowel quality and not the length in English: [bɪt] versus [biːt]. Viewed from a crosslinguistic perspective, it adds to the variability of interpreting transcriptions. In Swedish, there is a complementarity to vowel and consonant length in stressed syllables: if the vowel is short then the following consonant is long, but if the vowel is long then the following consonant is short. After a long debate on the subject, it was concluded that consonant length is 100% predictable from vowel length, whereas vowel length is not predictable from consonant length in a small percentage of contexts. Current procedure is to transcribe only the vowel length and not the consonant length leading to transcriptions such as *katten* "the cat" as [kʰatɛn], possibly surprising a non-native speaker who can hear the long [tː] in this word. English does not have a consonantal length contrast, but English-learning children may produce long consonants when reducing consonant clusters, e.g. *monkey* /mʌŋki/ as [mʌkːi]; but English speakers tend to ignore consonant length as irrelevant, and so such tokens are most often transcribed as short ([mʌki]), leading to possible transcription differences by native speakers of English versus native speakers of Italian, which has a consonant length contrast.

Addressing variability in description

In our crosslinguistic project, we have found it important to learn the language-specific conventions for IPA use for each language; together with the international partners, we have created a transcription conventions document for each language that reflects the key characteristics of the language but still allows for comparability across languages (Stemberger & Bernhardt, 2019). Acoustic analysis has been key for resolving conventional differences in use of the IPA. Videos on our crosslinguistic website provide guidelines and practice in transcription across languages (phonodevelopment.sites.olt.ubc.ca/Phonology). Using those videos and other websites for IPA training such as those noted above will enhance intra-observer reliability for transcription across languages.

Variability: Context

A second issue regarding variability concerns context: most speech sounds rarely occur on their own (exceptions being monosyllabic words containing only a vowel, e.g. French *eau* "water" [o] or "words" such as *shhh* [ʃː]). Most often, speech sounds are combined into syllables, words and sentences. A number of contextual factors can affect the phonetic realization of a speech sound, e.g. syllable/word position, surrounding segments, elicitation context (single word/phrase, morphological form) or rate/style of speech (casual/formal, discussed further in the next section). In speakers with inherent speech difficulties, a segment may be possible in only certain word positions, elicitation contexts, or morphological forms or sequences, e.g. [z] may be possible only in single words with monomorphemic codas (e.g. in "buzz" but not in "bees" or "a big zoo"). Segments in weaker prosodic positions, i.e. unstressed syllables, codas, clusters/diphthongs, often have lower amplitude and shorter duration than the same segment in strong prosodic positions, i.e. stressed syllables, onsets, singletons (Giles & Moll, 1975; Klatt, 1973); in early development and for speakers with inherent speech difficulty, such targets may show a higher proportion of mismatches than segments in strong prosodic positions (Bernhardt & Stemberger, 1998). Further, amplitude differences may affect the listener's perception; because shorter and quieter elements are less audible, they may be missed in noisy situations or recordings. Finally, rate or style of speech may facilitate or inhibit production of a particular speech sound. Charles (Chapter 8, Bernhardt & Stemberger, 2000) usually matched the target stop in word-initial liquid clusters when the word was uttered slowly (with or without an epenthetic vowel separating the consonant and glide) as in [ˈkeɪwʌ̃n]/[kəwejɔ̃n] for /ˈkɹeɪjæn/ 'crayon'. However, in rapid speech, the stop showed labial and continuant assimilation, e.g. [ˈfweɪjɔ̃n]. For both researchers and SLTs, it is important to elicit each segment in a variety of contexts. Further, it is important to ensure sufficient signal-to-noise ratio to hear the lower-intensity phones which tend to occur in weak prosodic positions.

Variability: Acceptability

A third challenge concerning variability is knowing whether an individual's production of a given speech sound/word falls in the acceptable range of variation for that speech sound/word in typical adult speech production. Depending on the language and region, there may be a wide or narrow set of alternative pronunciations. Slovenia, for example, has only 2 million people yet has 40+ sub-dialects in seven main dialectal regions (Greenberg, 2000). This compares with relatively fewer regional differences over the 21+ million native speakers of Canadian English over a huge land mass. Dialects of one language may vary considerably; for example, in Andalusian Spanish, codas are optional, /l/ and /r/ may interchange in certain words, coronal voiceless fricatives can be interdental or alveolar, medial consonant sequences such as /rt/ may be produced as geminate [tt], etc. Other languages or dialects may have less variation overall but still show reduction/deletion of vowels and weakening or dropping of medial or coda consonants in running speech (see *Journal of Phonetics*, *39*[3] for a set of papers on reduced pronunciations in casual speech in French, English, Dutch and German). Because speakers are more likely to use informal pronunciations in spontaneous conversational samples (Tucker & Ernestus, 2016), determining the range of variation will necessarily include collection of at least some conversational speech. More formal elicited data (such as single word speech sampling) can ensure coverage of the phonology of a language and make phonetic transcription easier because target words are known in advance. In clinical contexts, single-word tools have proven useful and reliable across languages (e.g. Masterson, Bernhardt, & Hofheinz, 2005), but are not necessarily representative of a speaker's casual everyday speech. Having both types of data can demonstrate the range of variation for speech targets, and, in comparison to similar data from adults of the area, help determine the level of acceptability of various pronunciations. If resources prohibit such data collection, family or community members or the research participant/ speech therapy client may be able to indicate whether the pronunciations of the participant/client fall within or outside the acceptable range of production for that community.

Variability: Summary

In summary, in order to evaluate speech data, one needs to know what is acceptable in a given language/dialect, and how the speech production of a client or research participant falls within that spectrum of variation across a range of contexts. For transcriptions, it is important to clarify how the symbols and diacritics of the IPA are being used to classify speech sounds, and whether and how acoustic or visual information has assisted the transcription. If a project or clinical assessment does not meet all of these methodological aims, limitations need to be stated in presentation of results.

We turn now to additional considerations concerning segments and word structure in the crosslinguistic context. The examples demonstrate the need for the researcher and SLT to learn as much as possible about: (a) the phonetic and word structure inventories of the child's language(s), and for the acquisitionist, (b) developmental timelines and patterns of acquisition across languages in both monolingual and bilingual/multilingual contexts.

Segments

Substitutions and the whole IPA

If a monolingual child used only the speech sounds in his or her language, the researcher or SLT might only need to learn the sections of the IPA relevant to that one language. But substitutions can arise that are not in the ambient language, e.g. palatal or lateral fricatives in a language like English that has none (Chapter 8, Bernhardt & Stemberger, 1998), or an English-type [ɹ] in a language with a trilled /r/ target (Pérez et al., 2018). Further, a bilingual/multilingual needs to acquire phones outside the researcher's/SLT's language, including phonetic variants of what are labeled as the same phones, as noted above for the English and Spanish affricate "ch." Learning the whole IPA allows the researcher or SLT: (1) to transcribe any segment with some degree of reliability, whether for a monolingual or bilingual; and (2) to determine the degree of interdependence of a bilingual/multilingual's segmental inventories. We return to a discussion of interdependence/independence of bilingual systems later in the chapter.

Segments: Developmental rate and mismatch patterns across languages

The types and frequencies of segments across languages can affect relative rate of acquisition and mismatch patterns, with phonetic complexity playing a notable but not exclusive role. Across languages, less articulatorily complex stops, nasals and glides are generally earlier-acquired than more complex fricatives/affricates and liquids, with the less complex segments often substituting for the more complex. However, crosslinguistic differences in frequency or phonetic details of particular targets can affect developmental timelines. For example, Pye, Ingram, and List (1987) observed earlier acquisition of the frequent affricate /tʃ/ in Quiché Mayan than in English. They attribute the earlier acquisition of the affricate in Quiché to its greater importance in the phonological system of Quiché Mayan than of English.

Differences in phonetic inventories of languages can also lead to different timelines for acquisition or type and frequency of mismatch patterns. Recent studies of one manner category, fricatives, in monolingual children with PPD in English, German, Icelandic and Bulgarian showed similarities reflecting articulatory complexity, but differences in mismatch patterns reflecting the inventories of the languages (Bernhardt et al., 2019; Bernhardt, Romonath, & Stemberger, 2014; Bernhardt, Másdóttir, Stemberger, Leonhardt, & Hansson, 2015). For example, the visible and articulatorily simple labiodental /f/ was in advance of other fricatives in all languages but Icelandic (for which /s/ was more advanced), whereas the lingual fricatives, especially /ʃ/, were generally less advanced (the Icelandic /s/ being an exception). Compared with the other groups, German children also showed a higher level of mastery for /v/, possibly because /v/ is a more frequent word-initial fricative in that language. Substitutions for fricatives were varied and included many of the same speech sounds across languages. However, frequency of substitution types to some extent mirrored the frequency of that phone in the language, i.e. more palatal fricatives and [ts] in German (segments occurring in the inventory), and more [h] substitutions in Icelandic (with its high proportion of [+spread glottis] consonants). One unexpected pattern was the frequent use of [θ] for /f/ in Icelandic (for which the /f/ was later-acquired than in the other languages), the opposite generally being true for English.

In terms of major places of articulation, labial place is often early-acquired across languages (Bernhardt & Stemberger, 1998), presumably because labiality is easy to observe visually, but this may depend on the manner category (as noted for Icelandic /f/ above). Across languages, dorsals and coronals vary in their rate of acquisition and direction of mismatches. In English, dorsal stops and nasals (velars) are often later-acquired than coronal stops and nasals, with "velar fronting" a common pattern (Bernhardt & Stemberger, 1998). Some languages with a higher proportion of dorsals (which may include fricatives) are reported to have a higher proportion of coronals appearing as dorsals (e.g. Japanese: Beckman, Yoneyama, & Edwards, 2003; Mandarin: Hua, 2006). Thus, frequency can affect direction of mismatch patterns for place categories that may substitute for one another.

Certain segments have more than one place of articulation, requiring complex coordination of articulators. The late-acquired English rhotic requires complex coupling of [Coronal] and [Dorsal] place and (at least word-initially) also [Labial] (Bernhardt & Stemberger, 1998). The /l/ shows different rates of acquisition depending on its complexity: "l" may be alveolar only ('light' /l/) or velarized at least in some word position. The simply alveolar lateral is often earlier-acquired than the velarized lateral of English and European Portuguese (e.g. Bernhardt & Stemberger,; Pye et al., 1987; Ramalho & Freitas, 2018). Other segments with secondary places of articulations show different trajectories of acquisition than their plain counterparts. In Arabic, the so-called "emphatics" (uvularized consonants) show later acquisition than their plain cognates (Ayyad, Bernhardt, & Stemberger, 2016), and in a typically developing Russian-English 3-year-old bilingual, fronting of the secondary velarization ("hard" consonants) was observed (Smatanova, 2002). In contrast, palatalized ("soft") consonants in Russian appear early and often substitute for other consonants (Zharkova, 2002). This is unlikely to be a frequency effect; Smirnova and Chistikov (2011) report token frequencies for the top 40 phonemes in Russian, and the velarized consonants are more frequent than the corresponding palatalized consonant in 14 out of 15 instances, with the only reversal being /lʲ/ in 17th place versus /l/ in 18th (though type frequency is a better predictor than token frequency). It is perhaps due to the finding that children may have a higher and more forward tongue-body position than adults (Gibbon, 1999) leading to a lack of velars and to the perception of a partial constriction in the palatal area.

The examples above demonstrate that there are crosslinguistic tendencies in phonetic/phonological acquisition reflecting complexity of articulatory form. However, there are also differences reflecting a phoneme's relative importance in the phonological system and its specific phonetic composition/realization. Knowing about these potential differences informs interpretation and analysis of individual phonological/phonetic profiles.

In the bilingual/multilingual case, if a child's phonological systems are more independent than interdependent, phonetic inventories and substitution patterns will reflect the specific languages with monolingual patterns such as those described above, and with minimal transfer or interference between the languages. If a child's two or more languages share a phonological system at least partially: (a) the phonetic inventories will be very similar (or even identical); (b) similar substitution patterns may appear in the two or more languages for similar segments; and/or (c) substitutions from the phonetic inventory of one language may appear in another. In the latter case, it may be difficult to distinguish mismatches that are borrowed across a bilingual's languages versus developmental mismatches within one language. For example, in a language such as English, flat (ungrooved) alveolopalatals with a high tongue body such as [ç], [ʐ], [t͡ɕ] or [d͡ʑ] are considered mismatches for the grooved (strident) sibilant fricatives and affricates /s, z, ʃ, ʒ, t͡ʃ, d͡ʒ/, and can be of clinical relevance if they are still present in 4-year-old children. However, some languages have alveolopalatals as phonemes (e.g. Mandarin, Japanese, Akan). These contrast with the grooved sibilants in those languages, but their presence in those languages potentially provides a source of substitutions for Mandarin, Japanese, and Akan monolingual children, and also for the other languages of children bilingual with English or other languages that lack alveolopalatals. Similarly, as noted above, in languages with the trilled /r/, young children can use the mismatch [ɹ]; this may be especially likely for children who are bilingual in English (e.g. Ball, Müller, & Munro, 2001).

Other aspects of speech production may be relevant in a bilingual context pertaining to specific conditions such as cleft palate or voice disorders. English-speaking children with cleft palates frequently use glottal, pharyngeal, and uvular substitutions for oral places of articulation (e.g. McWilliams, Morris, & Shelton, 1990) and such substitutions are often taken as an indication that there is a cleft palate; given that such "guttural" consonants are phonemes in languages such as Arabic, it is in principle possible that Arabic–English bilingual children might use them as mismatches even in their English, with or without a cleft palate. Children with voice disorders often use breathy and creaky voice in place of modal voice quality for vowels; languages such as Valley Zapotec (e.g. Chávez-Péon, 2010) have a phonemic contrast between modal (/a/), breathy (/a̰/) and creaky (/a̰/) vowels, Young Valley-Zapotec-speaking children bilingual with Spanish or English might in principle use breathy or creaky vowels in mismatches, generalized from Zapotec; there may be no voice disorder, but rather an over-generalized use of breathy or creaky voice. It would be important to disambiguate these differences in such cases.

Word structure

Word structure similarities and differences can also be observed across languages for development. Some languages have relatively simple word structure (minimal weaker contexts, i.e. unstressed syllables, codas, clusters, e.g. Mandarin, Japanese). Other languages have options for reducing structural complexity, e.g. Andalusian Spanish has optional codas; epenthesis is acceptable in clusters in Arabic (Ayyad, 2011). In the Granada Spanish corpus for our crosslinguistic project, 5-year-olds used a higher proportion of coda than the 3- and 4-year-olds in the sample, thus moving toward more complex structure after exposure to kindergarten and an introduction to reading. The Arabic children in Ayyad (2011) showed minimal use of word-initial clusters, with epenthesis allowing production of the segments. Coda deletion and cluster reduction were not mismatch patterns but extension of acceptable variants in the adult system (at a higher proportion than used by most adults in the community). These patterns underline the importance of learning about the adult range of variability for acceptable word structure in dialects/languages.

Another effect of simpler word structure for Granada Spanish and Mandarin concerns Whole Word Match (WWM, where the whole word must match the adult target). The Mandarin- and Granada Spanish-learning 4-year-olds with protracted phonological development (PPD) in Bernhardt and Stemberger (2017) had WWM scores in the range of 41%-39%, respectively, compared with scores of 11%–25% for languages with more complex structure: Icelandic, English, German and French (increasing order) (see also Bernhardt et al., 2020). Further replication of this potential trend is necessary.

Other differences concerning word structure concern coda use and multisyllabic words. The German cohort with PPD in the crosslinguistic study had a relatively higher use of codas than the English-speaking cohort, even though codas are equally important and relatively frequent in both languages (Major & Bernhardt, 1998; Romonath & Bernhardt, 2017). This might have a perceptual basis in that German requires glottal stop onsets to vowel-initial words, making word boundaries perhaps more salient to German-learning children than to English children, where glottal stops occur as onsets only after pauses. Finally, languages with higher proportion of di- and multisyllabic words than English (e.g. Spanish) showed earlier mastery of word length in spite of the complexity involved in production of multiple segmental sequences (Bernhardt, Hanson et al., 2015; Mason, 2018).

Developmental patterns for word structure, like those for segments, indicate crosslinguistic tendencies but also differences based on relative complexity of a language's word structure. Again, the importance of knowing about the word structure and its variants is important for a given language/dialect. A bilingual child may show reduced structure in the more complex of the two languages, or increased complexity of structure in the simpler language, depending on the relative dominance of the two languages and their independence/interdependence.

Treatment in the bilingual/multilingual context

For both segments and word structure, it is important for the SLT to try to determine whether a bilingual child's patterns are the same in both languages (i.e. there is less variability between the languages), or whether the problem is one of second language learning. If there are similar challenges in both languages, treatment effects may potentially transcend the language barrier (Holm & Dodd, 2001; Ray, 2002). If the two languages are more independent (and the more divergent the phonologies, the more likely this is), transfer to the untreated language or at least the parts of the phonological systems that do not overlap may be less likely. Some treatment reports have indicated faster change in the child's first language if treatment is provided in both (Gildersleeve-Neumann & Goldstein, 2015; Ramos & Mead, 2014). While therapy in the non-native language for the SLT might not be wholly possible, Rossouw and Pascoe (2018) chose a successful strategy of providing instruction in English and treatment stimuli in isiXhosa, the child's dominant language.

Conclusion

This chapter has addressed aspects of clinical phonetics in the crosslinguistic context. The value of learning about the phonology/phonetics of languages/dialects encountered and their range of variability is evident. Variability is a key feature for consideration, whether concerning acceptable variants of speech production in a community, description of speech phenomena, or developmental patterns for segments and word structure of languages across contexts. Crosslinguistic/multilingual research studies, although still sparse, are becoming more frequent in the literature. Furthermore, researchers and SLTs can now learn more about phonetics/phonology of different languages through various websites. The future of clinical phonetics will be necessarily global as patterns of migration result in increasing diversity across the world.

References

Ayyad, H.S. (2011). *Phonological development of typically developing Kuwaiti Arabic-speaking preschoolers*. Unpublished PhD dissertation, University of British Columbia.

Ayyad, H.S., Bernhardt, B.M., & Stemberger, J.P. (2016). Kuwaiti Arabic. Acquisition of singleton consonants. *International Journal of Language and Communication Disorders*, 51(5), 531–545.

Ball, J. & Bernhardt, B.M. (2008). First Nations English dialects in Canada: Implications for speech-language pathology. *Clinical Linguistics and Phonetics*, 22(8), 570–588.

Ball, M., Müller, N., & Munro, S. (2001). The acquisition of the rhotic consonants by Welsh-English bilingual children. *International Journal of Bilingualism*, 5(1), 71–86.

Bernhardt, B.M., Hanson, R., Pérez, D., Ávila, C., Lleó, C., Stemberger, J.P., Carballo, G., Mendoza, E., Fresneda, D., & Chávez-Peón, M. (2015). Word structures of Granada Spanish-speaking preschoolers with typical versus protracted phonological development. *International Journal of Language & Communication Disorders*, 50(3), 298–311. doi: 10.1111/1460-6984.12133.

Bernhardt, B.M., Ignatova, D., Amoako, W., Aspinall, N., Marinova-Todd, S., Stemberger J.P., & Yokota, K. (2019). Bulgarian consonant acquisition in children with typical versus protracted phonological development. *Journal of Monolingual and Bilingual Speech*, 1(2), 143–181.

Bernhardt, B.M., Másdóttir, T., Stemberger, J.P., Leonhardt, L., & Hansson, G.O. (2015). Fricative development in Icelandic and English-speaking children with protracted phonological development. *Clinical Linguistics and Phonetics*, 29(8-10), 642–665.

Bernhardt, B.M., Romonath, R., & Stemberger, J.P. (2014). A comparison of fricative acquisition in German and Canadian English-speaking children with protracted phonological development. In M. Yavaş (Ed.), *Unusual productions in phonology: Universals and language-specific considerations* (pp. 102–127). New York, NY: Psychology Press.

Bernhardt, B.H. & Stemberger, J.P. (2000). *Workbook in nonlinear phonology for clinical application*. Copyright reverted to authors. Available at http://phonodevelopment.sites.olt.ubc.ca under Test Materials/English.

Bernhardt, B.M. & Stemberger, J.P. (2017). Investigating typical and protracted phonological development across languages. In E. Babatsouli, D. Ingram & N. Müller (Eds.) *Crosslinguistic encounters in language acquisition: Typical and atypical development* (pp. 71–108). Bristol, UK: Multilingual Matters.

Bernhardt, B.M., Stemberger, J.P., Bérubé, D., Ciocca, V., Freitas, M.-J., Ignatova, D., Kogošek, D. LundeborgHammarström, I., Másdóttir, T., Ozbič, M., Pérez, D., & Ramalho, A.M., (2020). Identification of protracted phonological development across languages – the Whole Word Match and basic mismatch measures. In E. Babatsouli & M. Ball (Eds.) *An anthology of bilingual child phonology* (pp. 274–308). Bristol, UK: Multilingual Matters. doi.org/10.21832/BABATS8410

Bernhardt, B.M.H. & Stemberger, J.P. (1998). *Handbook of phonological development: From a nonlinear constraints-based perspective*. San Diego, CA: Academic Press.

Bohn, O.-S. & Flege, J.E. (1990). Interlingual identification and the role of foreign language experience in L2 vowel perception. *Applied Psycholinguistics, 11*(3), 303–328.

Chávez-Peón, M.E. (2010). *The interaction of metrical structure, tone and phonation types in Quiaviní Zapotec*. PhD dissertation, University of British Columbia.

Dodd, B., Holm, A., Crosbie, S., & McIntosh, B. (2006). A core vocabulary approach for management of inconsistent speech disorder. *Advances in Speech–Language Pathology, 8*(3), 220–230.

Duckworth, M., Allen, G., Hardcastle, W., & Ball, M. (1990). Extensions to the International Phonetic Alphabet for the transcription of atypical speech. *Clinical Linguistics and Phonetics, 4*, 273–280.

Esling, J. (2010). *IPA Charts [Internet]*; University of Victoria Canada, Department of Linguistics. Available from: http://web.uvic.ca/ling/resources/ipa/charts/IPAlab/.

Frost, D. (2011). Stress and cues to relative prominence in English and French: A perceptual study. *Journal of the International Phonetic Association, 41*(1), 67–84.

Gibbon, F.E. (1999). Undifferentiated lingual gestures in children with articulation/phonological disorders. *Journal of Speech, Language and Hearing Research, 42*(2), 382–97.

Gildersleeve-Neumann C., & Goldstein B. (2015). Crosslinguistic generalization in the treatment of two sequential Spanish–English bilingual children with speech sound disorders. *International Journal of Speech–Language Pathology, 17*(1), 26–40.

Giles, S.B. & Moll, K.L. (1975). Cinefluorographic study of selected allophones of English /l/. *Phonetica, 31*, 206–227.

Goldstein, B.A., & Gildersleeve-Neumann, C.E. (2015). Bilingualism and speech sound disorders. *Current Development and Disorders Reports, 2*, 237–244. https://doi.org/10.1007/s40474-015-0049-3.

Greenberg, M.L. (2000). *A historical phonology of the Slovene language*. Heidelberg, Germany: Universitätsverlag Carl Winter.

Hack, J.H., Marinova-Todd, S.H., & Bernhardt, B.M. (2012). Speech assessment of Chinese-English bilingual children: Accent versus developmental level. *International Journal of Speech-Language Pathology, 14*(6), 509–519.

Holm A. & Dodd B. (2001). Comparison of cross-language generalization following speech therapy. *Folia Phoniatrica et Logopaedica, 53*(3), 166–172. https://doi.org/10.1159/000052671.

International Phonetic Association. (1999). *Handbook of the International Phonetic Association: A guide to the use of the International Phonetic Alphabet*. Cambridge, UK: Cambridge University Press.

Isotalo, P. (2003). *Interactive IPA charts [Internet]*. University of California at Los Angeles USA, Phonetics Lab Archive. Available from: www.ipachart.com.

Klatt, D. (1973). Durational characteristics of word-initial consonant clusters in English. *Journal of The Acoustical Society of America, 53*, 379. doi: 10.1121/1.1982695.

Kochetov, A. & Colantoni, L. (2011). Coronal place contrasts in Argentine and Cuban Spanish: An electropalatographic study. *Journal of the International Phonetic Association, 41*, 313–342.

Ladefoged, P. & Johnson, K. (2014). *A course in phonetics* (7th ed.). Stamford, CT: Cengage.

Major, E. & Bernhardt, B. (1998). Metaphonological skills of children with phonological disorders before and after phonological and metaphonological intervention. *International Journal of Language and Communication Disorders, 33*, 413–444.

Mason, G. (2018). School-aged children's phonological accuracy in multisyllabic words on a whole word metric. *Journal of Speech, Language, and Hearing Research, 61*(12), 2869–2883.

Masterson, J., Bernhardt, B., & Hofheinz, M. (2005). A comparison of single words and conversational speech in phonological evaluation. *American Journal of Speech-Language Pathology, 14*(3), 229–241.

McWilliams, B., Morris, H., & Shelton, R. (1990). *Cleft palate speech*. Philadelphia, PA: Decker.

Miller, J.D., Engebretson, A.M., & Vemula, N.R. (1980). Vowel normalization: Differences between vowels spoken by children, women and men. *The Journal of the Acoustical Society of America, 68*, S33.

Pérez, D., Vivar, P., Bernhardt, B.M., Mendoza, E., Ávila, C., Carballo, G., Fresneda, D., Muñoz, J., & Vergara, P. (2018). Word-initial rhotic clusters in Spanish-speaking preschoolers in Chile and Granada, Spain. *Clinical Linguistics and Phonetics, 32*(5-6), 481–505. doi: 10.1080/02699206.2017.1359852 *phonodevelopment.sites.olt.ubc.ca.* Retrieved April 20, 2020.

Pye, C., Ingram, D., & List, H. (1987). A comparison of initial consonant acquisition in English and Quiché. In K. Nelson and A. van Kleeck (Eds.), *Children's Language, (Vol. 6,* pp. 175–190). Hillsdale, NJ: Erlbaum.

Ramalho A.M. & Freitas, M.-J. (2018). Word-initial rhotic clusters in typically developing children: European Portuguese. *Clinical Linguistics and Phonetics, 32*(5-6), 459–480.

Ramos E. & Mead, J. (2014). Dual language intervention in a case of severe speech sound disorder. *Revista de Investigacion En Logopedia, 4*(2), 93–111.

Ray J. (2002). Treating phonological disorders in a multilingual child: A case study. *American Journal of Speech-Language Pathology, 11*(3), 305–315.

Romonath, R. & Bernhardt, B.M. (2017). Erwerb prosodischer Wortstrukturen bei Vorschulkindern mit und ohne phonologische Störungen [Prosodic word structure acquisition in preschool children with and without phonological disorders]. *Forschung Sprache,* 1, 91–107.

Rossouw, K. & Pascoe, M. (2018, published online). Intervention for bilingual speech sound disorders: A case study of an isiXhosa-English-speaking child. *South African Journal of Communication Disorders, 65*(1), 566. doi: 10.4102/sajcd.v65i1.566

Smatanova, D. (2002). *A phonological analysis of a typically developing Russian-English bilingual 3-year-old. Unpublished MSc graduating paper,* School of Audiology and Speech Sciences, University of British Columbia.

Smirnova, N. & Chistikov, R. (2011). Statistics of Russian monophones and diphones. Paper presented at the 14th International Conference on Speech and Computer, Kazan, Russia.

Srebot-Rejec, T. (1973). Poskus kontrastivne analize slovenskega fonema /v/ z angleškim fonemom /v/ [Study of a contrastive analysis of the Slovene phoneme /v/ with the English phoneme /v/]. *Jezik in slovstvo, 19*(3), 89–93.

Stemberger, J.P. & Bernhardt, B.M. (2019). Transcription for speech-language pathology in the 21st century. *Folia Phoniatrica, 72,* 75–83. doi: 10.1159/000500701

Stow, C. & Dodd, B. (2003). Providing an equitable service to bilingual children in the UK: A review. *International Journal of Language and Communication Disorders, 38*(4), 351–377.

Toporišič, J. (2004). *Slovenska slovnica [Slovenian Grammar]* (4th ed.). Maribor: Založba Obzorja.

Tucker, B.V. & Ernestus, M. (2016). Why we need to investigate casual speech to truly understand language production, processing and the mental lexicon. *Mental Lexicon, 11*(3), 375–400.

Verdon, S., McLeod, S., & Wong, S. (2015). Reconceptualizing practice with multilingual children with speech sound disorders: People, practicalities and policy. *International Journal of Language and Communication Disorders, 50*(1), 48–62. https://doi.org/10.1111/1460-6984.12112.

Whalen, D.H. & Levitt, A.G. (1995). The universality of intrinsic F0 of vowels. *Journal of Phonetics, 23,* 349–366.

Werker, J.F., Gilbert, J.H.V., Humphrey, K., & Tees, R.C. (1981). Developmental aspects of cross-language speech perception. *Child Development, 52*(1), 349–355.

Zharkova, N. (2002). *Acquisition of the phonological system in child language: Experimental phonetic research.* Unpublished MA thesis, Department of Phonetics, State University of St. Petersburg, Russia.

8

CULTURAL AND MULTILINGUAL SOURCES OF PHONETIC VARIATION

Implications for clinical practice

Robert Allen Fox and Ewa Jacewicz

Introduction

Phonetic qualities of segments, vowels and consonants, vary greatly not only from speaker to speaker, language to language, social group to social group, but also geographically from region to region. Phonetic variation is omnipresent in daily interactions and its complexity has important consequences for clinical assessment and intervention. As demographics of world population change and global mobility creates new linguistic phonetic contact situations not only across parts of the English-speaking world but also across languages and dialects worldwide, clinical practice faces challenges as never before. We direct this chapter largely to practicing and aspiring clinicians with the aim to increase their awareness of such phonetic variation. We focus here on issues concerning American English (AE) spoken in the United States, but the specific examples discussed in this chapter are relevant to clinical work in the global multicultural speech community as a whole.

Clinicians in the United States who are completing appropriate, valid and ethical assessments of articulation and phonological disorders are faced with very significant variations in the speech patterns in different regions of the country (*regional dialects,* also termed *regional varieties*), different socio-cultural groups (*ethnolects*) and in non-native productions (*bilingual* and *foreign-accented* variations). These are the types of variations that clinicians should be cognizant of during clinical assessments, with the goal to appropriately and correctly differentiate speech-language *differences* from speech-language *disorders*.

The regional diversification of AE is of immediate relevance to clinicians providing speech-language services to speakers with distinct pronunciation patterns, which has important implications for clinical evaluation, diagnosis and treatment. Today, it is not uncommon for speech-language pathologists (SLPs) to seek employment in school districts or medical facilities across the United States, as the profession offers abundance of job opportunities and variety of experiences. Dialect contact is thus a realistic expectation in clinical work, and dialect awareness can have a profound impact on the success of clinical practice.

The need to recognize differences between speech delays/disorders and ethnicity-based norms (ethnolects) such as in African American English (AAE) also becomes pivotal in clinical assessment and intervention, and informed decisions are crucial in establishing an effective intervention plan for patients from different ethnic backgrounds. Guidelines and milestones for

African American speakers, especially for children in classrooms where instruction is in mainstream AE, must include appropriate criteria to separate linguistic differences and developmental targets. As it will be explicated below, the phonetic development of children who speak AAE and mainstream AE is expected to have different trajectories, which calls for greater sensitivity and discernment of SLPs and educators in interpretation of pronunciation and, relatedly, spelling patterns (Treiman & Bowman, 2015).

In addition, ongoing rapid demographic changes in the United States and worldwide have increased demand for clinical competence in the assessment of bilingual and multilingual patients. As illustrated in Figure 8.1, the number of foreign-born residents in the United States grew from 4.7 percent of the total population in 1970 to 12.9 percent in 2010 (U.S. Census Bureau, 2010), and the trend is still on the rise. Immigrants have long been attracted to big cities with many bilingual communities, and classrooms in urban schools tend to be increasingly multicultural and multilingual. In 2017, New York City alone was home to 3.1 million immigrants, the largest number in the city's history, comprising nearly 38 percent of the city population (MOIA Annual Report, 2018)

Adults learning their non-native languages later in life represent a particularly challenging case for SLPs who may encounter extensive variability in adults' productions as compared with bilingual children who learn the two languages early or simultaneously. The risk of

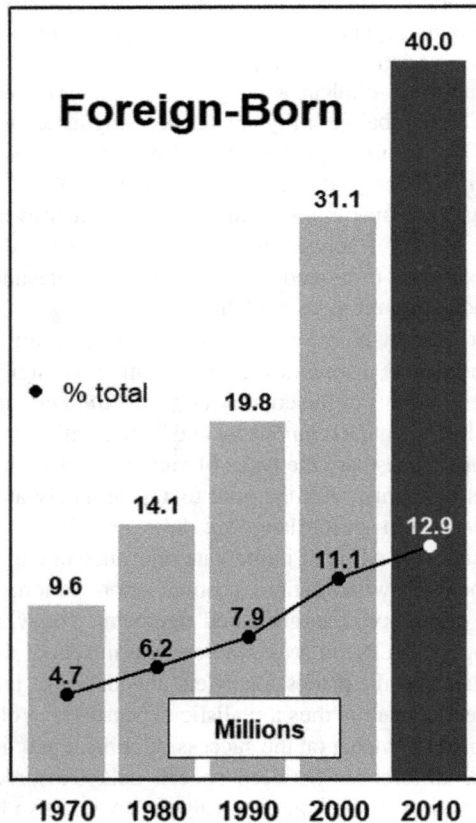

Figure 8.1 The rising trend of foreign-born US residents over the last five decades in millions and as a percentage of the total US population.

misdiagnosis increases for multilingual adults even if a more objective acoustic analysis is implemented. Distinguishing between early and late bilinguals is thus critical in selecting strategies for clinical work, particularly in treating patients with bilingual or multilingual aphasia, where it is uncertain which language is impaired and which language(s) should be the focus of interventions (Ijalba, Obler, & Chengappa, 2013).

The remainder of this chapter discusses phonetic variation coming from the three sources, regional dialect, ethnolect and bilingual/multilingual productions and considers potential challenges facing clinicians in making their assessment and treatment decisions. The overarching goal is to help SLPs recognize the non-disordered source of phonetic variation in their patients, and to encourage them to consult available research that can inform their clinical diagnosis. In a multicultural society, extensive phonetic variation is increasingly a norm rather than an exception and this dimension ought to be integrated with clinical objectives in treating speech communication disorders in children and adults.

Phonetic variation in regional dialects of American English

The field of communication disorders has increasingly recognized that monolingual children acquire the variety of their native language in which they are linguistically raised. In AE, the first systematic studies of the acquisition of local pronunciation patterns were conducted by sociolinguists (Roberts, 1997; Roberts & Labov, 1995). Fine-grained analyses of speech production data from young typically developing children growing up in Philadelphia showed that the children's speech represents features of the local regional variety (dialect). In the United States, these regional varieties are best documented in the work of Labov (Roberts, 1997; Roberts & Labov, 1995). According to the *Atlas of North American English* (Labov et al., 2006), differences in vowel production constitute the most salient single variable that diversifies AE into six major dialect areas illustrated in Figure 8.2. Each of these dialect regions spans several states, with the West and the South being geographically largest, followed by the

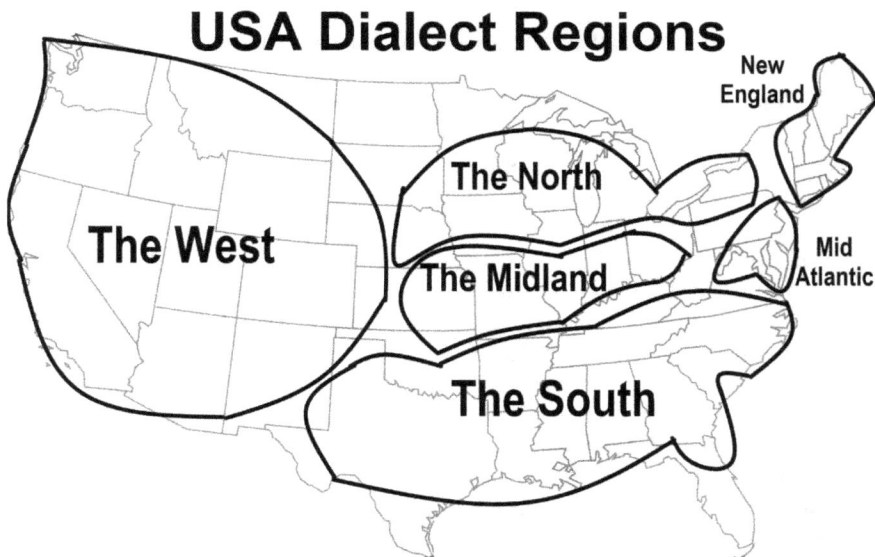

Figure 8.2   Map of dialect regions in the United States.

North and the Midland and finally by New England and Mid-Atlantic. Within each of these broad dialect regions, pronunciation patterns can also vary locally, defining smaller sub-regions and individual speech communities. Focusing on the pronunciation of vowels, we will now consider possible confusions and misinterpretations in clinical assessments of articulation and phonology that may arise as a result of the misalignment between the clinician's cultural and language background and the regional dialect of the patient.

The pronunciation of the low vowels /æ/, /ɑ/ and /ɔ/ is highly variable in contemporary AE, reflecting regional variation in the American vowel system. In particular, the low front /æ/ tends to be raised in the vowel space in the North such that the word *dad* can sound more like *dead* to people in the West or Midland because /æ/ in those regions is comparatively lower (Jacewicz, Fox, & Salmons, 2011a; Kendall & Fridland, 2017). The distinction between /æ/ and /ɑ/ is also influenced by regional variation and largely depends on how the perceptual boundary between the two vowels is located across dialects to preserve lexical contrast as in *pad-pod* or *sad-sod*. Even if no lexical contrast is involved and comprehension is not compromised, the vowel in *bath* or *apple* can be produced and perceived as more /æ/-like or more /ɑ/-like. This reflects the cross-regional permissible (and actual) phonetic ranges for the vowel categories /æ/ and /ɑ/. The relationship between the /ɑ/ and /ɔ/ vowels is complicated in yet another way. Namely, in some dialects both vowel phonemes can collapse into one phonetic category and thus the lexical contrasts such as *cot-caught* or *tot-taught* are lost. In sociolinguistic literature, this phonetic category overlap is called vowel merger, and the /ɑ/-/ɔ/ merger is termed the low back merger. This merger is widespread in AE except for the North and the South, however more recent reports converge in evidence that it is also spreading into these regions (Dinkin, 2011; Irons, 2007).

Given the extensive variability in the production of the three low vowels across the regions, clinical assessment can be challenging. For example, a SLP who moves from upstate New York (in the North) to central Ohio (in the Midland) may misrepresent the complete low back merger as a speech error, and a SLP from central Ohio may not only misperceive the raised Northern /æ/ as an /ɛ/ but also insist that the vowel in *apple* should be pronounced more /ɑ/-like. To give another example, it may also happen that *r*-less pronunciation of vowels in postvocalic positions (e.g. *Hampsha* for *Hampshire*) that is typical of eastern New England (Stanford, Leddy-Cecere, & Baclawski, 2012) can be interpreted as mispronunciations of /r/ by SLPs not familiar with this variety. Consequently, an older child whose family relocates from New Hampshire to the southern state of North Carolina can be diagnosed with a speech disorder because their *more* sounds like *maw* to a clinician born and raised in the South.

Clinical evaluation involves perceptual categorization of patients' productions by clinicians and, as indicated by the examples involving low vowels, SLPs judgements can be influenced by their own regional background. Recent research provided evidence that listeners from two dialect regions, the North and the Midland, also differ in their perception of nasality in vowels (Velik, Bae, & Fox, 2019). Presented with synthetic vowel stimuli with varying degrees of nasalization, listeners from the North rated them consistently as more nasal than listeners from the Midland. Importantly, the statistical difference in perception did not correspond to the nasalance scores (i.e. the ratio between nasal and total acoustic energy) that were similar in production of speakers from the two dialects. This suggests that clinicians from different regional backgrounds may perceive the level of patient's nasality differently, which has implications for their clinical decisions. However, an additional complication may potentially arise when a clinician from the North or Midland evaluates a patient from the South who does not make a phonetic distinction between /ɪ/ and /ɛ/ in prenasal position (in both production and perception). This merger, conditioned by a nasal, is a regional feature of the South and southern speakers may be insensitive to phonetic differences in *pin* and *pen* or *him* and *hem*. Will the clinician treat the merger as a speech error? If so, will she use her own nasality judgments in treating the "error?" Clearly, dialect contact can be a conundrum for the clinicians, and may lead to various misinterpretations unless dialect awareness is made explicit in clinical instruction in communication disorders.

Importantly, awareness of regional variation can also inform speech elicitation procedures in clinical practice. Consider, for example, the occurrence of conditioned vowel mergers (i.e. where the merger is conditioned by consonant that follows the vowel), which is relatively common across different dialect regions in the United States. An informed clinician may expect a loss of the tense versus lax distinction of the high front /i/-/ɪ/ and high back /u/-/ʊ/ vowels before /l/ in the Appalachian Mountains, Texas, the Midland or the West (Labov et al., 2006), and will elicit exemplars other than *peel – pill* or *full –fool* in assessments of vowel production accuracy in these regions. Frankly, this tense-lax contrast loss can be heard often outside of these regions in the speech of commentators on national sports talk radio shows. Some mergers are more restricted geographically, such as a merger of /æ/ and /e/ before /g/ in Wisconsin and Minnesota (Zeller, 1997). Consequently, pronunciation of *bag* as [beⁱg] or *tag* as [teⁱg] may be acceptable to a local clinician but not to SLPs relocating to these areas from other parts of the United States. Familiarity with the pre-velar merger can guide the creation of appropriate word lists, and representative exemplars of /æ/ and /e/ can be elicited in contexts other than the postvocalic /g/.

Variation in the degree of diphthongization in vowels is another regional feature that can be of clinical relevance in the assessment of vowel production by children and adults. Over the last decade, research in vowel acoustics has uncovered important regional differences in the dynamic structure of vowels. Regional varieties of AE were found to differ in their use of the audible diphthong-like changes in the time course of a vowel, known as vowel inherent spectral change (VISC) (Nearey & Assmann, 1986). These spectral variations, occurring not only in diphthongs but also in the majority of English monophthongs, coexist with dialect-specific vowel positions in the acoustic space and contribute to distinctiveness of regional dialects (e.g. Fox & Jacewicz, 2009; Jacewicz et al., 2011a). A large-scale study conducted in the North, Midland and South found that, within each regional variety, there are systematic differences in the way older and younger local speakers produce dynamics of monophthongs and diphthongs (Jacewicz & Fox, 2013; Jacewicz, Fox, & Salmons, 2011b). Overall, monophthongs of speakers in their 60s and 70s showed greater diphthongization than those of younger speakers and children. Dialects also differed in the degree of /u/-fronting, /æ/-raising, or /ɪ/-centralization, and these dialect-specific dispersion patterns were enhanced by vowel-specific amounts of VISC. Significant regional differences were also found in the temporal domain, indicating that dialects differ not only in their use of the vowel space and spectral dynamics but also in habitual articulation rate (Fox & Jacewicz, 2017; Jacewicz, Fox, & Wei, 2010).

The clinical importance of this work is that vowel error patterns in clinical assessments need to be interpreted with caution as some instances of fronting, backing, raising, lowering or diphthong reduction may represent regional and generational variation rather than vowel errors or disorders that are representative of the US population as a whole. To that end, the excellent summary of possible error patterns in children participating in the Memphis vowel project in the southern state of Tennessee (Pollock, 2013) needs yet to be confirmed in clinical work with children in other dialect regions. Also, socio-economic status and cultural background of the speakers (e.g. urban versus rural) is another dimension to consider in the assessment of vowel errors. It is known that the acquisition of the highly complex patterns of socio-indexical variation begins early, perhaps in the 3rd or 4th year, and continues into late adolescence (Docherty, Foulkes, Tillotson, & Watt, 2006; Smith, Durham, & Richards, 2013). Children from rural backgrounds may be aware of social influences on the local patterns, and may have acquired two forms for highly stigmatized vowel variants. For example, 8–10 year old children in the South utilized stylistic variation in the production of /ai/, producing a full diphthong in formal settings and a local monophthongal variant in spontaneous conversations (Jacewicz & Fox, 2019). Consequently, a clinician may expect variable productions from the same child, reflecting child's accommodation to the interlocutor with whom the child interacts during clinical evaluation.

Phonetic variation in an ethnolect (African American English)

Language variety spoken by a group of people sharing a common ethnic (as opposed to regional) background is termed an ethnolect. In the United States, the English variety spoken by many African Americans meets the criteria of an ethnolect because some of its features are common to all African Americans irrespective of geographic location, regional dialect or social context. Although African American English (AAE) is an ethnolect, it is by no means a monolithic variety. Rather, AAE is an ethnicity-based social variety with some stable features that are prevalent and perhaps uniform across the United States, and with some features that are specific to its vernacular form, termed African American Vernacular English (AAVE). As maintained by sociolinguists, features of AAE can be found in speech of middle-class African Americans whereas AAVE is spoken primarily by a working-class (Thomas, 2007; Wolfram & Schilling-Estes, 2006).

Variation in AAE speech patterns is largely attributable to a unique migration history of African Americans in the United States. The earliest ethnic concentrations were in the Chesapeake Bay and eastern Virginia encompassing the coastal regions of North and South Carolina, and the fertile farmlands of Georgia, Alabama and Mississippi. It is estimated that, in 1910, an overwhelming majority of African Americans lived in the South (about 90 percent), and regional features of southern dialects influenced the formation of the ethnolect. However, around the mid-twentieth century, large groups of African Americans moved to metropolitan areas in the North, including big cities such as Chicago, Detroit, New York or Philadelphia and gradually to other cities across the country. This massive exodus from the South is known as the great migration, and the basis for this relocation was primarily socio-economic: to find employment and to escape poverty and racial segregation. By 1970, almost half of African Americans lived in urban areas outside of the South. Given the migration history and the shift from the rural to urban life, African American speech contains not only ethnic but a blend of many regional pronunciation features found in other regional varieties of AE. In recent years, as economic situation improved in the South, many African Americans have relocated from the North back to the southern states (the movement is known as the reverse migration), but continue to maintain an urban life by concentrating their southern return to big cities such as Houston or Atlanta (see Wolfram & Thomas, 2002 and Rickford, 1999, for further readings).

A clinician working with African American patients must expect extensive variation in their speech and, given the historical context, some pronunciation features may vary between individuals even in the same geographic location. While we describe here the best known and documented phonological and phonetic variables, the summary is by no means complete, and a clinician may encounter many lesser known features reflecting the exposure to the northern and southern varieties of AE, and the nature and amount of this exposure may be unique to each patient. We focus in this chapter on the best known distinguishing phonetic features of AAE, most of which involving production of consonants. It needs to be emphasized that acoustic studies of consonantal variation in AAE are rare, and the published data are based primarily on impressionistic observations of individual researchers. However, a number of features are reported consistently by many scholars studying AAE, and we have chosen to center our discussion on these consistent findings.

All scholars agree that AAE has some degree of *r*-lessness in a syllable coda so that words *floor/four* can be produced as [flo:]/[fo:], [floə]/[foə] or [flou]/[fou]. In general, *r*-less pronunciation occurs predominantly in AAVE but it is also relatively common in speech of middle-class African Americans. The roots of *r*-lessness are thought to be historical, associated with English spoken in the plantation areas in the South. Also, migration to Northeast, including eastern New England and New York City metropolitan areas is another contributing factor, as these are the main dialect regions in the United States that have maintained *r*-less pronunciation. Labov, Cohen, Robins, & Lewis (1968) estimated that, in the 1960s, the *r*-lessness rate among African Americans in New York City was about 90 percent. A related feature of AAE is *l*-lessness, that is, a vocalization of the final [l] to schwa as in *feel* [fiə] or a complete deletion of [l] as in *pull* (see Thomas, 2007, for an extensive discussion).

The deletion of the word final stop consonants as a simplification of consonant clusters is another consistent AAE feature widely reported by sociolinguists (e.g. Gordon, 2000; Labov, 1972). As a result of this process, some words appear "unfinished" such as *des* for *desk*, *fas* for *fast*, *pas* for *past*, *breas* for *breast*, *ches* for *chest*, *ac* for *act*, etc. Also common is the deletion of word final consonants, especially voiced, even if they do not involve cluster reduction, e.g. *ma* for *mad* or *do* for *dog*. Naturally, consonant deletions in AAE have attracted attention of clinical researchers and SLPs as these are the types of productions that can signal developmental delays or disorders in children speaking mainstream varieties of AE. It was found that African American children residing in a predominantly African American community and speaking AAE as their primary language, showed a different order of acquisition of consonants and consonant sequences in words than their age-matched peers speaking mainstream AE (Pearson, Velleman, Bryant, & Charko, 2009). Explicit recommendations for SLPs working with AAE children were to first target the mastery of consonants in initial and then in medial word positions, as teaching new sounds in final position first would be a "misguided approach" (Velleman & Pearson, 2010).

Also common, although mostly in AAVE, are deletions of final /n/ so that the word *man* is produced with an open syllable and a heavily nasalized vowel. Variations in phonotactic patterns such as substitutions of /skr/ for /str/ are also relatively common, e.g. *skreet* for *street* or *skream* for *stream*. An interesting observation from fieldwork in Hyde County in coastal North Carolina was shared by Wolfram and Thomas (2002). Some of the AAVE speakers in their study mentioned that they were sent to special speech classes at school to "correct" pronunciation of the *skr*-cluster, referring to those classes as the "S-K-R-Club." As it is now recognized, such "corrections" can be inappropriate from the developmental point of view as they target ethnically based differences rather than speech disorders. No doubt, another inappropriate candidate for "correction" would be the metathesis *aks* for *ask* or *maks* for *mask*, which became a stereotypical feature of AAVE.

There are also systematic word final stop consonant voicing variations in AAE, including devoicing of the voiced stop (*bat* for *bad*) and a complete deletion of the voiceless stop (/kæ/ for *cat*) (Bailey & Thomas, 1998). Recent acoustic work examining these relations in greater detail showed that AAE speakers use the duration of the preceding vowel as the primary, most salient cue to the voicing status of the final consonant (Farrington, 2018; Holt, Jacewicz, & Fox, 2016). In particular, although vowels are longer before voiced stops than voiceless stops in all varieties of English, AAE speakers lengthen extensively the vowel preceding the devoiced stop to emphasize that the intended (and underlying) consonant was voiced and not voiceless. It appears that AAE utilizes temporal relations among vowels as one of the phonetic features marking the ethnic distinctiveness. This includes minimizing contrast between tense and lax vowels and prolonging durations of all vowels relative to the vowels in mainstream AE (Holt, Jacewicz, & Fox, 2015). The inherently longer AAE vowels are additionally affected by variable timing patterns across dialect regions in the United States.

The complexity of phonetic variation in AAE may seem overwhelming, yet our current focus on phonology does not even consider additional rich sources of variations in morphology and syntax. For many AAE children, linguistic interference can have a negative effect on literacy achievement as the correspondence of sound to letter may become overly complex (Labov & Baker, 2015). Therefore, an effective intervention needs to target specific types of phonological contexts, including those discussed above, to increase children's awareness of these discrepancies and help them cope with intense variability in speech.

Phonetic variation in bilingual and multilingual speakers

Until recently, the field of communication disorders in the United States attracted primarily monolingual AE speaking professionals, and about 90 percent of the current SLPs do not speak another language and lack specialized training in bilingualism. As the number of bilinguals is on the rise (given the significant demographic changes currently taking place in the United States), SLPs consider assessing and treating bilingual children as one of the greatest challenges in clinical practice. Under-diagnosis of speech sound disorders (SSD) in bilingual children is more frequent than in monolingual children (Stow & Dodd, 2005) and many bilinguals do not receive adequate intervention services. Recognizing these challenges, international projects and research studies have begun to support SLPs working with multilingual children with SSD.

Yavaş and Goldstein (1998) addressed this issue and more recently, specific recommendations were detailed in a tutorial article written by 27 experts in the field (McLeod, Verdon, & The International Expert Panel on Multilingual Children's Speech, 2017). The tutorial provides guidance and resources for SLPs to differentiate children with SSD from children with speech differences (bilingual or multilingual) and is addressed to clinicians who do not speak the language of their patients. For example, adaptation of speech assessments from one language to another is not recommended because languages differ in their segmental inventories (i.e. vowels, consonants and syllable types). Rather, clinicians may develop informal assessment tools using available phonetic resources and then work with a native speaker such as the child's family member. A useful strategy is to record single word productions by the child and then the same words by the family member, and compare the two using phonetic transcription or acoustic analysis. It is important to assess skills in all languages of the multilingual child as proficiency may differ by language.

Admittedly, phonetic transcription of non-native languages may be challenging for clinicians, and proficiency in narrow phonetic transcription is particularly helpful in the multilingual context.

Phonemes in the child's language may use different allophonic variants, which could be misdiagnosed as speech errors when only broad phonetic transcription is used. However, practice is needed to improve the transcribing skills in a foreign language and the tutorial refers clinicians to several websites that can improve their perception of non-native sounds. In general, diagnosis of SSD is difficult when working with multilingual children, and differentiation of SSD from accented speech production due to non-native language (or dialect of that language) can be challenging. The recommendations of the tutorial are concluded with a case study of a bilingual child speaking Cantonese and English who is assessed by a monolingual English clinician. The step-by-step assessment procedures and clinician's decisions are laid out in a comprehensive manner, leading to the diagnosis that intervention is needed in both of the child's languages.

Although acoustic analysis of speech can be of great help in clinical decision making, it is underutilized by SLPs because it requires expertise and is time consuming. However, clinicians can benefit from acoustic research studies with bilingual and multilingual children and adults, although research support is available only for selected languages and phonetic variables. A widely studied variable in bilinguals is voice onset time (VOT) differentiating voiced and voiceless stop consonants. Normative data about voicing development and use in either language of the bilingual were reported for Spanish-English (Fabiano-Smith & Bunta, 2012), Japanese-English (Harada, 2007), Greek-English (Antoniou, Best, Tyler, & Kroos, 2011), Korean-English (Lee & Iverson, 2011), Arabic-English (Khattab, 2000), French-English (Mack, 1990), among many others.

Vowel production in bilinguals has also been studied using acoustic analysis. Ideally, the developmental path of bilingual vowel spaces should be observed longitudinally but such studies are rare. A young Mandarin-English child in Yang, Fox, and Jacewicz (2015) was able to establish new native-like phonetic categories in English relatively quickly. However, bilinguals learning their second language in adulthood are unlikely to produce them in a native-like manner (e.g. Bohn & Flege, 1992). More complex interconnected relationships between the vowel systems have been reported longitudinally for adult multilingual speakers learning English as their third language (Kartushina & Martin, 2019). Importantly, frequency of language usage and switching habits influenced production of the native vowel targets that seemed to be changing as a function of language contact and switching events.

Conclusion

The above discussions of possible sources of phonetic variation are aimed to increase clinicians' awareness of pronunciation differences that can arise from regional, socio-cultural and multilingual uses of sound combinations. These various patterns are by no means deviant but represent lawful variation and social or cultural norms, and need to be recognized as such in the assessments of speech-language delays, phonological impairments, and various types of speech disorders. The present focus on AE serves illustrative purposes and is by no means exhaustive. Language or dialect contact situations of the types considered here arise not only in other parts of the English-speaking world including the British Isles, Canada, Australia and New Zealand, but are applicable to other languages, countries and cultures where clinical work is carried out and speech-language services are delivered. As population demographics change, clinicians treating bilingual or multilingual patients are expected to face challenges, as are the bilingual clinicians providing services across regional and socio-cultural groups. There is a need to develop effective strategies to guide the proper diagnosis and intervention amid cultural and linguistic diversity, and the demand for such new approaches is expected to intensify in years to come.

References

Antoniou, M., Best, C., Tyler, M., & Kroos, C. (2011). Inter-language interference in VOT production by L2-dominant bilinguals: Asymmetries in phonetic code-switching. *Journal of Phonetics, 39*, 558–570.

Bailey, G. & Thomas, E. (1998). Some aspects of African-American vernacular English phonology. In G. Bailey, J. Baugh, S. Mufwene, & J. Rickford (Eds.), *African-American English: Structure, history, and use* (pp. 85–109). New York, NY: Routledge.

Bohn, O.-S. & Flege, J. (1992). The production of new and similar vowels by adult German learners of English. *Studies in Second Language Acquisition, 14*, 131–158.

Dinkin, A. (2011).Weakening resistance: Progress toward the low back merger in New York State. *Language Variation and Change, 23*(3), 15–345.

Docherty, G.J., Foulkes, P., Tillotson, J., & Watt, D. (2006). On the scope of phonological learning: Issues arising from socially structured variation. In L. Goldstein, D. Whalen, & C. Best. (Eds.), *Laboratory phonology 8* (pp. 393–421). Berlin, Germany: Walter de Gruyter.

Fabiano-Smith, L. & Bunta, F. (2012). Voice onset time of voiceless bilabial and velar stops in 3-year-old bilingual children and their age-matched monolingual peers. *Clinical Linguistics & Phonetics, 26*(2), 148–163.

Farrington, C. (2018). Incomplete neutralization in African American English: The case of final consonant voicing. *Language Variation and Change, 30*, 361–383.

Fox, R.A. & Jacewicz, E. (2009). Cross-dialectal variation in formant dynamics of American English vowels. *Journal of the Acoustical Society of America, 126*, 2603–2618.

Fox, R.A. & Jacewicz, E. (2017). Reconceptualizing the vowel space in analyzing regional dialect variation and sound change in American English. *Journal of the Acoustical Society of America, 142*, 444–459.

Gordon, M.J. (2000). Phonological correlates of ethnic identity: Evidence of divergence? *American Speech, 75*, 115–136.

Harada, T. (2007). The production of voice onset time (VOT) by English-speaking children in a Japanese immersion program. *International Review of Applied Linguistics in Language Teaching, 45*(4), 353–378.

Holt, Y.F., Jacewicz, E., & Fox, R.A. (2015). Variation in vowel duration among Southern African American English speakers. *American Journal of Speech-Language Pathology, 24*, 460–469.

Holt, Y.F., Jacewicz, E., & Fox, R.A. (2016). Temporal variation in African American English: The distinctive use of vowel duration. *Journal of Phonetics and Audiology, 2*(2), 1–8.

Ijalba, E., Obler, L. K., & Chengappa, S. (2013). Bilingual aphasia: Theoretical and clinical considerations. In T.K. Bhatia & W.C. Ritchie (Eds.). *The handbook of bilingualism and mutlilingualism* (2nd ed., pp. 61–83). Oxford, UK: Blackwell Publishing.

Irons, T.L. (2007). On the status of low back vowels in Kentucky English: More evidence of merger. *Language Variation and Change, 19*, 137–180.

Jacewicz, E. & Fox, R.A. (2013). Cross-dialectal differences in dynamic formant patterns in American English vowels. In G. Morrison & P. Assmann (Eds.). *Vowel inherent spectral change* (pp. 177–198). New York, NY: Springer.

Jacewicz, E. & Fox, R.A. (2019). The old, the new, and the in-between: Preadolescents' use of stylistic variation in speech in projecting their own identity in a culturally changing environment. *Developmental Science, 22*, e12722.

Jacewicz, E., Fox, R.A., & Salmons, J. (2011a). Cross-generational vowel change in American English. *Language Variation and Change, 23*, 45–86.

Jacewicz, E., Fox, R.A., & Salmons, J. (2011b). Regional dialect variation in the vowel systems of typically developing children. *Journal of Speech, Language, and Hearing Research, 54*, 448–470.

Jacewicz, E., Fox, R.A., & Wei, L. (2010). Between-speaker and within-speaker variation in speech tempo of American English. *Journal of the Acoustical Society of America, 128*, 839–850.

Kartushina, N. & Martin, C.D. (2019). Third-language learning affects bilinguals' production in both their native languages: A longitudinal study of dynamic changes in L1, L2 and L3 vowel production. *Journal of Phonetics, 77* (2019) 100920, doi: 10.1016/j.wocn.2019.100920.

Kendall, T. & Fridland, V. (2017). Regional relationships among the low vowels of U.S. English: Evidence from production and perception. *Language Variation and Change, 29,* 245–271.

Khattab, G. (2000). VOT production in English and Arabic bilingual and monolingual children. *Leeds Working Papers in Linguistics, 8,* 95–122.

Labov, W. (1972). *Language in the inner city: Studies in the Black English vernacular.* Philadelphia, PA: University of Pennsylvania Press.

Labov, W. (1994). *Principles of linguistic change. I: Internal factors.* Oxford: Blackwell.

Labov, W. (1995). Can reading failure be reversed? A linguistic approach to the question. In V. Gadsden & D. Wagner (Eds.). *Literacy among African-American youth: Issues in learning, teaching, and schooling* (pp. 39–68). Cresskill, NJ: Hampton Press.

Labov, W. (2006). *The social stratification of English in New York City* (2nd ed.). Cambridge, UK: Cambridge University Press.

Labov, W. (2010). *Principles of linguistic change. III: Cognitive and cultural factors.* Oxford, UK: Blackwell.

Labov, W., & Baker, B. (2015). African American Vernacular English and reading. In S. Lanehart (Ed.), *The Oxford handbook of African American language* (pp. 617–636). Oxford, UK and New York, NY: Oxford University Press.

Labov, W., Ash, S., & Boberg, C. (2006). *Atlas of North American English: Phonetics, phonology, and sound change.* Berlin, Germany: Mouton de Gruyter.

Labov, W., Cohen, P., Robins, C., & Lewis, J. (1968). A study of the non-standard English of Negro and Puerto Rican speakers in New York City. *Report on cooperative research project 3288.* New York, NY: Columbia University.

Lee, S. A. S., & Iverson, G. (2011). Stop consonants of English–Korean bilingual children. *Bilingualism: Language and Cognition, 15,* 275–287.

Mack, M. (1990). Phonetic transfer in a French-English bilingual child. In P. H. Nelde (Ed.), *Language attitudes and language conflict* (pp. 107–124). Bonn, Germany: Dümmler.

McLeod, S., Verdon S., and The International Expert Panel on Multilingual Children's Speech (2017). Tutorial: Speech assessment for multilingual children who do not speak the same language(s) as the Speech-Language Pathologist. *American Journal of Speech-Language Pathology, 26,* 691–708.

MOIA Annual Report (2018). State of Our Immigrant City – Annual Report, March 2018. New York City, NY: Mayor's Office of Immigrant Affairs.

Nearey, T.M. & Assmann, P.F. (1986). Modelling the role of inherent spectral change in vowel identification. *Journal of the Acoustical Society of America, 80,* 1297–1308.

Pearson, B.Z., Velleman, S.L., Bryant, T.J., & Charko, T. (2009). Phonological milestones for African American English-speaking children learning mainstream American English as a second dialect. *Language, Speech, and Hearing Services in Schools, 40,* 1–16.

Pollock, K.E. (2013). The Memphis Vowel Project: Vowel errors in children with and without phonological disorders. In M.J. Ball & F.E. Gibbon (Eds.). *Handbook of vowels and vowel disorders* (pp. 260–287). New York, NY: Psychology Press.

Rickford, J.R. (1999). *African American Vernacular English: Features, evolution, educational implications.* Boston, MA: Wiley-Blackwell.

Roberts, J. (1997). Acquisition of variable rules: A study of (–t, d) deletion in preschool children. *Journal of Child Language, 24,* 351–372.

Roberts, J. & Labov, W. (1995). Learning to talk Philadelphian. *Language Variation and Change, 7,* 101–122.

Smith, J., Durham, M., & Richards, H. (2013). The social and linguistic in the acquisition of sociolinguistic norms: Caregivers, children, and variation. *Linguistics, 51*(2): 285–324.

Stanford, J., Leddy-Cecere, T., & Baclawski, K. (2012). Farewell to the founders: Major dialect changes along the East-West New England border. *American Speech, 87,* 126–169.

Stow, C. & Dodd, B. (2005). A survey of bilingual children referred for investigation of communication disorders: A comparison with monolingual children referred in one area in England. *Journal of Multilingual Communication Disorders, 3*(1), 1–23.

Thomas, E.R. (2007). Phonological and phonetic characteristics of African American Vernacular English. *Language and Linguistics Compass, 1,* 450–475.

Treiman, R. & Bowman, M. (2015). Spelling in African American children: The case of final consonant devoicing. *Reading and Writing, 28,* 1013–1028.

U.S. Census Bureau (2010). The American Community Survey, 2010 release. U.S. Department of Commerce.

Velik, K., Bae, Y., & Fox, R.A. (2019). Effects of regional dialect on oral-nasal balance and nasality perception. *Clinical Linguistics & Phonetics*, *33*(7), 587–600.

Velleman, S. & Pearson, B. (2010). Differentiating speech sound disorders from phonological dialect differences: Implications for assessment and intervention. *Topics in Language Disorders*, *30*(3), 176–188.

Wolfram, W. & Thomas, E.R. (2002). *The development of African American English*. Oxford, UK: Blackwell.

Wolfram, W., & Schilling-Estes, N. (2006). *American English: Dialects and variation* (2nd ed.). Oxford, UK: Blackwell.

Yang, J., Fox, R.A., & Jacewicz, E. (2015). Vowel development in an early Mandarin-English bilingual child: A longitudinal study. *Journal of Child Language*, *42*(5), 1125–1145.

Yavaş, M. & Goldstein, B. (1998). Phonological assessment and treatment of bilingual speakers. *American Journal of Speech-Language Pathology*, *7*, 49–60.

Zeller, C. (1997). The investigation of a sound change in progress: /ae/ to /e/ in Midwestern American English. *Journal of English Linguistics*, *25*, 142–155.

9

STYLISTIC VARIATION IN MISARTICULATIONS

Martin J. Ball, Orla Lowry, and Lisa McInnis

Introduction

The sociolinguistics revolution from the 1960s onward (e.g. Labov, 1966, and the overview presented in articles in Ball, 2005) showed, among many other things, correlations between linguistic and non-linguistic variables. These non-linguistic variables have included regional and social background, age, and sex of the speaker, and correlational studies have demonstrated the link between a speaker's membership of one or other of these groups and the likelihood of their producing a particular variant of a linguistic variable.

However, variable linguistic usage is not limited to inter-speaker differences, as intra-speaker variation has also been documented. In particular, stylistic variation has been widely studied in sociolinguistics, and the formalizing effect of reading from written texts is well-known (see Labov's, 1966, discussion of reading styles). Traditional assessments of children's speech using picture-naming tasks are similar to some extent to a single word reading task—shown by sociolinguists to be the most formal style speakers use. Indeed, older children are often asked to read word lists and reading passages, and these are the same formats used in sociolinguistic studies to investigate most formal styles. In recent decades, clinical phoneticians and speech-language pathologists have also laid stress on the need for examples of spontaneous speech as well as single word production (e.g. Grunwell, 1987).

Thus, current practice is similar to stylistic studies in sociolinguistics. It is therefore possible to study whether stylistic variation occurs in disordered speech data and, if it does, whether any of the variation might correlate with clinical variables (e.g. the so-called "therapy style" of speech used by both SLPs and their clients). In this chapter we examine a case of r-misarticulation and the range of variants that the clients uses for target /r/, and the styles in which they occur.

English approximant-r

The continuant-r, the most common realization of /r/ in varieties of English, can be produced in two different ways (Ball & Müller, 2005; Laver, 1994).[1] While both the two forms have very similar acoustic percepts, the tongue positions adopted in their articulation differ. The version normally described in textbooks on English is the variety we can label as a postalveolar approximant (sometimes termed apical-r or retroflex-r). The other variety is usually termed a bunched-r, and could perhaps be described as a "labial prevelar approximant with tongue tip retraction" into the tongue body (Laver, 1994, p. 301) although tracings from Delattre (1965; in Laver, 1994) suggest the constriction is closer to palatal. It seems that the choice between these forms is one of individual preference, though the bunched-r predominates in western American English. Apical-r is produced in the following way: the tongue tip is curled up toward, but not touching the alveolar ridge, and the front of the tongue is lowered. The back of the tongue is somewhat higher than the front, so there is a hollow in the body of the tongue. Air flows centrally over the tongue without turbulence. For the bunched-r the tongue dorsum is raised up toward the boundary between the hard and the soft palate and the tongue tip is drawn back into the body of the tongue. There may be some contact between the side rims of the tongue and the insides of the upper molar teeth, but air is allowed to flow freely over the center of the tongue without turbulence.

Evidence suggests that continuant-r is not only one of the last consonants of English to be acquired, but is also commonly misarticulated (Grunwell, 1987; Shriberg, 1993). However, despite this, there are comparatively few studies of r-misarticulations in the literature, and many that are available are primarily concerned with therapeutic issues (e.g. Brown, 1975; Bottell & Clark, 1986; McNutt, 1977), which is not the focus of this chapter. Flipsen, Shriberg, Weismer, Karlsson, and McSweeny (2001) and Shriberg Flipsen, Karlsson, and McSweeny (2001) are concerned with the basic acoustic characteristics of English /r/ and /ɝ/, and of commonly occurring substitutions of the latter (in this case, what the authors term "derhotacized" realizations, i.e. deletion of schwa off-glides).

Hagiwara, Fosnot, and Alessi (2002) describe a single case study of a child who presented with a misarticulated /r/. Impressionistically, the subject's realizations resembled [u], and acoustically the main point of interest was a greatly raised third formant. The misarticulation seemed to derive mostly from a banded lingual frenulum (tongue-tie), and this was eventually corrected surgically. The study then describes the post-surgical therapy, and the emergence of an acceptable adult-like /r/.

Heselwood and Howard (2002) discuss five cases of unusual /r/ realizations, including adults with acquired neurological disorders as well as children with articulation problems. Of the child cases, one realized target /r/ as an interdental lateral, while another assimilated plosives in plosive+ /r/ clusters to the labiality of the /r/. A Down's syndrome speaker usually realized /r/ as [j], while a cleft palate client used [w] and [u] for /r/. The authors note that all these results can be explained as compensatory articulations rather than as examples of phonological delay.

In this chapter we describe a case-study of a child with unusual realizations of target /r/, which seemed to co-vary with distribution in the word, and style of utterance. These realizations, too, do not seem to be simply a result of phonological delay; indeed, some of them appear to be articulations that result from inappropriate therapeutic intervention.

The study

Client background

The client we will call "Robert" was 9.8 at the time of recording, and he had received speech therapy since he was 3-years-old for a variety of articulation problems. His target accent was west Louisiana, which is rhotic and similar in many respects to eastern Texas. His main remaining articulation problem was reported to be with /r/. We collected a recording of his speech to see if we could throw light on the patterns of variable realization of target /r/ that had been noted by his clinician. In this region, a bunched-r is probably the commonest variety.

Data

Data were collected on tape using a variety of tasks:

- A 42-item word list containing /r/ in syllable initial and syllable final positions (both within word and word initial/final), and in singletons and clusters;
- A phonetically balanced reading passage (the Rainbow passage); and
- Spontaneous speech with a student clinician for about 20 minutes.

These speech samples were recorded in a quiet room using a good quality cassette tape recorder with an external microphone.

Transcription

Data were transcribed into the IPA by the authors. A relatively narrow transcription was used, differentiating between various approximants (including non-English ones) used by the client, and including duration information when this appeared excessive (but not normal allophonic length details). Inter- and intra-scorer reliability was high, being over 90% for both.

Results

Word list

The transcriptions of the 42-item word list are shown in Table 9.1.

Table 9.1 Transcription of word list

Target	Realization	Target	Realization
red	ɰːɛd	journal	dʒɑˠnəl
row	ɰːoʊ	word	wɜdˠ
rain	ɰːeɪn	eyebrow	aɪˠbᵊɹaʊ
right	ɰːaɪt	children	tʃɪldᵊɹən
root	ɰːut	january	dʒænjuɛwi
ground	gəɹaʊnd	bark	bɑk
breathe	bəɹɛθ	mirror	ˠmɪβ̞
green	gɰːin	water	ˠwɑɾə
orange	ɑβɪndʒ	your	jɔə
read	ɰːid	year	jɪə
robin	ɰːɑbɪn	labor	leɪbˠəɫ
rat	ɰːæt	car	kɑɹ
rib	ɰːɪb	core	kɔə
ring	ɰːɪŋk	pure	pjuə
turtle	tɜʔtl̩	poor	pɔ
therapy	θɛʊəpi	are	ɑ
shirt	ʃˠɜtˠ	doctor	dɑˠktə
operation	ɑpəβ̞eɪʃn	hair	hɛə
disorder	dɪsˠɔdˠəɫ	torn	tˠɔnˠ
parent	pˠɛəɰent	father	fɑðə
information	ɪnfɔmeɪʃən	mister	mɪstˠə

The word-list style of speech revealed different realizations of the target /r/:

- In word-initial position, Robert generally utilized a lengthened [ɥ] (often well over 300 ms);
- In medial position singleton /r/ was normally realized as an approximant (a variety of these were observed, including bilabial [β̞], labiodental [ʋ], and labiovelar [w]);
- In word final position, the commonest strategy (in both singletons and clusters) was deletion of the segment altogether; occasional glottal stop usage was also noted.
- Finally, we can note that word- and syllable-finally there was often a velarized voice quality throughout the syllable. This occasionally manifested itself in the use of a dark-l instead of the target /r/. This is clear evidence of an excessive tongue dorsum raising, which we presume to be the result of therapeutic intervention to teach the production of a bunched-r to Robert.

Rainbow passage

Robert's realizations of target /r/ during the reading of the Rainbow Passage were similar to those he used in the word list. For example, the prolonged [ɥː] is found initially, with the glides in initial clusters, and deletion realizations word-finally. Velarization was not noted, however, which suggests this is an aspect of the ultra-formal speech style Robert adopts in reading the Word List. The following shows just the realizations of /r/ in his reading of the Rainbow Passage ([Ø] represents deletion):

When the sunlight st[ɹ]ikes [ɥ]aind[ʋ]ops in the ai[ʔ], they act like a p[ʋ]ism and fo[Ø]m a [ɥ]ainbow. The [ɥ]ainbow is a division of white light into many beautiful colo[Ø]s. These take the shape of a long [ɥ]ound a[Ø]ch, with its path high above, and its two ends appa[ʋ]ently beyond the ho[ʋ]izon. The[ʔ]e is, acco[Ø]ding to legend, a boiling pot of gold at one end. People look, but no one eve[Ø] finds it. When a man looks fo[Ø] something beyond his [ɥ]each, his f[ʋ]iends say he is looking for the pot of gold at the end of the [ɥ]ainbow.

Spontaneous speech

In spontaneous speech, Robert generally used [ʋ] in prevocalic position, and deleted target /r/ in postvocalic position. There was little use of [ɥ] in prevocalic position, and there was no evidence of velarization in postvocalic position. We paid particular attention to sites of possible linking-r in the spontaneous speech sample. It was felt that Robert's usual strategy in this style of final /r/ deletion might be mitigated in those contexts where the following word begins with a vowel (as happens in many non-rhotic varieties of English such as Southern British Standard). Only one such context occurred in the Rainbow Passage ("there is, according to legend..."); and in this instance Robert used a glottal stop rather than outright deletion. However, this was a form he had also used elsewhere in word final position, so we did not consider this to be evidence of a linking-r phenomenon. We found in his spontaneous speech sample that Robert used a linking-r in two out of six possible contexts; the [ɹ] variant was the form used in both cases. This is of interest as in the word list style [ɹ] occurs twice as an intervocalic realization. This suggests that in his spontaneous speech he is able in a minority of instances to use a linking-r.

Table 9.2 Formant values in Hz for Robert and Author

	F1	*F2*	*F3*
Robert's [ɰ]	696.1	1232.5	2690.1
Author's [ɯ]	422.1	1910.8	2780.3
Author's [ɰ]	395.5	1939.9	2922.6
Author's [ɣ]	446.6	1304.0	2470.1

The nature of Robert's [ɰ]

The sound which we have transcribed as [ɰ] is an unusual realization of target /r/ in English. To ensure that our choice of symbol was appropriate, we undertook a spectrographic analysis of this approximant. The tokens used in the first three words in the Word List were chosen as representative, and the first three formants of the sound were measured midway through the segment, using the PRAAT speech analysis system (version 4.1.2). These values were then compared with those of the first author pronouncing Cardinal Vowel 16 (see Ball & Rahilly, 1999, for a description of the Cardinal Vowel system), the voiced velar approximant, and the voiced velar fricative. The figures are given in Table 9.2.

The expected formant values in children's speech are higher than those of adult males (Peterson & Barney, 1952); therefore, the higher value for Robert's F1 is expected compared to the first author's [ɯ] and [ɰ]. However, Robert does not display higher values for F2 and F3—indeed, they are lower. This would suggest that the sound he is producing is more centralized than those made by the first author, and perhaps also somewhat rounded. However, when the formant values for Robert's approximant are compared to the values of the first author's voiced velar fricative, we find a much closer fit (the F2 is still slightly less than expected). The first author's Cardinal Vowel 16 and voiced velar approximant were pronounced with the tongue in the highest, backest position possible, with the voiced velar fricative being articulated slightly forward of this. The figures suggest, therefore, that Robert is using a high back tongue position that can be characterized as advanced velar.

Discussion

While some of the substitutions observed (e.g. [ʋ], [w], deletion) are commonly reported for /r/ (Grunwell, 1987), the velar approximant (especially greatly prolonged) is not. The pervasive velarization to mark postvocalic-r is also atypical. It is interesting to consider what might be an underlying cause of these usage patterns.

In our opinion, the velar approximant is likely to be an artifact of therapy. If Robert was taught to produce a bunched-r (rather than an apical-r), this would account for the velar positioning of the tongue dorsum. Further, over-emphasis on the sound in training would account for the prolongation; and such over-emphasis might also underlie the velarization, this being the result of an attempt to introduce a postvocalic-bunched-r.

Interestingly, the prolongations and velarizations are largely absent from the spontaneous speech, again suggesting this is an artifact of careful "therapy-speech." The velarizations are also absent from the Rainbow Passage, suggesting that this usage is a marked or ultra-careful style.

The effects of style on the use of linguistic variables has, of course, been widely studied in the sociolinguistics literature, from such early investigations as Labov's classic study of New York English (1966) up to the present (Maclagan, 2005). Such work has demonstrated that different speaking tasks often produce different degrees of formality (in the sociolinguistics literature, formality is usually measured in terms of how close a speaker's realizations are to the "standard" or "educated" variety of their language). This is usually understood to derive, at least partly, from the amount of attention being paid to the task: reading a list of words focuses the speaker's attention on each individual word (thus promoting an overt regard for socially acceptable forms of pronunciation, for example). A reading passage also requires a fair amount of attention, but less so than a word list. Spontaneous speech requires a lesser degree of attention and so this type of speech is going to be less formal still (but even here, fully casual speech is difficult to access in any kind of interview situation, as the presence of an interviewer normally promotes a certain amount of formality).

In the case of Robert, it appears that the Word List and the Reading Passage operate as attention focusing contexts, just as in sociolinguistic studies. The standard to which Robert aspires in these formal contexts is "therapy speech": that is, in many instances, a prolonged velar approximant in initial position (probably mimicking the prolongations of the therapist) and a tendency to raise the tongue back in clusters and in word final position. This velarization is mostly absent from the slightly less formal Reading Passage (suggesting he only produces this feature when he is being extra careful in his speech), and tongue dorsum raising is mostly completely absent from his spontaneous speech. If, as we assume, the velar approximants and velarization are features of Robert's speech deriving from unsuccessful therapy (i.e. attempts to teach a bunched-r), then the simple substitution and deletion patterns of Robert's spontaneous speech probably represent his usage patterns pre-therapy. Robert's stylistic variation has allowed us to reconstruct his original /r/ realizations, for which we had no records.

Conclusion

As Robert could not originally produce a [ɹ], a motor approach to therapy was surely justified. It has had some success: in his word list style Robert does produce [ɹ] in a few instances. But it has also failed, in that he now produces many more instances of a prolonged velar approximant, and uses excessive velarization. The conclusion we must draw is that therapists should be aware of the different articulatory gestures that can produce an acceptable [ɹ], and if a bunched tongue shape proves problematic, an apical [ɹ] might be a better strategy to adopt.

Acknowledgements

Thanks to the client and his caregivers and to Stephanie Gary for her help with data collection.

Note

1 The remaining sections of this chapter are closely derived from Ball, Lowry & McInnis (2006).

References

Ball, M.J. (Ed.) (2005). *Clinical sociolinguistics*. Oxford: Blackwell.
Ball, M.J., Lowry, O., & McInnis, L. (2006). Distributional and stylistic variation in /r/-misarticulations: A case study. *Clinical Linguistics and Phonetics, 20*, 119–124.

Ball, M.J., & Müller, N. (2005). *Phonetics for communication disorders*. Mahwah, NJ: Lawrence Erlbaum.

Ball, M.J., & Rahilly, J. (1999). *Phonetics: The science of speech*. London, UK: Arnold, London.

Bottell, F., & Clark, J.E. (1986). /r/ misarticulation in children's speech. In *Proceedings of the First Australian Conference on Speech Science and Technology*, Canberra.

Brown, J.C. (1975). Techniques for correcting /r/ misarticulation. *Language Speech and Hearing Services in Schools, 6*(2), 86–91.

Flipsen, P., Shriberg, L., Weismer, G., Karlsson, H., & McSweeny, J. (2001). Acoustic phenotypes for speech-genetics studies: Reference data for residual /ɚ/ distortions. *Clinical Linguistics and Phonetics, 15*, 603–630.

Grunwell, P. (1987). *Clinical phonology* (2nd ed.). London, UK: Croom Helm.

Hagiwara, R., Fosnot, S., & Alessi, D. (2002). Acoustic phonetics in a clinical setting: A case study of /r/ distortion therapy with surgical intervention. *Clinical Linguistics and Phonetics, 16*, 425–441.

Heselwood, B.C., & Howard, S.J. (2002). The realization of English liquids in impaired speech: A perceptual and instrumental study. In F. Windsor, N. Hewlett, and L. Kelly (Eds.), *Investigations in clinical phonetics and linguistics* (pp. 225–241). New York, NY: Erlbaum.

Labov, W. (1966). *The social stratification of English in New York City*. Arlington, VA: Center for Applied Linguistics.

Laver, J. (1994). *Principles of phonetics*. Cambridge, UK: Cambridge University Press.

Maclagan, M. (2005). Regional and social variation. In M. J. Ball (Ed.), *Clinical sociolinguistics* (pp. 15–25). Oxford, UK: Blackwell.

McNutt, J. (1977). Oral sensory and motor behaviors of children with /s/ or /r/ misarticulation. *Journal of Speech and Hearing Research, 20*, 694–703.

Peterson, G., & Barney, H. (1952). Control methods in a study of the vowels. *Journal of the Acoustical Society of America, 24*, 175–184.

Shriberg, L. (1993). Four new speech and prosody-voice measures for genetics research and other studies in developmental phonological disorders. *Journal of Speech and Hearing Research, 36*, 105–140.

Shriberg, L., Flipsen, P., Karlsson, H., & McSweeny, J. (2001). Acoustic phenotypes for speech-genetics studies: an acoustic marker for residual /ɚ/ distortions. *Clinical Linguistics and Phonetics, 15*, 631–650.

10
ANALYZING PHONETIC DATA WITH GENERALIZED ADDITIVE MIXED MODELS

Yu-Ying Chuang, Janice Fon, Ioannis Papakyritsis,
and Harald Baayen

Introduction: A clinical example

To investigate the realizations of lexical stress by Greek speakers with dysarthria, Papakyritsis and Müller (2014) recorded and measured the productions of Greek words by five native speakers of Greek. Three speakers were diagnosed with dysarthria, the remaining two were controls. Each speaker completed a word repetition task, reading a total of 27 minimal pairs. These minimal pairs consisted of bisyllabic words that differed only in stress position, e.g. /ˈmilo/ *"apple"* and /miˈlo/ *"talk."* To quantify stress realizations, vowel duration and intensity of the two syllables were measured for each word. It was hypothesized that speakers with dysarthria have difficulty producing stress contrasts, resulting in smaller differences between stressed and unstressed syllables compared to control speakers.

In the dataset `clin`[1], stress position is specified in the column `stress`, with "SI" and "SF" indicating initial and final stress, respectively. In the column `group`, dysarthric and control participants are coded with "D" and "C." Vowel durations of the first and second syllables are provided in `dur1` and `dur2`. Hence, for words with initial stress (i.e. SI), `dur1` indicates the vowel duration of the stressed syllable, whereas for words with final stress (i.e. SF), it is `dur2` that refers to the vowel duration of the stressed syllable. With regards to intensity, `int1` and `int2` are the mean intensities of the first and second vowels. Since we are interested in the degree of contrast between stressed and unstressed syllables, following Papakyritsis and Müller (2014), we calculated duration and intensity ratios. That is, for a given word, we divided the vowel duration/intensity of the stressed syllable by the vowel duration/intensity of the unstressed syllable[2]. This gives us the response variables `durR` and `intR`, which are also available in the dataset.

```
> head(clin, 3)
  token stress subject group dur1  dur2  int1    int2    durR     intR
1 [celi]  SI      D1     D  0.291 0.262 56.791 51.977 1.110687 1.092618
2 [celi]  SI      D3     D  0.401 0.241 58.750 50.942 1.663900 1.153272
3 [celi]  SI      C1     C  0.140 0.086 74.027 61.278 1.627907 1.208052
```

Figure 10.1 presents the boxplots of duration and intensity ratios for control and dysarthric subjects when producing words with initial and final stresses. Larger ratios stand for greater

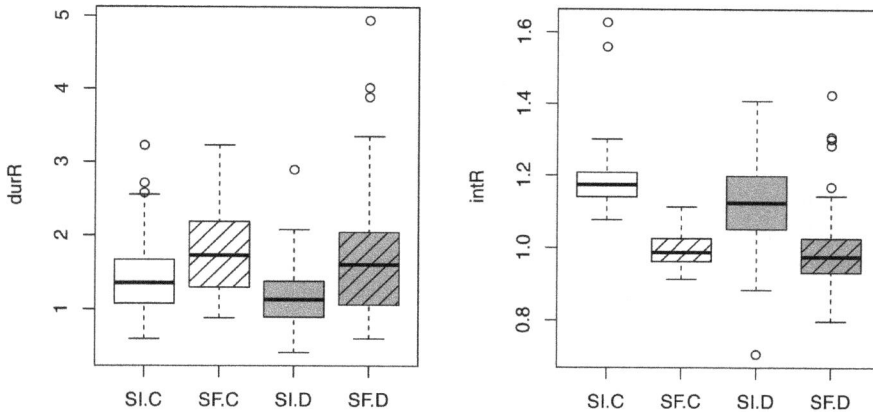

Figure 10.1 Boxplots of duration (left) and intensity (right) ratios for the four stress by group conditions.

contrasts between stressed and unstressed syllables. For duration (left panel), control participants show a larger stress contrast than dysarthric participants, more obviously so in stress-initial than stress-final words. The same holds for intensity (right panel), where between-group differences are also more pronounced in stress-initial words than stress-final words.

To evaluate the quantitative patterns in the data statistically, we fitted linear mixed models to durR (log-transformed) and intR separately, using the lme4 package in R. For both models, we included group and stress and their interaction as fixed-effect factors, as well as by-subject random intercepts. Model summaries are presented in Tables 10.1 and 10.2. For mathematical reasons, the lme4 package does not provide *p* values, but absolute values of the *t* statistics larger than 2 are good indicators of significance.

For duration ratios (Table 10.1), only the difference in stress position is supported. On the other hand, intensity ratios (Table 10.2) differ not only between stress positions, but also between participant groups, with dysarthric participants having a smaller intensity contrast for stress than control participants. Furthermore, the interaction effect indicates that for the

Tabel 10.1 Model summary for the effects of participant group and stress position, with duration ratio as the response variable

	Estimate	*Std. Error*	*t value*
(Intercept)	0.32	0.11	2.92
groupD	−0.22	0.14	−1.58
stressSF	0.22	0.07	3.03
groupD:stressSF	0.11	0.09	1.14

Tabel 10.2 Model summary for the effects of participant group and stress position, with intensity ratio as the response variable

	Estimate	*Std. Error*	*t value*
(Intercept)	1.19	0.02	61.10
groupD	−0.06	0.03	−2.41
stressSF	−0.20	0.02	−10.36
groupD:stressSF	0.06	0.03	2.31

dysarthric participants, the effect of stress position is reduced compared to that for the control participants, in line with the pattern shown in the right panel of Figure 10.1.

Although these analyses already captured the major trends in the data, there are further details that require attention. For example, while duration and intensity ratios clearly differ in the means between stress positions and participant groups, there are also differences in the variances. For duration ratios, stress-final words tend to have larger variances than stress-initial words, and intensity ratios appear to vary more for dysarthric participants than control participants. Canonical analysis of variance or the linear mixed model as implemented in lme4 cannot take such differences in variances into account. As will become clearer later, modeling the variance along with the mean is possible with generalized additive models, henceforth GAMs, which are the topic of this chapter.

GAMs can also help us refine the current analyses if we would have further information available. For instance, it would be useful to know the recording order of the words for each participant. This is because subjects' responses across the trials of an experiment are usually not independent of each other, which violates one of the core assumptions of the standard Gaussian regression model. This issue of inter-trial dependency can however be easily addressed with GAMs. Moreover, GAMs can model time-varying response variables. Take intensity for example. In the current dataset, we considered the mean intensity of the vowels. However, intensity actually changes over time, and instead of calculating the mean, we would have gained precision if we could have modeled how intensity changes over time. Given that dysarthric participants clearly show different mean intensities compared to control participants, it seems likely that there would also be qualitative differences between the intensity curves over time for the two participant groups. As these curves are usually nonlinear, analyses on the curves cannot be done with methods such as canonical anovas or linear models, which operate on the assumption of linearity.

As an example of a response variable that varies nonlinearly over time, consider the Mandarin pitch contour in Figure 10.2. This pitch contour realizes both lexical tones and an incredulous question intonation. The black solid line in the figure was obtained with the help of a GAM,

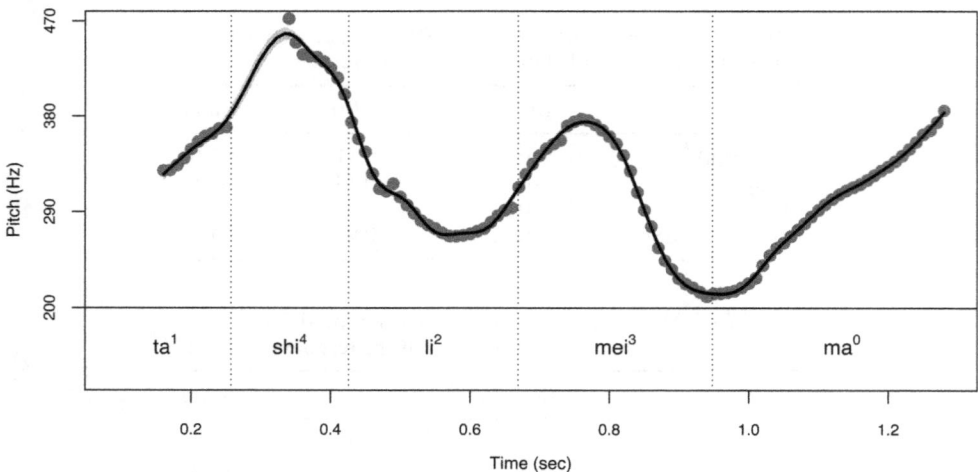

Figure 10.2 Pitch contour (grey dots) of the Mandarin question *ta¹ shi⁴ Li² Mei³ ma⁰* "Is she LiMei?". Dotted lines indicate syllable boundaries and the black solid line is the smooth curve obtained from GAM.

predicting pitch as a function of time. Accordingly, the dataset `mand` consists of the response variable `pitch` and the corresponding time points, `time`.

```
    pitch time
1 329.2815 0.16
2 329.7480 0.17
3 334.2271 0.18
4 340.9061 0.19
```

In R, to fit a GAM model, we use the `gam` function from the `mgcv` package (Wood, 2017). For the formula, we first specify the response variable, which is followed by the ~ symbol (which can be read as "modeled as a function of"), and that in turn is followed by the predictors. By applying the function `s()` to the predictor, we request the GAM to model pitch as a nonlinear smooth function of time. The simple model that we fit for this example is as follows.

```
mand.gam = gam(pitch ~ s(time), data = mand)
```

What the `s()` does is to build up wiggly curves (known as splines) from a set of simple wiggly curves called basis functions. By carefully assigning appropriate weights to basis functions, a wiggly trend in the data can be approximated as a weighted sum of basis functions.

The remainder of this chapter provides a tutorial on how to analyze phonetic data with GAMs. We present analyses for three example datasets, all of which address aspects of the phonetics of Taiwan Mandarin. Although these are not clinical data, the issues that arise in the analyses are similar to those that one might encounter when analyzing clinical data. For each analysis, we discuss the relevance of the methods that we illustrate for the analysis of clinical data.

The first dataset that we discuss contains response time data from an auditory priming experiment. With this dataset, we illustrate how to take into account subject-specific inter-trial dependencies, which can also be found in clinical experiments. For the second dataset, we look into the realizations of Mandarin high-level tones by different speaker groups in Taiwan. Like intensity, pitch contours vary with time. We will show how to work with numerical covariates, and how to take into account potential interactions with factorial predictors. The third dataset addresses the ongoing merging of two sets of sibilants in Taiwan Mandarin. As will be seen, GAMs can model response variables that vary not only with one single-dimensional predictor (e.g. time), but also with predictors of two or more dimensions (e.g. geographical coordinates of longitude and latitude, locations of sensors on the tongue in electromagnetic articulography, locations of electrodes in ERP studies, etc.).

Along with the analyses, we will introduce the basic concepts of GAMs. As the purpose of this tutorial is to illustrate how to use GAMs, we therefore focus primarily on application. It is also important to note that the approach that we take for the analyses presented here is exploratory, rather than confirmatory. One reason for this is that this allows us to introduce increasingly more intricate aspects of a GAM model step by step. The other reason is that the complexity of the data is such that it is difficult to predict in advance how exactly predictors interact and jointly shape a regression line or regression surface. Due to multiple testing inherent in exploratory data analyses, we will accept an effect as potentially replicable when its associate p value is less than 0.0001.

Example 1: Inter-trial dependencies

Individual variability is usually a major source of variance for behavioral data. This is true not only for non-clinical participants, but also for clinical ones. In the course of an experiment, subject responses are often differentially affected by factors such as familiarity, fatigue, or attention drift. Thus, in addition to effects induced by experimental manipulation, in the data there are also response patterns that are tied to individual subjects. These patterns are often nonlinear in time. By-subject random intercepts and slopes in the linear mixed model (LMM), therefore, are limited in this regard. The LMM can allow the intercept and slope of regression lines for individual subjects to vary, but it cannot handle the case in which functional relations are not linear but instead wiggly.

Sometimes the effects of central predictors of interest are also nonlinear. For example, lexical properties of the stimuli such as word frequency tend to have nonlinear effects on response times in lexicality decision tasks (Baayen et al., 2016). In clinical settings, it is also likely that some numeric predictors turn out to affect response variables in a nonlinear way. In longitudinal or cross-sectional studies where one traces the development or progress of clinical participants, age of participants, or the length of treatment received, can potentially have nonlinear effects on their performances. With GAMs, it is possible to discover whether nonlinear patterns are present in the data.

In the following example, we will be looking at response time data collected from an auditory priming experiment, conducted by Chuang (2017). The central question of this study is whether Taiwan Mandarin speakers recognize words with standard and variant pronunciations differently. Specifically, in Taiwan Mandarin, retroflex sounds (e.g. /ʂ/) undergo partial or complete deretroflexion, merging into their dental counterparts (e.g. /s/). Thus, while the standard pronunciation of the word *book* is [ʂu], the variant pronunciation of this word is [su]. The stimuli of this experiment were 30 retroflex-initial bisyllabic words which were produced either with retroflex or with deretroflexed pronunciations, coded as "standard" and "variant" respectively in the column `targetType` of the dataset `ret`. There were three priming conditions: the same word with retroflex pronunciation, the same word with deretroflexed pronunciation and a completely different word without any retroflex or dental sounds. In the `primeType` column, these conditions are referred to as "standard," "variant," and "control." To avoid the effect of speaker priming, primes and targets were produced by two different speakers. The `voice` column of `ret` specifies the speaker of the target word, "A" and "B." If the speaker of the target word is A, it also means that the speaker of the prime word is B and vice versa. Participants were instructed to perform auditory lexical decision on target words, and their response times (in millisecond) were recorded. In the `ret` dataset, only correct responses are included.

	subject	primeType	targetType	voice	RT	trial	word	targetP
1	S1	standard	variant	A	1062	1	shibai	0.3597897
2	S1	standard	standard	A	834	2	shanliang	0.4546521
3	S1	control	variant	A	1472	10	zhekou	0.3102893

We first excluded datapoints with RTs that are shorter than 300 ms and longer than 2500 ms, and log-transformed the raw RTs to ensure that model residuals better approximate normality. We used treatment coding, with "standard" as reference level for both `targetType` and `primeType`. For the baseline model, we fitted a GAM with `targetType`, `primeType` and `voice` as fixed-effect predictors. To take subject or item variability into account, we also included by-subject and by-word random intercepts. In GAMs, this is done by adding `bs = "re"` in the smooth term `s()`, where `"re"` stands for random effect. For this to work, it is essential that the pertinent random effect column in the dataset is encoded as a factor in R.

```
ret$subject = as.factor(ret$subject)
ret$word = as.factor(ret$word)
ret.gam0 = gam(logRT ~ targetType + primeType + voice +
                    s(subject, bs = "re") +
                    s(word, bs = "re"),
            data = ret)
```

A model summary is obtained as follows:

```
summary(ret.gam0)
```

The summary of model `ret.gam0` contains two parts.

```
Parametric coefficients:
                   Estimate Std. Error t value Pr(>|t|)
(Intercept)        6.822828   0.021024 324.527   <2e-16
targetTypevariant  0.075274   0.005840  12.888   <2e-16
primeTypecontrol   0.130702   0.007142  18.300   <2e-16
primeTypevariant  -0.012028   0.007131  -1.687   0.0918
voiceB             0.077066   0.005830  13.219   <2e-16

Approximate significance of smooth terms:
             edf Ref.df      F  p-value
s(subject) 45.94     47 42.990  < 2e-16
s(word)    22.60     29  3.609 2.22e-14


R-sq.(adj) =  0.516   Deviance explained = 52.9%
GCV = 0.023946   Scale est. = 0.023305   n = 2746
```

The first part of the summary reports parametric coefficients, just as in the summary of a linear regression model. According to this part of the summary, there is good evidence that RTs are longer if target words are produced with variant pronunciation (`targetTypevariant`). In addition, RTs are also longer when presented with a control prime (`primeTypecontrol`), because little priming can be induced by a totally different word. RTs however become shorter when prime words are produced with variant pronunciation (`primeTypevariant`), but the difference is not well supported. Finally, responses are slower for target words produced by speaker B (`voiceB`). This is due to the overall slower speaking rate of speaker B.

The second part of the summary reports statistics for the smooth terms. For this model, it is useful to have by-subject and by-word random intercepts, given that the p values for both effects are very small. The GCV score (0.0239) is an indication of the goodness of model fit. The lower the score, the better the model fit.

As a next step, we improve the model by taking further details of subject variability into account. Figure 10.3 displays RTs as a function of trial number in the experiment, for each subject separately. We can see that in addition to differences in intercepts, how RTs develop in the course of the experiment also differs substantially across subjects. S48, for example, becomes faster as the experiment proceeds. By contrast, S19 has the tendency to become slower. Staying for now with the LMM, we include by-subject random slopes for trial. To avoid that `trial` dominates prediction accuracy because of its larger scale as compared to other predictors, we first scaled it and created a new numeric variable `trialScaled`. The second smooth term in the formula of this model requests the by-subject random slopes for trial.

```
ret$trialScaled = as.numeric(scale(ret$trial, center = TRUE,
scale = TRUE))
ret.gam0a = gam(logRT ~ targetType + primeType + voice +
                s(subject, bs = "re") +
                s(subject, trialScaled, bs = "re") +
                s(word, bs = "re"),
            data = ret)
```

The GCV score of this model (0.0221) is lower than that of the previous model, indicating improved model fit. However, Figure 10.3 also shows that RT development is notably non-linear. For instance, S39 exhibits a convex pattern, whereas a concave pattern is found for S6. We therefore need **factor smooths** if we want our model to be more precise. A factor smooth fits a wiggly curve for each individual subject, and provides the nonlinear equivalent to the combination of random intercepts and random slopes in the linear mixed model. In model

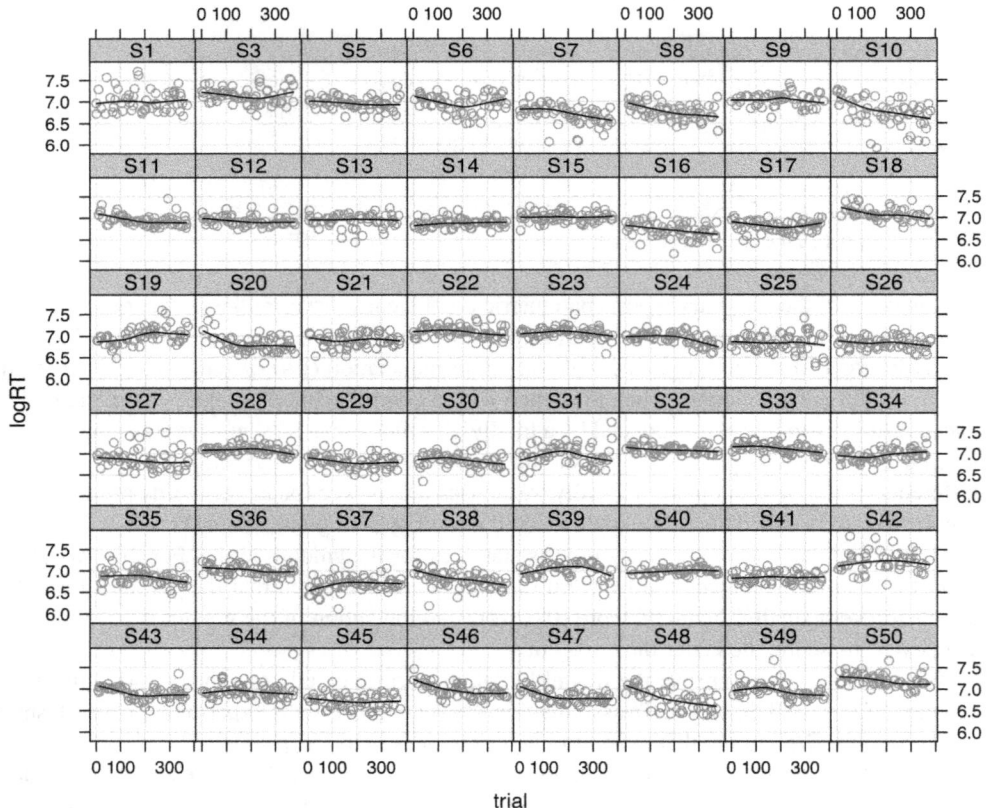

Figure 10.3 RTs across trials for each subject.

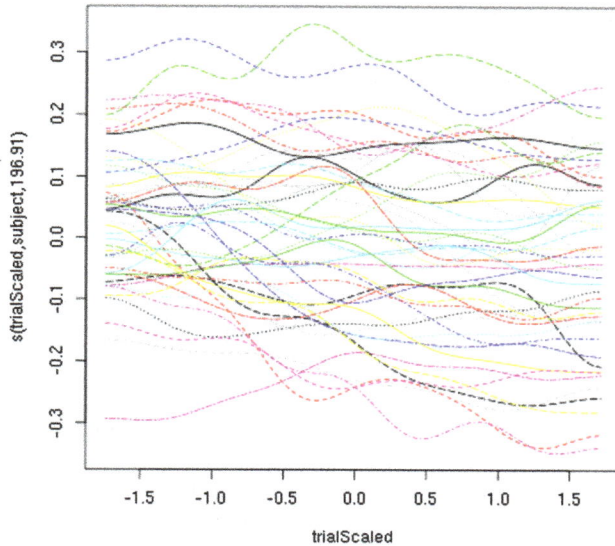

Figure 10.4 By-subject factor smooths from `ret.gam1`.

`ret.gam1`, a factor smooth was requested by specifying `bs = "fs"`. The directive `m = 1` enables shrinkage for the basis function for the linear tilted line. Thus, if there is no evidence of different linear slopes for the individual subjects, the coefficients of the linear basis function can be shrunk down all the way to zero. In this case, subject variability only involves intercepts, and the factor smooth has become functionally equivalent to a random effect with by-subject random intercepts.

```
ret.gam1 = gam(logRT ~ targetType + primeType + voice +
                    s(trialScaled, subject, bs = "fs", m = 1) +
                    s(word, bs = "re"),
               data = ret)
```

Figure 10.4 presents the fitted smooths for the subjects, all of which are clearly nonlinear across trials. The lower GCV score (0.0215) of this model indicates that the inclusion of the factor smooth has improved model fit.

Next we asked whether there are interactions among the factorial predictors. Of specific interest is whether RTs to variant target words are disparately influenced by different primes and different voices. We therefore built our next model including an interaction between `targetType` and `primeType`, and in addition an interaction between `targetType` and `voice`.

```
ret.gam2 = gam(logRT ~ targetType * primeType +
                    targetType * voice +
                    s(trialScaled, subject, bs = "fs", m = 1) +
                    s(word, bs="re"),
               data = ret)
---
```

```
Parametric coefficients:
                         Estimate Std. Error t value Pr(>|t|)
(Intercept)              6.838974   0.020115 339.990  < 2e-16
targetTypevariant        0.054803   0.010727   5.109 3.49e-07
primeTypecontrol         0.127271   0.009180  13.864  < 2e-16
primeTypevariant        -0.030184   0.009121  -3.309 0.000948
voiceB                   0.061979   0.008382   7.394 1.92e-13
targetTypevariant:
primeTypecontrol         0.005855   0.013186   0.444 0.657071
targetTypevariant:
primeTypevariant         0.037840   0.013173   2.873 0.004104
targetTypevariant:voiceB 0.015086   0.010781   1.399 0.161859
```

Model summary suggests that there is some hint of evidence that an upward adjustment of the intercept is needed when both the target and prime words are presented with variant pronunciations. The interaction between `targetType` and `voice`, on the other hand, does not seem to be necessary. Given that the GCV score (0.02149) remains practically the same as that of the model without interactions (`ret.gam1`), we should stay wary about the interpretation of these interaction effects.

In the next model we investigated the effect of a numeric predictor, `targetP`. This measure attempts to estimate the probability that a retroflex pronunciation activates the intended semantic field. When retroflexes are deretroflexed (e.g. /ʂu/→[su]), it is inevitable that more lexical candidates will emerge, because now in addition to words beginning with /ʂu/, words beginning with /su/ will be compatible with the acoustic input as well. Thus, the probability of obtaining the correct semantics is usually smaller for variant pronunciations than for standard pronunciations.

To explore whether the effect of targetP might be nonlinear, we included it in a smooth term. Since the interaction between `targetType` and `voice` was not significant, we left it out in the model shown here.

```
ret.gam3 = gam(logRT ~ targetType * primeType + voice +
                       s(targetP) +
                       s(trialScaled, subject, bs = "fs", m = 1) +
                       s(word, bs = "re"),
               data = ret)
---
```

```
Approximate significance of smooth terms:
                           edf  Ref.df     F  p-value
s(targetP)               5.078   5.816 2.745   0.0183
s(trialScaled,subject) 197.611 431.000 6.797  < 2e-16
s(word)                 21.736  29.000 3.581 2.53e-16
```

According to model summary, the effect of targetP is nonlinear, because the `edf`, denoting **effective degrees of freedom**, is larger than one. Before explaining `edf`, let's first visualize the effect. This can be done by using the `plot` function, as shown below. The directive `select` = 1 requests the first effect in the summary table for smooth terms to be plotted. To zoom in on

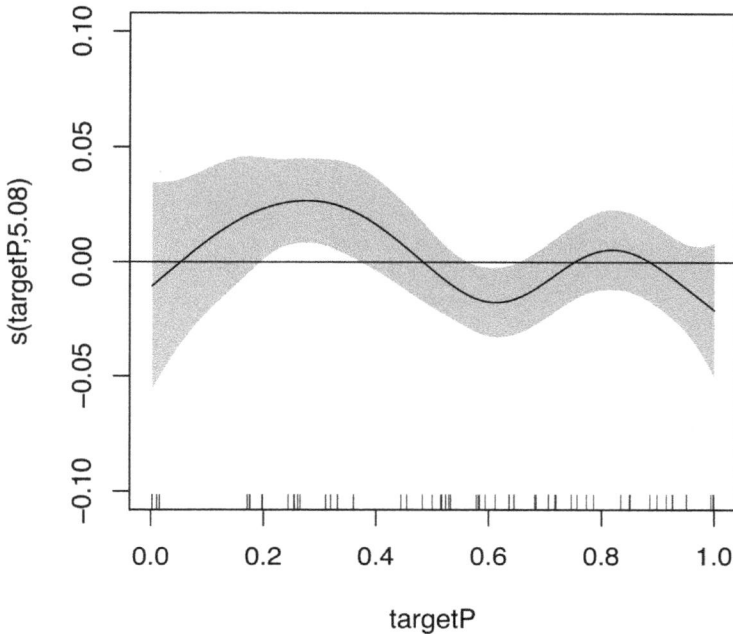

Figure 10.5 The effect of targetP from `ret.gam3`.

the effect, we set the range of the y-axis between –0.1 and 0.1. In addition, we added shading to the area of the confidence interval, and finally a horizontal line at zero.

```
plot(ret.gam3, select = 1, ylim = c(-0.1, 0.1), shade = TRUE)
abline(h=0)
```

As can be seen in Figure 10.5, the effect is indeed nonlinear, with a tendency of RTs to become shorter as the probability of obtaining the intended meaning increases. Note that the `plot` function visualizes the partial effect of `targetP`, i.e. the population intercept and the effects of other predictors are not included. This is why the curve is centered around the line y = 0.

Returning to the discussion of edf, we have mentioned previously that wiggly curves are modeled by assigning different weights to a set of basis functions. Usually approximating a more wiggly curve requires a larger number of basis functions. Unrestricted use of basis functions, however, may lead to overfitting. In fact, in such cases, models become unnecessarily complex. Under the assumption that simple models are to be preferred over complex ones, GAMs incorporate a mechanism that penalizes the weights of basis functions. Penalization may take the weight of a basis function completely to zero. The edf is the sum of the proportions of the unpenalized weights that are retained in the penalized weights. Since a larger edf typically implies more basis functions are used, its magnitude is a rough indicator for the degree of wiggliness of the smooth.

Given that the support for the effect of targetP is only minimal ($p = 0.018$), we need to be cautious and refrain ourselves from jumping into conclusions. We therefore went on to further examine whether targetP interacts with other factors. In the next model, we added the directive `by = voice` to the smooth term of `s(targetP)`. This requests two separate smooths, one for each voice.

```
ret.gam4 = gam(logRT ~ targetType * primeType + voice +
                    s(targetP, by = voice) +
                    s(trialScaled, subject, bs = "fs", m = 1) +
                    s(word, bs = "re"),
            data = ret)
---
                       edf   Ref.df      F  p-value
s(targetP):voiceA    4.327    5.100  1.404  0.22028
s(targetP):voiceB    7.545    8.313  3.010  0.00212
```

The model summary suggests that, apparently, the effect of targetP is only present for voice B, but not for voice A. This explains why the effect of targetP is not well supported when both voices are considered together in model `ret.gam3`. The visualization of the two effects is presented in Figure 10.6. In the left panel, the confidence interval always includes zero, indicating that there is no significant effect anywhere. By contrast, in the right panel, there is only a small portion of the curve where the confidence interval includes zero, suggesting that the effect is better supported.

Although now the downward trend for voice B is clearer, the curve is still uninterpretably wiggly. In fact, the high degree of wiggliness is likely to be a technical artifact. The values of targetP are sparsely distributed, as can be seen from the rugs on the x-axis. Given that there are only 30 target words, and that each word comes with two pronunciations (standard *vs.* variant), there are at most 60 unique values for targetP. When there are many datapoints with the same targetP value, as is the case in the present experiment in which 48 subjects responded to each target token, the GAM is presented with substantial evidence about where the mean should be for each stimulus. As a consequence, it does its best to bring the predictions as close as possible to the observed values. This then leads to overfitting. To remedy this, we brought down the

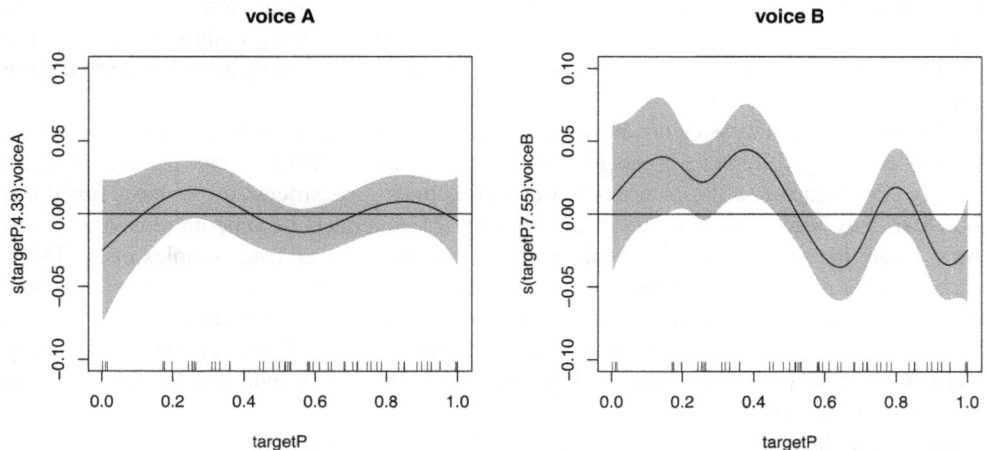

Figure 10.6 The effects of targetP for voice A (left) and voice B (right) from `ret.gam4`.

number of basis functions used to fit the curves. The default number of basis functions is ten. In the following model, we set this number to four by specifying k = 4.

```
ret.gam5 = gam(logRT ~ targetType * primeType + voice +
                  s(targetP, by = voice, k = 4) +
                  s(trialScaled, subject, bs = "fs", m = 1) +
                  s(word, bs = "re"),
            data = ret)
---
                      edf Ref.df      F  p-value
s(targetP):voiceA    1.00      1  0.031  0.86110
s(targetP):voiceB    1.00      1  8.658  0.00328
```

Now the effects of targetP for both voices are practically linear, as shown in Figure 10.7. The linearity of the effects can also be read off their edfs, both of which are equal to one. Because the first two basis functions of the spline are a horizontal line and a tilted line (the counterparts of the intercept and slope of a standard linear regression model), an edf value close to or equal to one means that in addition to the intercept (the first basis function, which is already represented in the parametric part of the summary), only one additional basis function is needed, which is the basis function for the tilted line. In other words, the GAM has detected, when restrained from overfitting, that the effect is linear rather than nonlinear.

In summary, the analysis of this dataset illustrated how to use factor smooths to model the nonlinear random effect for individual subjects. In addition, we introduced how to request smooths for different levels within a given factorial factor. We also noted that we should be cautious about smooths that are excessively wiggly, as they might be artifacts resulting from sparsely represented numerical predictors in repeated measurement experimental designs. This issue can be addressed by adjusting the number of basis functions.

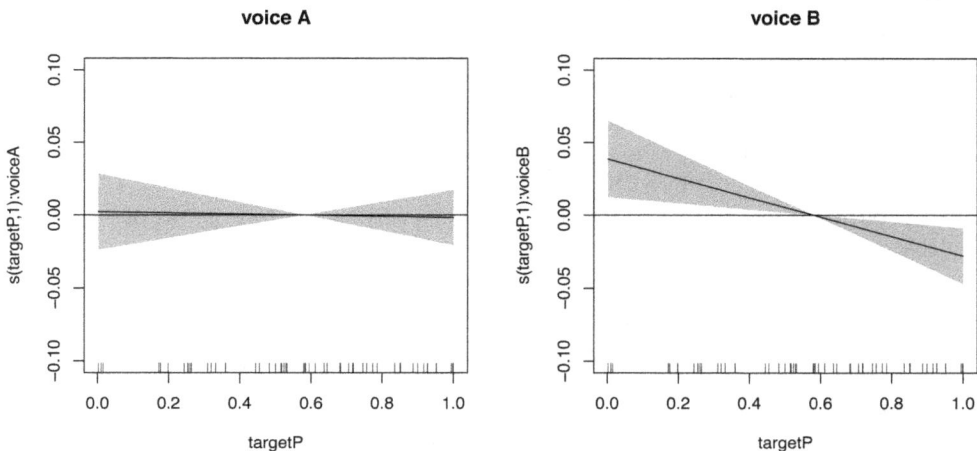

Figure 10.7 The effects of targetP for voice A (left) and voice B (right) from ret.gam5.

Example 2: Time-varying response variables

In phonetics, a lot of features that we measure change over time. These include pitch, intensity and formants. Tongue positions traced by electromagnetic articulography, and signals recorded by EEG electrodes are also dynamic in nature. As discussed previously in the analysis of the introductory clinical example, when it comes to these measurements, it has been a common practice to pre-process the data, e.g. by calculating the mean, range, or maximum/minimum values, and then use these aggregated data as input for statistical analyses. By doing so, we however run the risk of missing out on potentially interesting aspects of the data. For example, participants with dysarthria might have intensity profiles for stressed and unstressed syllables that are very different from those of control speakers, which might be characterized by less abrupt changes in intensity. Fine-grained details such as these cannot be brought to light by the traditional ways of data analysis.

The dataset of the next example consists of the F0 measurements of the high-level tone, or Tone 1 (henceforth T1) of Mandarin. Speakers were sampled from two regions in Taiwan, Taipei and Taichung, which are two metropolitan cities located in northern and central Taiwan, respectively. Of interest is whether T1 realizations differ between the two speaker groups. A clinical parallel to the present between-group comparison is a comparison between a control group of healthy speakers and a group of clinical participants. With the present dataset, we will illustrate how to model wiggly curves for different speaker groups (the levels of a factorial predictor), as well as how to ascertain whether, and if so, where, the contours of two groups are significantly different. In other words, we can use GAMs to model the curves of any response variable separately for control and clinical groups. We can also set the model up in such a way that we can compare two curves directly and find out where in the curves the two speaker groups differ significantly. Finally, we will discuss how to take the variances of different speaker groups, in addition to the means, into account in GAMs. From the perspective of clinical phonetics, it is conceivable that speakers with an impairment, due to lack of control, produce data with greater variability as compared to a control group. Failure to take such differences in the variance into account may introduce inflated *p* values. GAMs provide a flexible way for dealing with unequal variances.

For the current dataset, Fon (2007) recorded 25 native speakers of Taiwan Mandarin. Thirteen speakers (six males, seven females) were from Taipei, and 12 (six males, six females) were from Taichung. Stimuli were 24 bisyllabic words, and the target T1 syllables occur in either the first (P1) or the second (P2) position of the bisyllabic words. The adjacent preceding or following syllable carried one of the four lexical tones (T1, T2, T3, T4). In total, the manipulation of position and adjacent tone gave rise to eight different tonal contexts (specified in the column context). By way of example, the word *bing³gan¹* "cookie" has the target syllable *gan¹* in P2, and is preceded by a T3 syllable, and hence the context coding is "P2.T3." To capture the pitch contour of T1, the F0 values at ten equally-spaced time points of each target syllable were measured.

	subject	sex	location	word	tarSyll	position	adTone	context	time	pitch
1	CWQ	M	TAICHUNG	bandai	ban	P1	T4	P1.T4	1	161.8738
2	CWQ	M	TAICHUNG	bandai	ban	P1	T4	P1.T4	2	159.1713
3	CWQ	M	TAICHUNG	bandai	ban	P1	T4	P1.T4	3	156.3541

Figure 10.8 presents T1 realizations in the eight different contexts by the four speaker groups (broken down by sex and location). In general, females have higher pitch values than

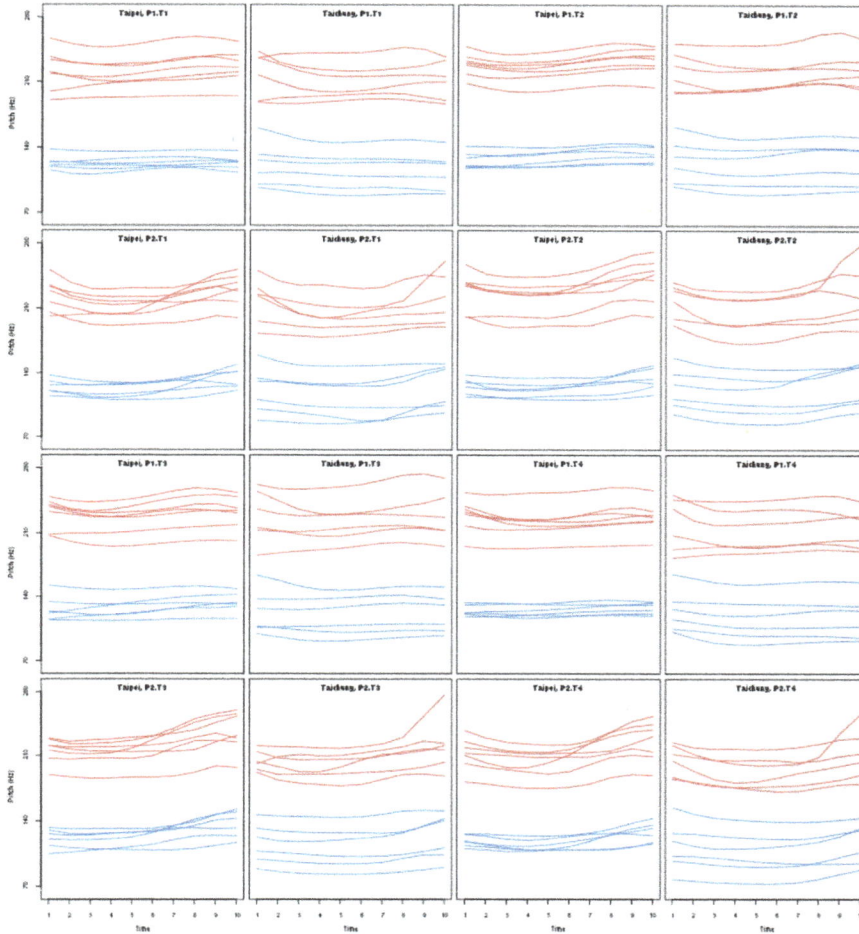

Figure 10.8 T1 contours of different contexts for individual male (blue) and female (red) subjects.

males, as expected. Interestingly, T1 is not really a "level" tone as canonically described. Instead, it is featured by a final rise, as is clearly visible especially for females and for word-final positions (P2).

Before fitting models, we centered `time`. Time is a numeric variable ranging from one to ten in normalized time. Centering was implemented because the model intercept, the y-coordinate where the regression line hits the y-axis, is not interpretable, since pitch at time 0 does not make sense. We centered `time` so that the intercept now will represent the mean pitch in the middle of the target syllables. We fitted our first model with `sex`, `location` and `context` as fixed-effect factors, along with a smooth for the variable of scaled time (`timeScaled`). In addition, we also requested a by-subject factor smooth for `timeScaled` (i.e. a wiggly line for each subject) and random intercepts for word. Also note that here we used `bam` instead of `gam`. This is because when working with a large dataset, `bam` works more efficiently at minimum cost of accuracy. In addition, with the directive `discrete` set to TRUE, covariates are binned in a mathematically principled way to enable faster estimation of the model's coefficients.

```
tone$timeScaled = as.numeric(scale(tone$time, center =
TRUE, scale = FALSE))
tone.gam0 = bam(pitch ~ sex + location + context +
                    s(timeScaled) +
                    s(timeScaled, subject, bs = "fs", m = 1) +
                    s(word, bs="re"),
              data = tone, discrete = TRUE)
---
```

```
Parametric coefficients:
                   Estimate Std. Error t value Pr(>|t|)
(Intercept)         123.505       6.337  19.489  < 2e-16
sexF                 98.017       7.156  13.698  < 2e-16
locationTAICHUNG     -8.739       7.156  -1.221   0.2220
contextP2.T1         -1.196       1.163  -1.028   0.3040
contextP1.T2          6.371       1.163   5.476 4.52e-08
contextP2.T2          2.295       1.163   1.973   0.0486
contextP1.T3          7.601       1.163   6.533 6.99e-11
contextP2.T3         -1.943       1.163  -1.670   0.0950
contextP1.T4          2.108       1.163   1.812   0.0701
contextP2.T4         -9.670       1.163  -8.312  < 2e-16
```

```
Approximate significance of smooth terms:
                        edf  Ref.df       F  p-value
s(timeScaled)         5.677   6.567   27.66  < 2e-16
s(timeScaled,subject) 119.356 225.000 150.77        1
s(word)              13.698  16.000    5.95 3.89e-16
```

```
R-sq.(adj) =  0.973   Deviance explained = 97.4%
fREML =  21572   Scale est. = 73.039    n = 6000
```

According to model summary, pitches have to be adjusted upward for females, unsurprisingly. While the effect of location is not supported, context shows up with several well-supported contrasts. With respect to the smooth terms, the overall contour of T1, as shown in Figure 10.9, indeed has a dipping curvature. The by-subject factor smooth, on the other hand, is not significant, indicating that inter-subject variability is not substantial.

There is, however, one serious problem for this model. When we apply the autocorrelation function to the residuals of the model, we obtain the plot presented in the left panel of Figure 10.10.

```
acf(resid(tone.gam0))
```

It suggests that there is still structure remaining in the residuals, violating the crucial modeling assumption that the residuals are independent of each other. That is, residuals at time t are correlated with residuals at preceding time steps t_lag. At shorter lags, autocorrelations are strongest. This autocorrelation is inevitable, since given physical constraints, the vibration of vocal folds at time t cannot be completely independent of that at time $t-1$. One strategy to deal

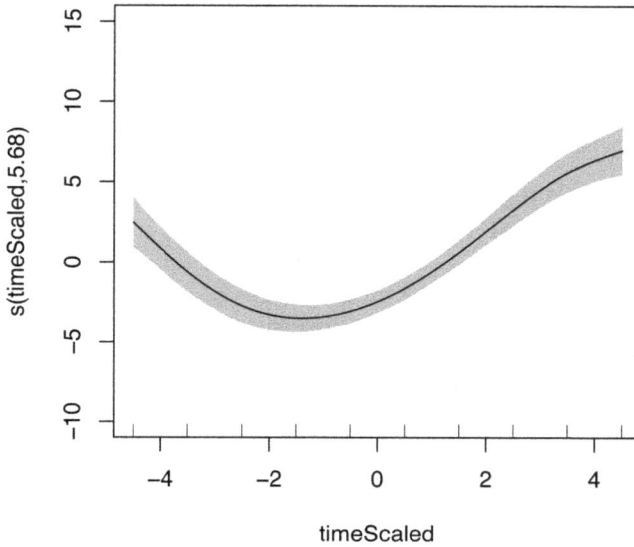

Figure 10.9 Partial effect of timeScaled from `tone.gam0`.

with autocorrelated residuals is to incorporate an AR(1) process in the model. This correction process assumes that the error at time t is the sum of a proportion ρ of the preceding error at time $t-1$ and Gaussian noise. Adding an AR(1) component to our model requires that we add a further variable to the dataframe. The required variable specifies the beginning of each production (i.e. time 1) with the logical value `TRUE`, and all the others with the value `FALSE`. We now fit a new model with the AR(1) process incorporated, setting `rho` to 0.8, the approximate value at lag 1 in the left panel of Figure 10.10.

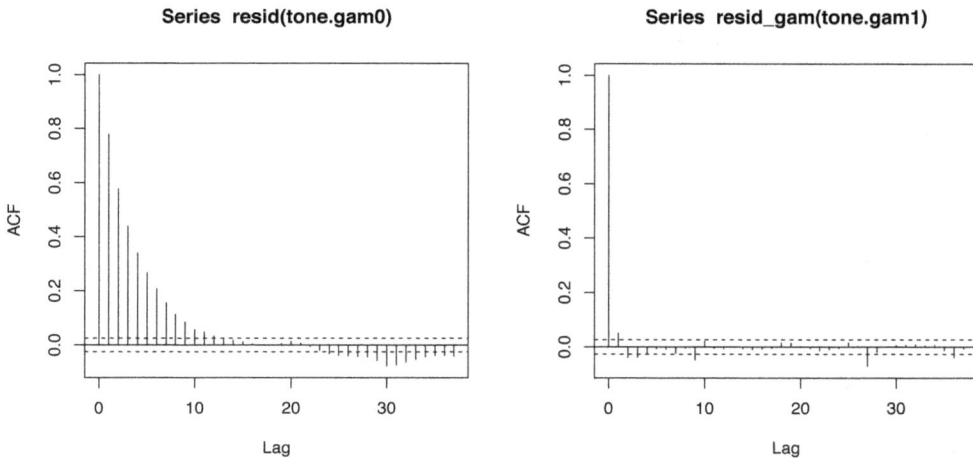

Figure 10.10 Autocorrelation functions fitted to models `tone.gam0` (left) and `tone.gam1` (right). Lag indicates the number of time steps preceding a given time t.

```
tone$AR.start = FALSE
tone$AR.start[tone$time==1] = TRUE
tone.gam1 = bam(pitch ~ sex + location + context +
                        s(timeScaled) +
                        s(timeScaled, subject, bs = "fs", m = 1) +
                        s(word, bs = "re"),
                data = tone, discrete = TRUE,
                AR.start = tone$AR.start, rho = 0.8)
```

To inspect the residuals, this time we used the `resid_gam` function from the `itsadug` package (van Rij et al., 2017). This function discounts the part of residuals that has been taken care of by the AR(1) process.

As shown in the right panel of Figure 10.10, autocorrelation in the errors has been successfully eliminated.

```
acf(resid_gam(tone.gam1))
```

To further examine the effect of `context`, we fitted a new model and requested a separate smooth for each context. In order to compare the model fit of this model with that of the previous model, we used the method of maximum likelihood estimation with the directive `method = "ML"`. It is important that we cannot use the method of (fast) restricted maximum likelihood estimation, i.e. (f)REML, if the models to be compared have different fixed-effect structures.

```
tone.gam2 = bam(pitch ~ sex + location + context +
                        s(timeScaled, by = context) +
                        s(timeScaled, subject, bs = "fs", m = 1) +
                        s(word, bs = "re"),
                data = tone, AR.start = tone$AR.start, rho = 0.8,
                method = "ML")
```

After also refitting the previous model with maximum likelihood estimation, we can now compare the model fits.

```
compareML(tone.gam1, tone.gam2)
---
Chi-square test of ML scores
-----
      Model     Score Edf Difference      Df  p.value Sig.
1 tone.gam1 16925.54  15
2 tone.gam2 16578.79  29     346.752  14.000  < 2e-16  ***
```

Model fit has improved substantially by allowing each combination of position and lexical tone to have its own smooth (as indicated by the lower ML score). Figure 10.11 clarifies that T1 is realized very differently when in P1 compared to when in P2. Furthermore, tonal contours are also clearly depending on the tones of preceding and following syllables.

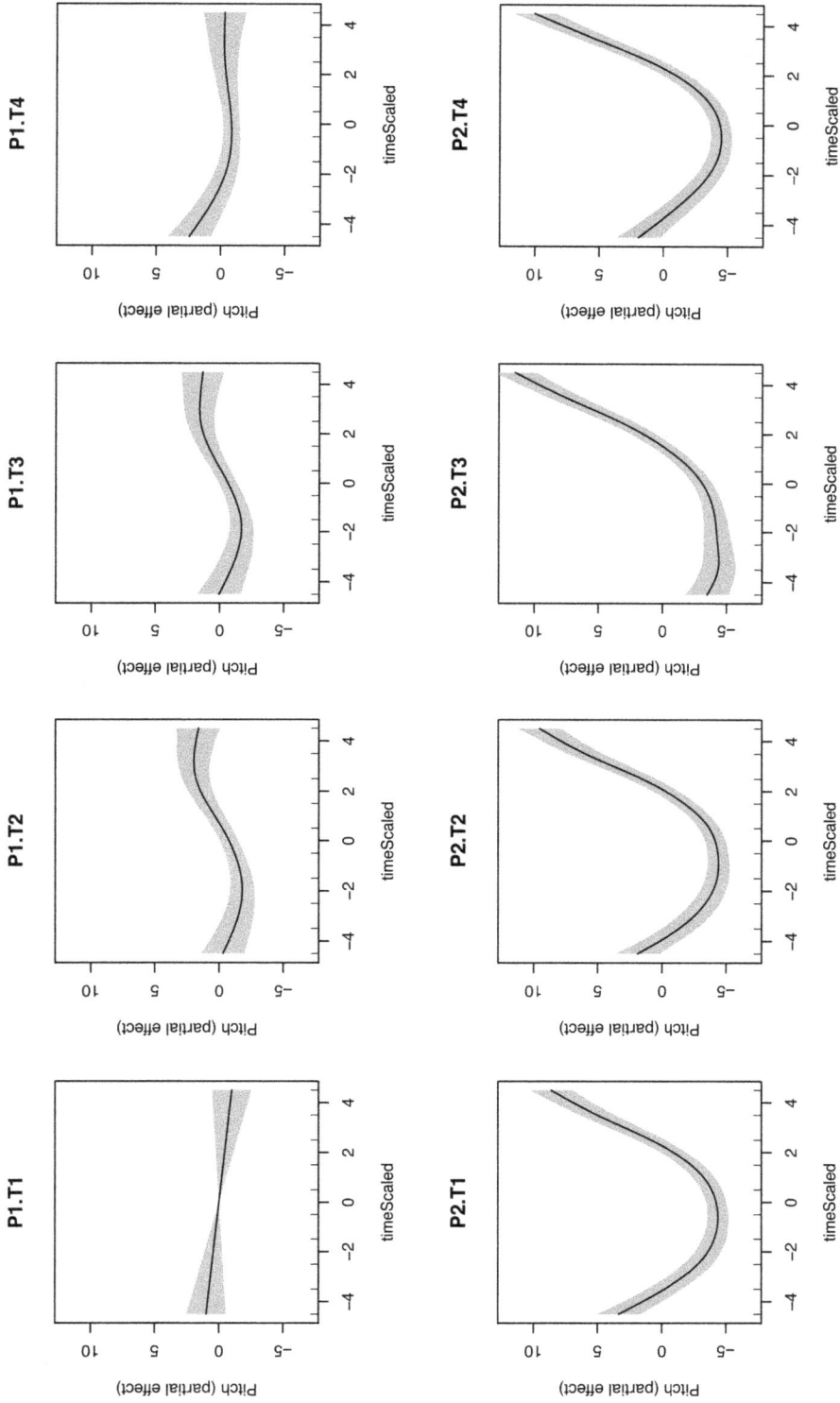

Figure 10.11 Partial effects of pitch contours for different contexts from tone.gam2.

Although T1 looks very different for several of the eight contexts, it can however not be straightforwardly inferred from the model where pairs of contours are significantly different. For example, in the contexts of "P2.T2" and "P2.T3" (lower mid panels, Figure 10.11), the T1 contour in the "P2.T3" context appears to start lower than that in "P2.T2," suggesting a clear influence from preceding tones. However, we do not know whether this difference is statistically supported. To address this issue, we can build a **difference curve**.

By way of example, to zoom in on this particular contrast, we first subsetted the data to include only the pertinent datapoints. We then transformed the variable context into a numeric variable, with the reference level "P2.T2" coded as 0 and the contrast level "P2.T3" coded as 1. A new model was fitted, in which we included not only a smooth for the general effect of timeScaled, but also a smooth for the difference between the reference and the contrast levels. What this second smooth term does is to provide a corrective curve for the datapoints that fall under the contrast level. In this way, we obtain a difference curve for the two levels.

```
toneP2 = droplevels(tone[tone$context=="P2.T2"
|tone$context=="P2.T3", ])
toneP2$contextNum = as.numeric(toneP2$context)-1
toneP2.gam = bam(pitch ~ sex + location +
                s(timeScaled) +
                s(timeScaled, by = contextNum) +
                s(timeScaled, subject, bs = "fs", m = 1) +
                s(word, bs = "re"),
            data = toneP2, discrete = TRUE,
            AR.start = toneP2$AR.start, rho = 0.8)
```

The difference curve for the present example is shown in the left panel of Figure 10.12. T1 contours are always lower when following T3 than when following T2: the entire curve lies under the x-axis. To better understand the difference curve, we plotted the fitted values for the two contexts in the right panel of Figure 10.12. The difference is greater at the beginning and gradually attenuates toward the end, which also indicates that the difference decreases

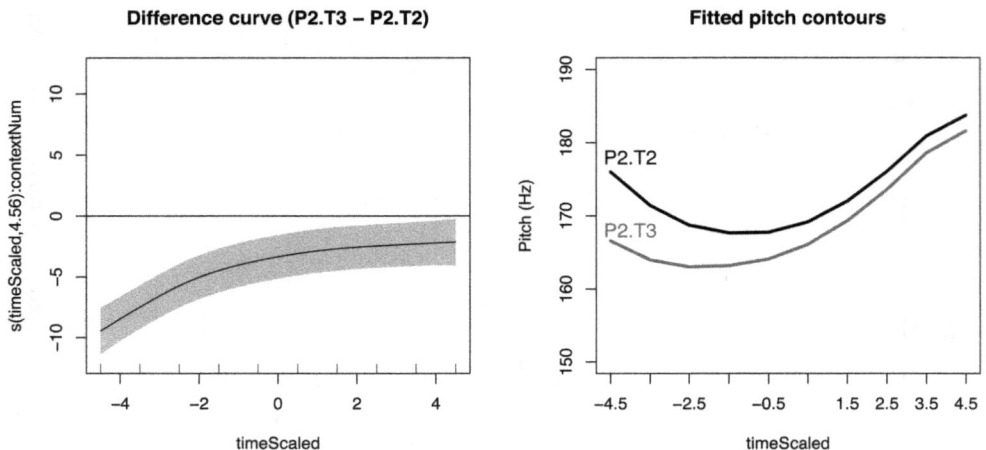

Figure 10.12 Difference curve between "P2.T2" and "P2.T3" contexts (left) and the predicted pitch values for the two contexts (right) obtained from toneP2.gam.

Difference curve (P1.T3 – P1.T2)   **Fitted pitch contours**

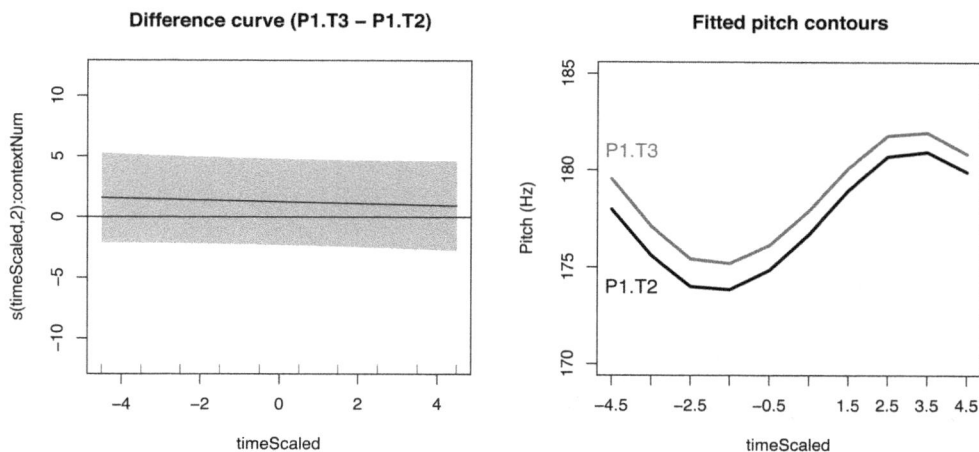

Figure 10.13 Difference curve between "P1.T2" and "P1.T3" contexts (left) and the predicted pitch values for the two contexts (right) obtained from model `toneP1.gam`.

over time. Importantly, the confidence interval of the difference curve never contains zero, suggesting that even at the endpoint in time, the small remaining difference is still significant.

With the same method, we can also examine whether the contours of "P1.T2" and "P1.T3" are significantly different. Detailed code is provided in the supplementary material. The difference curve (left panel, Figure 10.13) is a straight line above zero, since "P1.T3" has higher predicted pitch values than "P1.T2" for all time points (right). Notably the confidence interval of the difference curve always contains zero, a clear indicator that there is no real difference between these two contexts.

In addition to the effect of context, we were interested in variation in different subject groups. Thus, we further asked whether the effect of context interacts with sex or location. The next model now has two additional interactions: one between `sex` and `context`, and the other between `location` and `context`.

```
tone.gam3 = bam(pitch ~ context * (sex + location) +
                s(timeScaled, by = context) +
                s(timeScaled, subject, bs = "fs", m = 1) +
                s(word, bs = "re"),
            data = tone, AR.start = tone$AR.start,
            rho = 0.8, method = "ML")
```

Using `compareML()`, we observed a substantial improvement of model fit. Including by-sex or by-location smooths for each context, however, did not significantly improve model fit. This clarifies that in terms of tonal shape, we do not have sufficient statistical evidence supporting cross-dialect or cross-gender variation.

So far `tone.gam3` is our best model. But now we have to subject `tone.gam3` to model criticism, to clarify whether this model is actually appropriate for our data. We first checked whether residuals of this model follow a normal distribution using a quantile-quantile plot.

```
qq.gam(gam.tone3)
```

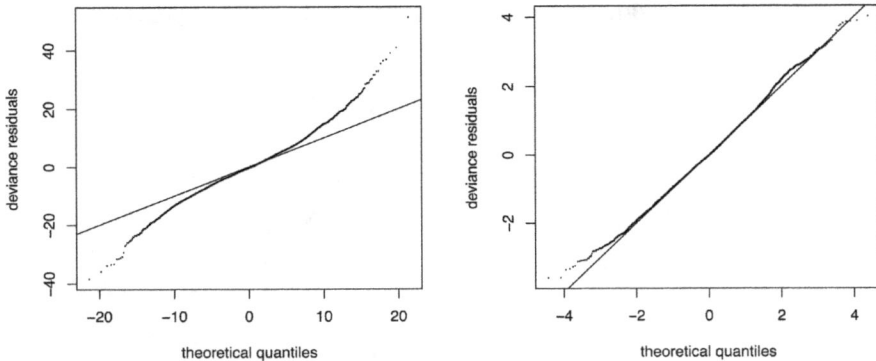

Figure 10.14 Quantile-quantile plots for the residuals of models `tone.gam3` and `tone.gam3a`.

This plot is presented in the left panel of Figure 10.14. Ideally, the residuals should fall on the black solid line, an indication that they follow a normal distribution. However, we see that the distribution of the residuals clearly has two heavy tails, indicative of a t distribution. We therefore modeled the data with a scaled-t distribution, which transforms the residuals back to normality. In the model specification we thus added `family = "scat"`, which gave us `tone.gam3a`:

```
tone.gam3a = bam(pitch ~ context * (sex + location) +
                    s(timeScaled, by = context) +
                    s(timeScaled, subject, bs = "fs", m = 1) +
                    s(word, bs = "re"),
              data = tone, AR.start = tone$AR.start,
              rho = 0.8, method = "ML", family = "scat")
```

The quantile-quantile plot for the residuals of `tone.gam3a` is presented in the right panel of Figure 10.14. It is clear that now the distribution of errors is much closer to a normal distribution.

A further way to carry out model criticism is to run the function `gam.check()`, which provides further useful information about residuals. For example, Figure 10.15 presents one of the plots output by `gam.check()`. It is clear that the residuals cluster into two groups. Given that `sex` is the most powerful linear predictor, the two clusters could roughly be considered as belonging to males and females. This scatterplot tells us that residuals spread out more for females (cluster on the right) than for males (cluster on the left). In other words, the model is still problematic, as it violates the assumption of homogeneity of variance for residuals. Indeed, as also shown in Figure 10.8, Taipei males in particular, show much less variability than Taichung males and females in general.

GAMs can directly model the variance, in addition to the mean. This can be achieved by using the Gaussian location-scale model, with the specification of `family = "gaulss"`. Since we are now modeling not only the mean but also the variance, we need to specify two formulae, one for each. Combined into a list, the first formula is similar to the one of model `tone.gam3`. The second formula is for the variance, which includes an interaction between `sex` and `location`. We also removed the random effect of by-subject factor smooth in the first formula, because subject variability coincides with the effect of `sex` × `location` on variances to a substantial extent.

Resids vs. linear pred.

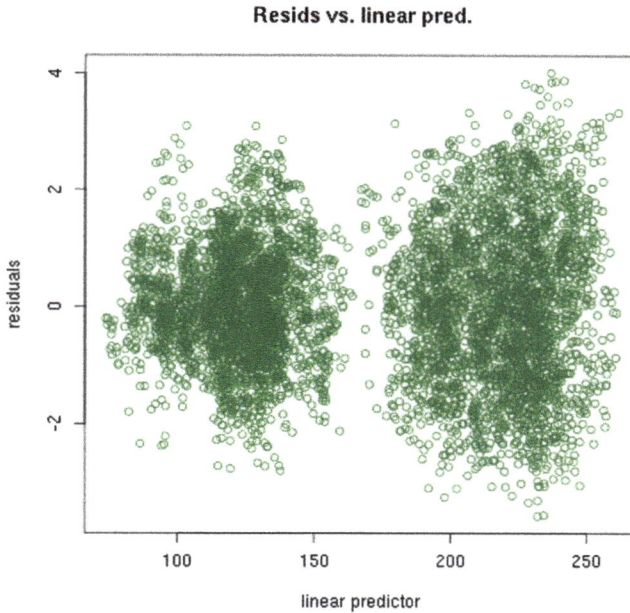

Figure 10.15 One of the output plots given by gam.check() for tone.gam3a.

```
tone.gam4 = gam(list(pitch ~ context * (sex + location) +
                     s(timeScaled, by = context) +
                     s(word, bs = "re"),
                ~ sex * location),
           data = tone, family = "gaulss")
---
```

```
Parametric coefficients:
                        Estimate Std. Error z value Pr(>|z|)
(Intercept)            123.68768    0.78478 157.608  < 2e-16
contextP2.T1             1.80746    1.10982   1.629 0.103396
...                          ...        ...     ...      ...
(Intercept).1            2.27445    0.01878 121.100  < 2e-16
sexF.1                   0.59782    0.02565  23.308  < 2e-16
locationTAICHUNG.1       0.81179    0.02657  30.557  < 2e-16
sexF:locationTAICHUNG.1 -0.62281    0.03687 -16.891  < 2e-16
```

The summary of the parametric predictors now contains two parts. The first part presents the results for modeling the mean, which is similar to the results of model tone.gam3. The second part is the results for modeling the variance. All three predictors reach significance, confirming our observation that the variance indeed differs across speaker groups. The downside of using the Gaussian location-scale model, however, is that autocorrelation is no longer under control. Here we have to wait for further development of GAMM theory and implementation.

In summary, the analyses of pitch contours for this dataset illustrated how GAMs can be used to model time series of acoustic measurements. In particular, we addressed the issue of

129

autocorrelation. We also introduced difference curves, which are useful to track the difference between the curves of two contrast levels. Finally, we showed how model criticism can lead to the selection of a different "family" to fine-tune the model better.

Example 3: Interacting covariates

While some response variables vary with time, as shown in the previous tone example, others vary across location. Unlike time, which is represented by one numeric predictor, location has to be represented by at least two numeric predictors, e.g. x and y coordinates. Thus, instead of wiggly curves, now we have to deal with wiggly three-dimensional surfaces. A straightforward application of this in phonetics is the study of dialectal variation. Speakers of the same language but from different locations often pronounce words differently. To investigate how pronunciation variations are distributed geographically, we can use GAMs to predict pronunciation by fitting a nonlinear surface projected from geographical coordinates, i.e. longitude and latitude.

In clinical phonetics, more and more attention is directed to the issue of language variation and its potential impact on clinical assessment and treatment (see Chapters 7 and 8 for detailed discussion). The technique introduced here provides a tool that can be used not only to study dialectal variation, but also to study the consequences of dialectal variation for the speech of geographically diversified control and clinical speaker groups. Other applications within clinical phonetics are the positions of sensors on the tongue in electromagnetic articulography. For instance, when sensor positions on the midsaggital plane are considered as a function of time, then tongue height can be modeled with a regression surface predicted from sensor location and time, while contrasting one or more clinical speaker groups with a control group (for an example of such an analysis, see Tomaschek et al., 2018).

As mentioned previously, retroflex sibilants are merging with dental sibilants in Taiwan Mandarin. However, the degree of merging is heterogeneous across Taiwan. In some areas, the retroflex-dental distinction still persists, whereas in other areas, sibilants are merged to a greater or lesser extent. In order to investigate how sibilant realizations differ geographically, a total of 323 participants from 117 different locations of Taiwan were recruited (Chuang et al., 2019). As shown in Figure 10.16, a large number of the participants are from the north, comprising the urban and suburban areas of Taipei, the capital city. From central to southern Taiwan, we only had participants from the western side of the country (between the two big cities of Taichung and Kaohsiung). This is because the eastern part is mountainous and sparsely populated. For each geographical location, we obtained its longitude and latitude coordinates.

Stimuli were 15 retroflex-initial and 15 dental-initial words. The production of these words was elicited by means of a picture-naming task. For each sibilant, we measured its centroid frequency, which was calculated based on a 30-ms spectral slice extracted from the middle of the frication part of the sibilant. Centroid frequency is generally considered a good index for sibilants' place of articulation: the more anterior the articulation, the higher the centroid frequency. Thus, dental articulation results in higher mean centroid frequency values compared to retroflex articulation. The pertinent information can be found in the dataset `mer`.

```
  Subject Word gender   vowel sibilant centfreq longitude latitude minflu
1      S1   W1      m unrounded    D  6310.199  121.5717 25.03062      6
2      S2   W1      m unrounded    D  5245.757  121.4871 25.06282      1
3      S3   W1      m unrounded    D  7276.224  121.5317 24.93039      5
```

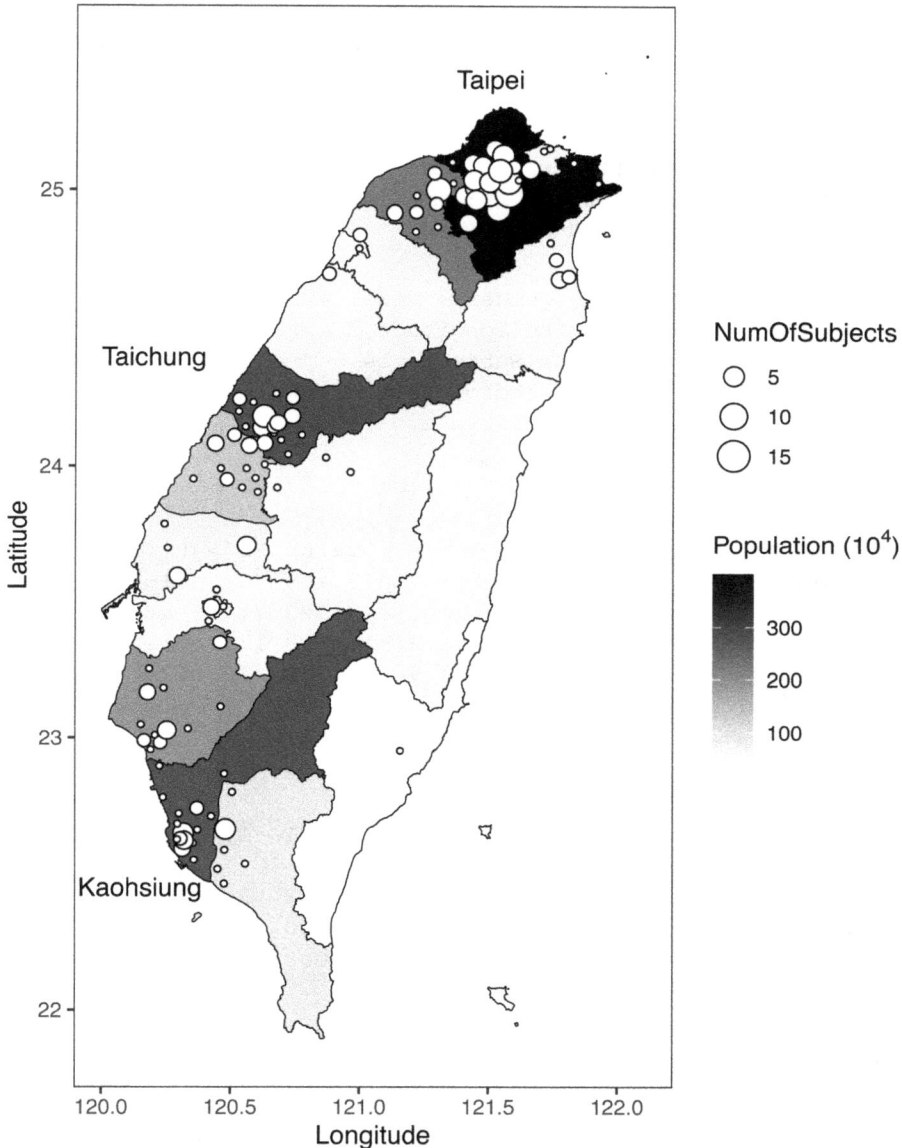

Figure 10.16 The geographical distribution of population in Taiwan, and the participants in this study.

We first fitted a model with three factorial predictors as fixed effects. In addition to `sibilant`, we also included `gender` and `vowel`, the latter of which specifies whether the sibilant is followed by a rounded or an unrounded vowel. Males' sibilants in general have lower centroid frequencies because vocal tract length is usually longer for males than for females. Similarly, when sibilants are followed by rounded vowels, the vocal tract is lengthened due to anticipatory coarticulation of lip protrusion. This leads to the lowering of centroid frequencies as well.

To inspect the effect of geography, since a geographic location is determined simultaneously by two predictors, longitude and latitude, we need **tensor product smooths**. Just as splines fit a wiggly curve for the effect of a single predictor, tensor product smooths fit a wiggly surface for the joint effect of two or more predictors. The pertinent function for tensor product smooths in GAMs is te(). For the present dataset, a wiggly surface is projected from longitude and latitude. In addition, we added by = sibilant in the specification of the tensor product smooth, to request two wiggly surfaces, one for each sibilant category. This model includes by-subject and by-word random intercepts as well.

```
mer.gam0 = bam(centfreq ~ gender + vowel + sibilant +
                    te(longitude, latitude, by = sibilant) +
                    s(Subject, bs = "re") +
                    s(Word, bs = "re"),
            data = mer, discrete = TRUE)
---
```

```
Parametric coefficients:
                 Estimate Std. Error t value Pr(>|t|)
(Intercept)        6252.8      143.9  43.446  < 2e-16
genderf             317.9       59.1   5.379 7.67e-08
vowelunrounded      759.3      112.2   6.769 1.37e-11
sibilantR         -1185.5      583.9  -2.030   0.0424
```

```
Approximate significance of smooth terms:
                         edf   Ref.df      F   p-value
te(longitude,latitude):
sibilantD              3.001    3.001  1.446     0.227
te(longitude,latitude):
sibilantR             15.058   16.259  5.593  1.47e-12
s(Subject)           295.054  323.000 23.399     0.317
s(Word)               28.322   29.000 56.137   < 2e-16
```

```
R-sq.(adj) =  0.543   Deviance explained = 55.8%
fREML =  86336   Scale est. = 6.2616e+05   n = 10613
```

The table of parametric coefficients shows that centroid frequencies are higher for females and for sibilants followed by unrounded vowels, as expected. The effect of sibilant, on the other hand, is not very well supported, presumably because of merging. With regards to the effect of geography, there is also evidence supporting that retroflex (but not dental) realizations differ across regions. Before visualizing this effect, we first check the **concurvity** of the model. Concurvity is a concept similar to collinearity in linear regression. It occurs when predictors are highly correlated with one another. When there is high correlation among the predictors, coefficient estimates become inaccurate, and it becomes unclear what the unique contribution of a predictor to the model fit is. The concurvity of the model can be obtained with the function concurvity():

```
concurvity(mer.gam0)
---
```

	para	te(longitude,latitude):sibilantD
worst	1	1
observed	1	1
estimate	1	1

	te(longitude,latitude):sibilantR	s(Subject)	s(Word)
worst	1	1.0000	1.0000
observed	1	0.0700	0.0114
estimate	1	0.0824	0.1065

Concurvity values are bounded between zero and one, with larger values indicating high concurvity. The fact that the estimates of the two tensor product smooths are both one suggests a serious concurvity problem of this model. The problem results from the high correlation between the effect of geographical location and the by-subject random effect. Given that for half of the locations we have only one participant, the effect of geographical location is inevitably closely tied to the random effect of subject. To remedy this, we left out the by-subject random intercept, an effect which also turned out to be not statistically supported in model mer.gam0.

To visualize the regression surfaces, we use the vis.gam function. This function produces a contour plot of the fitted values. The output contour plots for dentals and retroflexes, overlaid with the map of Taiwan, are presented in Figure 10.17. More coding details are colder in the supplementary material. Warmer colors represent higher centroid frequencies, whereas colder colors represent lower centroid frequencies. We can immediately see that, as expected, dentals (left) have higher centroid frequencies than retroflexes (right). In addition, geographical differentiation is more prominent for retroflexes than dentals as it is the realization for retroflex sounds that varies substantially across regions. Specifically, people in central Taiwan (the area

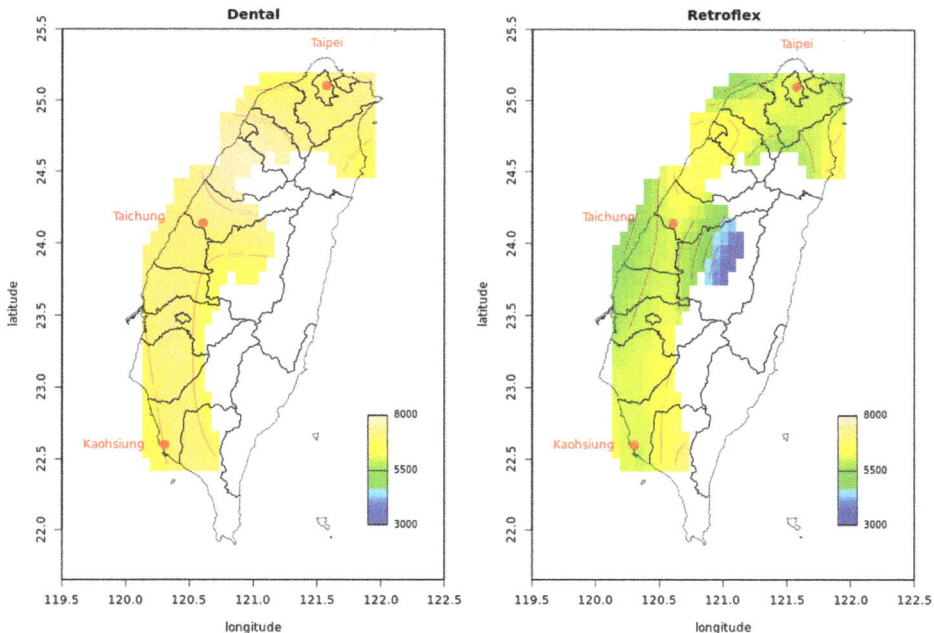

Figure 10.17   The effect of geography on dental (left) and retroflex (right) sibilants from mer.gam0.

near Taichung) have very retroflexed productions, and there are a few places (the yellow areas) where people have almost dental-like, or deretroflexed productions, indicating a high degree of merging.

Figure 10.17 shows that centroid frequencies vary geographically in ways that differ between dental and retroflex sibilants. This leads to the question of where across the country the dental and retroflex realizations are most similar (i.e. high degree of merging). We can investigate this by setting up a model with a difference surface, which will be predicted by the geographical coordinates (longitude and latitude). Similar to the difference curve described earlier for pitch contours, we first transformed `sibilant` into a numeric variable. Next in the formula we specified two tensor products. The first one is for the reference sibilant category (dental), while the second one is for the difference surface (retroflex – dental).

```
mer$sibNum = as.numeric(ifelse(mer$sibilant=="D", 0, 1))
mer.gam1 = bam(centfreq ~ gender + vowel +
                         te(longitude, latitude) +
                         te(longitude, latitude, by = sibNum) +
                         s(Word, bs = "re"),
               data = mer, method = "ML")
```

Figure 10.18 presents the partial effects of the two tensor product smooths. The left panel shows the contour plot of the reference level (i.e. dental). The numbers on the contour lines are the predicted partial effect for centroid frequency. Since partial effects exclude intercepts and the effects of other predictors, we therefore observe the "pure" effect of geography. For example, Taichung is located around the contour line of zero. To the east of Taichung, the number gradually decreases (from –500 to –1,000). This indicates that the centroid frequency

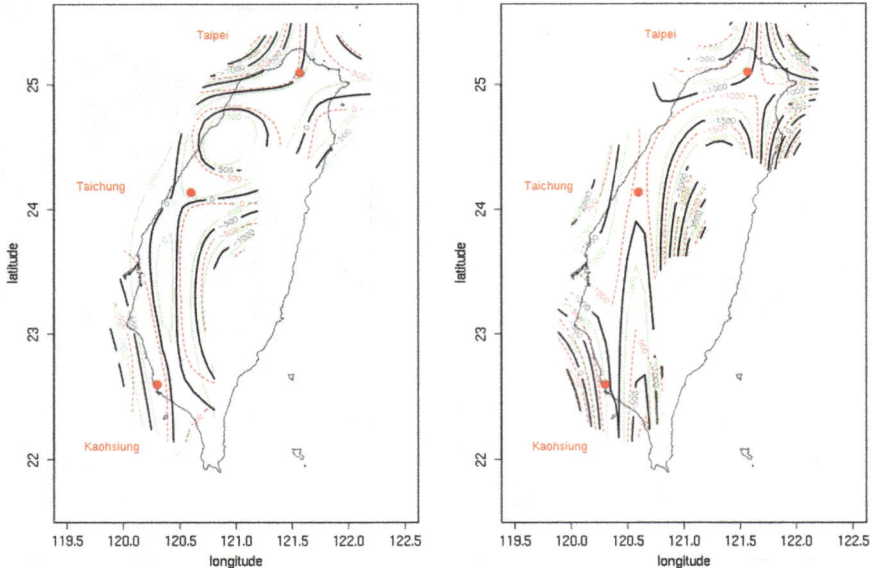

Figure 10.18 Contour plots of the partial effects of the reference dental sibilants (left) and the difference surface (right) obtained from `mer.gam1`. One SE (standard error) confidence regions are indicated by green dotted and red dashed lines for the upper and lower bounds of the interval respectively.

predicted for dental sibilants decreases to the east. The contour plot in the right panel presents the magnitude of the difference in centroid frequencies between the two sibilants (retroflexes – dentals). Given that retroflexes have lower centroid frequencies than dentals, more negative values thus indicate a larger difference and less merging. Notably, speakers from central Taiwan (to the east of Taichung) keep the production of the two sibilants most distinct (the predicted difference in centroid frequencies can be as large as 3,000 Hz). As this is the location of the former capital of Taiwan, speakers from that region appear to preserve retroflexion to a greater extent. In addition, we found that the degree of merging for the three major cities in Taiwan is fairly similar (all located around the –1,000 contour lines). This could be a consequence of urbanization. Since the population of these cities is all composed of speakers from different regions across the country, extensive interactions among different dialectal or ethnic groups could have led to a new variety that is specific to urban areas. However, we will need more data to verify this hypothesis.

One frequently asked question regarding sibilant merging in Taiwan Mandarin is to what extent the degree of merging is subject to the influence of Min, another major substrate language spoken in Taiwan. Like Mandarin, Min also has the three dental sibilants. However, unlike Mandarin, it lacks all of the three retroflex counterparts. Merging, essentially deretroflexion, is thus often regarded as a negative transfer from Min. The question of interest is whether Min fluency has an effect on sibilant merging. Specifically, we ask whether highly fluent Min speakers deretroflex more when speaking Mandarin, and also whether knowledge of Min interacts with the geographic effect.

In the `mer` dataset, the column `minflu` provides our participants' self-reported ratings of Min speaking fluency. The ratings range from one (low fluency) to seven (high fluency). In the next model, we included a tensor product for `minflu` and the two geographical coordinates, and further requested separate wiggly surfaces for the two sibilant categories. We fitted the model with the maximum likelihood method to enable model comparisons.

```
mer.gam2 = bam(centfreq ~ gender + vowel + sibilant +
                    te(longitude, latitude, minflu, by = sibilant) +
                    s(Word, bs = "re"),
            data = mer, method = "ML")
```

Compared to `mer.gam0` (refitted with `method = "ML"`), `mer.gam2` clearly has better model fit. To visualize the interaction of longitude and latitude by Min fluency, we plotted separate maps for different levels of Min fluency. Given that most of our participants have Min proficiency ratings between three and six, we therefore focused on these four fluency levels.

Figure 10.19 presents the effect of the four-way interaction, with the predicted surface for dentals in the upper row, and the predicted surface for retroflexes in the bottom row. Columns are tied to Min fluency, increasing from three (left) to six (right). At all Min fluency levels, the distinction between the two sibilants is still retained. Dental realizations are comparatively stable, whereas retroflex realizations vary across Min fluency levels to a much greater extent. Generally speaking, speakers from the center of Taiwan have more retroflexed pronunciation, but typically for speakers with mid-to-high Min fluency. On the other hand, for speakers from northern Taiwan (areas with latitude above 24.5), the realization of retroflexes becomes more dental-like with increasing Min fluency, consistent with the hypothesis of negative Min transfer. Interestingly, our analysis clarifies that this influence is region-specific.

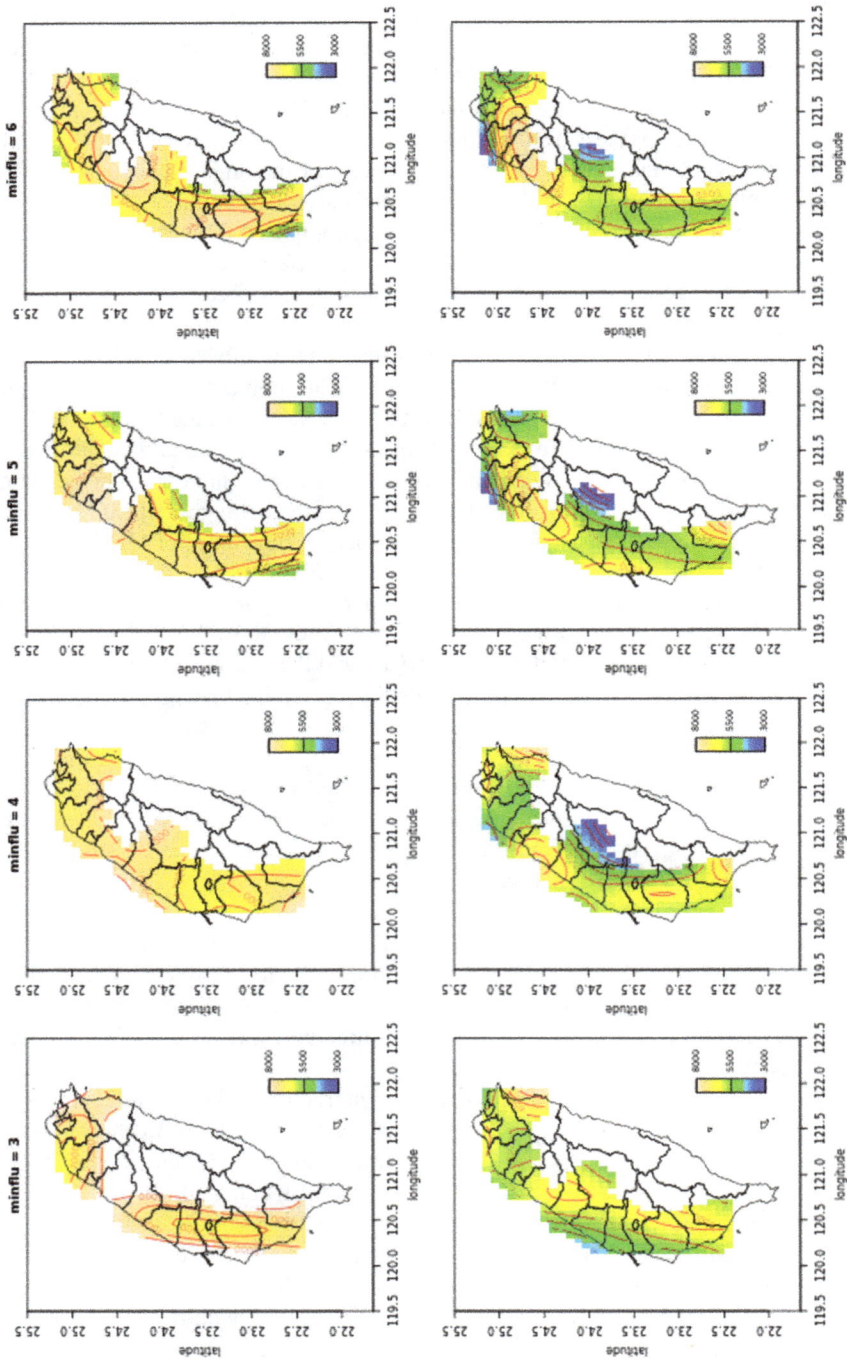

Figure 10.19 The effect of geography on dentals (upper panels) and retroflexes (lower panels), conditioned on Min fluency levels.

In summary, we have shown how to analyze the geographical distribution of sociophonetic variation with GAMs. Instead of using categorical variables that distinguish different geographical locations, we showed that directly working with geographical coordinates provides us with novel and powerful ways of studying variation. Specifically, tensor product smooths are available for modeling nonlinear interactions between two or more predictors, enabling dialectal variation to be studied in conjunction with other phonetic or social variables in considerable detail.

Conclusion

The goal of this chapter has been to introduce GAMs to the clinical phonetician. GAMs, which are rapidly gaining popularity in phonetics in general due to their versatility, are a promising tool also for the analysis of data from clinical phonetics.

As we have only provided a basic introduction to the main concepts of GAMs in this chapter, we refer the interested reader to Wood (2017) for a detailed exposition of the mathematics underlying GAMs and discussion of a wide range of examples of application to empirical data. A general, non-technical introduction to the mathematical concepts underlying GAMs is provided by Baayen et al. (2017) and Wieling (2018).

Introductions to GAMs focusing specifically on application to phonetics are Wieling et al. (2016) and Baayen and Linke (2020). Wieling et al. (2016) used GAMs to analyze tongue movement data obtained with electromagnetic articulography, investigating the difference in articulatory trajectories between two Dutch dialects. Baayen and Linke (2020) analyzed the distribution and occurrence of pronunciation variants, extracted from the Buckeye corpus, with GAMs. A GAM analysis on eye-tracking data collected for the perception of Cantonese tones can be found in Nixon et al. (2016).

Quantile GAMs (QGAMs, Fasiolo et al., 2020) provide an extension of the GAM framework that makes it possible to study how the quantiles of the distribution of a response variable depend on a set of predictors. As QGAMs are distribution-free, they are especially useful for datasets for which models that build on the assumption that the residual errors should be independently and identically distributed turn out to be inappropriate. For this reason, Tomaschek et al., (2018) turned to QGAMs for modeling tongue movements registered with electromagnetic articulography.

Notes

1 The datasets and the supplementary material for this chapter are available at https://osf.io/5wf4v/.
2 For one dysarthric participant (D2), the duration and intensity of the first and second syllables, instead of vowels, were measured, because the vowels could not be reliably identified. We do not expect this difference to skew the results, since instead of using raw duration and intensity data, we calculated the ratios and used them as our response variables. Moreover, statistical results are qualitatively similar irrespective of whether D2 is included or excluded. We therefore retained the data of D2 in the analyses.

References

Baayen, R. H. and Linke, M. (2020). An introduction to the generalized additive model. In Paquot, M. and Gries, S. T., editors, *A practical handbook of corpus linguistics*. Springer, Berlin.

Baayen, R. H., Milin, P., and Ramscar, M. (2016). Frequency in lexical processing. *Aphasiology*, 30(11), 1174–1220.

Baayen, R. H., Vasishth, S., Kliegl, R., and Bates, D. (2017). The cave of shadows: Addressing the human factor with generalized additive mixed models. *Journal of Memory and Language*, 94, 206–234.

Chuang, Y.-Y. (2017). *The effect of phonetic variation on word recognition in Taiwan Mandarin.* PhD thesis, National Taiwan University, Taipei.

Chuang, Y.-Y., Sun, C.-C., Fon, J., and Baayen, R. H. (2019). Geographical variation of the merging between dental and retroflex sibilants in Taiwan Mandarin. In *Proceedings of the 19th International Congress of Phonetic Sciences*, pages 472–476, Melbourne. Australasian Speech Science and Technology Association.

Fasiolo, M., Wood, S. N., Zaffran, M., Nedellec, R., and Goude, Y. (2020). Fast calibrated additive quantile regression. *Journal of the American Statistical Association*, 1–11.

Fon, J. (2007). The effect of region and genre on pitch range of Tone 1 in Taiwan Mandarin. Technical Report NSC95-2411-H-002-046-, National Science Council, Taipei, Taiwan.

Nixon, J. S., van Rij, J., Mok, P., Baayen, R. H., and Chen, Y. (2016). The temporal dynamics of perceptual uncertainty: Eye movement evidence from Cantonese segment and tone perception. *Journal of Memory and Language*, 90, 103–125.

Papakyritsis, I. and Müller, N. (2014). Perceptual and acoustic analysis of lexical stress in Greek speakers with dysarthria. *Clinical linguistics & phonetics*, 28(7-8), 555–572.

Tomaschek, F., Tucker, B. V., Fasiolo, M., and Baayen, R. H. (2018). Practice makes perfect: The consequences of lexical proficiency for articulation. *Linguistics Vanguard*, 4, 1–13.

van Rij, J., Wieling, M., Baayen, R. H., and van Rijn, H. (2017). itsadug: Interpreting time series and autocorrelated data using GAMMs. R package version 2.3.

Wieling, M. (2018). Analyzing dynamic phonetic data using generalized additive mixed modeling: a tutorial focusing on articulatory differences between L1 and L2 speakers of English. *Journal of Phonetics*, 70, 86–116.

Wieling, M., Tomaschek, F., Arnold, D., Tiede, M., Bröker, F., Thiele, S., Wood, S. N., and Baayen, R. H. (2016). Investigating dialectal differences using articulography. *Journal of Phonetics*, 59, 122–143.

Wood, S. (2017). *Generalized Additive Models: An Introduction with R* (2nd Ed.). CRC Press, Boca Raton, FL.

PART III

Phonetic transcription
Introduction

Part III of the *Manual* contains six chapters on phonetic transcription. The ability to transcribe speech into phonetic symbols has long been, and still is, the gold standard for speech-language pathologists and clinical phoneticians wishing to make a record of disordered speech. Since the beginning of interest in speech disorders among phoneticians and the beginning of the profession of speech therapy the International Phonetic Alphabet (IPA, 1999) has been the only accepted form of phonetic transcription.

However, it was not perhaps a foregone conclusion that IPA would be the transcription method for clinical phoneticians. Indeed, an earlier system came out of the study of hearing impairment, in the form of Bell's *Visible Speech* (Bell, 1867). In Bell's system, phonetic symbols are created out of a set of sub-symbol shapes. For consonants, these correspond to phonetic features such as place and manner of articulation, voicing and resonance. The vowel symbols consisted of a basic vowel symbol with additions to mark tongue and lip position. Such a system could be very useful for a reader unfamiliar with how to produce a spoken text from traditional written symbols, once they had learnt what each aspect of the composite symbols referred to in articulatory terms. However, as a transcription system there are drawbacks. It takes time to deconstruct a sound phonetically and then draw the relevant combination of sub-symbols and put them together into a correct composite. A trained phonetician does not need to transcribe speech sounds into composite symbols; instead, an arbitrary system such as are found in many alphabetic writing systems will be sufficient. Even in reading Visible Speech, the fact that many aspects of the composite symbols are similar in shape is likely to interfere with the ease of interpretation of the written text. Nevertheless, out of interest, had Visible Speech become the transcription of choice in phonetics or clinical phonetics, the name of this book would be written thus: Әꞇʊꟺꞁꞁꙍ ꞁꝫ ꝙꙍꞁʊꞁꝙꞁꙍ ꝫꞁʊꞁꝙꞁꙍꙅ.

Another phonetically based alphabet, devised by Ronald Kingsley Read (1964), as winner of a competition organized by George Bernard Shaw, is the Shavian (or Shaw) alphabet. While the symbols are unitary (unlike with Visible Speech), the size and direction the symbols are pointing do represent many phonetic features (especially in the case of the consonants). Unfortunately, the grouping of symbols together into families of similar shapes does make reading the system problematic (at least initially) as one criticism is that they look too similar. Putting the title of this book into Shavian would produce the following: ꟾ𐑦𐑣𐑦𐑒 𐑮 𐑛𐑰𐑝𐑦𐑛𐑮𐑒 𐑪𐑮𐑛𐑦𐑒𐑕.

The phoneticians who founded the International Phonetic Alphabet towards the end of the nineteenth century opted for a system of symbols based on the Latin alphabet, with additions. This alphabet has evolved and expanded over the years and was adopted by speech and language pathologists/therapists in most jurisdictions during the twentieth century. It is this system and derivatives from it, that is the focus of the chapters in this part of the book. Our *Manual of Clinical Phonetics* in the IPA system is /ˈmænjʊəl əv ˈklɪnɪkl̩ ˈfənɛtɪks/.

There are six chapters in the part. Catia Cucchiarini and Helmer Strik discuss the nature of phonetic transcription in the first of these. This is followed by an account of the International Phonetic Alphabet (IPA) by Michael Ashby and Patricia Ashby, and then a discussion of how to transcribe disordered speech (partly through the use of the Extensions to the IPA - extIPA) by Martin Ball. Jill Titterington and Sally Bates's chapter deals with issues surrounding teaching and learning phonetic transcription, particularly transcribing disordered speech. Martin Ball then looks at the debate within clinical transcription about whether to transcribe what the client says (using the full range of IPA and extIPA symbols) or what the client was trying to say (using diacritical marks to denote how the actual speech differed from the intended speech). The final chapter rounds off the section by providing numerous examples of disordered speech with sample transcriptions, from the files of the authors: Martin J. Ball, Nicole Müller, Marie Klopfenstein and Ben Rutter.

Phonetic transcription is a foundational skill for speech-language pathologists and clinical phoneticians. The chapters in this section examine the background, development and use of transcription, and provide the resources needed to learn and employ it in the clinic and speech laboratory.

References

Bell, A. M. (1867). *Visible speech. The science of universal alphabetics*. London: Simkin, Marshall, & Co.
IPA (1999). *The handbook of the International Phonetic Association*. Cambridge: Cambridge University Press.
Read, K. (1964). *Shaw-Script; a quarterly in the Shaw alphabet*. Worcester: Kingsley Read.

11

THE NATURE OF PHONETIC TRANSCRIPTION

Catia Cucchiarini and Helmer Strik

Introduction

A phonetic transcription can be defined as the written representation of a speech utterance through specially developed symbols usually organized in a phonetic alphabet. More precisely, a phonetic transcription is the result of an auditory, and often partly visual, analysis of an utterance into a linear sequence of discrete units of speech represented by phonetic symbols. In turn, phonetic symbols are defined by parameters that are mainly articulatory, although some auditory categories are also used (Cucchiarini, 1993). This definition is limited to the transcription of segmental phenomena in speech. The analysis and transcription of suprasegmental aspects of speech is beyond the scope of this chapter and is addressed in Chapter 5.

The development of specially designed symbols for representing the sounds of speech has a long tradition that goes back to ancient Indian phoneticians who studied the sounds of Sanskrit (Allen, 1953) and Greek scholars who developed the first alphabetic system with distinct symbols for consonants and vowels (Allen, 1981). In later years various transcription systems were developed such as Robert Robinson's Vox Vivenda (Robinson, 1617), Francis Lodwick's Universal Alphabet (Lodwick, 1686), the phonetic alphabet devised by Pitman and Ellis (Pitman, 1847), the transcription system developed by Brücke (Brücke, 1863), Alexander Melville Bell's Visible Speech (Bell, 1867), the system presented by Otto Jespersen in *The Articulations of Speech Sounds* (Jespersen, 1889), and Henry Sweet's Organic Alphabet (Sweet, 1890).

Many of these phonetic transcription systems are segmental, in the sense that they are linear representations of speech in terms of segments or units of sound. Analphabetic transcriptions like Jespersen's *The Articulations of Speech Sounds* (1889) may include complex symbols intended to illustrate the articulators involved in the production of speech sounds. Alphabetic transcriptions, on the other hand, tend to contain one symbol for each speech segment. They can be iconic if the symbols evoke characteristics of the speech production mechanism, like Bell's Visible Speech (Bell, 1867) and Sweet's Organic Alphabet (Sweet, 1890).

In general, transcriptions based on the Romanic alphabet have been preferred because they are easier to use and are less anchored in theories of speech production because the relationship between phonetic symbols and speech sounds is completely arbitrary.

While many of these phonetic representation systems were originally developed for educational purposes, for instance to illustrate the correct pronunciation of sounds in different languages, in later years they were employed as research tools in phonetics and dialectology to describe unknown languages and dialects for linguistic investigation. The phonetic alphabet developed by Pitman and Ellis (Pitman, 1847) formed the basis of the International Phonetic Alphabet (IPA, 1949) (see Chapter 12) and was mainly used in phonetic studies. The transcription systems used in dialectology, on the other hand, differed according to the research tradition. French dialectologists relied on a system originally developed by Rousselot (Gardette, 1968). A modified version of the system elaborated by Ascoli was used in a survey of Italian and Swiss dialects by Jaberg and Jud (1928), while German scholars adopted the alphabet of the review "Theutonista." Apparently, comparability between languages was considered less important than comparability between studies of the same dialect or language (Francis, 1983, p. 92).

In many linguistic disciplines, phonetic transcriptions have been used to obtain written records of speech data that were subsequently employed as a basis for research. In early times, phonetic transcriptions were made instantaneously by fieldworkers while interviewing their informants and were the only recordings of speech material. For this reason, it was important to have systems that were easy to learn and to use.

Although nowadays, speech material can be easily recorded through various mobile devices, symbolic notations of speech are still employed for research purposes in various fields of linguistics, including phonetics, phonology, dialectology, sociolinguistics, second language acquisition, speech pathology, studies of language development and language disorders and even speech technology. For instance, phonetic transcriptions have been extensively used to compile multipurpose speech corpora to be used in speech technology to train systems for automatic speech recognition and speech synthesis and for scientific research and application development in general. Well-known examples are TIMIT (Zue, Seneff, and Glass, 1990), Switchboard (Godfrey, Holliman, and McDaniel, 1992), Verbmobil (Hess, Kohler, and Tillman, 1995), the Spoken Dutch Corpus (Oostdijk, 2002), the Corpus of Spontaneous Japanese (Maekawa, 2003), Buckeye (Pitt, Johnson, Hume, Kiesling, and Raymond, 2005) and "German Today" (Brinckmann, Kleiner, Knöbl, and Berend, 2008).

The way in which transcriptions are realized and the level of detail they contain vary considerably depending on the aim for which transcriptions are made. In any case, it is important to realize that a phonetic transcription, whatever the type, is always the result of an analysis or classification of speech material. Far from being the reality itself, transcription is an abstraction from it (Cucchiarini, 1993).

Types of phonetic transcription

Transcriptions that are made according to the principles of the IPA may be of different types. Abercrombie (1964, 1967) distinguished between systematic transcriptions, which are analyses based on phonological knowledge, and impressionistic transcriptions, those based on general phonetic categories (Catford, 1974) without reference to the phonological system. Impressionistic transcriptions can be made when transcribing an unknown language or subphonemic characteristics or different varieties of a known language (Abercrombie, 1967; Knowles, 1978).

Systematic transcriptions can differ depending on their degree of explicitness. Nowadays the terms broad, narrow and acoustic are more commonly used to indicate transcriptions with varying degree of explicitness: (Delais-Roussarie, and Post, 2014; Gibbon, Moore, and Winski, 1997)

a. Broad phonetic or phonemic: contains the minimum number of symbols required to indicate the distinctive segments of a language (one phoneme one symbol).
b. Narrow phonetic transcription (allophonic): some phonemes may be denoted by more than one symbol, thus providing information about their allophonic realizations.
c. Acoustic phonetic transcription: very detailed transcription indicating different phases in production (e.g. aspiration, glottal closure, burst).

In addition, the advent of computers led to the introduction of a series of machine-readable phonetic alphabets, which are often referred to as computer phonetic alphabets (CPAs). Many different CPAs have been proposed and used. In the European project "Speech Assessment Methods" (SAM), "SAM Phonetic Alphabet" (SAMPA) was established through a consultation process among international speech researchers (Wells, J. C., 1997) [http://www.phon. ucl.ac.uk/home/sampa/]. SAMPA became a standard in Europe, and essentially is a mapping between symbols of the International Phonetic Alphabet and ASCII codes. Its extended version X-SAMPA aimed at covering all symbols of the IPA Chart to provide machine-readable phonetic transcriptions for every known human language.

ARPABET was developed by the Advanced Research Projects Agency (ARPA) and consists of a mapping between the phonemes of General American English and ASCII characters. Worldbet (Hieronymus, J., 1994.) is a more extended mapping between ASCII codes and IPA symbols intended to cover a wider set of the world languages. Many other computer-readable phonetic alphabets exist in addition to those mentioned above (see e.g. Draxler, 2005; Gibbon, Moore, and Winski, 1997; Hieronymus, 1994; Wells, 1997; and https://en.wikipedia. org/wiki/ Comparison_of_ASCII_encodings_of_the_International_Phonetic_Alphabet).

Degree of detail in phonetic transcription

How detailed a phonetic transcription should be depends mainly on the purpose for which the transcription is made (Cucchiarini, 1993; Delais-Roussarie, and Post, 2014). Nevertheless, the issue of how much detail should be captured in phonetic transcription has been a topic of discussion in the literature. Early scholars emphasized that transcriptions should record only what is linguistically relevant without excessive information (Bloomfield, 1933; Grønnum-Thorsen, 1987; Ladefoged, 1975; Rischel, 1987). Chomsky and Halle (1968) stated that fine-grained transcriptions are useless to linguists, who are interested in the structure of language and not in the minute details of speech. Kelly and Local (1989), on the other hand, stressed the importance of detailed transcriptions of speech arguing that linguistic knowledge should constitute the result of the investigation and not its starting point (Kelly and Local, 1989). As a matter of fact: "It is not possible to use a phonemic transcription when you do not know the phonology" (Ball, 1991, p. 60; see also Bloch, and Trager, 1942, p. 37), so in this case it is impossible to make a transcription that indicates only linguistically relevant properties because these still have to be discovered. According to Kelly and Local (1989) transcribers working with unknown languages should not gain information about the language beforehand, but should try to make detailed recordings based on their knowledge of the speech production mechanism. The relevant information about the structure of that specific language would then be distilled out of these preliminary notes. They emphasize the importance of recording phonetic details because they think it is not possible to know in advance what is going to be relevant as "the relevance and 'distinctiveness' of features depend, to a large extent, on the particular aspect of analysis which is being pursued at any given time" (Kelly and Local, 1989, p. 118).

Chomsky and Halle also criticized the use of fine-grained transcriptions on the ground that it is actually impossible to record tiny details of speech in a consistent manner:

> even the most skillful transcriber is unable to note certain aspects of the signal, while commonly recording in his transcriptions items for which there seems to be no direct warrant in the physical record (Chomsky and Halle, 1968, p. 293).

Variability in phonetic transcription

Over the years, various researchers have pointed out that detailed phonetic transcriptions are likely to be inconsistent (Hammarström, 1958; Shockey and Reddy, 1974), and that this might be problematic for linguistic research. Bloomfield (1933, p. 84) had questioned the objectivity of detailed transcriptions, which he considered to be determined by "accidental and personal factors" and Bloch and Trager (1942, p. 36–7) stated that "the completeness of any transcription depends entirely on the accident of the writer's background: no two listeners, regardless of their competence, will ever transcribe all utterances exactly alike."

That phonetic transcriptions could be influenced by the native language of fieldworkers or their previous experience emerged from analyses made by Hotzenkocherle (1962) in his survey of Swiss German dialects and by Ringaard (1964) in one of his surveys of Danish dialects who observed that "the narrow transcriptions of the phoneticians do not tell us so very much about the actual dialectal realizations of the phonemes, but tell us more about the fieldworkers themselves, about their native pronunciations and about their confusion when coming to new regions" (Ringaard, 1964, p. 501).

In spite of these findings, the use of phonetic transcription as a means of recording speech seemed to be generally taken for granted, as aptly observed by Abercrombie (1965, p. 109) "The ideal trained phonetician is thus looked on as being in some way like a recording machine—his hearing of sounds automatically produces a transcription in the same way as the cutting head makes a groove in the wax. But the fact is that a transcription is not a simple record of an utterance, it is a generalization about an utterance. The utterances are the original basic facts. The field-worker's transcriptions are the first processing, the first analysis, of these facts they are not the facts themselves."

Various studies have indeed shown that phonetic transcriptions of the same utterance can differ, either when they are made by different transcribers (between-subjects variation) or when they are made by the same transcriber at different times or under different conditions (within-subjects variation). The factors influencing the transcriptions can vary from those related to the transcriber like native language, knowledge of the language to be transcribed and experience to those concerning the speech material, like language variety, speech style and length of the utterances (Amorosa, Benda, Wagner, and Keck, 1985; Henderson, 1938; Laver, 1965; Oller, and Eilers. 1975; Pye, Wilcox, and Siren. 1988; Shriberg and Lof. 1991; Ting, 1970; Wester, Kessens, Cucchiarini, and Strik. 2001; Witting, 1962).

The scientific status of transcription as a research tool was questioned by Pierrehumbert (Pierrehumbert, 1990), who suggested that although fine phonetic transcription had been useful in the past, it had now been supplanted by improved research techniques that provide quantitative representations of various phonetic phenomena (articulator movements, articulator excitation, acoustic waves).

For linguistics and other disciplines that employ transcription to obtain data for further research, the existence of discrepancies between transcriptions is problematic because it affects the reliability of phonetic transcription as a research tool. Various authors have indeed addressed the issues of reliability and validity with respect to phonetic transcription (Van Borsel, 1989; Cucchiarini, 1993, 1996; Kerswill, and Wright. 1990; Oller and Eilers. 1975; Pye, Wilcox, and Siren. 1988; Strik, and Cucchiarini. 2014; Vieregge, and Cucchiarini. 1988, Vieregge, and Cucchiarini. 1989).

Concern about the value of phonetic transcription as a research tool was particularly evident in clinical linguistics. In disciplines like speech pathology and child phonology, auditory analysis still constitutes an important instrument of data collection (Ball, 1991; Ball, Rahilly, and Tench, 1996; Howard, and Heselwood, 2002; Stemberger, and Bernhardt, 2019). These data are used as a basis for speech assessment, therapy, and the evaluation of treatment effectiveness. This explains why the issue of transcription reliability has received considerable attention in clinical linguistics, as already exemplified by the review in Shriberg and Lof (1991).

The process of phonetically transcribing speech

A description of the stages involved in transcribing speech was provided by Almeida and Braun (1985), who identified the following stages: listening, imitating, sensing and coding. (Cucchiarini, 1993) suggested a slightly modified description of the process with the following stages: perceiving, imitating, sensing and coding.

Various researchers underlined that when making a phonetic transcription, it is necessary to focus on the phonetic shape of the utterance rather than on its semantic aspect (Catford, 1974; Kelly, and Local, 1989; Vieregge, 1987), but when the transcriber is familiar with the language it is almost impossible to analyze the phonetic shape of an utterance without being influenced by its meaning.

In principle, the contribution of the visual ("face") modality to phonetic transcription is limited to those movements that can be seen. For the rest, it is a form of indirect observation: the transcriber analyses a spoken utterance to derive information about the movements that produced that utterance. Inferring movements from auditory sensations is something a transcriber has to learn by imitating the sounds (Catford, and Pisoni, 1970; König, 1988) until the imitation sounds like the original utterance. Through sensing transcribers try to feel in their own vocal tract which articulatory movements produced the utterance (also known as proprioception) and finally they can select the phonetic symbols that best represent the sounds in question (coding).

In general, the stages of imitating and sensing can be skipped by highly experienced phoneticians transcribing languages they know. (Catford, 1977, p. 5) effectively describes this capacity of trained phoneticians to experience "a kind of 'empathic' immediate awareness of the organic movements going on in the speaker's vocal tract."

Nowadays phonetic transcriptions are generally made by using specially developed tools that allow to listen to the speech while simultaneously looking at visual, graphical representations (oscillogram, spectrogram, fundamental frequency, formant curves, etc.) while producing the transcriptions in a tier-based structure. This thus is a different contribution of the visual modality to the transcription process, than the one mentioned earlier that referred to actually "seeing" the articulators. Well known examples of such systems are ELAN (Sloetjes, Wittenburg, and Somasundaram, 2011), Praat (Boersma, and Weenink, 2013), EXMARaLDA (Schmidt, and Wörner, 2009) and ANVIL (Kipp, 2014). Phonetic transcriptions made with these tools are therefore the results of both auditory and visual analyses of acoustic representations.

Even when using these more advanced tools, making phonetic transcriptions is still extremely time-consuming and costly. Producing phonetic transcriptions from scratch can take up to 50–60 times real time. This factor obviously depends to a large extent on the type of speech that has to be transcribed: it is lower for well-articulated read speech, and higher for more "difficult types of speech" such as spontaneous speech (esp. conversations with many speakers and overlapping turns), non-native and pathological speech. For these reasons, researchers have been looking for ways of making this process more efficient (Van Bael, Boves, van den Heuvel, and Strik, 2007; Binnenpoorte, and Cucchiarini, 2003; Binnenpoorte, Goddijn, and Cucchiarini, 2003). This was particularly necessary when compiling large speech corpora such as TIMIT (Zue, Seneff, and Glass, 1990), Switchboard (Godfrey, Holliman, and McDaniel, 1992), Verbmobil (Hess, Kohler, and Tillman, 1995), the Spoken Dutch Corpus (Oostdijk, 2002), the Corpus of Spontaneous Japanese (Maekawa, 2003), Buckeye (Pitt, Johnson, Hume, Kiesling, and Raymond, 2005) and "German Today" (Brinckmann, Kleiner, Knöbl, and Berend, 2008).

One way of obtaining phonetic transcriptions more efficiently has been by trying to at least partly automatize this process (Van Bael, Boves, Heuvel, and Strik, 2007; Cucchiarini and Strik, 2003; Kessens and Strik, 2004). For example, in cases in which an orthographic transcription (verbatim transcription) is available, a simple grapheme-phoneme conversion procedure can be applied so that strings of graphemes are replaced by corresponding strings of phonetic symbols. If a pronunciation dictionary is available, this can be done through a lexicon-look-up procedure in which each individual word is replaced by its phonological representation in the pronunciation dictionary (Binnenpoorte, 2006). For words not present in the pronunciation dictionary, or for all words if a pronunciation dictionary is not available, it is possible to use a grapheme-phoneme conversion algorithm (Binnenpoorte, 2006). If grapheme-phoneme conversion is used, the resulting transcription cannot be considered an auditory analysis of a speech utterance, as no human listening to the speech signal is taking place during the transcription process.

Another procedure that has been adopted to speed up the process of producing phonetic transcriptions is that of asking transcribers to correct an example transcription taken from a lexicon or a dictionary, which they can edit and improve after having listened to the corresponding speech signal. For example, this procedure was used for compiling large corpora like Switchboard and the Spoken Dutch Corpus. Transcribers were asked to verify an example transcription rather than transcribing from scratch (Goddijn, and Binnenpoorte, 2003; Greenberg, Hollenback, and Ellis, 1996). Although such a check-and-correct procedure may be attractive in terms of cost reduction, it has been suggested that it may bias the resulting transcriptions toward the example transcription (Binnenpoorte, 2006). In addition, the procedure is still rather time-consuming as manual verification can take up to 15 minutes for one minute of speech recorded in formal lectures and 40 minutes for one minute of spontaneous speech (Demuynck, Laureys, and Gillis, 2002).

Alternatively, phonetic transcriptions can be obtained automatically through Automatic Speech Recognition (ASR) (Van Bael, Boves, Heuvel, and Strik, 2007; Kessens, and Strik, 2004; Strik, and Cucchiarini, 2014). In this case previously trained acoustic phone models of the speech sounds (phones) to be identified are used. If no orthographic transcription is available, a transcription can be obtained by means of phone recognition. However, the number of errors in such a transcription is generally rather high, and thus no high-quality transcriptions can be obtained in this way, see, e.g. Stemberger & Bernhardt (2019). If orthographic transcriptions are available, an option is to first generate pronunciation variants and next apply "forced alignment" to select the pronunciation variants that best match the audio signal (Van Bael, Boves, Heuvel, and Strik, 2007; Binnenpoorte, Cucchiarini, Strik, and Boves, 2004; Strik, and Cucchiarini, 2014; Wester, Kessens, Cucchiarini and Strik, 2001).

The advantages of producing phonetic transcriptions automatically or semi-automatically become really evident when it comes to annotating large speech corpora, because this makes it easier to achieve uniformity in transcription and because automatic methods allow to transcribe large amounts of data, which would not be feasible through manual phonetic transcriptions. However, the question may arise as to whether the resulting annotations are indeed phonetic transcriptions in the sense of "an auditory, and often partly visual, analysis of an utterance into a linear sequence of discrete units of speech represented by phonetic symbols," as in these cases there is actually no auditory or partly visual analysis by a human expert. ASR-based transcriptions are obtained without the intervention of human experts, so they might fit the definition of phonetic transcription as the procedure of "assigning a label to a portion of the speech signal" (Delais-Roussarie, and Post, 2014, p. 48), but probably not that of auditory analysis of an utterance.

Nevertheless, ASR-based phonetic transcriptions can be useful in many research situations. For instance, they can function as some sort of benchmark or element of comparison so that transcribers can identify possible errors due to disattention or bias or solve possible doubts or disagreements between different transcribers.

Finally, we would like to add some practical information and suggestions based on the lessons we learned after having been involved in several phonetic transcription projects at our department. First of all, one should consider whether to involve expert transcribers or lay people. Experts are of course likely to produce more accurate annotations (Munson, Johnson, and Edwards, 2012) but for some tasks, e.g. intelligibility annotation, it can be useful to use lay people in view of representativity and generizability issues. In general, for phonetic transcription experts are to be preferred because this is a special technique that lay people normally will not master and that therefore requires specialized training (Shriberg, Hinke, and Trost-Steffen, 1987; Shriberg, Kwiatkowski, and Hoffmann, 1984) (see also Chapter 14). These "experts" could be speech professionals, such as phoneticians or speech therapists, or "speech students." The latter are usually carefully selected students, often from a phonetics class, who have followed a training and are known to have "a good ear" to work accurately. These students first receive some training for the specific transcription task they have to accomplish.

Furthermore, it is good to have a clearly defined procedure which is specified in a transcription protocol. When transcribers have doubts, they can make notes, and at regular intervals they can get together to discuss the problematic cases (Shriberg, Hinke, and C. Trost-Steffen, 1987, Shriberg, Kwiatkowski, and Hoffmann, 1984). When decisions are made, they can be added to the protocol. The goal here is obviously to try to be consistent. It is advisable to check the level of consistency, by measuring the degree of intra-transcriber and inter-transcriber agreement. For examples, specific protocols and quality checking procedures were established in the Dutch language speech corpora compilation initiatives such as the Dutch Spoken Corpus (Oostdijk, 2002) and the JASMIN-CGN Corpus containing speech of children, non-natives and elderly people (Cucchiarini, Driesen, Hamme, and Sanders, 2008; Cucchiarini, and Hamme, 2013).

An important decision is also what annotation scheme should be used, for instance the symbol set. For native, non-pathological speech one of the many existing CPAs could be used.

However, for transcriptions of atypical speech, such as non-native and pathological speech an existing CPA might not suffice (see also Chapter 13). For instance, when annotating non-native, second language (L2) speech, specific symbols might be required to indicate inter-language speech sounds. For pathological speech, dedicated symbol sets have been designed (Chapter 13) as existing CPAs might not be sufficient to describe all the phenomena occurring in pathological speech utterances.

Conclusion

In this chapter we have introduced and discussed the nature of phonetic transcription. We started from a definition of this notion limited to transcribing segmental units of speech, as suprasegmental phenomena will be addressed in Chapter 5. We proceeded to a brief histor-ical overview of the use of phonetic transcription in linguistic research. We saw that various alphabets have been proposed and used over the years and that different ways of produ-cing phonetic transcriptions have been suggested. From the times in which fieldworkers made phonetic transcriptions instantaneously while interviewing their informants, we have moved to computer phonetic alphabets and very specialized tools that allow to make phon-etic transcriptions while having access to visual representations of the speech signal and to information about, e.g. VOT, segment duration, frication and glottalization. More recently, semi-automatized and automatized methods of producing phonetic transcriptions through ASR technology have come within reach. These innovations have not only changed the procedures to obtain phonetic transcriptions, but possibly also the nature of phonetic tran-scription itself.

References

Abercrombie, D. (1964). *English phonetic texts*. London: Faber and Faber.

Abercrombie, D. (1965). *Studies in phonetics and linguistics*. London: Oxford University Press.

Abercrombie, D. (1967). *Elements of general phonetics*. Edinburgh: Edinburgh University Press.

Allen, W. S. (1953). *Phonetics in ancient India*. London: Oxford University Press.

Allen, W. S. (1981). The Greek contribution to the history of phonetics. In R. E. Abher & E. J. A. Henderson (Eds.), *Towards a history of phonetics* (pp. 115–122). Edinburgh: Edinburgh University Press.

Almeida, A., & Braun, A. (1985). What is transcription? In W. Kürschner & R. Vogt (Eds.), *Grammatik, Semantik, Textlinguistik* (pp. 37–48). Tübingen: Niemeyer.

Amorosa, H., von Benda, U., Wagner, E. & Keck, A. (1985). Transcribing phonetic detail in the speech of unintelligible children: A comparison of procedures. *International Journal of Language & Communication Disorders, 20*(3), 281–287.

Ball, M. J. (1991). Recent developments in the transcription of nonnormal speech. *Journal of Communication Disorders, 24*(1), 59–78.

Ball, M. J., Rahilly, J. & Tench, P. (1996). *The phonetic transcription of disordered speech*. San Diego: Singular Publishing.

Bell, A. M. (1867). *Visible Speech: The science of universal alphabetics*. London: Simpkin, Marshal.

Binnenpoorte, D. (2006). *Phonetic transcriptions of large speech corpora*. Ph.D. dissertation, Radboud University Nijmegen, the Netherlands.

Binnenpoorte, D., & Cucchiarini, C. (2003). Phonetic transcription of large speech corpora: how to boost efficiency without affecting quality. *Proceedings of 15th ICPhS, Barcelona, Spain,* 2981–2984.

Binnenpoorte, D., Cucchiarini, C., Strik, H. & Boves, L. (2004). Improving automatic phonetic transcrip-tion of spontaneous speech through variant-based pronunciation variation modelling. *Proceedings of the 4th International Conference on Language Resources and Evaluation*. European Language Resources Association (ELRA), Lisbon, Portugal. 681–684.

Binnenpoorte, D., Goddijn, S. & Cucchiarini, C. (2003). How to improve human and machine transcriptions of spontaneous speech. *Proceedings of ISCA IEEE Workshop on Spontaneous Speech Processing and Recognition (SSPR), Tokyo, Japan.* 147–150.

Bloch, B. & Trager, G. L. (1942). *Outline of linguistic analysis.* Baltimore, MD: Waverly Press.

Bloomfield, L. (1933). *Language.* London: Unwin (9th Reprint, 1969).

Boersma, P. & Weenink, D. (2013). Praat: Doing phonetics by computer [Computer Program]. *Glot International,* 5 (9/10): 341–345.

Brinckmann, C., Kleiner, S., Knöbl, R. & Berend, N. (2008). German today: An areally extensive corpus of Spoken Standard German. *Proceedings of the 6th International Conference on Language Resources and Evaluation, LREC 2008, Marrakech, Marocco.*

Brücke, E. W. (1863). Über eine neue Methode der phonetischen Transscription. *Sitzungsberichte der Philosophisch-Historischen Classe der Kaiserlichen Akademie der Wissenschaften Wien,* 41, 223–285.

Catford, J. C. (1977). *Fundamental problems in phonetics.* Edinburgh: Edinburgh University Press.

Catford, J. C. (1974). Phonetic fieldwork. In A. Sebeok (Ed.), *Current trends in linguistics* (pp. 2489–2505). The Hague: Mouton.

Catford, J. C., & Pisoni, D. B. (1970). Auditory vs. articulatory training in exotic sounds. *The Modern Language Journal,* 54(7), 477–481.

Chomsky, N., & Halle, M. (1968). *The sound pattern of English.* New York: Harper and Row.

Cucchiarini, C. (1993). *Phonetic transcription: A methodological and empirical study.* PhD Thesis, University of Nijmegen.

Cucchiarini, C. (1996). Assessing transcription agreement: Methodological aspects. *Clinical Linguistics and Phonetics,* 10(2), 131–155.

Cucchiarini, C., Driesen, J., Van Hamme, H. & Sanders, E. (2008). Recording speech of children, non-natives and elderly people for hlt applications: The JASMIN-CGN corpus. *Proceedings of the 6th International Conference on Language Resources and Evaluation, LREC 2008, Marrakech, Marocco.*

Cucchiarini, C., & Van Hamme, H. (2013). The JASMIN speech corpus: Recordings of children, non-natives and elderly people. In P. Spyns & J. Odijk (Eds), *Essential speech and language technology for Dutch* (pp. 43–59). Springer, Berlin, Heidelberg.

Cucchiarini, C., & Strik, H. (2003). Automatic phonetic transcription: An overview. *Proceedings of 15th ICPhS, Barcelona, Spain,* 347–350.

Delais-Roussarie, E., & Post, B. (2014). Corpus annotation and transcription systems. In J. Durand, U. Gut, & G. Kristoffersen (Eds), *Handbook of corpus phonology* (pp. 46–88). Oxford: Oxford University Press.

Demuynck, K., Laureys, T. & Gillis, S. (2002). Automatic generation of phonetic transcriptions for large speech corpora. *7th International Conference on Spoken Language Processing, ICSLP 2002.* Denver, Colorado.

Draxler, C. (2005). WebTranscribe - an extensible web-based speech annotation framework. *Proceedings of the 8th International Conference on Text, Speech and Dialogue (TSD 2005), Karlovy Vary, Czech Republic,* 61–68.

Francis, W. N. (1983). *Dialectology, an introduction.* London: Longman.

Gardette, P. (1968). *Atlas linguistique et ethnographique du Lyonnais. Vol IV Exposé méthodologique et tables.* Paris: Centre National de La Recherche Scientifique.

Gibbon, D., Moore, R. & Winski. R. (1997). *Handbook of standards and resources for spoken language systems.* Berlin: Mouton de Gruyter.

Goddijn, S., & Binnenpoorte, D. (2003). Assessing manually corrected broad phonetic transcriptions in the spoken Dutch corpus. *Proceedings of 15th ICPhS, Barcelona, Spain,* 1361–1364.

Godfrey, J. J., Holliman, E. C. & McDaniel, J. (1992). SWITCHBOARD: Telephone speech corpus for research and development. *ICASSP, IEEE International Conference on Acoustics, Speech and Signal Processing – Proceedings, San Francisco, California.*

Greenberg, S., Hollenback, J. & Ellis, D. (1996). Insights into spoken language gleaned from phonetic transcription of the switchboard corpus. *International Conference on Spoken Language Processing, Philadelphia, PA.*

Grønnum-Thorsen, N. (1987). Suprasegmental transcription. In A. Almeida & A. Braun (Eds.), *Probleme der phonetischen Transkription* (pp. 79–109). Wiesbaden: Franz Steiner Verlag.

Hammarström, G. (1958). Representation of spoken language by written symbols. *Miscellanea Phonetica*, *3*, 31–39.

Henderson, F. M. (1938). Accuracy in testing the articulation of speech sounds. *Journal of Educational Research*, *31*, 348–56.

Hess, W., Kohler, K. J. & Tillman, H. G. (1995). The Phondat-Verbmobil speech corpus. *Proceedings of Eurospeech-95, Madrid, Spain*, 863–866.

Hieronymus, J. (1994). *ASCII phonetic symbols for the world's languages: Worldbet.* AT&T Bell Laboratories, Technical Memo. New Jersey: Murray Hill.

Hotzenkocherle, R. (1962). *Sprachatlas der Deutschen Schweiz*. Bern: Francke Verlag.

Howard, S. J., & Heselwood, B. C. (2002). Learning and teaching phonetic transcription for clinical purposes. *Clinical Linguistics and Phonetics*, *16*(5), 371–401.

IPA (1949). *The principles of the International Phonetic Association.* London: International Phonetic Association.

Jaberg, K. & Jud, J. (1928). *Der Sprachatlas als Forschungsinstrument: Kritische Grundlegung und Einführung in den Sprach- und Sachatlas Italiens und der Südschweiz*. Halle (Saale): Niemeyer.

Jespersen, O. (1889). *The articulations of speech sounds represented by means of analphabetic symbols.* Marburg: Elwert.

Kelly, J., & Local, J. (1989). *Doing phonology.* Manchester: Manchester University Press.

Kerswill, P. & Wright, S. (1990). The validity of phonetic transcription: Limitations of a sociolinguistic research tool. *Language Variation and Change*, *2*(3), 255–275.

Kessens, J. M., & Strik, H. (2004). On automatic phonetic transcription quality: Lower word error rates do not guarantee better transcriptions. *Computer Speech and Language*, *18*(2), 123–141.

Kipp, M. (2014). ANVIL: The video annotation research tool. In J. Durand, U. Gut, & G. Kristoffersen (Eds.), *Handbook of Corpus Phonology* (pp. 420–436). Oxford: Oxford University Press.

Knowles, G. O. (1978). The nature of phonological variables in Scouse. In P. Trudgill (Ed.), *Sociolinguistic Patterns in British English* (pp. 80–90). London: Arnold.

König, W. (1988). Zum Problem der engen phonetischen Transkription. *Zeitschrift für Dialektologie und Linguistik*, *55*, 155–178.

Ladefoged, P. (1975). *A course in phonetics.* New York: Harcourt Brace Jovanovich.

Laver, J. D. M. H. (1965). Variability in vowel perception. *Language and Speech*, *8*(2), 95–121.

Lodwick, F. (1686). An essay towards an universal alphabet. *Philosophical Transactions*, *16*, 126–137.

Maekawa, K. (2003). Corpus of spontaneous Japanese: Its design and evaluation. *Proc. of ISCA and IEEE Workshop on Spontaneous Speech Processing and Recognition, Tokyo, Japan.*

Munson, B., Johnson, J. M. & Edwards, J. (2012). The role of experience in the perception of phonetic detail in children's speech: A comparison between speech-language pathologists and clinically untrained listeners. *American Journal of Speech-Language Pathology*, *21*(2), 124–139.

Oller, D. K., & Eilers, R. E. (1975). Phonetic expectation and transcription validity. *Phonetica*, *31*(3-4), 288–304.

Oostdijk, N. H. J. (2002). The design of the Spoken Dutch Corpus. In P. Peters, P. Collins & A. Smith (Eds.), *New Frontiers of Corpus Research* (pp. 105–112). Amsterdam: Rodopi.

Pierrehumbert, J. (1990). Phonological and phonetic representation. *Journal of Phonetics*, *18*(3), 375–394.

Pitman, I. (1847). The English phonotypic alphabet. *The Phonotypic Journal*, *6*(61).

Pitt, M. A., Johnson, K., Hume, E., Kiesling, S., & Raymond, W. (2005). The Buckeye corpus of conversational speech: Labeling conventions and a test of transcriber reliability. *Speech Communication*, *45*, 89–95.

Pye, C., Wilcox, K. A. & Siren, K. A. (1988). Refining transcriptions: The significance of transcriber 'errors'. *Journal of Child Language*, *15*(1), 17–37.

Ringaard, K. (1964). The phonemes of a dialectal area, perceived by phoneticians and by the speakers themselves. *Proceedings of the Vth International Congress of Phonetic Sciences, Münster*, 495–501.

Rischel, J. (1987). Phonetic transcription in fieldwork. In A. Almeida & A. Braun (Eds), *Probleme der phonetischen Transkription*. (pp. 57–77). Wiesbaden: Franz Steiner Verlag.

Robinson, R. (1617). *The art of pronunciation.* London: Nicholas Oakes.

Schmidt, T., & Wörner, K. (2009). EXMARaLDA - Creating, analysing and sharing spoken language corpora for pragmatic research. *Pragmatics*, *19*, 565–582.

Shockey, L., & Reddy, R. (1974). Quantitative analysis of speech perception: Results from transcription of connected speech from unfamiliar languages. Paper Presented at the Speech Communication Seminar, Stockholm.

Shriberg, L. D., Hinke, R. & Trost-Steffen, C. (1987). A procedure to select and train persons for narrow phonetic transcription by consensus. *Clinical Linguistics and Phonetics*, *1*(2), 456–465.

Shriberg, L. D., Kwiatkowski, J. & Hoffmann, K. (1984). A procedure for phonetic transcription by consensus. *Journal of Speech and Hearing Research*, 27(3), 456–65.

Shriberg, L. D., & Lof, G. L. (1991). Reliability studies in broad and narrow phonetic transcription. *Clinical Linguistics and Phonetics*, *5*, 225–279.

Sloetjes, H., Wittenburg, P. & Somasundaram, A. (2011). ELAN - Aspects of interoperability and functionality. *Proceedings of the Annual Conference of the International Speech Communication Association, INTERSPEECH,* Florence, Italy.

Stemberger, J., & Bernhardt, B. M. (2019). Phonetic transcription for speech-language pathology in the 21st century. *Folia Phoniatrica et Logopaedica*, *72*(2), 75–83.

Strik, H., & Cucchiarini, C. (2014). On automatic phonological transcription of speech corpora. In J. Durand, U. Gut, & G. Kristoffersen (Eds.), *Handbook of Corpus Phonology* (pp. 89–109). Oxford: Oxford University Press.

Sweet, H. (1890). *A primer of phonetics.* Oxford: Clarendon Press.

Ting, A. (1970). *Phonetic transcription: A study of transcriber variation.* Report from the Project on Language Concepts and Cognitive Skills Related to the Acquisition of Literacy, Madison, University of Wisconsin.

Van Bael, C., Boves, L., van den Heuvel, H., & Strik, H. (2007). Automatic phonetic transcription of large speech corpora. *Computer Speech and Language*, *21*(4), 652–668.

Van Borsel, J. (1989). The reliability of phonetic transcriptions: A practical note. *Child Language Teaching and Therapy*, *5*, 327–333.

Vieregge, W. H. (1987). Basic aspects of phonetic segmental transcription. In A. Almeida & A. Braun (Eds.), *Probleme der phonetischen Transkription* (pp. 5–55). Wiesbaden: Franz Steiner Verlag.

Vieregge, W. H., & Cucchiarini, C. (1988). Evaluating the transcription process. In W. A. Ainsworth & J. N. Holmes (Eds.), *Proceedings of Speech '88, Edinburgh*, 73–80.

Vieregge, W. H., & Cucchiarini, C. (1989). Agreement procedures in phonetic segmental transcriptions. In M. E. H. Schouten & P. Th. van Reenen (Eds.), *New methods in dialectology* (pp. 37–45). Dordrecht: Foris.

Wells, J. C. (1997). SAMPA computer readable phonetic alphabet. In D. Gibbon, R. Moore & R. Winski (Eds.), *Handbook of standards and resources for spoken language systems (Part IV, section B).* Berlin: Mouton de Gruyter.

Wester, M., Kessens, J. M., Cucchiarini, C. & Strik, H. (2001). Obtaining phonetic transcriptions: A comparison between expert listeners and a continuous speech recognizer. *Language and Speech*, *44*(3), 377–403.

Witting, C. (1962). On the auditory phonetics of connected speech: Errors and attitudes in listening. *Word*, *18*(1–3), 221–248.

Zue, V., Seneff, S. & Glass, J. (1990). Speech database development at MIT: Timit and beyond. *Speech Communication*, *9*, 351–356.

12

THE IPA

Michael Ashby and Patricia Ashby

Introduction

The International Phonetic Alphabet (IPA) provides the academic community with a universal standard notation for the phonetic representation of languages. It is used in any context where the need arises to specify the pronunciation of a sound, word, phrase, or longer sequence—for example, to indicate the pronunciations of words in a dictionary, to take down speech when documenting a language in fieldwork, or to transcribe texts for the teaching of languages.

It was developed by, and remains in the care of, the International Phonetic Association (also IPA), which was established in 1886 and defines its goal as the promotion of "the scientific study of phonetics and the various practical applications of that science." The idea of creating such an alphabet, independent of the pronunciation and writing system of any particular language, dates back many centuries, and in the past numerous competing systems were devised (Kemp, 2006). But only the IPA has secured widespread and enduring adoption. IPA symbols are incorporated in the Unicode Standard, and can therefore be displayed, processed and printed with computers and mobile devices worldwide.

Linguistic relevance and abstractness

The IPA does not aim to symbolize every possible human vocal sound. It deals only with linguistically relevant sounds. To merit inclusion in the alphabet, a sound must function as an essential contrastive unit (a phoneme) in at least one language. Nor does the IPA set out to represent the recognizable individual characteristics of particular speakers. IPA transcriptions are therefore abstract in the sense that one representation can serve equally well for an indefinite number of speakers who are "saying the same thing." Finally, the IPA does not provide comprehensively for pronunciations that are in any way atypical. Those who have speech disorders commonly employ types of sound and sound modifications, different from any of those included in the basic alphabet. The IPA may form the essential basis for work in the transcription of disordered speech, but it requires considerable augmentation to do this adequately (see Chapter 13, this volume).

Sources of symbols

The IPA takes as its starting point the letters of the basic Latin alphabet, assigning them sound values that are widely familiar across languages. But the aim is to provide a separate symbol for every sound used distinctively in any human language, and 26 letters are not enough to represent even the forty-or-so distinct sounds used in English. Many further symbols are therefore required, and they have been obtained in a wide variety of ways. Some are drawn from the Extended Latin alphabet, and are already employed in the writing systems of certain languages; examples are [æ] and [ð]. (Note that by convention, square brackets are used around phonetic symbols, to demarcate them from ordinary text). A further small number of symbols, such as [ɸ] and [ɣ], are based on letters from the Greek alphabet (though the values attached to the symbols are not necessarily Greek sounds). Certain symbols have been made by inventing new shapes, such as [ŋ], [ɥ]. The new shapes mostly look like existing Latin letters, and have some visible feature in them that suggests relationships among sounds. In a few cases, small capital Latin letters are used, with different meanings from the lowercase ones; for example, [r] and [ʀ] stand for different sounds, as do [n] and [ɴ]. But apart from those used in this way as phonetic symbols, there are no capitals in the IPA, and no systematic use is made either of text effects such as **bold** and *italic*.

Each phonetic symbol has an approved form (any complete Unicode font will include its own version of that form), and is assigned a unique "Unicode code point," which is a four-digit hexadecimal number, preceded by "U+." For example, the symbol shape æ has the code point U+00E6. Quite apart from the sound which a symbol represents, the symbol also often has a name for convenient reference. For example, phoneticians usually call æ "ash." Symbols also have official Unicode names. The Unicode name for æ is LATIN SMALL LETTER AE.

The IPA chart

The alphabet is presented in the form of a chart (familiarly known as "the IPA chart"), which fits conveniently onto a single page—see Figure 12.1.

To begin with, a basic division is made between Consonants and Vowels. The Consonants are further subdivided into Pulmonic and Non-Pulmonic; these terms refer to the air stream mechanism which is employed.

At the head of the chart, the Pulmonic Consonants are arranged in an array or matrix, which is the most familiar and characteristic feature of the chart. The columns correspond to places of articulation, arranged with the most front (bilabial) at the left and progressing to the most back (glottal). The rows of the array correspond to so-called "manners" of articulation, arranged in a sequence from the most closed (plosive), through intermediate degrees of intermittent closure (trill) and partial closure (fricative) to the most open, approximant. The cells created by the intersection of the places and the manners represent sound classes such as velar plosives, palatal fricatives, and so on. The third essential classificatory term in traditional phonetic taxonomy—voice vs. voicelessness—is represented by placing symbols in the left or right of the cells of the grid, voiceless on the left and voiced to the right. In this way a large proportion of the most common pulmonic consonants encountered in human languages are accommodated in the array.

Where a cell is left empty, it means that no symbol has been agreed for the sound-type in question. An example is "palatal lateral fricative." There is no difficulty in making a sound which fits this description; the implication of leaving the cell empty is that the sound has not hitherto been attested with contrastive function in a language, so no dedicated symbol has yet

THE INTERNATIONAL PHONETIC ALPHABET (revised to 2020)

CONSONANTS (PULMONIC) © ⊕ ⊜ 2020 IPA

	Bilabial	Labiodental	Dental	Alveolar	Postalveolar	Retroflex	Palatal	Velar	Uvular	Pharyngeal	Glottal
Plosive	p b			t d		ʈ ɖ	c ɟ	k ɡ	q ɢ		ʔ
Nasal	m	ɱ		n		ɳ	ɲ	ŋ	N		
Trill	ʙ			r					R		
Tap or Flap		ⱱ		ɾ		ɽ					
Fricative	ɸ β	f v	θ ð	s z	ʃ ʒ	ʂ ʐ	ç ʝ	x ɣ	χ ʁ	ħ ʕ	h ɦ
Lateral fricative				ɬ ɮ							
Approximant		ʋ		ɹ		ɻ	j	ɰ			
Lateral approximant				l		ɭ	ʎ	ʟ			

Symbols to the right in a cell are voiced, to the left are voiceless. Shaded areas denote articulations judged impossible.

CONSONANTS (NON-PULMONIC)

Clicks		Voiced implosives		Ejectives	
ʘ	Bilabial	ɓ	Bilabial	ʼ	Examples:
ǀ	Dental	ɗ	Dental/alveolar	pʼ	Bilabial
ǃ	(Post)alveolar	ʄ	Palatal	tʼ	Dental/alveolar
ǂ	Palatoalveolar	ɠ	Velar	kʼ	Velar
ǁ	Alveolar lateral	ʛ	Uvular	sʼ	Alveolar fricative

OTHER SYMBOLS

ʍ Voiceless labial-velar fricative
w Voiced labial-velar approximant
ɥ Voiced labial-palatal approximant
H Voiceless epiglottal fricative
ʕ Voiced epiglottal fricative
ʡ Epiglottal plosive

ɕ ʑ Alveolo-palatal fricatives
ɺ Voiced alveolar lateral flap
ɧ Simultaneous ʃ and x

Affricates and double articulations can be represented by two symbols joined by a tie bar if necessary.

t͡s k͡p

VOWELS

Front — Central — Back

Close: i • y   ɨ • ʉ   ɯ • u
ɪ Y   ʊ
Close-mid: e • ø   ɘ • ɵ   ɤ • o
ə
Open-mid: ɛ • œ   ɜ • ɞ   ʌ • ɔ
æ   ɐ
Open: a • ɶ   ɑ • ɒ

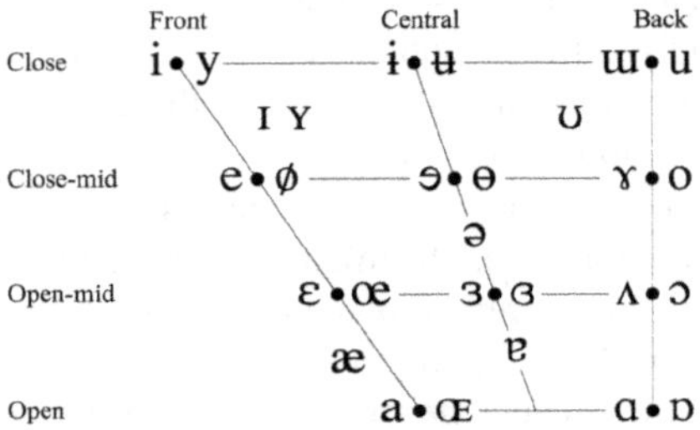

Where symbols appear in pairs, the one to the right represents a rounded vowel.

SUPRASEGMENTALS

ˈ	Primary stress	ˌfoʊnəˈtɪʃən
ˌ	Secondary stress	
ː	Long	eː
ˑ	Half-long	eˑ
̆	Extra-short	ĕ
ǀ	Minor (foot) group	
ǁ	Major (intonation) group	
.	Syllable break	ɹi.ækt
‿	Linking (absence of a break)	

DIACRITICS

̥	Voiceless	n̥ d̥		̤	Breathy voiced	b̤ a̤		̪	Dental	t̪ d̪
̬	Voiced	s̬ t̬		̰	Creaky voiced	b̰ a̰		̺	Apical	t̺ d̺
ʰ	Aspirated	tʰ dʰ		̼	Linguolabial	t̼ d̼		̻	Laminal	t̻ d̻
̹	More rounded	ɔ̹		ʷ	Labialized	tʷ dʷ		̃	Nasalized	ẽ
̜	Less rounded	ɔ̜		ʲ	Palatalized	tʲ dʲ		ⁿ	Nasal release	dⁿ
̟	Advanced	u̟		ˠ	Velarized	tˠ dˠ		ˡ	Lateral release	dˡ
̠	Retracted	e̠		ˤ	Pharyngealized	tˤ dˤ		̚	No audible release	d̚
̈	Centralized	ë		̴	Velarized or pharyngealized	ɫ				
̽	Mid-centralized	e̽		̝	Raised	e̝ (ɹ̝ = voiced alveolar fricative)				
̩	Syllabic	n̩		̞	Lowered	e̞ (β̞ = voiced bilabial approximant)				
̯	Non-syllabic	e̯		̘	Advanced Tongue Root	e̘				
˞	Rhoticity	ɚ a˞		̙	Retracted Tongue Root	e̙				

Some diacritics may be placed above a symbol with a descender, e.g. ŋ̊

TONES AND WORD ACCENTS

LEVEL			CONTOUR		
e̋ or ˥	Extra high		ě or ˇ	Rising	
é ˦	High		ê ˆ	Falling	
ē ˧	Mid		e᷄ ˏ	High rising	
è ˨	Low		e᷅ ˎ	Low rising	
ȅ ˩	Extra low		e᷈ ˜	Rising-falling	
↓	Downstep		↗	Global rise	
↑	Upstep		↘	Global fall	

Typefaces: Doulos SIL (metatext); Doulos SIL, IPA Kiel, IPA LS Uni (symbols)

Figure 12.1 IPA Chart, http://www.internationalphoneticassociation.org/content/ipa-chart, available under a Creative Commons Attribution-Sharealike 3.0 Unported License.

been called for. Certain other empty cells refer to articulatory impossibilities, and we may be confident that they will never be encountered in a human language. An example is "pharyngeal nasal." By definition, nasal consonants depend on the diversion via the open velum of airflow which is prevented by a complete closure from flowing outward via the oral cavity; a pharyngeal closure, even supposing it can be achieved, is upstream from the velum, rendering the nasal airway unreachable. Areas of the chart which indicate "impossible" articulations are shown shaded.

By contrast with the consonant array, symbols for Vowels are displayed in a different way. They are shown as points arranged around and within a quadrilateral shape which is placed below and aligned to the right of the consonant grid. This quadrilateral represents the "vowel space," which, as explained below, may variously be interpreted in articulatory, auditory or acoustic terms.

Thus, the alphabet assumes a phonetic framework which includes a binary voicing choice, a number of airstream mechanisms, various places and manners of articulation, and the vowel quadrilateral. The separate aspects of this underlying phonetic framework are discussed further in the sections which follow.

Place of articulation

More information on the places of articulation which form the columns of the IPA's consonant grid can be found in any phonetics manual, and needs to be studied in conjunction with a simple diagram of the organs of speech. The terms for places which appear on the chart are of various kinds. The first two, Bilabial and Labiodental, specify both the location along the vocal tract where the articulation occurs (the "passive" articulator) and the moving articulator which forms the articulation (the "active" articulator). Most of the others name only the "passive" articulator (the relevant point on the upper surface of the oral cavity), it being implied that the active articulator will be that portion of the tongue lying opposite on the lower surface of the cavity. So, for example, it is assumed that velar sounds will be made with the back of the tongue as the active articulator. Glottal is again unlike the others, in that the two vocal folds act together in the articulation, and when approaching or closing they move horizontally and laterally.

Though certain place labels are unproblematic and long-established (everyone agrees what "bilabial" or "velar" mean, for instance), phonetics manuals do show some differences in the list of places of articulation they recognize, and likewise somewhat different sets of places have been specified at different times in successive versions of the IPA. For example, at one time the chart had separate columns both for fricatives [ʃ ʒ], which were called "palato-alveolar," and for [ɕ ʑ], which were called "alveolo-palatal." In the current version of the chart, neither of these "places" is accorded a column. The symbols [ʃ ʒ] are still on the chart, but the sounds are analyzed as postalveolars, while the alveolo-palatals are removed from the main consonant chart and placed under "Other symbols."

For many sound types, an adequate specification of "place" in fact requires explicit mention of the active articulator. So [ʃ], for example, may be called "lamino-postalveolar," where "lamino-" means formed with the tongue blade, whereas [ɹ] is "apico-postalveolar" (made with the tongue tip). The resulting more complex labels do not lend themselves so readily to labeling the columns in an array, and on the whole the IPA has tended to adopt names for places which specify the passive point of articulation along the upper surface of the mouth, but do not attempt to capture the whole of a characteristic articulatory configuration. A notable exception to this is however provided by Retroflex, which might more accurately be termed "apico-prepalatal" (or in some cases, "sub-apico-prepalatal"). Retroflex names a tongue configuration (tongue tip curled, and displaced somewhat rearwards) rather than a unique "place" in the simple sense.

A consideration which has undoubtedly influenced the choice of "places" which are allocated separate columns on the chart is the number of occupied cells which will result from the intersection of a column with the various manners. The greater the number of occupied cells in a column, the greater the descriptive efficiency of the array. It is noticeable that no fewer than six of the manners in the Retroflex column are occupied, a greater number than any other place with the sole exception of Alveolar. By contrast, if the "palato-alveolar" or "alveolo-palatal" columns are included on the chart, only the fricative manner is occupied in either of them.

Finally, it may be noted that phoneticians and phonologists commonly make use of a number of broader "place" categories (e.g. labial, coronal, dorsal) which are not explicitly recognized on the chart. For the most part, these are largely equivalent to groupings of two or more adjacent "places" in the narrow sense. Thus, "labial" covers both labiodental and bilabial, and "dorsal" is equivalent to palatals plus velars. But the "natural classes" of place evidenced in particular languages may not entirely coincide with groupings captured on the present IPA chart. In English, for instance, the consonant [w] patterns with bilabials [p b m] in assimilatory processes, though the very natural phonetic motivation for this is not evident from the chart.

Manners of articulation

The situation with manners of articulation is not unlike that noted for places, and again one or more phonetics manuals should be consulted. The arrangement of all manners along a one-dimensional scale of degrees of openness is certainly open to debate. For instance, trills and taps are currently placed near the top of the grid, below plosives and nasals, but above fricatives. The rationale for this is that trills and taps involve one or more complete closures. Trills, for instance, can be seen as intermittent closures. But they might equally be regarded as interrupted openings, and therefore placed lower down the chart, nearer to the approximants—and trills and taps resemble approximants in that (when voiced) they typically have no friction noise.

The vowel space

Vowels are all relatively open articulations, but their distinct auditory qualities are clearly brought about by articulatory differences of some sort. In a vowel such as [i], the arch of the tongue body is well forward in the mouth, beneath the hard palate, whereas in [u] the arch occurs toward the back, beneath the velum. And whereas both [i] and [u] have the tongue body relatively high in the oral cavity (close to the palate), the vowel [a] requires it to be lowered well away from the palate. The labels Front, Central and Back resemble "places of articulation," and indeed what is called Front in relation to vowels corresponds to what is termed Palatal in consonants. The degrees of height (Close, Close-mid, Open-mid, Open) similarly continue the notion of manners increasing in openness. The placing of the quadrilateral below the consonant array is also consistent with that suggestion, and indeed in some earlier versions of the chart the vowel space was more explicitly linked to the consonant array on both the place and the manner dimensions.

Though all the labels around the quadrilateral vowel space appear to refer to articulation, phoneticians usually have only limited evidence about the articulation of a particular vowel, relying instead on auditory judgment to place a given vowel in the vowel space. The IPA vowel quadrilateral is effectively identical with the Cardinal Vowel system, devised by Daniel Jones in 1917 and described in numerous later publications. Jones recorded his Cardinal Vowels (on three separate occasions through his life) to serve as reference points for phoneticians learning the system. The eighteen vowel symbols arranged in pairs at nine dots on the periphery of the

IPA quadrilateral are identical with the symbols for Cardinal Vowels. The remaining 10 IPA vowel symbols do not represent Cardinal Vowel qualities.

Vowels can be subjected to acoustic analysis, and estimates obtained of their characteristic formant frequencies (particularly $F1$ and $F2$). When those values are plotted on appropriate scales, the result is a formant space which is not too different from the conventional shape of the vowel space. The proposal that the vowel quadrilateral, supposedly showing the articulation of vowels, in truth represents the arrangement of vowels in formant space is especially associated with Peter Ladefoged (1925–2006), whose ideas were influential at the time of the last comprehensive revision of the alphabet, in 1989.

The IPA does not attempt to further specify the nature of the distinction between Consonants and Vowels, though the implication is that vowels are by default syllabic, and consonants non-syllabic. A diacritic is provided meaning "syllabic," to be attached to consonants, as in [n̩], indicating a "syllabic [n]," heard in one common pronunciation of the English word "garden." Also provided is a diacritic with the meaning "non-syllabic"; it is a small subscript arch. The understanding is that this would only be applied to vowel symbols, as in [e̯], which is the example shown on the chart.

Thus, the alphabet appears to take for granted both the vowel/consonant distinction and syllabicity itself. By implication, the fundamental categories "vowel," "consonant" and "syllable" are presented as phonetic entities, though difficulties arise in the precise definition of all three. Interestingly, all three have in the past been seen by some as phonological constructs (i.e. notions which emerge only on account of the sound patterns of particular languages) rather than natural phonetic classes.

An even more basic assumption behind the IPA is the idea that speech can be represented as a sequence (or string) of non-overlapping units—speech sounds, or "segments." The segment is a problematic notion, since neither the acoustic signal nor instrumental registrations of articulatory activity invariably show clear divisions corresponding to segments. Some have maintained that it, too, is an artificial product of linguistic experience—specifically, knowledge of the ordinary alphabet. At the same time, the segment is a powerful idea which appears indispensable as a descriptive tool.

Airstream mechanisms

The outward flow of lung air (the "egressive pulmonic" airstream) is the basis of speech in all languages, and the only airstream mechanism that can power vocal fold vibration (voice). Certain languages supplement it with "non-pulmonic" airstreams—that is, articulatory manoeuvres that produce short-term compressions or rarefactions effected in the vocal tract itself and of sufficient duration to power single consonant segments. The non-pulmonic sound types found in languages are "ejectives," "implosives" and "clicks," and each of these is given a column in the small table on the chart.

Ejectives, symbolized with a following apostrophe ['], are the commonest of the non-pulmonic classes in languages, and are made with the egressive glottalic airstream. The compression is produced by raising the glottis, which is held closed to form what is effectively a piston. It follows that ejectives must always lack vocal fold vibration (voicing). Stops such as [k'] are relatively common; fricatives, such as [s'], rather less so. The Implosives, also found fairly widely in languages, reverse this action to produce a potentially inward-flowing (ingressive) glottalic airstream, but almost all are "voiced"—since the descending glottis is in its vibrating rather than fully-closed state, and the pulmonic airstream continues in use concurrently with the glottalic. Implosives have symbols featuring a "hook top": [ɓ, ɗ, ɠ, ...]. Only stop-like articulations are found, and the symbols are based on those for voiced pulmonic plosives.

Clicks, which are found as linguistic sounds in relatively few languages, are a class apart. They are powered by totally enclosing a volume of air in the mouth, and enlarging that volume by tongue movement, to bring a significant reduction in pressure. The enclosed volume is invariably bounded at the back by the tongue in contact with the velum (hence the term ingressive velaric airstream); at the front, the closure may be completed by the lips or by the tongue tip and blade in various configurations. Sudden opening of this enclosure at the front causes a sharp noise. According to the place where the front closure is formed and released, clicks are categorized as bilabial, dental, (post)alveolar, palato-alveolar and alveolar lateral, as listed on the chart. Basic clicks are of course voiceless, but because clicks are formed entirely within the mouth ahead of the velum, independently of the rest of the vocal tract, it is possible to add a wide range of simultaneous "accompaniments," including voicing, aspiration, voice-plus-nasality, glottal closure and others. More than a dozen such accompaniments have been documented in accounts of click languages (Nakagawa, 1996). Strictly, even the basic voiceless clicks are necessarily accompanied by a simultaneous [k], and it is now the general practice to write all clicks with an accompaniment: [k͡ʘ, g͡ʘ, ŋ͡ʘ], etc. There is a sense, then, in which it could be claimed that the click symbols shown on the chart represent rather less than a complete segment.

"Other symbols"

This section contains all the remaining letter-like symbols which will not fit into the current version of the consonant array. It was formerly called "Other sounds," and also provided a home for ejectives, implosives and clicks before a separate "Non-pulmonic" consonants section was added.

Sounds may have two (and in principle more than two) simultaneous places of articulation. Most such double articulations have to be written with paired symbols linked with a tie-bar above, as in [k͡p], the symbol for a voiceless labial-velar plosive. The only dedicated symbols provided for double articulations are [ʍ w ɥ ɫ], and all of these are placed in "Other symbols," as is the tie-bar itself.

All three of the sounds recognized by the IPA as having the epiglottal place of articulation, are also placed in this section: [ʜ ʢ ʡ]. It is worth observing that [ʡ], the epiglottal plosive, is not specified as either voiced or voiceless, it being argued that a voiced epiglottal stop is a physical impossibility (Laufer, 1991). Inconsistently, the glottal stop—to which the same argument applies even more obviously—is included on the main chart, and implicitly shown as voiceless.

The alveolo-palatal fricatives [ɕ ʑ] have already been mentioned above in connection with place of articulation. The term "alveolo-palatal" is retained, though without explanation of its meaning. The remaining "other symbol" is [ɺ], a voiced alveolar lateral flap.

Overall, the system of phonetic classification underlying the arrangement of letter-like symbols on the chart should not be taken as a definitive solution to the problems of phonetic classification, or even as entirely consistent in itself. But it does have the merit of permitting the alphabet to be displayed efficiently, in a way which leaves very little in the way of miscellaneous residue.

Uses of the consonant array

It is interesting to note that in accounts of the phonetics and phonology of particular languages, authors routinely adapt the rows and columns of the consonant matrix to suit the language, whereas the vowel diagram is retained unchanged, however sparsely it may be populated. Looking no further than the IPA's own *Handbook* (IPA, 1999), the consonant array in the very first "Illustration"—Peter Ladefoged on American English (pages 41–44)—adds a row for the Affricate manner. It is placed near the top of the array, between Plosive and Nasal. The following Illustration—Hayward & Hayward on Amharic (pages 45–50)—retains the Affricate row in that position, and adds further rows (at the bottom of the array) for "Ejective Stop," "Ejective Affricate" and "Ejective Fricative," as well as an extra Place column, "Labialized Velar," which is rather surprisingly placed to the right of Glottal. Progressing to the third Illustration—Thelwall & Sa'adeddin on Arabic (pages 51–54)—we again find a row for Affricate, though now placed below the row of fricatives. By contrast, all three accounts reproduce exactly the same quadrilateral figure on which the vowels are plotted, even though both Amharic and Arabic each have only a single open vowel (near central), and their vowel systems both clearly invite a triangular arrangement, rather than a quadrilateral. Examples could be multiplied, but enough has been said to establish that the IPA's consonant array is a fairly flexible paradigm. The more accounts of specific languages we examine, the more variations we encounter. On the other hand, the vowel quadrilateral embodies a specific theoretical model and is reproduced without change.

Diacritics

Returning to the chart, below "Other symbols" is a tabular display of 31 "Diacritics" (various small marks used above, below or otherwise along with a symbol to modify its meaning). The apostrophe which is used to indicate "ejective," might also reasonably be regarded as a "diacritic." Most of the diacritical marks are located centrally on the symbol carrying them, appearing directly above, below or though the symbol, as seen in [ã a̱ ɫ], but nine occupy some space to the right of the base symbol, and seven of these are recognizable as superscript versions of full symbols. Careful experimentation in keyboarding the diacritics with various fonts will reveal, however, that the superscripts provided as diacritics are not necessarily identical in size, heaviness and positioning with the regular superscript versions of the corresponding symbols. The dedicated diacritic superscripts are commonly somewhat larger, and positioned rather lower relative to the base symbol.

The diacritics are organized loosely into groups according to their functions. Voice, place, and manner may all be affected. Some diacritics specify glottal state, others indicate small adjustments in place of articulation or position in the vowel space. Five diacritics grouped together in the center column indicate secondary articulations—simultaneous articulatory adjustments in which a rather open approximation at the secondary place is superimposed upon a closer consonantal constriction elsewhere.

For a full discussion of types of diacritic, (see Ball, 2001). He reminds us that in some cases, diacritics provide the only means of symbolizing sound types which have phonemic status in a language. For instance, the basic chart provides no symbols for voiceless sonorants, yet voicing contrasts in sonorants are found in some of the world's languages. Burmese, for example, contrasts voiced and voiceless nasals at four places of articulation (Watkins, 2001). The voiceless ones must be symbolized [m̥, n̥, ɲ̊, ŋ̊], making use of the "voiceless" diacritic.

All of the superscript letter diacritics currently included on the chart are written to the right of the base symbol (though this should emphatically not be interpreted as meaning that their effect is necessarily restricted to, or audible only in, the "offglide" from the sound indicated). Keating, Wymark, and Sharif (2019) have recently pointed out that although all three of pre-nasalization, pre-aspiration and pre-glottalization are known to mark phonemic contrasts in at least some languages, there are no officially approved IPA devices for marking these properties (there is no shortage of improvised methods, which are mostly immediately transparent to the phonetically-aware reader). Keating et al. (2019) propose to symbolize these effects with super-script diacritics placed to the left of the symbol concerned.

Finally, at the bottom right of the chart are Suprasegmentals—marks indicating stress, length and phrasing—and Tones and word accents. Many of these are plainly diacritical marks, though the layout of the chart may seem to suggest otherwise. In fact the IPA's *Handbook* explicitly refers to them as diacritics (IPA, 1999). The IPA has always deprecated the use of diacritics in general, and avoided their use wherever possible, but the marking of "length, stress and pitch" has regularly been the first example in a list of justifiable applications of diacritics. Perhaps at work under the surface is an unspoken implication that the true diacritics are "quality modifiers" for segments. Indeed, in earlier editions of the chart, they were termed "Modifiers."

Though "length, stress and pitch" are grouped together by long tradition on the chart, it may reasonably be asked in what sense length is "suprasegmental." The long and half-long marks apply straightforwardly to the single segment they follow.

It is worth pointing out that the IPA has no approved marks for notating intonation (as distinct from tone). The IPA does not specify or endorse any scheme for impressionistically sketching pitch in intonation patterns. Early writers on intonation simply improvised with wavy lines drawn above the text (Klinghardt and Klemm, 1920, p. 162), and a century later, analysts approaching the problem afresh have been obliged to do the same (Ward, 2019).

Change and development

The IPA has grown and evolved over more than 120 years of international collaboration, with new symbols being added by consultation and consensus when new sounds were encountered in languages that had not previously been described—though not at a steady rate, and not always promptly. The most recent symbol to be adopted was for the voiced labiodental flap [ⱱ], added in 2005. By that time, evidence for a contrastive labiodental flap had been in print for a century, though it was not widely known or easily accessible. Olson and Hajek (1999) published exten-sive evidence from more than 60 languages, but still a further six years were to elapse before a formal proposal was put to a vote of the IPA Council and accepted (Nicolaidis, 2005). The IPA has frequently been described as "conservative"—a characterization not disputed by the Association, but rather claimed as a beneficial stabilizing influence (IPA, 1999).

The principle of "one symbol per distinctive sound" operates even more strongly in the other direction, and stipulates that a symbol should not be redundantly added to the alphabet if evi-dence of its contrastive status is lacking. This is to prevent over-enthusiastic embellishment of the chart with "possible" but redundant sound-types. This prohibition has not always operated so consistently in the past: the symbol [ɱ] for the labiodental nasal was added to the chart in 1926, though the earliest report of contrastive use in a language was apparently not published until 1975 (Ladefoged & Maddieson 1996). In time, considerably more support came to light (Hajek, 2009).

The extensive literature on particular languages and language families no doubt contains indications of numerous instances of unsuspected contrasts and phonetic rarities that have never come to the attention of phoneticians. There is no automatic mechanism by which they will do so. Besides, though the basic principle of the phoneme is readily illustrated with robust examples from English (IPA, 1999), the question of the phonemic status of problematic sounds in little-known languages is not always so easily decided. How are we to proceed, for instance, if the putative contrast is found in only a handful of words, or in a sub-part of the lexicon, such as ideophones?

The development of the IPA is not always in the direction of enlargement. Symbols and diacritics can be removed, as well as added. For example, dedicated symbols for voiceless implosives were introduced in 1989, but withdrawn again in 1993 following further debate and discussion. So the "hooktop" shapes for voiceless implosives [ɓ, ɗ, ʄ, …] joined a growing collection of obsolete phonetic symbols, knowledge of which may be required in interpreting older literature. It should be clarified that the contrastive status of voiceless implosives in at least a small number of languages was never in doubt—and the evidence has since become stronger and more extensive (Mc Laughlin, 2005). The debate was about whether dedicated symbols were mandated, rather than use of the "voiceless" diacritic.

Conclusion

The IPA is a powerful and valuable tool—arguably the single most important tool we have for describing human language. But its purpose and limitations should always be kept in mind. Contrary to what is sometimes mistakenly stated and believed, the IPA does not (and could not) provide means of representing "every shade of sound." The alphabet was designed for "practical linguistic needs" (IPA, 1949: 1) such as recording unwritten languages, teaching pronunciation and developing orthographies. The IPA and the phonetic framework which underlies it should not be regarded as immutable, and should not be permitted to straightjacket approaches to speech undertaken with different purposes in mind.

Further information

The most authoritative and up-to-date reference for the IPA's alphabet is on the Association's webpages at https://www.internationalphoneticassociation.org/

The IPA makes the chart available for free download (under a Creative Commons license) in many forms. See https://www.internationalphoneticassociation.org/content/ipa-chart

Particularly valuable are the "tooltip" versions in which, when the tooltip is moved over a symbol in the chart, a popup window appears, containing the phonetic description of the sound represented, the name of the symbol, the Unicode code point, and other details. An interactive clickable version additionally provides recordings of each sound from a number of phoneticians. Many historical versions of the chart are also provided for reference.

For an account of the IPA in relation to Unicode, see the relevant sections of the latest account of the Unicode Standard (The Unicode Consortium, 2019, pp. 296–297).

The IPA's *Handbook* (IPA, 1999). Handbook of the International Phonetic Association: A guide to the use of the International Phonetic Alphabet. Cambridge: Cambridge University Press.) aims to be a complete "user's manual" for the alphabet. It remains invaluable, but it should be remembered that it was prepared more than 20 years ago, so the version of the chart which it incorporates lacks the latest revisions.

The most up-to-date examples of the alphabet in use are to be found in the numerous accounts of particular languages ("Illustrations") regularly published in the IPA's journal, *The Journal of the International Phonetic Association* (*JIPA*): https://www.cambridge.org/core/journals/journal-of-the-international-phonetic-association

A reference work on phonetic symbols—their forms, origins and functions, and not restricted to present or former IPA symbols—is Pullum and Ladusaw (1996).

References

Ball, M.J. (2001). On the status of diacritics. *Journal of the International Phonetic Association, 31,* 259–264.

Hajek, J. (2009). Labiodental ɱ in Drubea. *Oceanic Linguistics, 48,* 484–487.

IPA. (1949). *The principles of the International Phonetic Association.* London, UK: International Phonetic Association.

IPA. (1999). *Handbook of the International Phonetic Association: A guide to the use of the International Phonetic Alphabet.* Cambridge, UK: Cambridge University Press.

Keating, P., Wymark, D., & Sharif, R. (2019). Proposal for superscript diacritics for prenasalization, preglottalization and preaspiration. *Journal of the International Phonetic Association.* [Published online at https://doi.org/10.1017/S0025100319000057]

Kemp, J.A. (2006). Phonetic transcription: History. In K. Brown & A.H. Anderson (Eds.), *Encyclopedia of language and linguistics* (2nd ed., pp. 396–410). Amsterdam, The Netherlands: Elsevier.

Klinghardt, H. & Klemm, G. (1920). *Übungen im englischen Tonfall.* Cöthen: Otto Schulze.

Ladefoged, P. & Maddieson, I. (1996). *The sounds of the world's languages.* Oxford, UK: Blackwell.

Laufer, A. (1991). Does the 'voiced epiglottal plosive' exist? *Journal of the International Phonetic Association, 21,* 44–45.

Mc Laughlin, F. (2005). Voiceless implosives in Seereer-Siin. *Journal of the International Phonetic Association, 35,* 201–214.

Nakagawa, H. (1996). A first report on the click accompaniments of ǀGui. *Journal of the International Phonetic Association, 26,* 41–54.

Nicolaidis, K. (2005). IPA News. *Journal of the International Phonetic Association, 35,* 261–262.

Olson, K.S. & Hajek, J. (1999). The phonetic status of the labial flap. *Journal of the International Phonetic Association, 29,* 101–114.

Pullum, G. & Ladusaw, W. 1996. *Phonetic symbol guide.* 2nd ed. Chicago: University of Chicago Press.

The Unicode Consortium. (2019). *The Unicode Standard, Version 12.1.0.* Mountain View, CA: The Unicode Consortium.

Ward, N.G. (2019). *The prosodic patterns of English conversation.* Cambridge, UK: Cambridge University Press.

Watkins, J.W. (2001). Burmese. *Journal of the International Phonetic Association, 31,* 291–295.

13

TRANSCRIBING DISORDERED SPEECH

Martin J. Ball

Introduction

The consonant section of the IPA chart shown in Chapter 12 only includes bare symbols, although more complex symbols are derivable through reference to the diacritics section of the chart. Clinical phoneticians often need to be able to transcribe complex sounds, and thus a more elaborated version of the IPA consonant chart would be useful. For example, the IPA chart has columns for dental, alveolar, and postalveolar places of articulation, yet these three are only filled with symbols for the fricative row, for the other manners of articulation the three columns are merged into one. As clinical phoneticians often need to distinguish between these places of articulation in obstruents other than fricatives, the consonant section of the IPA chart has to be read in conjunction with the diacritics section to do this. Another example involves release mode in plosives. Voiceless plosives on the consonant section of the IPA chart are shown as unaspirated (actually, due to the regrettable lack of a diacritic to mark unaspirated in the IPA, these bare symbols probably are meant to denote "unspecified as to release type"). A fuller representation could include both unaspirated and aspirated symbols, this distinction often being important for clinical phoneticians. Finally, the consonant section of the IPA chart does not include affricates or non-pulmonic consonants, these all being relegated to other parts of the chart.

Esling (2010) illustrates a fuller consonant chart (see Figure 13.1). This is solely based on the IPA chart, but displays the consonants on a full page (other sounds such as vowels, and suprasegmentals are excluded). With a full chart devoted to consonants, the various consonant types referred to above can be included; thus, there are dental, alveolar, and postalveolar nasals and plosives as well as fricatives; unaspirated and aspirated voiceless plosives; affricates, implosives, ejectives and clicks. There are also some voiceless approximants (e.g. some of the rhotics), but not the laterals. This chart can be useful for clinical phoneticians, but, as noted below, it will not fulfill all their requirements in terms of a symbol system to denote disordered speech.

As noted in Chapter 12, the IPA was not designed to transcribe disordered speech and, although much of the speech encountered in the clinic can be denoted by IPA symbols, there may well be sounds in disordered speech that do not occur in natural language (or very rarely so) and, thus, have no symbols in the IPA system. There have been a number of attempts to

CONSONANTS

	Bilabial	Labiodental	Dentolabial	Linguolabial	Dental	Alveolar	Postalveolar	Retroflex	Alveolo-palatal	Palatal	Velar	Uvular	Pharyngeal/ Epiglottal	Glottal
Plosive	pʰ p b	p̪ b̪	p͆ b͆	t̼ d̼	t̪ʰ t̪ d̪	tʰ t d	t̠ʰ t̠ d̠	ʈʰ ʈ ɖ	ȶʰ ȶ ȡ	cʰ c ɟ	kʰ k ɡ	qʰ q ɢ	ʡ	ʔ
Nasal	m̥ m	ɱ̊ ɱ	m̥͆ m͆	n̼̊ n̼	n̪̊ n̪	n̊ n	n̠̊ n̠	ɳ̊ ɳ	ȵ̊ ȵ	ɲ̊ ɲ	ŋ̊ ŋ	ɴ̥ ɴ		
Trill	ʙ̥ ʙ			r̼̊ r̼	r̪̊ r̪	r̥ r	r̠̊ r̠					ʀ̥ ʀ	ʜ ʢ	
Tap or Flap	ⱱ̟	ⱱ				ɾ̥ ɾ ɺ		ɽ̊ ɽ				ɢ̆	ʡ̆	
Fricative	ɸ β	f v	f͆ v͆	θ̼ ð̼	s̪ z̪ θ ð	s z	s̠ z̠ ʃ ʒ	ʂ ʐ	ɕ ʑ	ç ʝ	x ɣ ɧ	χ ʁ	ħ ʕ	h ɦ
Lateral fricative				ɬ̼ ɮ̼	ɬ̪ ɮ̪	ɬ ɮ	ɬ̠ ɮ̠							
Approximant	β̞ ʍ ɥ w	ʋ		ɹ̼	ð̞	ɹ̥ ɹ		ɻ̊ ɻ		ʝ̞ j ɥ	ɣ̞ ʍ ɰ w	ʁ̞	ʕ̞	
Lateral approximant				l̼	l̪	l	l̠	ɭ		ʎ	ʟ			
Affricate	pɸ bβ	p̪f b̪v	p͆f͆ b͆v͆	t̼θ̼ d̼ð̼	t̪s̪ d̪z̪ t̪θ d̪ð	ts dz	t̠s̠ d̠z̠ tʃ dʒ	ʈʂ ɖʐ	tɕ dʑ	cç ɟʝ	kx ɡɣ	qχ ɢʁ	ʡħ ʡʕ	
Lateral affricate						tɬ dɮ								
Implosive	ɓ̥ ɓ					ɗ̥ ɗ		ᶑ̊ ᶑ		ʄ̊ ʄ	ɠ̊ ɠ	ʛ̥ ʛ		
Ejective	pʼ	fʼ			θʼ t̪θʼ	tʼ sʼ ɬʼ tsʼ tɬʼ	ʃʼ tʃʼ	ʈʼ ʂʼ ʈʂʼ	tɕʼ	cʼ çʼ cçʼ	kʼ xʼ kxʼ	qʼ χʼ qχʼ		
Click	ʘ				ǀ	ǃ ǁ				ǂ				

Figure 13.1 An elaborated phonetic chart of consonants based on the IPA chart.

Source: Esling, 2010. Reproduced with permission of Wiley Publishers.

overcome these limitations, including, for example Shriberg and Kent's system (first described in Shriberg & Kent, 1982). We discuss some of the shortcomings of their proposals in Chapter 14, and will not discuss their system further here. Another early attempt to create clinically useful phonetic symbols was devised by the Phonetic Representation of Disordered Speech group (PRDS, 1980, 1983). This was a group of mainly British clinical phoneticians, and many of their suggestions have survived into the current extIPA system to be described later in this chapter.

A drawback of the PRDS system was that it lacked international recognition. However, The International Phonetic Association Congress held in Kiel in August 1989, had a mandate to revise the IPA. To this end a number of working parties were established. One of these was dedicated to the transcription of disordered speech. The participants in this working party produced a number of proposals that have been adopted by the Association as constituting part of the Extensions to the IPA, with other sections being added over time. A description of the original extIPA system is given in Duckworth, Allen, Hardcastle, and Ball (1990), and the most recent revisions to the system are reported in Ball, Howard, and Miller (2018).

The symbols and diacritics included on the extIPA chart are included due to requests from clinicians and phoneticians working with disordered speech data. However, those devising symbols for disordered speech try and avoid providing them for rare usages, instead concentrating on providing symbols for atypical speech sounds that occur relatively frequently in clinical data.

As well as symbols for segmental aspects of disordered speech, clinical phoneticians have also devised a method of transcribing aspects of typical and non-typical voice quality, and these are briefly described later in this chapter. However, we turn first to an examination of the extIPA system.

Extensions to the IPA for disordered speech (extIPA)

This description of the extIPA ([ɛkˈstaɪpə]) symbols is based on the current (2015) revision as described in Ball et al. (2018), and shown in Figure 13.2 in its 2020 re-arranged chart.

Consonant table

As on the IPA Chart (see Figure 12.1), the top part of the chart is dominated by a consonant table. Following IPA conventions, this table is constructed with place of articulation across the top, and manner of articulation down the side, creating a series of "boxes" at the intersections of the rows and columns. Also, as on the IPA consonant table, where there are two symbols in any one box, that on the left is voiceless, that on the right is voiced. Where a box has only a single symbol, its position at the left or at the right identifies its voicing status. There are also shaded boxes which, as with the IPA chart, denote that this particular articulation is deemed to be impossible to make. Empty boxes are either articulations for which an ordinary IPA symbol exists, or articulations which have no symbol in either the IPA or the extIPA.

Places of articulation

The place of articulation columns include many of the places found on the IPA chart but also some that are not. The former are, of course, not disordered but some combinations of these places with specific manners are. The non-IPA places of articulation are labioalveolar (lower lip articulating against the upper alveolar ridge), dentolabial (upper lip to lower teeth), bidental

extIPA SYMBOLS FOR DISORDERED SPEECH

CONSONANTS (other than those on the IPA Chart)

©①② ICPLA 2020

	bilabial	labio-dental	labio-alveolar	dento-labial	bidental	linguo-labial	inter-dental	alveolar	retroflex	palatal	velar	velo-pharyng.	(upper) pharyng.
Plosive		p̪ b̪	p̺ b̺	p̼ b̼			t̪ d̪	t̺ d̺					Ꝙ ꞯ
Nasal		m̥̪ m̪	m̥̺ m̺				n̥̪ n̪	n̥̺ n̺					
Trill						r̼		r̺				ʩ̥ ʩ	
Fricative median		f̪ v̪	f̺ v̺	h̪ h̺		θ̼ ð̼	θ̪ ð̪	θ̺ ð̺				ʩ̥ ʩ	
Fricative lateral				ꞎ̪ ꞎ̺	ꞎ̼ ꞎ̼		ꞎ ꞎ	ꞎ ꞎ	ꞎ ꞎ				
Fricative lat. + med.								ls lz					
Fricative nasal	m̥̃ m̃	m̥̪̃ m̪̃					ñ̥̺ ñ	ñ̥̪ ñ̪	ñ̥ ñ	ñ̥ ñ			
Approxt. lateral						l̼	l̺						
Percussive	ʬ				¡								

DIACRITICS

♀	labial spreading	s̯ ᵊ	ȏ, ȍ	denasal, partial denasal	m̄ n̄	♀	main gesture offset right	s̹
♀	strong articulation	f̬	ȏ	fricative nasal escape	v̬ ð̬	♀	main gesture offset left	s̜
♀	weak articulation	ʋ	ȏ	velopharyngeal friction	s̞ ʒ̞	♀	whistled articulation	s̪
\	reiteration	p\p\p	↓	ingressive airflow	p↓	◌◌	sliding articulation	θs

CONNECTED SPEECH, UNCERTAINTY ETC.

(.) (..) (...) (1.3s)	short, medium, long, 1.3-second pause
f, ff	loud(er) speech: [{f lavd f}, {ff lavdə ff}]
p, pp	quiet(er) speech: [{p kwaɪət p}, {pp kwaɪətə pp}]
allegro	fast speech: [{allegro fast allegro}]
lento	slow speech: [{lento sloʊ lento}]
cresc(endo), rall(entando), etc. may also be used	
⊙ Ⓒ Ⓖ Ⓕ Ⓛ	indeterminate: sound, consonant, glide, fricative, lateral,
Ⓝ Ⓟ Ⓡ Ⓢ Ⓣ	nasal, voiceless plosive, rhotic, sibilant, tone/stress,
Ⓥ Ⓚ σ ⓑ etc.	nasal vowel, click, syllable; probably [b], etc.
( )	silent articulation, e.g. (ʃ), (m)
(( ))	extraneous noise, e.g. ((2 sylls)) or ((2σ))

VOICING

◌̥	pre-voicing	̬t
◌̬	post-voicing	z̬
◌̰	post-creak etc.	a̰
◌̥	partial devoicing	z̰ ʒ̰
◌̥	initial partial devoicing	z̰ ʒ̰
◌̥	final partial devoicing	z̰ ʒ̰
◌̬	partial voicing	s̬
◌̬	initial partial voicing	s̬
◌̬	final partial voicing	s̬
◌=	unaspirated	p=
ʰ◌	pre-aspiration	ʰp

OTHER SOUNDS

ɹ̈ ï	apical-r, bunched-r (molar-r)
s̺ z̺	laminal fricatives (incl. lowered tongue tip)
kꞎ cꞍ dꞎ	[k, c, d] with lateral fricated release etc.
tˡˢ dˡᶻ	[t, d] with lateral and median release
tʰ̪	[t] with interdental aspiration
tʰʰ or tʰː	[t] with long aspiration

ʞ ꝗ ᶇ	velodorsal oral and nasal stops
ꞎ	sublaminal lower alveolar percussive
ǃ¡	alveolar click with sublaminal percussive release
◌r̼	buccal interdental trill (raspberry)
t̼θ d̼ð	linguolabial affricates etc.
*	sound with no available symbol

Figure 13.2 The extIPA Chart. ©ICPLA. (Reproduced with permission).

(upper and lower teeth), linguolabial (tongue tip to upper lip), velopharyngeal (articulation at the velopharyngeal port where the soft palate meets the upper pharynx wall), and upper pharyngeal (tongue back retracted into the upper pharynx). Labioalveolar articulations are only possible in speakers with overbites such that attempts at biblabial or labiodental articulations will result in this labioalveolar contact. The symbols are formed by adding the extIPA alveolar diacritic to symbols for labial consonants (the IPA surprisingly has no diacritic for alveolar place of articulation; the extIPA diacritic was designed to suggest the upper and lower edge of the alveolar ridge). Dentolabial articulations may also be found termed "reverse labiodentals" and use the IPA dental diacritic above the symbol rather than below to denote that this is the "reverse" of the usual articulation. Linguolabials are found in a very few natural languages (see IPA, 1999) as well as in disordered speech, and the diacritic used in this column is an official IPA one. Velopharyngeal and upper pharyngeal articulations have dedicated extIPA symbols for articulations made at these places (though see below for a diacritic to denote accompanying velopharyngeal friction).

Manner of articulation

The manner of articulation rows have just three atypical types: lateral+median fricative, nasal fricative and percussive. The first has both central and lateral grooving such that air escapes along both channels. They have only been reported at the alveolar place and have been given dedicated symbols (a combined l+s and l+z). The nasal fricatives are not to be confused with nasalized fricatives, and need to have audible nasal air escape to be assigned to this manner. The symbols consist of nasal stop symbols with the extIPA diacritic for audible nasal air escape added to them; voiceless versions are denoted by adding the IPA voicelessness diacritic to the relevant symbol. Percussives involve the rapid striking of one semi-rigid or rigid articulator against another. Symbols are provided for just two of these: bilabials and bidentals, in each case using a pair of relevant IPA diacritics one above the other. Percussives are probably produced most often with a simultaneous glottal stop and, if this is required to be symbolized, the IPA conventions for showing double articulation can be utilized.

The novel extIPA symbols

Many of the symbols shown in the consonant table are, of course, normal IPA symbols differentiated by one of the diacritics described above. These include all the labioalveolar, dentolabial, linguolabial and interdental symbols, and most of the labiodental, and alveolar symbols. The first totally novel extIPA symbols are those for the upper pharyngeal stops. Echoing the IPA symbols for uvular stops ([q, ɢ]), these are a small capital-Q and a reverse, inverted, small capital-G [ꞯ, ↄ].

The velopharyngeal trills and fricatives involve new symbols (albeit with the IPA voicing diacritic to denote the voiced versions). The symbols are constructed out of the IPA [f] and [ŋ] to suggest the involvement of the velum and the fricative nature of the resultant sounds. The trill symbols have an added horizontal wavy line to suggest the trilled nature of these sounds; trill: [fŋ͌], fricative: [fŋ].

The lateral fricative row of the extIPA chart includes some non-IPA symbols (although these have been used before unofficially by phoneticians working with a variety of non-European languages). Symbols are now provided for voiceless and voiced retroflex lateral fricatives ([ꞎ, 𝼅]), and voiceless lateral fricatives at the palatal and velar places of articulation ([ʎ̝̊, ʟ̝̊]); with voiced symbols shown by use of the IPA voicing diacritic. Lateral fricatives at other atypical places of articulation (linguolabial and interdental) are transcribed with the addition of the diacritics described above ([l̼, ꞎ], [l̪͆, ꞎ̪͆]).

Novel extIPA symbols are also provided for the lateral+median fricatives and the percussives, and these were described earlier.

Diacritics

The next section of the chart illustrates some dozen extIPA diacritics. Some of these supply ways of symbolizing aspects of articulation found in both typical and disordered speech but which have no way of being shown via IPA diacritics or symbols. Examples include the diacritics for lip spreading, ingressive airflow, and whistled articulation of sibilants. Others are mainly or solely aimed at transcribing disordered speech. These include the diacritics for weak and strong articulations, reiteration, denasal, fricative nasal air escape, accompanying velopharyngeal friction, left and right offset gestures, and sliding articulation.

The notion of denasal is somewhat problematic because, if a sound is totally denasal, then an oral symbol should be used (the devisors of extIPA do not support transcribing by target, see Chapter 15). The diacritic, therefore, would seem to be of use to denote partial denasalization. If transcribers wish to make this clear, then the use of parentheses around the diacritic accomplishes this and echoes the use of such parentheses in the phonation diacritics elsewhere on the chart.

The sliding articulation diacritic differs from the others in that it is placed below two symbols. Its use is to denote the rapid movement of the articulators from one position to a neighboring one within the timing slot for a single segment.

Connected speech and voicing

Connected speech and uncertainty

Below the diacritics section of the extIPA chart, to the left, is a section showing ways of transcribing aspects of connected speech and uncertainty in transcription. The connected speech items cover aspects of pausing, loudness, and tempo. While the notations for pausing are self-explanatory, it is worth pointing out that the symbols for loudness and tempo introduce a novel way of transcribing prosodic information (that is, phonetic characteristics that extend over more than one segment). This is the labeled brace (see also the section on the VoQS symbols later in this chapter). The braces are placed around the stretch of segments over which the prosodic feature operates, and also the braces are "labeled" by adding the prosodic symbol to the right of the opening brace and to the left of the closing one. Thus, [ˈðɪs ɪz {$_f$ ˈlaʊd $_f$} ˈspitʃ] ("this is loud speech") illustrates a change from normal loudness to louder speech, but just on the word "loud" itself.

Uncertainty in transcription is shown by using a circle. An empty circle means that the transcriber thinks there was a segment, but is unsure whether it was a vowel or consonant; a circle around V or C denotes that the sound was assumed to be a vowel or a consonant but no further details can be made out. Circles can be placed around abbreviations for manners or places of articulation, or voicing, or around specific phonetic symbols, all meaning that the transcriber was uncertain of the information placed within the circle.

At the end of this section are conventions for transcribing silent articulations (also known as "mouthings"), and extraneous noises (such as someone knocking on the door part-way through a recording session).

Voicing

The symbols in this section are all concerned with phonation and its timing. By using the IPA diacritic for voice and placing it to the left or right of the relevant symbol, extIPA allows the marking of pre- or post-voicing. Also, by using the diacritic-in-parentheses strategy referred to earlier, partial voicing or devoicing can be shown and, if required, the use of a single round bracket can indicate whether this is at the beginning or end of the segment concerned. Finally, extIPA allows the marking of an unaspirated plosive (the diacritic here was long used unofficially, though the IPA itself does not allow for the unambiguous transcription of non-aspiration), or a pre-aspirated plosive (by simply moving the IPA aspiration diacritic to be in front of the symbol rather than after it).

Other sounds

The final section of the extIPA chart is a collection of a dozen or so other symbols that do not easily fit elsewhere. The first two show extIPA recommendations for transcribing apical versus molar-r (also known as retroflex versus bunched). The apical version is to be transcribed using the IPA apical diacritic, the second using the IPA centralization diacritic. The third example illustrates the recommended way of transcribing [s] and [z] that are produced with the tongue blade rather than the tip (using the IPA laminar, or blade, diacritic). These laminar sibilants are often found with the tongue lowered to articulate with the lower alveolar ridge behind the lower front dentition. There is no specific recommendation on how to show this in transcription, but a combination of the laminar diacritic and the lowering mark would suffice: [s̪˕].

The next several examples illustrate various unusual release types for plosives: lateral fricated release, lateral and median release, and interdental release, all using relevant extIPA symbols as release diacritics.

The second column of 'other sounds' starts with the symbols for velodorsals (where the soft palate is the active articulator against a static and passive tongue dorsum). These are reversed versions of the usual velar symbols for oral and nasal stops. Next are the sublaminal percussive click (tongue tip struck downwards against the lower alveolar ridge), and the so-called 'cluck-click' of an alveolar click followed immediately by the sublaminal percussive click. A way of transcribing the buccal interdental trill (or 'rasp-berry') is shown, combining the buccal airstream symbol from the VoQS chart (see below), and the trill symbol with interdental diacritics.

Then we have an illustration of atypical affricates, in this case a linguolabial affricate; the suggestion of the 'etc' being that others could be shown in a similar manner using the IPA linking mark above the relevant symbols. The very last symbol—the asterisk—is the recommendation for transcribing a sound for which no symbol exists; the asterisk is then repeated at the end of the transcription with a verbal description of the sound produced.

Possible extra symbols

There have been symbols proposed either as alternatives for current IPA and extIPA symbols or as additions for sounds not so far covered. These include:

- Labiodental stops (using Africanist symbols): [ꝑ, Ꝓ];
- Alveolo-palatal sounds: [t̠, d̠, n̠, l̠] as well as IPA [ɕ, ʑ];
- Miscellaneous: [ɭ̆] for a retroflex lateral flap, [ʁ] for an epiglottal trill.

The main area lacking adequate symbols, though, is the approximant category. Symbols are provided for lateral, rhotic, and semi-vowel approximants, but very few for "weak fricative" approximants often encountered clinically (as in dysarthric speech); also, using the lowering diacritic results in symbols that are difficult to read. The IPA has [ʋ] for a "weak" version of [v] but it can be argued that [j] and [ɥ] should be restricted to semi-vowels as they are not identical to weak fricative versions of [ʝ] and [ɣ]. Suggested in Ball, Rahilly, Lowry, Bessell, and Lee (2020) are: [β̞, ð̞, ɹ, ɹ̠, j̞, ʎ̝, ʁ̞, ʕ̞], for bilabial, dental, alveolar, postalveolar, palatal, velar, uvular and pharyngeal approximants, respectively. It is possible that some, or all, of the symbols mentioned in this section could be incorporated into future iterations of the extIPA chart.

Voice quality symbols (VoQS)

The extIPA chart shown in Figure 13.2 provides a method of marking prosodic information in phonetic transcription through the use of labeled braces. However, that chart illustrates the concept only with symbols for loudness and tempo, even though this approach could clearly be used for a variety of other features. A range of suprasegmental phonetic characteristics that are usually subsumed under the heading of voice quality would seem to be ideal additions to the labeled brace convention. An initial set of voice quality symbols (abbreviated to VoQS, [vɑks]/[vɒks]) was drawn up by Ball, Esling, and Dixon (1995, 2000), and a revision, adding more categories, was undertaken recently (Ball, Esling, & Dixon, 2018). The current, 2016, chart is given in Figure 13.3.

Sections of the VoQS chart

In this part of the chapter, the main sections of the VoQS chart will be described and the symbols suggested for the different voice quality types described.

The chart is divided into several sections corresponding to different ways of contributing to voice quality (it should be noted that a particular speaker may use more than one of these to produce a multi-source voice quality). The topmost section is devoted to non-typical airstream types that contribute to the speaker's voice quality. Two of these are pulmonic ingressive speech (see examples in Chapter 15), that is, speech produced on an airstream that is the reverse of the usual pulmonic egressive air, and the buccal airstream: speech produced by expanding the cheeks and filling them with air and then expelling that air by contracting the cheeks thus increasing the air pressure. The sound often termed a "raspberry" is typically made using this airstream. The other two symbols denote airstreams that can be produced by speakers who have undergone laryngectomy (see Chapter 6). Depending on the type of laryngectomy, it may be possible for speakers to use air taken into the esophagus. This can be expelled past the sphincter at the pharyngoesophageal junction, thus causing phonation-like vibration. Alternatively, in certain types of laryngectomy, lung air can be used via a valve linking the trachea and the esophagus, to exit through the pharyngoesophageal junction. Symbols are provided for both esophageal and tracheoesophageal speech.

The next section contains symbols to denote phonation types. Several of these are official IPA symbols but, whereas the IPA mandates their use on individual symbols, the VoQS system allows them to be marked over a stretch of speech.[1] In this section most of the voice quality symbols consist of "V" (for "voice") with the relevant IPA, extIPA, or VoQS diacritic added. There are exceptions to this, however. Four basic phonation types of modal voice, whisper, creak, and falsetto are shown by V, W, C, and F. This allows modifications of these (such as

VoQS: Voice Quality Symbols

Airstream Types

ⅅ	buccal airstream	↓	pulmonic ingressive speech
Œ	œsophageal airstream	Ю	tracheo-œsophageal speech

Phonation Types

V	modal voice F falsetto	W whisper	C creak
V̤	whispery voice V̰ creaky voice	V̥ breathy voice V! harsh voice
F̤	whispery falsetto F̰ creaky falsetto	F! harsh falsetto C! harsh creak
V̤!	harsh whispery voice	V̰! harsh creaky voice
V̰̤	whispery creaky voice	V̰̤! harsh whispery creaky voice
F̰̤	whispery creaky falsetto	F̰̤! harsh whispery creaky falsetto
V̪	slack/lax voice	V̬ pressed phonation / tight voice
V‼	ventricular phonation	V̤‼ diplophonia
V̤‼	whispery ventricular phonation	Vᴧ aryepiglottic phonation
ʍ	spasmodic dysphonia	И electrolarynx phonation

Larynx Height

L̝	raised-larynx voice	L̞	lowered-larynx voice

Supralaryngeal Settings
Labial settings, lingual settings, state of the velum, jaw and tongue settings

Vᵒᵉ	labialized voice (open rounded)	Vʷ	labialized voice (close rounded)
V̜	spread-lip voice	Vᵛ	labio-dentalized voice
V̺	linguo-apicalized voice	V̻	linguo-laminalized voice
Vˤ	retroflex voice	V̪	dentalized voice
V̠	alveolarized voice	V̠ʲ	palato-alveolarized voice
Vʲ	palatalized voice	Vˠ	velarized voice
Vʁ	uvularized voice	Vˤ	pharyngealized voice
V̞ˤ	laryngo-pharyngealized voice	Vᴴ	faucalized voice
Ṽ	nasalized voice	V̰	denasalized voice
J̞	open-jaw voice	J̝	close-jaw voice
J̪	right offset-jaw voice	J̺	left offset-jaw voice
J̟	protruded-jaw voice	Θ	protruded-tongue voice

Labeled braces and numerals mark degree and combinations of voice quality:

['nɔˑməl 'vɔɪs {3V! 'vɛ.ɪ 'haʃ 'vɔɪs 3V!} {L̝ 1V! 'lɛs 'haʃ 'vɔɪs wɪð 'ɹeɪzd 'læ.ɹɪŋks 1V! L̝}]

Figure 13.3 The VoQS Chart. (© Martin J. Ball, John Esling, and Craig Dickson.

Source: Reproduced with permission.

harsh voice or whispery creak) to be readily denoted by adding diacritics to these capital letters. (Voiceless phonation is assumed to be shown at the segmental level, however, breathy voice is denoted by using the IPA diacritic for breathy, attached to V.)

Lax and tight voice (also known as slack and pressed phonation) are denoted using extIPA diacritics with capital-V, while various combinations of ventricular and aryepiglottic phonation types use the double exclamation mark (ventricular) and the double-A (aryepiglottic) as diacritics. Finally, in the phonation types, there are dedicated symbols for spasmodic dysphonia and for electrolarynx phonation; the former a type of voice disorder, the latter another voice-producing mechanism (an externally handheld device that produces a buzz) for speakers who have undergone a laryngectomy.

The next section of the chart contains just two entries, both denoting voice quality derived from larynx height. Using the IPA raising and lowering diacritics on a capital-L, the effect of speaking with either a raised or lowered larynx can be transcribed.

The largest section of the chart is devoted to ways of denoting voice quality derived from supralaryngeal settings. The first subsection is for voice quality derived from differing labial settings, the second mainly for lingual settings[2], the third for oral/nasal distinctions, and the final subsection mainly for jaw settings. Most of these use relevant IPA and extIPA diacritics added to the V symbol. Exceptions to the V symbol include J for the jaw settings and Θ for protruded tongue voice.

At the bottom of the chart, there is an illustration of how to use these symbols with the labeled brace convention and, also, how to denote degrees of a particular voice quality (e.g. somewhat harsh through to very harsh). Clearly not all the symbols are amenable to the use of numerals (it is difficult to see how one could have a slightly falsetto phonation). The example also shows how two or more VoQS symbols can be used together to denote combined voice qualities (in this case harshness and larynx height). It would be satisfying if one could restrict such combinations to voice qualities from different part of the chart (i.e. a voice quality from one (sub)section could only combine with one from another). This is often the case; for example, nasalized voice cannot simultaneously be denasal; raised larynx speech cannot simultaneously be lowered larynx speech. However, this restriction does not always hold as left or right offset jaw could combine with open jaw or protruded tongue, and linguo-apicalized voice could combine with alveoralized voice, and so forth. Nevertheless, the sections and subsections are generally a good guide as to which voice quality types can co-occur and which cannot.

It could be argued that some of these symbols are unlikely to be used with the labeled brace system as they are permanently "on" for a speaker. In particular, the esophageal and tracheoesophageal airstreams would be used all the time by certain speakers, as might some of the phonation types in certain voice disorders. In such cases, of course, the VoQS symbol can be placed at the beginning and end of the entire transcription as a reminder to the reader of the voice type used by the speaker.

Transcribing intonation

Intonation, along with other suprasegmental aspects of speech, is described in Chapter 5, and in Chapter 12 the lack of IPA conventions for transcribing intonation is noted. Various notation types are discussed in Chapter 5, but some of these are inapplicable to disordered intonation. Notations, such as the ToBI system (Pierrehumbert, 1980), or even the O'Connor and Arnold system (O'Connor & Arnold, 1971) have a set number of intonation units designed around a specific language or language variety. Disordered intonation often involves tone units, tone placements, and tone movements that are outwith the norm for the target language variety and

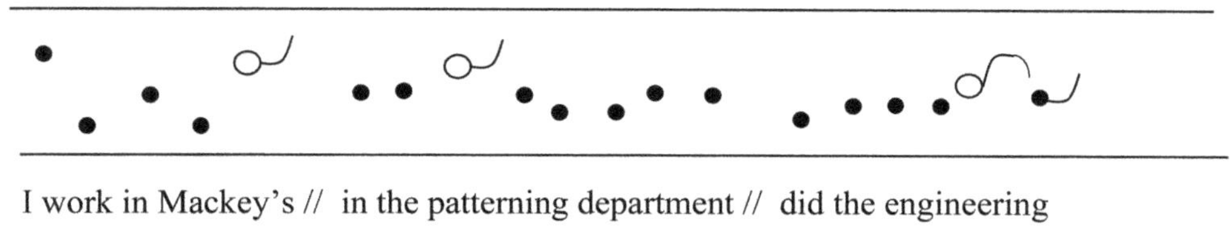

I work in Mackey's // in the patterning department // did the engineering

Figure 13.4　Intonation pattern display of speaker with hearing impairment.

Source: From Rahilly, 1991; reproduced with permission of the author.

thus may prove difficult to capture via notations designed for the typical speech prosody of that variety.

So-called "tadpole" or "musical stave" notation (Müller, 2006) may well be the best way to transcribe disordered intonation. Here, large dots represent stressed syllables and small dots unstressed syllable and, where relevant, "tadpole tails" denote the direction and extent of any pitch movement. We can illustrate this with an example from Rahilly (1991), where a postlingually hearing impaired adult male uttered the following phrase: "I work in Mackey's, in the patterning department, did the engineering." We display this intonation pattern using stave (tadpole) notation, in Figure 13.4.

While the division into three tone units is what might be expected, the high rises in the first two units and the rise-fall-rise in the last are definitely unusual, both in terms of the location of the pitch movements (e.g. in the first tone unit it is one what would be expected to be an unstressed syllable), and their direction and extent.

Conclusion

In this chapter we have looked at current standards of transcription of segmental and supra-segmental aspects of disordered speech. These are not set in stone, however, and—just as in the case of the International Phonetic Alphabet itself—are subject to revision. In revisions, symbols may be withdrawn (if the speech behavior they denote turns out to be extremely rare), changed (perhaps to avoid confusion with other symbols), or added to (if newly discovered atypical sounds are described in the literature and need to be transcribed). It is likely, therefore, that both the extIPA and VoQS symbol systems will be subject to further revision. The methods of transcribing intonation described in this chapter, being mainly iconic, are presumably suffi-cient to denote any unusual pitch contours and, thus, unlikely to need to be changed or added to.

Notes

1　In such cases, it is assumed that voiceless symbols still denote voiceless sounds, but that voiced symbols are produced with the relevant phonation type denoted by the VoQS symbol.
2　The exception to this is the symbol for faucalized voice (where the faucal pillars are drawn closer together), as there is not specific lingual usage here.

References

Ball, M.J., Esling, J., & Dickson, C. (1995). The VoQS System for the transcription of voice quality. *Journal of the International Phonetic Association, 25*, 71–80.
Ball, M.J., Esling, J., & Dickson, C. (2000). Transcription of voice. In R.D. Kent & M.J. Ball (Eds.), *Voice quality measurement* (pp. 49–58). San Diego, CA: Singular Publishing.

Ball, M.J., Esling, J., & Dickson, C. (2018). Revisions to the VoQS system for the transcription of voice quality. *Journal of the International Phonetic Association, 48*, 165–171.

Ball, M.J., Howard, S.J., & Miller, K. (2018). Revisions to the extIPA chart. *Journal of the International Phonetic Association, 48*, 155–164.

Ball, M. J., Rahilly, J., Lowry, O., Bessell, N., & Lee, A. (2020). *Phonetics for speech pathology* (3rd ed.). Sheffield, UK: Equinox.

Duckworth, M., Allen, G., Hardcastle, W.J., & Ball, M.J. (1990). Extensions to the International Phonetic Alphabet for the transcription of atypical speech. *Clinical Linguistics and Phonetics, 4*, 273–280.

Esling, J. (2010). Phonetic notation. In W.J. Hardcastle, J. Laver, & F.E. Gibbon (Eds.), *The handbook of phonetic sciences* (2nd ed., pp. 678–702). Chichester, UK: Wiley-Blackwell.

IPA (1999). *Handbook of the IPA*. Cambridge: Cambridge University Press.

Müller, N. (Ed.), (2006). *Multilayered transcription*. San Diego, CA: Plural Publications.

O'Connor, J.D. & Arnold, G.F. (1971). *Intonation of colloquial English: A practical handbook* (2nd ed.). London, UK: Longmans.

Pierrehumbert, J. (1980). *The phonology and phonetics of English intonation*. PhD thesis, MIT. Distributed 1988, Indiana University Linguistics Club.

PRDS (1980). The phonetic representation of disordered speech. *British Journal of Disorders of Communication, 15*, 217–223.

PRDS (1983). *The phonetic representation of disordered speech: Final report*. London, UK: King's Fund.

Rahilly, J. (1991). *Intonation patterns in normal hearing and postlingually deafened adults in Belfast*. Unpublished PhD thesis, Queen's University of Belfast.

Shriberg. L. & Kent, R.D. (1982). *Clinical phonetics*. New York, NY: Wiley.

14

TEACHING AND LEARNING CLINICAL PHONETIC TRANSCRIPTION

Jill Titterington and Sally Bates

Introduction

Seventy per cent of speech and language therapists' (SLTs') pediatric caseloads in the United Kingdom are impacted by speech sound disorder (SSD) (Dodd, B., 2005) and a large proportion of the adult population receiving SLT services experience disorders of motor speech and/ or voice (Duffy, 2013). The high incidence of SSD in SLT caseloads highlights the importance of clinical phonetics for SLTs and is mirrored by findings that phonetics and phonology are the predominant areas of research published in the journal of *Clinical Linguistics & Phonetics* (Crystal, 2002; Perkins, 2011).

Clinical phonetic transcription is recognized as a highly specialist skill requiring many hours of practice to develop and maintain (Knight, Bandali, Woodhead, & Vansadia, 2018): it is a unique component of the SLT's role. The accuracy and reliability of phonetic transcription directly informs the analysis of disordered speech and subsequent clinical decision making, thus underpinning ethical use of SLT time (e.g. Ball & Rahilly, 2002; Howard & Heselwood, 2002; Rahilly, 2011; Stemberger & Bernhardt, 2019; UK and Ireland's Child Speech Disorder Research Network (CSDRN), 2017; Bates, Titterington with the CSDRN, 2017). Clearly then, the ability of entry level SLTs to produce good-quality phonetic transcriptions with a high level of accuracy and consistency (Müller and Damico, 2002) should be the goal of all pre-registration training. This chapter considers: (1) how teaching and learning for pre-registration SLT programs could (and to some extent does) address the challenges posed by the expectations inherent in such a goal and; (2) will specifically review a solution-focused investigation into managing some of the key challenges identified.

Section One

Expectation 1: Professional standards, underpinned by quality assurance, guarantee expertise in clinical phonetic transcription by newly qualified SLTs

Background: Across the world, accredited pre-registration programs for SLTs have a set of competency/proficiency-based standards for newly qualified practitioners supported by curriculum guidance. These standards inform the teaching and learning of all subjects covered in the SLT curriculum. In the United Kingdom, general details are provided about the competency levels to be attained in clinical transcription prior to graduation, e.g. the Health and Care Professions Council (HCPC) Standards of Proficiency (SOP) standard: "14.7 [.] to describe and analyse service users' abilities and needs using, where appropriate, phonetic transcription, linguistic analysis, instrumental analysis and psycholinguistic assessment" (Health & Care Professions Council (HCPC), 2014; Standards of Proficiency for Speech and Language Therapists, 2014). In other countries such as Australia and the United States, competencies to be attained are specified in a similarly broad manner[1]. This relatively non-prescriptive approach across all these countries (and potentially globally) means that the quality standards used to specify curricular content and subsequent clinical competencies/proficiencies in phonetic transcription are not specific.

Challenge: How can adequate entry level skills in clinical phonetic transcription be guaranteed without detailed baseline competencies?

The lack of detail about baseline competencies required of newly qualified SLTs in phonetic transcription results in a lack of consensus across programs with regard to the fundamental components of an effective and efficient pedagogic and clinical experience to best support learning of phonetic transcription. This lack of consensus and consequent variation in teaching and learning of phonetic transcription impacts on: the number of hours devoted to practice in transcription; how skill levels are set and assessed; the experience students receive; and subsequent parity in the skill level achieved by students graduating from different institutions. Indeed, there is some concern that this lack of standardization and benchmarking of competencies leads to the reality that "expertise cannot be assumed" (Powell, 2001).

These concerns extend to SLTs in practice when knowledge and skills developed during pre-registration training can be difficult to maintain without periods of revision and when certain skill areas may be tapped infrequently (Knight, Bandali, Woodhead & Vansadia, 2018; Stemberger & Bernhardt, 2019). This is particularly the case when SLTs are increasingly working with multilingual clients and may not be familiar with the speech sounds, phonetic inventory and phonotactics of each child's target language (Stemberger & Bernhardt, 2019). SLTs often report a lack of post-registration opportunities for further learning in clinical phonetics to maintain their skills and build expertise which further compounds the issue of maintaining core competencies/proficiency standards once SLTs are in the workplace (Knight, Bandali, Woodhead, & Vansadia, 2018; Nelson, Mok, and Eecen, 2019).

Solutions: Opportunities could be created to agree and develop a benchmark of core competencies/proficiency standards to be attained in phonetic transcription for pre-registration SLT programs. Ideally this would be agreed at an international level; perhaps through an organization such as the *International Association of Logopedics & Phoniatrics.*

Once in the workplace, SLTs have the option to maintain and build their skills through independent revision of IPA symbols (perception and production) and participate in tutorials supporting revision online (see Stemberger & Bernhardt, 2019 for a list and discussion of these). However, in the main, these tools do not provide the supported, applied and active learning environment that therapists have identified as being most useful (Knight, Bandali, Woodhead, & Vansadia, 2018, Nelson, Mok, & Eecen, 2019). Consequently, the development of the benchmarks, guidance and/or standards proposed above could be extended to support maintenance and development of clinical phonetic transcription skills for SLTs post-registration both in more generalist and specialist settings (such as cleft lip and palate and hearing impairment where more support and training opportunities are generally in place).

Such benchmarks could also support the development of newer fields of speciality in clinical phonetic transcription such as for multilingual children with SSD. The outcome of this work would be the development of a layered, accountable and transparent approach to the development of clinical phonetic transcription skills. This would specify proficiency standards/competency levels for: new graduates; postgraduate generalists; and then postgraduate specialists supported by continuing professional development opportunities.

Expectation 2: All entry-level graduates possess the requisite level of skill in phonetic transcription to support differential diagnosis, selection of targets/ intervention approaches and monitoring of client progress in intervention

While expectation one highlights the need for a competency-based framework to support skill development and maintenance in phonetic transcription, here, we discuss challenges and possible solutions around setting such standards. Different areas are important to consider and include: (a) skills in broad and narrow transcription and; (b) the level of skill achieved in instrumental/ technological analysis.

What should the requisite level of skill be for broad versus narrow transcription?

Background: There has been much debate about the value of a production versus target philosophy toward clinical phonetic transcription (i.e. Howard & Heselwood, 2002; Rahilly, 2011; see Chapters 15 and 16 of this volume). Rahilly (2011) talks about "…the imperative to be led by actual production, rather than misled by expectations" where narrow transcription captures the reality of an individual's speech productions and broad transcription captures the generality of what an individual produces. Indeed, the benefits of narrow over broad transcription have been clearly demonstrated by Ball and colleagues (e.g. Ball and Rahilly, 2002; see Chapters 15 and 16 of this volume) and reduce the likelihood of over- or under-recognizing issues with speech accuracy.

Challenge: As transcriptions become more detailed and narrow, they become less reliable (see Powell, T. (2001) and transcribers generally have less confidence as speech becomes more unintelligible and less predictable (Ramsdell, Kimbrough Oller, & Ethington, 2007). Knight et al. (2018) found that 45% of her sample of 759 UK SLTs used a mixture of narrow and broad transcription while 41% used only broad transcription. SLTs appeared to use narrow transcription when they worked with specialist caseloads, i.e. cleft lip and palate or hearing impairment but otherwise felt they did not have the time or confidence to use it. This is an important finding and may reflect several key issues: (1) pre-registration training may not be comprehensive enough to support SLTs to use narrow transcription in practice; (2) student SLTs may not experience narrow transcription being used (and may not have the opportunity to use it themselves) when on clinical placement; (3) SLTs who provide predominantly screening and review (as in some triage systems) may rely predominantly on broad transcription; (3) SLTs may not have the time and confidence to use narrow transcription effectively within more generalist clinical settings.

Solutions: Phonetic transcription is a skill that has to be learnt. As with any skill, we become more confident and able with practice; it therefore follows that increased skill level can be attained with increased hours of practice. Indeed, this accords with Howard and Heselwood's (2002) recommendations that the time required to develop adequate skills in phonetic transcription should be raised from 100 hours (as recommended previously) to 700 hours! This is a challenge because many pre-registration programs at undergraduate and postgraduate levels are now 3 and 2 years long, respectively. Considering the outcomes of the Royal College of Speech and Language Therapists' (RCSLT, 2017) curriculum guidelines online conversation ($n = 1,383$ participants) there is also a strong drive to increase hours of clinical placement, and time on non-linguistic skills such as leadership, resilience and time management. These are all important of course, but this focus tends to result in less face-to-face time for teaching students clinical phonetic transcription.

Ensuring that students receive sufficient hours across SLT programs to practice and develop their skills of phonetic transcription at pre-registration level would increase confidence and skill in both broad and narrow transcription. To overcome the challenge of shorter programs with dense teaching and clinical placement, online learning opportunities can be used to supplement face-to-face teaching (see Knight, Bandali, Woodhead, & Vansadia, 2018; Nelson, Mok, & Eecen, 2019). These online learning opportunities may utilize current resources available (see Stemberger & Bernhardt, 2019) and/or involve developing bespoke online learning mapped to specific teaching and learning outcomes (see Titterington & Bates, 2018). Developing suitable online materials to support learning of phonetic transcription can be challenging when considering IT issues such as software use and future proofing, and also of course data protection issues around use of speech recordings from clients. However, support from IT departments, collaboration with others teaching clinical phonetics within and across countries, adherence to GDPR and clinical governance guidelines will hopefully help drive the development of useful resources to support the teaching and learning of phonetic transcription worldwide.

In order to maximize learning for students from these online tools (which are invariably used independently by students), understanding about the pedagogy of online learning that best supports phonetic transcription needs to be further investigated and developed. Research into this area has been promising to-date. For example, Knight (2010) supported 30 undergraduate SLTs in their learning of phonetic transcription by using podcasts. The students enjoyed the experience and reported that it increased their confidence for their final piece of transcription coursework. Titterington and Bates' (2018) study particularly considered the importance of student engagement and motivation for independent online learning when aiming to increase hours of phonetic transcription practice. These findings have implications for how online learning could be used to optimally support student learning of phonetic transcription and will be considered in more depth under section 2.

Importantly, this increase in hours of transcription practice should extend to ensuring that students experience clinical placement with specialists in SSD and have consequent opportunities to practice skills of narrow transcription within the context of clinical placement. Indeed, the use of consensus transcription techniques could support student learning in this context as long as the potential "pitfall" noted by Stemberger and Bernhardt (2019) of "two wrongs do not make a right" is avoided. These approaches could increase student skill and confidence in their use of narrow transcription. Importantly, they could also support student appreciation of differences between narrow transcriptions of the same data and potential issues around inter-transcriber reliability (see Chapter 16 of this volume).

While the number of hours of transcription practice are important; where the teaching and learning for phonetic transcription is situated within a SLT program also needs consideration. This is particularly important when considering the fade in learning that can happen if there is a gap between acquiring a skill and using it (Knight, Bandali, Woodhead, & Vansadia, 2018; Stemberger & Bernhardt, 2019). Modules teaching phonetic transcription skills are often situated in the first year of SLT programs and some consideration must be given to the possibility of either distributing the learning across the whole program and/or providing revision sessions in final year. Good practice would be a program that integrates phonetic transcription practice across modules and within all placement opportunities as appropriate (supporting deep learning, Biggs, 2003).

As well as ensuring that students have repeated, regular opportunities for transcription practice, it is valuable to consider the recommendations made for expectation one; where a layered, accountable and transparent approach to the development of clinical phonetic transcription skills would release the pressure of acquiring high-level skills in narrow transcription at the pre-registration level. Instead, an agreed series of benchmarked competencies could be laid out to support progression and development of clinical phonetic transcription skills from entry level right through to the postgraduate specialist level. Indeed, this approach to building skills across a SLTs career sits well with the reality that many entry-level SLTs will never need to use phonetic transcription in their clinical work.

It is also important to acknowledge the perspective that it may not always be necessary or indeed possible for SLTs to take a narrow approach to transcription. Stemberger and Bernhardt (2019) discuss the importance of the purpose of transcription driving the choice of broad or narrow transcription. They argue that a broad transcription may suffice when screening, or assessing generalization post-intervention. Indeed, when considering the phonological nature of the majority of the SLT's caseload presenting with SSD, broad transcription clearly has a valid place in clinical phonetic transcription. However, it is important to note as Stemberger and Bernhardt (2019) also argue; that narrow transcription provides important insight into a child's erred realizations thereby better supporting selection of appropriate targets, interventions and the monitoring of progressive change during therapy. Stemberger and Bernhardt (2019) also discuss the thorny issue of transcribing the speech of the multilingual caseload where children with SSD may speak a non-native language to the SLT. Here the expectation of narrow transcription is even more challenging for the SLT. Indeed, initially (once the target IPA system and an appropriate form of assessment has been identified (see McLeod and Verdon, 2014), Stemberger and Bernhardt (2019) suggest SLTs adopt an approach which considers how well the child's realizations match the adult target, venturing into more detailed transcription once the SLT is more familiar with the child's speech productions and target language. This is to help compensate for the biases that may arise when a native speaker of one language phonetically transcribes a different language, potentially resulting in inaccuracies. These are important issues for consideration when developing teaching and learning of clinical phonetic transcription.

What should the level of skill be for instrumental analysis of speech?

Background: Ideally, instrumental analysis of speech combines phonetically transcribed speech data captured through transcriber perception with speech data recorded and analyzed using instruments/technology in multi-tiered transcription. This provides greater information about less visible parts of the oral structure and musculature, and supports layering of segmental, voice and prosodic information, for example in the case of an individual with partial glossectomy of the tongue (see Howard & Heselwood, 2011). Furthermore, the ability to transcribe prosodic aspects of speech (particularly intonation, which can be difficult for some to perceive) can be greatly supported by instrumental analysis. Fundamentally from a teaching and learning perspective, instrumental analysis can add to the depth of student learning about both speech perception and production.

Challenge: Applying phonetic knowledge and skills to instrumental analysis of speech can be complex, time consuming and costly. While some instrumental tools for the analysis of speech and voice production are expensive, tools are increasingly becoming available that offer a wide range of free features, e.g. Praat (Boersma & Weenink, 2007). Whether an instrumental tool is free or not (or indeed accessible within the constrained software products approved within the UK's NHS IT systems), the time it takes to complete and interpret an acoustic analysis or evaluate lingual function using the electropalatograph for instance; is generally a resource not available to most clinicians. When the emphasis in teaching clinical transcription skills for entry level SLTs must be to support them to reach optimal skills of impressionistic phonetic transcription with clinical populations in the first instance, it seems that instrumental analysis may be the poor cousin. Fundamentally, the auditory perception of speech directly influences how it is understood; "speech works by sounding how it does regardless of how it is produced" (Howard & Heselwood, 2011). This places impressionistic phonetic transcription at the center of the SLTs core skills underpinning effective speech assessment.

Solutions: Despite this, there is no doubt that judicious use of instrumental analysis is important for particular presentations of SSD and caseloads. Analysis showing that a speaker's communicative intention does not match the transcriber's perception will inform diagnosis and intervention (Howard & Heselwood, 2011). Furthermore, intonational patterns can be difficult for many to perceive and its impressionistic transcription is plagued by different transcription approaches. These factors can lead to unreliability which can be resolved through the use of instrumental analysis. This is important for certain populations who have difficulties with prosody such as individuals with hearing impairment or autism spectrum disorder (Ball & Rahilly, 2002). Consequently, pre-registration training must at least, encompass the core basics of acoustic phonetics (taught with the support of instrumental tools for the analysis of speech and voice) in order to develop fundamental understanding and insight into the physiological processes underpinning speech production. Entry level SLTs can build on this understanding to make use of instrumental tools in their analysis of speech depending on what is available and expected within their own clinical setting.

Expectation 3: Teaching and assessment is underpinned by good pedagogical practice which motivates students to fully engage with learning clinical phonetic transcription

Background: Acquiring competency in clinical phonetic transcription requires an approach that supports deep rather than surface learning (Ashby & Ashby, 2013). Deep learning is the process of learning for transfer, meaning it allows a student to take what is learned in one situation, i.e. the classroom, and apply it to another, i.e. the clinical context. It involves translating declarative knowledge (i.e. factual information stored in memory) into functional knowledge (i.e. an understanding of how information can be adapted and applied practically) (Biggs & Tang, 2011). In addition to technical competence, effective use of phonetic transcription as a clinical tool also requires an appreciation of its potential limitations and an ability to integrate this understanding with knowledge and skills gained in other subject areas, e.g. phonetic and phonological analysis, and principles of assessment and remediation for individuals with SSD.

Deep learning results from students taking ownership of their learning and actively engaging with learning opportunities specifically designed to achieve the intended learning outcomes. Motivation and, in particular, what Biggs and Tang (2011) describe as *intrinsic* motivation is fundamental to this process. According to Biggs and Tang's (2011) expectancy-value theory of motivation, intrinsic motivation occurs when students find completion of the task itself rewarding. This is in contrast to *extrinsic* motivation, where students receive some kind of external reward for completing the task. Both types of motivation have an important role to play in supporting student engagement with learning.

*Challenge: Teaching and learning clinical phonetic transcription is a "threshold concept" (see (*https://www.heacademy.ac.uk/knowledge-hub/threshold-concepts*, 2019)*

Students must learn to think about speech in an entirely new way, focusing on the form of utterances rather than propositional content and suspend the knowledge they have been refining throughout their school years about written word forms and spelling patterns. As they progress in their training, they are also asked to suspend belief in the notion of sounds (and indeed spoken words) as discrete, invariant units and embrace the concept of speech as a dynamic, fluid phenomenon characterized by overlapping articulatory gestures. Historically, at the point when students are developing competence in narrow phonetic transcription, they must then face the fact that impressionistic transcriptions are open to debate and disagreement, and thus move away from the perspective of knowledge being absolute. This, coupled with the many hours of practice required to develop and maintain skill levels and the potential "problems and pitfalls" encountered along the way (see Howard & Heselwood, 2002) can make clinical phonetics an unpopular subject among some students (Knight, 2010). A key challenge for the tutor, therefore, is how to engender and sustain student motivation.

Solutions: Students who found learning phonetic transcription to be easier in Knight et al.'s (2018) survey cited "having a good teacher" as key. Although we do not fully understand as yet what makes good teachers of phonetics (Knight, Bandali, Woodhead, & Vansadia, 2018), we do know that good teaching is underpinned by good pedagogy.

Creating an environment which supports deep learning necessitates taking a student-centred, outcomes-based approach in which both teaching and assessment methods are constructively aligned with the desired learning outcomes (Biggs, 2003). Learning outcomes must be specified in terms of both the skill-set to be developed and, importantly, the context in which it is to be used, i.e. they must be clearly functional. In other words, teaching and assessment methods must be relevant to the real-life skills that students will need in practice. Students are more likely to engage in and benefit from the learning opportunities provided if they understand the clinical value and importance of phonetic transcription. Our research has shown that this is essential in supporting the development of both intrinsic and extrinsic motivation in students (Titterington & Bates, 2018).

Clinical relevance can be highlighted by using pseudo and authentic clinical data and through activities which require students to integrate and apply theoretical knowledge in a clinically meaningful way. For example, by asking students to use their knowledge of consonant and vowel classification to identify phonological processes and atypical speech patterns, or to generate minimal pairs targeting specific phonological contrasts for use in assessment or remediation. Approaching the same concepts (e.g. distinctive feature analysis) through a variety of activities assists retention as well as helps students structure their knowledge.

Ideally, opportunities to apply knowledge and skill in clinical phonetics should be woven throughout professional placement and, where possible, other modules as appropriate (Howard & Heselwood, 2002; Knight et al., 2018).

Ear training and speech production exercises can also be made more clinically meaningful by drawing students' attention to the parallels between their own experience and that of a client faced with the task of learning new motor patterns. Nonsense words incorporating non-system sounds and/or sound sequences which are either made-up, or "borrowed" from another language, are particularly useful in highlighting the challenges involved.

As in the clinical context, tasks may be "stepped-up" by asking students to produce longer and/or more complex sequences. Applying phonological processes to tongue twisters as for example, in the case of /ʃi sɛlz si ʃɛlz ɒn ðə si ʃɔ/ → [ti tɛlz ti tɛlz ɒn də ti tɔ] and asking students to produce these in turn as part of a "Mexican wave" is a fun and effective way of targeting several core skill areas. Error analysis can also give students valuable insight into the psycholinguistic processes underpinning speech production and increase understanding of key concepts such as phonetic and phonological contrast, phonetic similarity and top-down vs. bottom-up processing.

Establishing a supportive, safe environment is necessary if students are to fully engage in practical activities of this type. Students should therefore have the opportunity to meet regularly in small groups. Small class sizes help defray anxiety about performing in front of their tutor and peers and help build and strengthen peer relationships. This is particularly important at the start of the course and with less confident students. Small class size supports responsive teaching. It allows the tutor to monitor student engagement and performance, identify where individual students are experiencing difficulty and provide additional explanation and support as appropriate. Just as in the clinical context, individually tailored explicit feedback on performance and appropriately targeted praise for specific behaviors can also help build student understanding and confidence. As Lemov (2015) notes, "the more actionable the thing you reinforce, the more students can replicate their success." Responsive teaching can thus minimize the risk of a student developing a negative mindset toward the subject and losing motivation. Smaller class sizes also allow students to achieve a higher response density in perception/production work, thereby also increasing the number of auditory models available. Input from multiple speakers supports listeners in generalizing learning and developing more robust phonetic categories in long-term memory (Clopper & Pisoni, 2004).

Quality of input is also of importance and relates to scaffolding techniques and the introduction of activities in a graded fashion, progressively increasing the difficulty and/or task demands. For example, when introducing non-system or unfamiliar sound contrasts, start with focused auditory stimulation followed by detection (e.g. when does the sound change?), discrimination (e.g. same-different) and finally identification. Increase task demands by targeting the sound in different word positions, in nonsense words and in longer, more articulatorily complex words (real or nonsense). Build confidence discriminating and transcribing typical speech data before targeting real clinical data. Pseudo-clinical data can provide a useful transition here. In all cases, it is important that teaching and assessment reflects the cultural and linguistic diversity that students may encounter in clinical practice.

Section Two

A solution-focused investigation into increasing hours of practice of phonetic transcription

Titterington and Bates (2018) attempted to address the key issue identified in this chapter around increasing hours of phonetic transcription practice (see paper for specific detail: doi: 10.1080/02699206.2017.1350882). Ulster University (where the first author works) provides a 3-year undergraduate SLT degree program. Prior to the study, pre-registration SLT students received a total of 48 hours of face-to-face teaching in semester one; falling well below the 100 (never mind the 700) hours recommended by Howard and Heselwood (2002). In an attempt to address this in light of intense teaching and clinical placement in the program, online learning was utilized. Two resources were used: Webfon (WF) (Bates, Matthews, & Eagles, 2010) and; the Ulster Set (Titterington, unpublished). WF[2] is a universally accessible website supporting learning and maintenance of phonetic transcription skills. The Ulster Set is a series of 5 online quizzes developed to focus on Ulster vowels accessed via the University's virtual learning environment (VLE). The final assessment for the module involved phonetic transcription of single words produced by a typically developing 3-year-old. The study investigated associations between engagement with WF, performance on the Ulster set, and marks for the final transcription coursework. It also considered how the students perceived and engaged with the online learning opportunities provided.

All students enrolled in the module were female and gave informed consent to participate ($n = 27$, mean age: 19.5 (SD: 1.4)). The module was delivered as usual and required attendance at all face-to-face practical sessions/lectures. Online learning involved completion of 10 weekly homework tasks on WF after which students posted a response to "sparks" (questions posed by the lecturer) on the VLE's discussion board (DB). In addition, students completed the Ulster Set online quizzes weekly from week 6 of the 12-week semester. Each Ulster Set quiz contributed 1% to the final module mark for phonetic transcription (5% in total). On completion of the final transcription coursework, students completed a questionnaire investigating their perception and engagement with the online learning resources.

Students who posted most to the "sparks" about WF did better on the Ulster Set (rho =.44, $p =.03$ (n = 26)), and students who did better on the Ulster Set also did better on the final transcription coursework (Pearson' r = .48, $p = .01$ (n = 26)). Students completed 100% of the Ulster Set quizzes compared to 88.15% (SD: 15.7%) of the WF "sparks." Both online resources were perceived to be intrinsically motivating to the students and the additional contribution of the Ulster Set to final coursework marks provided valued extrinsic motivation. Student quotations highlight these findings (Titterington & Bates, 2018): *"Good to be tested on accents similar to our own – think will help for placement"* and *"I found it helpful that I was given a mark for each quiz as it gave me a marker on my progress."* This is important learning for all of us wishing to increase hours of phonetic transcription practice using online resources. To use these resources successfully, online tasks must be constructively aligned with learning outcomes (be intrinsically motivating) and contribute to overall module marks (be extrinsically motivating) thereby reaching a threshold of valence to optimize student engagement and benefit.

These findings add to our knowledge and understanding about how best to use online opportunities to support student learning of phonetic transcription. Further investigation is required to identify the type of tasks and amount of time needed to optimize independent online learning of phonetic transcription for SLTs.

Conclusion

This chapter considers the expectations and challenges of teaching and learning clinical phonetic transcription to a requisite level of skill thereby supporting effective clinical practice. Possible solutions put forward include the importance of collaborative work (preferably internationally) that will agree core benchmark competencies for entry level SLTs and map out a path in professional development supporting maintenance and further development of specialist skills as appropriate. Increasing hours of practice in phonetic transcription to support skill development, developing core skills in acoustic phonetics to support future work with instrumental speech analysis, and the use of sound pedagogical approaches to teaching, learning and assessment are also discussed. How to best engage students with teaching, learning and assessment is particularly considered when striving to optimize the potential of independent online learning.

We are not suggesting that SLTs currently qualifying from degree programs have inadequate skills for effective phonetic transcription in the workplace. However, it is important to highlight the constraints that many lecturers in clinical phonetics face around the delivery of a suitable level of teaching and learning to support sufficient attainment of transcription skills within the current environment. There is much work to be done to continue building on the historical foundation of the importance of phonetic transcription within the pre-registration SLT curriculum. Pedagogic research can add weight to thinking around this area. Furthermore, positive change for the future can be supported and driven by good collaborative working across higher education institutes, with professional and regulating bodies and across countries. Such collaborative work is vital to support clinical phonetic transcription skills as one of the unique selling points of SLTs working with clients who have speech difficulties.

Notes

1 See Speech Pathology Australia's (SPA) (2017) competency-based occupational standards for entry-level Speech Pathologists (CBOS); S. Arnott (SPA) (personal communication, October 3, 2019), and the 2020 American Speech-Language-Hearing Association (ASHA, 2020) certification standards underpinned by the Council on Academic Accreditation in Audiology and Speech-Language Pathology's (CAA) accreditation standards for speech-language pathology curricula (CAA, 2019); D. Recor (ASHA) (personal communication, October 29, 2019).
2 Since the writing of this chapter, WebFon is unfortunately no longer accessible. For the interest of the reader: a series of weekly online tasks have subsequently been developed integrating other online resources such as Seeing Speech (https://www.seeingspeech.ac.uk/) and Phonetic Flashcard (https://www.phon.ucl.ac.uk/home/johnm/flash/flashin.htm) with synthesised clinical speech data and group exercises. As with WebFon, these revised online weekly tasks require weekly responses to "sparks" posted on the Discussion Board.

References

American Speech-Language-Hearing Association (ASHA). (2020). *Standards and Implementation Procedures for the Certificate of Clinical Competence in Speech-Language Pathology.* https://www.asha.org/Certification/2020-SLP-Certification-Standards/. (Accessed online 29/10/19).
Ashby, M.G. & Ashby, P. (2013). Phonetic pedagogy. In M.J. Jones & R.-A. Knight (Eds.), *Bloomsbury companion to phonetics* (pp. 198–207). London, UK: Bloomsbury.
Ball, M.J. & Rahilly, J. (2002). Transcribing disordered speech: The segmental and prosodic layers. *Clinical Linguistics & Phonetics*, 16(5), 329–344, doi: 10.1080/02699200210135866.
Bates, S., Matthews, B., & Eagles, A. (2010). *Webfon: Phonetic transcription self-study programme.* Plymouth, UK: University of St Mark and St John. Retrieved from http://elearning.marjon.ac.uk/ptsp/.
Bates, S. & Titterington, J. with the Child Speech Disorder Research Network. (2017). *Good practice guidelines for the analysis of child speech.* Retrieved from Bristol Speech and Language Therapy Research Unit website: (https://www.nbt.nhs.uk/bristol-speech-language-therapy-research-unit/bsltru-research/guidelines-relating-clinical).
Biggs, J.B. (2003). *Teaching for quality learning at university* (2nd ed.). Buckingham, UK: Open University Press/Society for Research into Higher Education.
Biggs, J. & Tang, C. (2011). *Teaching for quality learning at university* (4th ed.). Maidenhead, UK: Open University Press.
Boersma P. & Weenink, D. (2007). *Praat: Doing phonetics by computer.* Version 6.0.46 [software]. www.fon.hum.uva.nl/praat/. (Accessed 20/11/19).

Clopper, C.G. & Pisoni, D.B. (2004). Effects of talker variability on perceptual learning of dialects. *Language and Speech*. 47(3), 207–238. doi: 10.1177/00238309040470030101

Council on Academic Accreditation in Audiology and Speech-Language Pathology. (2019). *Standards for Accreditation of Graduate Education Programs in Audiology and Speech-Language Pathology*. https://caa.asha.org/wp-content/uploads/Accreditation-Standards-for-Graduate-Programs.pdf. (Accessed 29/10/19).

Crystal, D. (2002). Clinical Linguistics and Phonetics' first 15 years: An introductory comment. *Clinical Linguistics & Phonetics*, 16(7), 487–489.

Dodd, B. (2005). *The differential diagnosis and treatment of children with speech disorders* (2nd ed.). London, UK: Whurr.

Duffy, J. (2013). *Motor speech disorders: Substrates, differential diagnosis, and management*. (3rd ed.). Elsevier.

Health & Care Professions Council (HCPC). (2014). *Standards of proficiency for speech and language therapists*. London, UK: HCPC.

Howard, S.J. & Heselwood, B.C. (2002). Learning and teaching phonetic transcription for clinical purposes. *Clinical Linguistics & Phonetics*, 16(5), 371–401. doi:10.1080/02699200210135893.

Howard, S. & Heselwood, S. (2011). Instrumental and perceptual phonetic analyses: The case for two-tier transcriptions. *Clinical Linguistics & Phonetics*, 25(11-12), 940–948. doi: 10.3109/02699206.2011.616641.

Knight, R.-A. (2010). Sounds for study: Speech and language therapy students' use and perception of exercise podcasts for phonetics. *International Journal of Teaching and Learning in Higher Education*. 22, 269–276. Retrieved from http://www.isetl.org/ijtlhe/

Knight, R.-A., Bandali, C., Woodhead, C., & Vansadia, P. (2018). Clinicians' views of the training, use and maintenance of phonetic transcription in speech and language therapy. *International Journal of Language and Communication Disorders*, 53(4), 776–787. doi: 10.1511/1460-6984.12381.

Lemov, D. (2015). *Teach like a champion 2:0: 62 techniques that put students on the path to college*. San Francisco, CA: John Wiley & Sons Inc.

McLeod S. & Verdon S. (2014). A review of 30 speech assessments in 19 languages other than English. *American Journal of Speech Language Pathology,* 23(4), 708–23. doi: 10.1044/2014_AJSLP-13-0066.

Müller, N. & Damico, J.S. (2002). A transcription toolkit: Theoretical and clinical considerations. *Clinical Linguistics & Phonetics*, 15(5), 299–316. doi: 10.1080/02699200210135901.

Nelson, T.L., Mok, Z., & Eecen, K.T. (2019). Use of transcription when assessing children's speech: Australian speech-language pathologists' practices, challenges, and facilitators. *Folia Phoniatrica et Logopaedica*. Published online Sept 24, 2019. doi: 10.1159/000503131.

Perkins, M.R. (2011). Clinical linguistics, its past present and future. *Clinical Linguistics & Phonetics*, 25(11–12): 922–927.

Powell, T. (2001). Phonetic transcription of disordered speech. *Topics in Language Disorders*, 21(4), 52–72.

Rahilly, J. (2011). Transcribing speech: Practicalities, philosophies and prophesies. *Clinical Linguistics & Phonetics*, 25(11-12), 934–939. doi:10.3109/02699206.2011.601391.

Ramsdell, H.L., Kimbrough Oller, D., & Ethington, C.A. (2007). Predicting phonetic transcription agreement: Insights from research in infant vocalizations. *Clinical Linguistics & Phonetics*, 21(10), 793–831. doi: 10.1080/02699200701547869.

Royal College of Speech and Language Therapists. (2018). *Curriculum guidance for the pre-registration education of speech and language therapists*. London, UK: RCSLT.

Royal College of Speech and Language Therapists. (January 2017). Professional Practice and Policy Committee Meeting Papers. *Appendix 8a: Workshops to inform the update of the RCSLT Curriculum Guidelines* (findings from online conversation with members). London, UK:Royal College of Speech and Language Therapists.

Shriberg, L.D. & Lof, G.L. (1991). Reliability studies in broad and narrow transcription. *Clinical Linguistics & Phonetics*, 5(3), 225–279.

Speech Pathology Australia. (2017). *Competency-based occupational standards for speech pathologists: Entry; evel*. The Speech Pathology Association of Australia Ltd. ABN 17 008 393 440.

Stemberger, J.P. & Bernhardt, B.M. (2019). Phonetic transcription for speech-language pathology in the 21st Century. *Folio Phoniatrica et Logopaedica*. Published online Sept 24, 2019. doi: 10.1159/000500701.

Titterington, J. (unpublished). The "Ulster set." Belfast, Ireland: Ulster University. Retrieved from https://learning.ulster.ac.uk/webapps/blackboard/content/listContentEditable.jsp?content_id=_3253270_1&course_id=_255731_1&mode=reset

Titterington, J. & Bates, S. (2018). Practice makes perfect: The pedagogic value of independent online phonetic transcription practice for speech and language therapy students. *Clinical Linguistics & Phonetics*, 32(3), 249–266. doi: 10.1080/02699206.2017.1350882

UK and Ireland Child Speech Disorder Research Network. (2017). *Good practice guidelines for transcription of children's speech samples in clinical practice and research*. Retrieved from Bristol Speech and Language Therapy Research Unit website: (https://www.nbt.nhs.uk/bristol-speech-language-therapy-research-unit/bsltru-research/guidelines-relating-clinical).

15

TRANSCRIBING

By target or by realization?

Martin J. Ball

Introduction

It has been stressed on many occasions that a detailed phonetic transcription of disordered speech is a vital first step in accurate diagnosis and relevant intervention in the clinic (for example, Ball, Rahilly, and Tench, 1996; Buckingham and Yule, 1987; Carney, 1979; Howard and Heselwood, 2002; see also the following chapter of this book).[1] Phoneticians and speech pathologists have long used the International Phonetic Alphabet (IPA) as their primary resource in transcribing speech—whether disordered or not. The current *Handbook of the IPA* (IPA, 1999) describes the alphabet and its use. However, clients being assessed in the speech clinic may use sounds that are, in some cases, not found in natural language at all. There have over the years been various developments of symbol systems to capture these atypical sounds (see Chapter 13 of this volume, and the description in Ball et al., 1996). Duckworth et al. (1990) describe the drawing up of the extended IPA (extIPA) to transcribe atypical speech sounds, and this system now has the approval of the IPA and was included in the 1999 *Handbook*. The recent revision of the system is described in Chapter 13 above.

The main competitor to the extIPA symbol system within speech pathology is the system developed by Shriberg and Kent from the early 1980s on (edition referred to here: 2003). This system (henceforth SK) includes some novel and extremely helpful (to the learner) features, such as the categories of diacritic placement around the main symbol (e.g. stress, nasality and lip diacritics above the main symbol; tongue and sound source diacritics below; and off-glide and stop release diacritics above and to the right).

Transcription philosophies

Apart from some differences in choice of symbols and choice of atypical speech behaviors to symbolize, the main difference between the approaches of those who utilize IPA and extIPA and the recommendations for use by Shriberg and Kent (2003) for the SK system lies in what one might term *transcription philosophies*. Shriberg and Kent specifically urge their readers to be aware of the intended target pronunciation before they start transcribing. They say, "when intended targets are unknown, transcription is almost impossible," and further, "clinicians must attempt to determine, word-for-word, what the child intended to say at the time the sample is obtained" (Shriberg and Kent, 2003, p. 138). This approach will be classed as *transcribing by target*. Interestingly, the authors do note that other research has pointed out the dangers of this approach. Howard and Heselwood (2002, p. 393) summarize these, and note, "it's crucial to understand some of the ways in which a native speaker–hearer's perceptual system will constrain perception of speech data." In particular they point to *phonemic false evaluation* (see also Buckingham and Yule, 1987), where listeners place speech sounds into their own internalized phonemic categories, due to the influence of categorical hearing. Predictions of expected speech sounds through knowing the intended target form also have a part to play in producing unreliable transcriptions. Howard and Heselwood (2002, p. 395) note, "the effects of listener expectations are extremely robust," and refer to a study by Ingrisano, Klee, and Binger (1996) which demonstrated that transcribers who knew the intended target were influenced by this and transcribed what they thought they heard.

It is common, therefore, for many clinical phoneticians to *transcribe by production*, and this author's experience is that, while admittedly difficult with highly unintelligible clients, it is not "almost impossible" to transcribe them without knowing the intended target (indeed, this is a task given to graduate students when the speech samples are spontaneous with no known targets).

These two different transcriber philosophies have consequences for the symbol systems themselves. Because in many instances SK requires the use of the phonetic symbol for the target sound, a range of diacritics are then needed to show the absence of a particular articulatory feature, or a change to a particular articulatory feature. Usually, in IPA and extIPA these characteristics are denoted by the use of a different symbol for the sound in question. Further, because several target sounds may be altered in disordered speech to the same realization, this may result under SK conventions in the use of two notably different transcriptions for the same sound, a practice against the principles of the IPA (see IPA, 1999). Another important result of this approach is that using diacritics to show that some feature is missing may leave it unclear as to what the actual production of the sound was. While the initial transcriber may, of course, retain a percept of the realization, no-one else looking at the transcription will. While it is true that any transcription system is likely to miss some aspects of a sound's production, at least the IPA and extIPA attempt to show that production. See, for example, some of the SK diacritics that show a sound is different (e.g. lateralization and frictionalized stops below). Finally, and least importantly, some SK diacritics are used with other meanings in the IPA, although often the different usage is disambiguated through the position that the diacritic is used in. In the following section, some of the points raised here are illustrated.

Examples of differences between IPA/extIPA and SK

In the following subsections a series of transcriptional differences between the IPA (and extIPA) approach and the SK approach are examined, and where appropriate any ambiguities arising from the different transcriptional practices are noted.

Rounded and unrounded vowels

As research has demonstrated (see reviews in Ball and Gibbon, 2002, 2013), a range of vowel errors has been identified in disordered speech. Among these are monophthongization of diphthongs, and movement toward corner vowels. Also possible are the unrounding of target rounded vowels and the rounding of target unrounded vowels. If either of these last two patterns is found, a transcriber of clinical speech samples has to decide how to denote them. If you wish to emphasize the production (and thus to follow the IPA route), there are symbols provided by the IPA for front rounded and back unrounded vowels (i.e. [y, ø, œ, ɶ] and [ɑ, ʌ, ɤ, ɯ]). However, an alternative approach is to emphasize the target in the transcription. The SK system, therefore, recommends that vowels produced with lip-rounding the opposite from what would be expected for the intended target should be transcribed with the symbol for the target together with the IPA diacritics for more or less rounding. So, a high front rounded vowel for English target /i/ would be transcribed as [iʾ] and a high back unrounded vowel for English target /u/ would be transcribed as [uᶜ].

A problem arises between IPA and SK usage of these diacritics. As noted, the IPA defines them as "more" and "less" rounded, whereas the SK usage is to denote opposite rounding from that of the symbol to which they are attached. Of course, the positioning of the diacritics differs: IPA mandates their use beneath a vowel symbol, SK as superscripts to the right of the symbol. Nevertheless, there is clearly potential for confusion here unless it is clearly stated which usage is intended.

Lateral fricatives

Alveolar lateral fricatives are found in several languages (see, for example, Ladefoged and Maddieson, 1996), including Welsh and Zulu. In the clinic, they may also be encountered for target sibilant fricatives, sometimes described as "lateral lisps." The IPA provides symbols for voiceless and voiced alveolar lateral fricatives ([ɬ, ɮ]). Again, the SK approach is to consider the target sound first and then add a diacritic to it. So, for lateral realizations of target /s, z/ one finds [s̬, z̬]. Moreover, if, as can also happen, the lateral fricative is being used for target postalveolar fricatives, then the lateralization diacritic is added to those symbols: [ʃ̬, ʒ̬]. This is potentially confusing as it is possible to make postalveolar lateral fricatives (there are no IPA symbols for them, but extIPA has adopted a set of symbols for various lateral fricatives, see Ball and Rahilly, 1999, and Chapter 13 above). So the SK symbols [ʃ̬, ʒ̬] could denote either target postalveolars realized as alveolar lateral fricatives, or target postalveolars realized as postalveolar lateral fricatives. Matters are further complicated in that the same diacritic is used by the IPA to denote non-syllabic vowels, though in a mixed IPA and SK transcription ambiguity would be unlikely.

Retroflex fricatives

Apart from their use in a range of other languages, retroflex fricatives may be found in some accents of English. For example, Northern Irish English has retroflex fricatives following the retroflex approximant [ɻ], so "papers" may be realized as ['pʰeəpəɻz̺]. Retroflex realizations of alveolar and postalveolar target fricatives may also be encountered in the clinic. The IPA approach is to transcribe these in terms of the production, thus [ʂ, ʐ]. As was seen in the case of the lateral fricatives, the SK approach is to highlight the target. Therefore, retroflex realizations of target /s, z/ will be transcribed as [s̺, z̺], whereas retroflex realizations of target /ʃ, ʒ/ will be transcribed as [ʃ̺, ʒ̺] (SK give the example of English "harsher" as an instance when a retroflex realization of a target postalveolar fricative might occur as a normal variant due to the influence of the r-sounds). While on this occasion there is no ambiguity as to the nature of the articulation, the end result of this strategy is to have different transcriptions to denote the same sounds. This is of course perfectly possible if one transcribes via the target rather than via the production, but would normally be considered something to be avoided if only because the visual representation suggests something different from the auditory impression.

Frictionalized stops

By this term SK denote what phoneticians would normally call affricated stops. These occur naturally in some dialects of English (for example, Liverpool English has affricated fortis stops in some contexts), and may also occur in speech disorders, characterized by Shriberg and Kent (2003: p. 197) as having "a gradual, rather than a sudden, movement away from the closure." Interestingly, Shriberg and Kent (2003) do not equate these sounds with affricates, but the above description seems to correspond with the notion of affricated stops (rather than full affricates) as described, for example, by Clark and Yallop (1990). The SK system transcribes these "frictionalized," or affricated, stops through the use of a diacritic beneath the relevant stop symbol: [ţ, ķ, p̩]. This usage, however, hides potentially important information concerning the nature of the fricative release of these stops. So, whereas affricated release of a velar stop would usually be also velar, affricated release of bilabial stops could be bilabial or labiodental, and of alveolar stops could be dental, alveolar, or postalveolar, as illustrated here with the fortis stops of English: [kˣ, tˢ, tᶿ, tˢ, pᶠ, pᶲ]. Shriberg and Kent (2003) point out that the use of frictionalized stops in disordered speech may signal the beginning of the development of fricatives; all the more useful, then, for someone looking at a transcription to be able to tell whether the affricated part of the stop corresponds with the relevant fricative type for that context. The diacritic used in the SK system also clashes with the IPA usage (where it is used to mark mid-centralized vowels). However, the IPA uses the diacritic above vowel symbols whereas SK uses it beneath stop symbols, so the likelihood of confusion here is slight.

Derhoticization

In this and the subsequent subsection, two examples of marking the absence of a phonetic characteristic proposed in the SK system are examined. The most difficult to grasp is the notion of derhoticization. Shriberg and Kent (2003, p. 118) define it thus: "a *derhoticized* sound is an /r/ consonant or an r-colored vowel that is significantly lacking in *r*-ness (rhotic or retroflex quality) but does not fall into another phonemic category of English." There are, in my opinion, several difficulties with this definition. First, one has to assume that when the authors use "/r/ consonant" they mean a target /r/, for otherwise if an /r/ lacks *r*-ness it cannot be a rhotic. Second, the definition invokes phonemic categories although one would assume that transcription at this level is phonetic rather than phonemic (i.e. we have to assume that the /r/ target is [ɹ] rather than a trill). Finally, the definition is noted to apply only to English, and so begs the question of whether one could use this diacritic with languages other than English that a client might use.

As noted above, an advantage of the SK system is that often it allows one to mark in a transcription the target sound that the client has misarticulated. However, in this specific case, the disadvantage of marking derhoticization is that the resultant transcription does not show what sound the client used instead. So, one could imagine that a target apical variety of English /r/, made with no tongue tip raising or retroflexion, could result in a [j] realization; a target bunched /r/ with the tongue pulled slightly too far back could result in a [ɰ] (see Ball, Lowry, and McInnis, 2006, and Chapter 9 for an example of just that realization). Shriberg and Kent (2003) refer to a sound between /r/ and /w/. This could well be a labiodental approximant, which occurs frequently in the clinic, and if so could be transcribed with [ʋ]. Also, the SK diacritic ([ɹ̆]) is used in the IPA to denote a short segment (albeit usually above the symbol), so again confusion might arise in a mixed IPA and SK transcription.

Non-labialized consonant

This category is included in the SK system among various lip symbols (Shriberg and Kent, 2003, p.116). The definition states that the listed diacritic should be used with consonants that are "not articulated with a constriction or narrowing, of the lips." However, as this would apply to a large number of consonants, it becomes clear that the authors mean that it is only to be used with target labial consonants: "If a speaker fails to narrow and protrude the lips for the /w/ in *weed*, the non-labialization symbol would be appropriate" (Shriberg and Kent, 2003, p.116). The IPA approach would be to transcribe such a sound with the IPA symbol for a velar (i.e. non-labial velar) approximant. So, the SK system would give us [wʷ], while the IPA would use [ɯ̽]. While there is no ambiguity in this instance of disagreement between SK and IPA norms, one might wish that the SK diacritic had a more useful definition. Defined simply as non- labialized does not imply necessarily that the sound has lip-spreading (just that it lacks lip constriction and protrusion). So, while the symbols available to transcribers of either tradition are suitable to capture sounds such as a non-labial velar approximant without recourse to a diacritic, SK does not (although extIPA does) provide the transcriber with the means to denote a consonant made with lip-spreading. This might, for example, be a case where a spread-lip mouth shape was used where normal coarticulatory effects would make one expect a lip-rounded shape (e.g. [t̺] where one might expect [tʷ] in a word like "two"), or simply to mark that the expected coarticulatory effect of lip-spreading has in fact taken place in a word like "tea."[2]

Trills

This final subsection will consider the SK method of transcribing trills. Best practice in the narrow transcription of English (e.g. Ball and Müller, 2005) suggests that the IPA symbol for a postalveolar central approximant, [ɹ], should be used to transcribe the normal realization of English /r/, and that [r] be used only for trill realizations in English or in other languages that a client might use. (In fact, in Ball and Müller, 2005, it is recommended that /ɹ/ be used for English at the phonemic transcription level exactly to avoid the complications encountered with the SK proposals.) Because SK retain [r] at the phonetic as well as the phonemic levels for the English approximant-r, they are forced to provide a diacritic for trills (though not for taps, where the normal IPA tap symbols are used).

So, whereas in IPA a trilled-r is [r], in SK it is [r̝]. Shriberg and Kent (2003, p. 119) also suggest that this diacritic be used when transcribing languages other than English that use trills. However, if a trill is the default value for a rhotic consonant, it would seem more sense to use [r] (if apical) as the trill symbol, and [ɹ] for any approximant realization that might be found in normal or disordered speech.

Conclusion

Transcribing by production has long been the tradition within clinical phonetics as practiced by phoneticians. It is probably true, however, that where possible transcription by target may well be the choice of the clinician confronted by unintelligible speech. However, it is not always possible to know the target of each and every word, so to some extent transcription by production has to be undertaken unless large amounts of useful speech data are to be ignored. The IPA and extIPA approach to transcription can be understood to be production-based. The SK system, on the other hand, is overtly target-based and the authors of the system feel that this is the only realistic way to proceed. The result of this, however, as has been shown above, is that in some instances the SK system produces unclear transcriptions. While the two approaches may well be able to co-exist, some thought might be given as to how the insights of SK (such as diacritic placement categories) might be used to improve the IPA/extIPA approach, the avoidance of target symbols with diacritics might be adopted by SK to avoid the uncertain transcriptions that have been highlighted. Such a move would not mean that SK users would have to change to transcribing via the production (much as that might be welcomed by many phoneticians), but that, for example, a lateral fricative is transcribed as a lateral fricative, not as a fricative with added lateralization.

Notes

1 This chapter is adapted from Ball (2008).
2 It is true that SK does mark some features not covered by IPA/extIPA. These include "inverted lip," and different diacritics to mark fronted and retracted in consonants as opposed to vowels. The first is rare according to the authors, while the second would appear unnecessary.

References

Ball, M.J., & Gibbon, F. (Eds.) (2002). *Vowel disorders*. Woburn, MA: Butterworth Heinemann.
Ball, M.J., & Gibbon, F. (Eds.) (2013). *Handbook of vowels and vowel disorders*. London, UK: Psychology Press.
Ball, M.J., & Müller, N. (2005). *Phonetics for communication disorders*. Mahwah, NJ: Erlbaum.
Ball, M.J., & Rahilly, J. (1999). *Phonetics. The science of speech*. London, UK: Edward Arnold.
Ball, M.J., Lowry, O., & McInnis, L. (2006). Distributional and stylistic variation in/r/-misarticulations: A case study. *Clinical Linguistics and Phonetics, 20*, 119–124.
Ball, M.J., Rahilly, J., & Tench, P. (1996). *The phonetic transcription of disordered speech*. San Diego, CA: Singular Publishing.
Buckingham, H., & Yule, G. (1987). Phonemic false evaluation: Theoretical and clinical aspects. *Clinical Linguistics and Phonetics, 1*, 113–125.
Carney, E. (1979). Inappropriate abstraction in speech assessment procedures. *British Journal of Disorders of Communication, 14*, 123–135.
Clark, J., & Yallop, C. (1990). *An introduction to phonetics and phonology*. Oxford, UK: Blackwell.
Duckworth, M., Allen, G., Hardcastle, W., & Ball, M.J. (1990). Extensions to the International Phonetic Alphabet for the transcription of atypical speech. *Clinical Linguistics and Phonetics, 4*, 273–280.
Howard, S.J., & Heselwood, B.C. (2002). Learning and teaching phonetic transcription for clinical purposes. *Clinical Linguistics and Phonetics, 16*, 371–401.
Ingrisano, D., Klee, T., & Binger, C. (1996). Linguistic context effects on transcription. In T. W. Powell (Ed.), *Pathologies of speech and language: Contributions of clinical phonetics and linguistics* (pp. 45–46). New Orleans, LA: ICPLA.
IPA (1999). *Handbook of the International Phonetic Association*. Cambridge, UK: Cambridge University Press.
Ladefoged, P., & Maddieson, I. (1996). *The sounds of the world's languages*. Oxford, UK: Blackwell.
Shriberg, L., & Kent, R. (2003). *Clinical phonetics*, 3rd ed. Boston, MA: Allyn & Bacon.

16

EXAMPLES OF NARROW PHONETIC TRANSCRIPTION IN DISORDERED SPEECH

Martin J. Ball, Nicole Müller, Marie Klopfenstein, and Ben Rutter

Introduction

In this chapter we explore examples of unusual realizations of targets in disordered speech and thus the need for narrow phonetic transcription. The chapter is adapted from Ball, Müller, Klopfenstein, and Rutter (2009), with the section on non-pulmonic egressive sounds adapted from Ball and Müller (2007).

The majority of US phonetics texts aimed at speech language pathology (SLP) students work through the phonetics of English before turning (if at all) to non-English sounds (see, for example, Calvert, 1992; Edwards, 2002; Garn-Nunn & Lynn, 2004; Shriberg & Kent, 2002; and Small, 2004). This is also the way that most transcription courses operate: starting with English and turning only later to other sounds. There are clear drawbacks to this approach, especially if non-English sounds are ignored, or only dealt with in a cursory manner. While some speech clients may show only "substitution" realizations (i.e. using another sound of the language for the target sound), many do not and use sounds not found in the language in question, or indeed, use atypical sounds not found in natural language at all.

Restricting transcription training to the sounds of one language will not equip students to deal with these latter cases, and speech-language pathologists who have not been trained in narrow phonetic transcription will be unable to record such clients' speech in a way that reflects their patterns of speech production. This may lead to over- or under-evaluation of their phonological abilities (see discussion in Ball, Rahilly, & Tench, 1996 and Ball & Rahilly, 2002) and inaccurate characterization of their motor abilities.

However, simply introducing a transcription system to students does not ensure it will be used successfully. As described in Shriberg and Lof (1991), when highly detailed transcriptions are required, inter-transcriber reliability drops. This might be overcome to some extent if the problems derived from phonemic listening are tackled during the training of phonetic transcription. Howard and Heselwood note (2002: p. 393): "it's crucial to understand some of the ways in which a native speaker-hearer's perceptual system will constrain perception of speech data." They describe two particular problems that arise from phonemic listening. First, they point to phonemic false evaluation (see also Buckingham & Yule, 1987). Phonemic false evaluation is where listeners place speech sounds into their own internalized phonemic categories, due to the influence of categorical hearing.

Second, predictions of expected speech sounds through knowing the intended target form also have a part to play in producing unreliable transcriptions. Howard and Heselwood (2002: p. 395) note: "the effects of listener expectations are extremely robust." They refer to a study by Ingrisano, Klee, and Binger (1996) which demonstrated that transcribers who knew the intended target were influenced by this and transcribed what they thought they heard.

One way to address these problems of phonemic listening is to introduce students in transcription classes first to nonsense words that contain both non-English as well as English sounds, so that word meaning does not interfere with listening [this approach is advocated for example in Ball and Müller (2005)]. From the authors' experience, teaching transcription via an English-first approach has led to the following examples (among others) of phonemic listening:

- The Southern British Standard vowel /ɒ/ transcribed as General American /ɑ/
- The General American sequence /ɑɹ/ often transcribed as /ɔɹ/ in southwest Louisiana
- The Southern British Standard non-rhotic /ə/ for final "-er" is often transcribed as General American rhotic/ɚ/.

The question whether students need to learn to transcribe non-English or even atypical speech sounds was addressed in Ball, Müller, Rutter, and Klopfenstein (2009); Ball, Müller, Klopfenstein and Rutter (2010); and Rutter, Klopfenstein, Ball and Müller (2010). In this chapter, we provide further examples from clinical data of the importance of narrow phonetic transcription. We will illustrate this importance in two main sections below: pulmonic egressive sounds and non-pulmonic egressive sounds.

Pulmonic egressive sounds

We provide five different cases to illustrate the need for narrow transcription of pulmonic egressive sounds. We give some examples from the following:

- A severely disfluent client
- A child with progressive hearing loss
- Repair sequences in dysarthric speakers
- A child with idiosyncratic velar articulations
- An adult with progressive speech degeneration

These cases were chosen because they illustrate a range of speech cases, both adult and child, both developmental and acquired, and because they allow us to demonstrate a range of different symbolizations. In these transcriptions we use the International Phonetic Alphabet (IPA), the Extended IPA (extIPA) and the Voice Quality Symbols system (VoQS) (see Ball & Müller, 2005, and Chapter 13 for descriptions of these).

Examples

Example of disfluent speech

The example given here is based on the fuller account of Ball and Local (1996). A male, NS, aged 24 at the time of recording, presented with severe stuttering behaviors which had been present since childhood. In spontaneous speech he used excessive struggle behaviors and facial grimacing. His speech was characterized by part-word repetitions of plosives and fricatives and severe blocking on word initial sounds. He had particular difficulty in initiating voicing at sentence boundaries, due to an intermittent ingressive gasp of air or intrusive nasal snort. The data shown in the transcriptions below come from a reading passage, adapted from an article about the football World Cup tournament in Spain.

The transcription (using extIPA and VoQS conventions[1]) illustrates NS's strategies to get beyond a series of repetitions. It allows us to see:

- The use of creaky voice at the onset of repetitions (example (1))
- Use of a velopharyngeal fricative ([fŋ], examples (2) and (3))
- Changes in loudness during repetitions [examples (2) and (3)]

(The use of ejectives and of pulmonic ingressive sounds with this client is described later in this chapter.)

1. [ð\ð:ə̰ {V̰[ə\ə\ə]V̰} ˈhwəɹld ˈkʌp]   (*the World Cup*)
2. [ðə tˢˈ\tʲ (.) {ₚ tˈ\tˈₚ} fŋ\{_f fŋ\fŋ _f}\ˈtŏpˈ ˈneʃənz]   (*the top nations*)
3. [ɪnˑ ə̰ {_pp tʰəʃ\ĭ̃ʰə\təʃ _pp}\ˈtʉɹnəmənt]   (*in a tournament*)

While the extIPA symbols provide us with a means of transcribing the velopharyngeal fricative ([fŋ]), and the VoQS system allows us to transcribe degrees of loudness and the use of pulmonic ingressive airflow, the majority of the non-normal realizations in these transcriptions are transcribable through the use of standard IPA symbols. However, if the transcriber had not been taught, for example, how to transcribe ejective consonants, then the client's pattern of ejective use at repetition sites would be completely missed. Information on the use of ejectives and of pulmonic ingressive speech adds to our knowledge of this client's abilities as regards breath support for speech, and the use of the VoQS symbols for loudness further illustrate possible breath control problems during extended periods of repetition.

Child with hearing loss

These data are based on transcriptions collected by the third author in the Speech and Hearing Clinic of the University of Louisiana at Lafayette. The participant was JF, a girl aged 10;10 at the time of recording, with progressive hearing loss that was first identified and treated at 5;0. She had a profound hearing loss in her right ear, moderate-to-severe hearing loss in her left ear, and wore a hearing aid in her left ear. Evaluating clinicians consistently identified problems in the production of fricatives and affricates across initial, medial and final word positions. The data are from spontaneous speech samples collected by the third author.

JF produced fricatives that match the place of articulation of a preceding fricative or the release of a preceding affricate. An example of this can be seen in (4):

4. [ˈtʃiʃkʰeɪkˀ] (*cheesecake*)

In the production of "shoes," the final fricative was produced with a sliding articulation, indicating that the subject might have been having trouble placing the tongue in the correct position or producing the correct type of channel (5):

5. [ʃɪˑusʃ] (*shoes*)

The ability to mark these "sliding articulations," using the subscript arrow convention of the extIPA system, may also be a mark of a move away from the fricative repetition strategy that JF had adopted. Sliding articulations involve a change of articulatory place within the timing slot of a single segment (rather than one fricative followed by another within a fricative cluster), and the ability to show this subtle change in articulation is important in charting progress for this client in fricative realization.

Repair sequences in dysarthria

The examples here are based on the work of the fourth author (Rutter, 2008). C was 41 at the time of recording. She is a white female from Louisiana. She was diagnosed with multiple sclerosis (MS) at the age of 21 after going into a coma for a period of six months. The progression of MS post coma was extremely rapid, and she now suffers from reduced speech intelligibility, locomotor and general muscular deficits, and myodesopsia. Her MS is currently in the secondary progressive stage. Her problems are generally due to spasticity of the muscles. She also has unilateral paralysis of the oral structures, which causes sagging and drooling. Various phonetic problems were identified that were likely to produce a repair, and there were prosodic characteristics as well as segmental ones. To illustrate the fine phonetic detail found in repair sequences, we include two sample transcriptions here taken from spontaneous speech recorded by the fourth author. Self-repairs in C's data did on occasion have an interregnum that ran for some period of time and were sometimes filled by silence. The following fragment serves as an example (6). The trouble source is the word "questions" which in its first production lacks any frication at the end of the first syllable and is produced with hypernasality.

6. C: I'll ask you a few questions [kw̃ẽʔn̩s]

    (0.25 s) questions [kwestʃn̩s]

The repaired form has the correct friction and lacks the hypernasality. The ability to transcribe glottal stop and nasality is required to capture the subtle phonetic changes that occur at this self-repair. C also produced the second fragment to be looked at here (7). On one occasion the number of repair attempts reached four before it was signaled as being successful. The original trouble source, "it runs too fast," is produced by C as follows:

7. C: it runs too fast? [ɨʔ ɹʌ̃n̩ṣu fæs]

Phonetically, the original trouble source is characterized by weak overall articulation and minimal contact for the target /t/ in "too." Rather, during the fricative [ṣ] the tongue advances but never achieves complete closure. There is zero closure at the end of the word "fast," and so no final plosive is achieved. Again, we see that narrow transcription is needed to capture the characteristics of this utterance that initiated a repair sequence between C and her interlocutors. The study from which these data come (Rutter, 2008) aimed to investigate what fine phonetic details differentiated between the clients' misunderstood utterances, and their repaired, clear speech. A comparison of successful and failed repair attempts could also be particularly insightful in revealing those techniques that seem to bring about successful communication in this client group.

Child with idiosyncratic velar articulations

A fuller account of this case is found in Ball, Manuel, and Müller (2004). T was aged 3;10 at the time of the recording of his spontaneous speech and showed the following characteristics in his highly unintelligible speech:

- Virtually no use of tongue tip or blade for articulation, which we termed deapicalization
- Back of the tongue typically raised toward the soft palate giving a velarized voice quality
- Typically a hypernasalized voice quality, though some hyponasal speech also occurred
- Velic movements against his tongue back functioned as crypto-articulations, which we have termed velodorsal articulations

The velarized and hypernasal voice quality can be shown nonlinearly through the use of the VoQS bracketing convention. However, the velodorsal articulation needs new symbols, e.g., [ʞ][2]. These aspects of T's speech can be seen in the transcription in (8) where the VoQS braces mark nasalized and velarized voice quality:

8. {Ṽˠ [ʞæ̃ʇ] Ṽˠ} (*cat*)

Ball et al. (2004) used videofluorography to investigate T's atypical articulations. Nevertheless, an ability to use narrow phonetic transcription and the extIPA and VoQS systems was necessary in order to record the findings in accessible form.

Progressive speech degeneration

Ball, Code, Tree, Dawe, and Kaye (2004) investigated a client with progressive speech degeneration. CS was a right-handed 63-year-old male at the time of testing. He first noticed speech problems 8 years previously when he was 55 years old. He became unintelligible some 6 months after testing and almost mute, managing only the occasional utterance a few months later. A motor speech examination demonstrated no significant motor weakness or sensory loss, no apparent dysarthria, although it is impossible to rule out some dysarthric impairment, despite an absence of clear motor or sensory weakness. He had clear problems initiating laryngeal and oral movement (for example, coughing and producing vowels on command). In summary, CS showed particular problems with initiation of laryngeal, tongue and lip movements; little or no apparent groping and searching; problems with control of voicing; and coordination of laryngeal with oral articulation. However, his performance on articulatory tasks was inconsistent and highly variable, ruling out a significant dysarthric element. The absence of groping and searching in CS suggests he does not have a "typical" apraxia of speech, and the assumption was that his speech resembled most closely the cortical anarthria of the opercular syndrome. However, he did not have agrammatism, aphasia or cognitive decline at the time of testing but did have accompanying progressive apraxias. Among CS's speech characteristics are:

- Selective denasalization (see example (9))
- Lateral addition to word final /-u/ (see example (10))
- Labial addition to initial /ɹ-/ (see example (11))
- Loss of aspiration in fortis plosives over time (see example (12))

We can see these features in the transcriptions which include data from spontaneous speech, word lists, and reading passages:

9. [tʃɪd] *chin*, [bɔ], *more*, [spoʊk] *smoke*, [bɑdæwə] *banana*, and [læɡəwɪs] *language*
10. [kɹul] *crew*, [skɹul] *screw*, [ɹul] *rue*
11. [bɹæp], [pɹæp] *rap*, [bɹɪɡ] *rig*, [pɹeɪ], [fɹeɪ] *ray*, [fɹul] *rue*, [pɹæŋ] *rang*, [fɹæt] *rat*, [tɹaɪp] *ripe*
12. time 1: [tʰu] *two*, [kʰoʊt˺] *coat*; time 2: [p˭æk˺] *pack*, [k˭æp˺] *cap*.

While only the items in (12) require the use of narrow phonetic transcription to capture the presence versus absence of aspiration, the other three sets of examples clearly illustrate the need to avoid transcribing with the intended target in mind. As the data recorded here were mostly in the form of read word lists or standard passages, the target form without the denasalization, without the added final lateral, or without the added initial labial consonant might well be expected from transcribers who have not been able to move beyond phonemic listening.

Non-pulmonic egressive sounds

Generally, non-pulmonic egressive speech has not been given much attention as possible substitutions for pulmonic egressive targets in disordered speech. In this section we review the small set of studies that have reported on its use in disordered speech, suggesting that, at the very least, speech pathology students do need to be aware of these groups of sounds and that they may occur clinically.

Examples

Pulmonic ingressive speech

In impaired speech, pulmonic ingressive speech has been reported for people with stuttering (see Ball & Rahilly, 1996), disordered child phonology (for example, Gierut & Champion, 2000; Grunwell, 1981; Ingram & Terselic, 1983) and cochlear implant users (Chin, 2003). The client reported above under "dysfluent speech" (see also Ball & Rahilly, 1996) was, as noted previously, a male, aged 24 at the time of recording. He presented with severe stuttering behaviors which had been present since childhood. In spontaneous speech he used excessive struggle behaviors and facial grimacing. His speech was characterized by part-word repetitions of plosives and fricatives, and severe blocking on word-initial sounds. He had particular difficulty in initiating voicing at sentence boundaries, due to an intermittent ingressive gasp of air or intrusive nasal snort. Ingressive airflow was also found in other situations, and some of these are illustrated in (13)–(15) (see Ball, Code, Rahilly, & Hazlett, 1994, for a description of conventions). Part of this transcript was given in (1)–(3) above, but the following include examples of ingressive speech.

13. [ð\ð:ə̰ {V̰[ə\ə\ə]V̰]} ˈhwəɹld ˈkʌp ˈf̃\faɪnəlz əv ˈnaɪntin eəti {↓ ˈtʉ ↓}] (*the world cup finals of nineteen-eighty two*)
14. [p\pɹəv\ˈvɪnʃəl {ₚt'\t'ₚ}\{ₚₚt'\t'ₚₚ} (.) t'\t' {ₚₚt'\t'ₚₚ} fŋ\fŋ\{↓ ˈtãũnz ↓}] (*provincial towns*)
15. [wɪð ðə s'\s'\s'\ˈ\s'{↓ɛmi ˈfaɪnəlz ↓}] (*with the semi-finals*)

As can be seen from these transcriptions, the client often uses ingressive speech on syllables immediately following a dysfluency (as the examples of "towns", and "emi finals" following the four repetitions of an ejective [s']). He also uses pulmonic ingressive speech where there are no dysfluencies (the "two" in the first sentence). It may well be that the use of an ingressive airstream in these latter instances is a way of avoiding the dysfluencies that the client often shows on syllable-initial /t/, or an indication that the timing of breath support for speech is disrupted.

Unlike in this example, the reported use of pulmonic ingressive speech in child speech disorders is restricted to one or two ingressive sounds, rather than the use of an ingressive airflow for entire syllables or words. Grunwell (1981) described a 6;3-year-old child with disordered phonology who, among other atypical realizations, used a voiceless ingressive lateral fricative in final position of words whose adult target forms contained final sibilant fricatives. Among the examples she provides are those listed in (16) (transcription conventions are those of extIPA, as described in Ball & Müller, 2005, rather than the original).

16. Target   Realization
    dish   [dɪɬ↓]
    bus   [bʌɬ↓]
    match   [baɬ↓]

Ingram and Terselic (1983) also observed ingressive sounds used for final target fricatives in a client aged 4;1. In this instance, the sound produced was a pulmonic ingressive alveolar fricative, and the targets were /s, z, ʒ, f/. Examples can be seen in (17) (again, transcription conventions are those of extIPA, rather than the original).

17. Target   Realization
    rouge   [wus↓]
    rough   [wʌs↓]
    vase   [beɪs↓]

Gierut and Champion (2000) report on a 4;5 boy with disordered phonology who uses a "voiceless ingressive fricative with no identifiable point of articulation" (p. 606) for target postvocalic sibilants. Examples are shown in (18), where the ingressive sound is transcribed as [h↓].

18. Target   Realization
    bus   [bʌh↓]
    nose   [noʊh↓]
    fish   [fɪh↓]
    catch   [kɛh↓]
    page   [peɪh↓]

Whereas the child phonology studies reviewed here all report pulmonic ingressive sounds being used for target fricatives, the example given in Chin (2003) of speech by a cochlear implant user is of pulmonic ingressive nasals in free variation with pulmonic egressive nasals, normally in word initial position. Typical examples of this usage are *moon* [m↓ūd] and *mad* [m↓æd].

Clicks

Clicks are made on a velaric ingressive airtsream (see Ball & Müller, 2005). Several studies describe clicks replacing target pulmonic sounds: Howard (1993), where a cleft palate client used bilabial clicks; Bedore, Leonard, and Gandour (1994), where clicks were used for target fricatives; and Heselwood (1997), who reported on nasalized clicks used for target sonorants. Howard (1993) describes a 6-year-old girl whose cleft palate had been repaired at the age of 2;2. She had a range of unusual sounds, including a bilabial click as one realization of target /p/, and representative examples can be seen in (19).

19. Target   Realization
    pig   [ʘɪʔʰ]
    tap   [ʔæʔʘ]
    zip   [ʄɪʔʘ]

Unlike the common pattern of pulmonic ingressive use for target sibilants, the few studies reporting click usage do not show a consistent pattern of target replacement. Bedore et al. (1994), unlike the Howard (1993) study, describe the use of a dental click for target sibilants. The client was a girl of 4;4, and typical examples of her realizations are shown in (20).[3]

20. Target   Realization
    ones   [wənl̩]
    shark   [lɑɹk]
    treasure   [twɛlɚ]
    match   [mæl̩]

Heselwood (1997) illustrates yet another pattern of click use. The client was a severely dysfluent young male adult with Down syndrome, who used both click and non-click realizations of certain target English phonemes. The click realizations were manifestations of dysfluency, occurring after a pause. Some examples are given in (21).

21. Target sound   Realization
    /j, l, ɹ, n/   [ŋ͡ǂ]
    /w/   [ŋ͡ːʘʷ]
    /m/   [ŋ͡ːʘ]
    /t/   [ǂ] (alternate transcription [k͡ǂ][4])
    /f/   [ʘ̥] (alternate transcription [k͡ʘ̥])
    /d, g, ð/   [g͡ǂ]

Gibbon (2006) notes that click usage is a common characteristic of the speech of clients with velopharyngeal incompetence (cf. Howard, 1993, discussed earlier). She reports on the case of a Scottish-English-speaking 14-year-old girl with velocardiofacial syndrome, who presented with ongoing velopharyngeal incompetence, albeit having a normal palatal arch. This client used a dental click for target /d/ and a palatal click for target /k, g/ in all positions in word structure, and examples of her usage can be seen in (22), although the author did not provide full-word transcriptions.

22. Target   Click used
    daddy   [ǀ]
    cake   [ǂ]
    bag   [ǂ]
    lego   [ǂ]

Gibbon speculates that the client's use of clicks is an active learned strategy to "capitalize on negative pressure for the production of plosion" (Peterson-Falzone, Hardin-Jones, & Karnell, 2001, p.170), because the velopharyngeal incompetence makes it impossible for her to build oral pressure using a normal pulmonic airstream. Clicks provide plosion in the presence of velopharyngeal incompetence. Support for this reasoning came from the results of therapy, when the clicks were replaced by weak plosives.

Ejectives

Other than the pulmonic ingressive and velaric ingressive airstreams, the remaining non-pulmonic egressive airstreams are rarely reported in the clinical literature. We noted above the use of ejectives in the speech of a severely dysfluent adult male (see examples in (14) and (15)). Ejectives are made on a glottalic egressive airtsream (see Chapter 1, and Ball & Müller, 2005). Chin (2002) reports on one cochlear implant user who sometimes realized target post-vocalic voiceless plosives as ejectives. Examples are shown in (23).

23. Target   Realization
    boot   [bʏt']
    socky [ʂɑk'i]
    sock   [sɑk']
    pig   [bɪk']

Nicolaides (2004) reported on consonant production in Greek by speakers with hearing impairment. For target [k] and [c] one of her four participants used [k'], although ejectives were not used by the other participants or for other target consonants.

We should be aware, however, that ejectives are more common in normal speech than may be realized. We often hear final lenis stops in English realized as ejectives, especially when stressed (e.g. *that's that* [ˈðæts ˈðæt']). This can be particularly the case in artificially stressed "therapy talk," and it can be an illuminating experience for student clinicians to hear how unlike the canonical target sounds their emphatic realizations actually are.

Implosives

Implosives are produced on a glottalic ingressive airstream (see Ball & Müller, 2005). In natural language they are usually voiced (through the addition of some voiced pulmonic egressive airflow). Implosive usage in disordered speech is rarely reported outside the hearing-impaired population. One exception to this is Shahin (2006), who describes the speech characteristics of three Arabic speakers with cleft palate. All three speakers used a voiceless velar implosive ([ƙ]) for target /k/. Shahin feels that the implosive realizations could be a result of an intended glottal reinforcement of the /k/.

Other recently reported instances of implosives are found in Higgins, Carney, McCleary, and Rogers (1996) and Pantelemidou, Herman, and Thomas (2003), both of which deal with hearing-impaired speakers. Higgins et al. (1996) refer to studies by Monsen (1976, 1983) that describe implosive usage in hearing impaired clients. Their study investigated the speech of four children (two boys and two girls) between the ages of 6;6–9;2. All were cochlear implant users, and all used implosives at least some of the time. This usage was inconsistent, however, and the example is given of the phrase *bye bye baby* uttered by one of the subjects where the target /b/s of the *bye bye* are implosives, while the target /b/s of *baby* are plosives.

The study investigated whether implosive usage was related to the following vowel context, and also looked at the effects of therapy on implosive use. Rather than rely on impressionistic transcription, this study used an air pressure sensing tube that the speaker had inserted behind the lips. All tokens contained bilabial plosive targets only. While the presence of the pressure sensing tube might have had an effect on the naturalness of speech, certain patterns did emerge. Two of the clients showed a preference for implosives before low vowels, but this was not the case with the other two. Two subjects used implosives more often for target /b/ than for target /p/, and with one subject there was a preference for implosives before front vowels. Finally, one subject used implosives very commonly for both /p/ and /b/ targets with no noticeable patterning.

Pantelemidou et al. (2003) describe a case study of a female aged 8;9 who had been fitted with a cochlear implant 3 years previously. For target /g/ the client often produced an implosive, described as either a pharyngeal or a velar implosive.

Finally, we can note that data collected by the authors on the speech of a profoundly deaf adult female shows common usage of implosives. Examples are given in (24).

24. Target   Realization
    man   [ɓɜ̃n]
    down   [ɗʒ̃]
    clipboard [ɗəˈɓũə]
    found   [ɓãũn]

Discussion

The majority of clinical phonetic transcriptions consist of the writing down of symbols at the segmental level. This implies that speech is segmentable into tidy, discrete units. Although this clearly has some validity at the phonological level of analysis, we know that in terms of speech production, the segment is only a convenient fiction. The boundaries of phonetic activity (such as voicing, friction, nasal air flow, etc.) do not all coincide at a single moment in time: speech sounds have "ragged edges" between each other. This is difficult to show in a linear transcription, although some aspects can be shown in a narrow transcription through the use and placement of certain diacritics (such as those for voiced and voiceless, and for nasalization). Indeed, many of the diacritics used in the extIPA system (see Chapter 13, Ball & Müller, 2005; Ball, Howard & Miller, 2018) are specifically designed to record coarticulatory effects that transcend "segment" boundaries (see, especially, those for phonation effects). While it is possible to adopt parametric phonetic diagramming (see Ball, 1993; Ball, Rahilly, Lowry, Bessell, & Lee, 2020) to tease out different phonetic parameters and their alignment in time, for the most part segmental transcription, with the added flexibility of diacritics to denote coarticulation, will suffice for both clinical and non-clinical phonetic transcription.

There are, however, other aspects of the speech signal that are not amenable to any kind of segmental or subsegmental transcription. Prosodic features such as pitch, voice quality, loudness and tempo cannot be reduced to writing within the same-sized space as is used for a vowel, a fricative or a plosive. Suprasegmental characteristics of speech extend over several segments, syllables and phrases. To transcribe them, therefore, we need written devices that can likewise be spread over a greater or smaller number of segmental symbols. The VoQS system advocates the use of labeled braces, as described in note 1 below. Another approach is to use a multilayered transcription system as illustrated by Müller (2006).

There are competing tensions in the phonetic transcription of disordered speech. First, there is the need to produce as accurate a transcription as possible to aid in the analysis of the speech of the client being investigated which, in many cases, will inform the patterns of intervention that will be planned in remediation (as we have illustrated above). Opposed to this requirement is the problem of reliability: it can be argued that the more detailed a transcription is, the less reliable it tends to be, as the more detailed symbols there are, the more likelihood there is for disagreement about which symbol to employ.

Although it can be demonstrated that narrow transcriptions of disordered speech are important if we are to avoid misanalysis of clients' abilities (see Ball et al., 1996;), there is also evidence to suggest that narrow phonetic transcription—as opposed to broad—may produce problems of reliability. Transcription reliability has two main exponents: inter-judge and intra-judge reliability. Inter-judge reliability refers to measures of agreement between different transcribers when dealing with the same speech data. Agreement measures usually involve one-to-one comparison of the symbols and the diacritics used, or refinements such as "complete match," "match within one phonetic feature," and "non-match." Intra-judge reliability refers to measures of agreement between first and subsequent transcriptions of the same material by the same transcriber.

In order for narrow transcriptions to be trusted as bases for analysis and remediation, it is important that issues of reliability are considered. However, as Shriberg and Lof (1991) noted, at that time barely three dozen studies from the 1930s onward had addressed this issue. Their own study was based on a series of transcriptions of different client types undertaken for other purposes over several years. They used a series of different transcriber teams to under-take broad and narrow transcriptions of the data, and then compared results across consonant symbols, vowel symbols and diacritics. Overall, there is a good level of agreement (inter- and intra-judge) with broad transcription, but on most measures narrow transcription does not produce acceptable levels of reliability.

This study is clearly an important one, but suffers from the fact that the data used were not primarily intended for such an investigation, that the symbols utilized lacked the recent developments toward a comprehensive set for atypical speech sounds, and that access to acoustic instrumentation was not available (we return to this point below).

Cucchiarini (1996) offers a critique of the whole methodology of transcription agreement exercises (and therefore of reliability measures as reported in the literature). She points out that traditional percentage agreement scores do not reflect the range of discrepancies that might occur between two transcribers. For example, the difference between [d̪] and [tˀ] is much less than that between [d] and [b] However, percentage agreement scoring systems are generally not sophisticated enough to take this into account. Cucchiarini also notes that broad transcription (where the number of symbols to be compared between transcribers is less than with narrow transcription) increases the likelihood of chance agreement. She notes that an agreement of 75% when transcribers have to choose between two symbols, and 75% when choosing between four is considerably different but is not usually reflected in accounts of transcription agreement. Finally, she makes the valid point that transcription alignment is often neglected in reliability reports. We may well find that a word is transcribed with different numbers of symbols by different transcribers. Conventions need to be agreed on in such cases; clearly a strict one-to-one alignment of symbols could mean that two transcriptions would have a very low agreement factor if one transcriber had an extra symbol early in the word in question.

A tendency has developed in reliability studies to oversimplify the broad-narrow transcription division. On one side are the "full" symbols of the IPA, whereas on the other are all the diacritics. The implication is that diacritics are all the same, all equally difficult to learn to use, and only useful for the transcription of perceptually non-salient sound differences. However, a brief study of the variety of diacritics found on the IPA chart demonstrates that this is a false view. Some diacritics have equivalent status to full symbols (e.g. voiceless sonorants need a diacritic, voiceless obstruents have symbols). Others represent perceptually clear distinctions (nasalized vowels as opposed to oral ones). On the other hand, less perceptually clear distinctions to do with fine degrees of segment duration, stop release types and precise vowel qualities are also shown through diacritics. Finally, although implosives and clicks have dedicated symbols in the IPA, ejectives use the pulmonic egressive symbols with an added diacritic.

From this discussion, we see again the importance of fine-grained analyses of transcriber agreement and the danger of simplistic conclusions telling us that diacritics and specialized symbols for atypical speech are too difficult to learn, and that their use leads to unreliable transcriptions. Clearly, avoiding all diacritics and specialist symbols may have the effect of producing transcriptions that are reliable between transcribers but grossly inaccurate as regards what the speaker said.

Shriberg and Lof (1991) conclude their study by pointing to a future combination of instrumental phonetic description with impressionistic transcription (see also Ball, 1988) to overcome the problems of narrow transcription reliability. This development has now been reported for some clinical phonetics cases, for example Klee and Ingrisano (1992) and Ball and Rahilly (1996). Recent software development also highlights the growing use of computer technology as an aid to speech analysis and transcription.

Turning to non-pulmonic egressive sounds, the review above has shown that these sounds are encountered in disordered speech and, thus, deserve to be included in courses on phonetic theory and in transcription training sessions. The review has also shown that some patterns do emerge for the various non-pulmonic-egressive sound types. Findings to date indicate that pulmonic ingressive speech appears to be restricted to single ingressive consonants in disordered child phonology (often used for target fricatives), whereas with dysfluent speech we can find one or more syllables spoken ingressively. The exception to this pattern was Chin's (2003) cochlear implant client who used ingressive nasals. With clicks, studies were divided between the speech of clients with cleft palate or other forms of velopharyngeal incompetence, the dysfluent speech of a client with Down's syndrome, and disordered child phonology. All the cases reported were restricted to the use of only one or two click types, though the choice of click varied between the cases. Ejectives were reported in the speech of a dysfluent client, and of various hearing-impaired clients and users of cochlear implants. Implosives too are characteristic of hearing impaired and cochlear implant speakers, although one instance of a cleft palate client was reported.

We would like to encourage this combination of impressionistic and instrumental description in transcription and in transcription training. However, print-outs from acoustic and articulatory instrumentation are not always easy to read or to integrate between systems (for example, combining spectrograms with ultrasound). There will continue to be a need, therefore, to use information derived from instrumentation to refine transcriptions that are accessible to the clinician who is not a specialist in the instruments used, and to allow data from a variety of sources to be combined.

Conclusion

Clinical experience shows that clients in the speech clinic (whether children or adults) do not restrict themselves to the sounds of their target language. The examples we have given in this article have demonstrated the importance of detailed, narrow transcriptions if we wish to capture the fine-grained phonetic information that will be important in a description of highly unintelligible clients. Buckingham and Yule (1987, p. 123) note "without good phonetics, there can be no good phonology," and we would add that, in clinical terms, without good phonetics there can be no reliable intervention plan. We need, therefore, to emphasize the importance of training student clinicians in fine-grained phonetic description. As noted above, this may well be in conjunction with training in instrumental phonetics (rather than solely in articulation courses). The marrying together of acoustic and articulatory measurement with detailed transcription is surely the way forward in the description of disordered speech.

Notes

1 The VoQS system provides for the marking of prosodic features over strings of segments through the use of marked braces; so {V̰[ə\ə\ə]V̰} denotes a repeated schwa produced with creaky voice. Loud and quiet are marked with musical conventions (*f(f)* and *p(p)*) and ingressive speech with ↓.
2 This is not the symbol used in Ball et al. (2009), but the amended version described in Ball, Howard, and Miller (2018).
3 The symbol for the vowel and for the rhotic in the *shark* example has been changed from the original to better reflect the pronunciation.
4 So-called plain clicks can be transcribed with just the click symbol as was done in the source work, but some phoneticians prefer to add the symbol for a doubly-articulated [k] as plain clicks do also involve a velar closure as explained in Ball and Müller (2005). This applies to the following example also.

References

Ball, M.J. (1988). The contribution of speech pathology to the development of phonetic description. In M. J. Ball (Ed.), *Theoretical linguistics and disordered language* (pp. 168–188). London, UK: Croom Helm.

Ball, M.J. (1993). *Phonetics for speech pathology* (2nd ed.). London, UK: Whurr.

Ball, M.J., Code, C., Rahilly, J., & Hazlett, D. (1994). Non-segmental aspects of disordered speech: developments in transcription. *Clinical Linguistics and Phonetics, 8*, 67–83.

Ball, M.J., Code, C., Tree, J., Dawe, K., & Kay, J. (2004). Phonetic and phonological analysis of progressive speech degeneration: a case study. *Clinical Linguistics and Phonetics, 18*, 447–462.

Ball, M.J., Howard, S.J., & Miller, K. (2018). Revisions to the extIPA chart. *Journal of the International Phonetic Association, 48*, 155–164.

Ball, M.J. & Local J. (1996). Advances in impressionistic transcription of disordered speech. In M.J. Ball & M. Duckworth (Eds.), *Advances in clinical phonetics* (pp. 51–89). Amsterdam, The Netherlands: John Benjamins.

Ball, M.J., Manuel, R., & N. Müller (2004). Deapicalization and velodorsal articulation as learned behaviors: A videofluorographic study. *Child Language Teaching and Therapy, 20*, 153–162.

Ball, M.J. & Müller, N. (2005). *Phonetics for communication disorders*. Mahwah, NJ: Erlbaum.

Ball, M.J. & Müller, N. (2007). Non-pulmonic egressive speech sounds in disordered speech: a brief review. *Clinical Linguistics and Phonetics, 21*, 869–874.

Ball, M.J., Müller, N., Klopfenstein, M., & Rutter, B. (2010). My client's using non-English sounds! A tutorial in advanced phonetic transcription. Part 2: Vowels and Diacritics. *Contemporary Issues in Communication Sciences and Disorders, 37*, 103–110.

Ball, M.J., Müller, N., Klopfenstein, M., & Rutter, B. (2009). The importance of narrow phonetic transcription for highly unintelligible speech: Some examples. *Logopedics Phoniatrics Vocology, 34*, 84–90.

Ball, M.J., Müller, N., Rutter, B., & Klopfenstein, M. (2009). My client's using non-English sounds! A tutorial in advanced phonetic transcription. Part 1: Consonants. *Contemporary Issues in Communication Sciences and Disorders, 36,* 133–141.

Ball, M.J. & Rahilly, J. (1996). Acoustic analysis as an aid to the transcription of an example of disfluent speech. In M.J. Ball & M. Duckworth (Eds.), *Advances in clinical phonetics* (pp. 197–216). Amsterdam, The Netherlands: John Benjamins.

Ball, M.J. & Rahilly, J. (2002). Transcribing disordered speech: The segmental and prosodic layers. *Clinical Linguistics and Phonetics, 16,* 329–344.

Ball, M.J., Rahilly, J., Lowry, O., Bessell, N., & Lee, A. (2020). *Phonetics for speech pathology*(3rd ed.). Sheffield, UK: Equinox.

Ball, M.J., Rahilly, J., & Tench, P. (1996). *The phonetic transcription of disordered speech.* San Diego, CA: Singular Publishing.

Bedore, L., Leonard, L., & Gandour, J. (1994). The substitution of a click for sibilants: A case study. *Clinical Linguistics and Phonetics, 8,* 283–293.

Buckingham, H. & Yule, G. (1987). Phonemic false evaluation: Theoretical and clinical aspects. *Clinical Linguistics and Phonetics, 1,* 113–125.

Calvert, D. (1992). *Descriptive phonetics,* (2nd ed.). New York, NY: Thieme.

Chin, S. (2002). Aspects of stop consonant product by pediatric users of cochlear implants. *Language, Speech, and Hearing Services in Schools, 33,* 38–51.

Chin, S. (2003). Children's consonant inventories after extended cochlear implant use. *Journal of Speech, Language, and Hearing Research, 46,* 849–862.

Cucchiarini, C. (1996). Assessing transcription agreement: Methodological aspects. *Clinical Linguistics and Phonetics, 10,* 131–155.

Edwards, H. (2002). *Applied phonetics* (3rd ed.). San Diego, CA: Singular Publishing Group.

Garn-Nunn, P. & Lynn, J. (2004). *Calvert's descriptive phonetics.* New York, NY: Thieme.

Gibbon, F. (2006). Current perspectives on clinical applications of EPG. *Keynote Presentation at the 11th Meeting of ICPLA,* Dubrovnik, Croatia.

Gierut, J. & Champion, A. (2000). Ingressive substitutions: Typical or atypical phonological pattern? *Clinical Linguistics and Phonetics, 14,* 603–617.

Grunwell, P. (1981). *The nature of phonological disability in children.* London, UK: Academic Press.

Heselwood, B. (1997). A case of nasal clicks for target sonorants: A feature geometry account. *Clinical Linguistics and Phonetics, 11,* 43–61.

Higgins, M., Carney, A., McCleary, E., & Rogers, S. (1996). Negative intraoral air pressures of deaf children with cochlear implants: Physiology, phonology, and treatment. *Journal of Speech and Hearing Research, 39,* 957–967.

Howard, S. (1993). Articulatory constraints on a phonological system: A case study of cleft palate speech. *Clinical Linguistics and Phonetics, 7,* 299–317.

Howard, S. & Heselwood, B. (2002). Learning and teaching phonetic transcription for clinical purposes. *Clinical Linguistics and Phonetics, 16,* 371–401.

Ingram, D. & Terselic, B. (1983). Final ingression: A case of deviant child phonology. *Topics in Language Disorders, 3,* 45–50.

Ingrisano, D., Klee, T., & Binger, C. (1996). Linguistic context effects on transcription. In T.W. Powell (Ed.), *Pathologies of speech and language: contributions of clinical phonetics and linguistics*(pp. 45–46). New Orleans, LA: ICPLA.

Klee, T. & Ingrisano, D. (1992). *Clarifying the transcription of indeterminable utterances. Paper presented at the annual Convention of the American Speech-Language-Hearing Association,* San Antonio, November 1992.

Monsen, R. (1976). The production of English stop consonants in the speech of deaf children. *Journal of Phonetics, 4,* 29–41.

Monsen, R. (1983). General effects of deafness on phonation and articulation. In I. Hochberg, H. Levitt, & M. Osberger (Eds.), *Speech of the hearing impaired: research training and personnel preparation* (pp. 23–34). Baltimore, MD: University Park Press.

Müller, N. (Ed.) (2006). *Multilayered transcription.* San Diego, CA: Plural Publishing.

Nicolaides, K. (2004). Articulatory variability during consonant production by Greek speakers with hearing impairment: An electropalatographic study. *Clinical Linguistics and Phonetics, 18,* 419–432.

Pantelemidou, V., Herman, R., & Thomas, J. (2003). Efficacy of speech intervention using electropalatography with a cochlear implant. *Clinical Linguistics and Phonetics, 17,* 383–392.

Peterson-Falzone, S., Hardin-Jones, M., & Karnell, M. (2001). *Cleft palate speech* (3rd ed.). St. Louis, MO: Mosby.

Rutter, B. (2008). *Acoustic properties of repair sequences in dysarthric conversational speech: an interactional phonetic study.* Unpublished Ph.D. dissertation, University of Louisiana.

Rutter, B., Klopfenstein, M., Ball, M.J., & Müller, N. (2010). My client's using non-English sounds! A tutorial in advanced phonetic transcription. Part 3: Prosody and unattested sounds. *Contemporary Issues in Communication Sciences and Disorders, 37,* 111–122.

Shahin, K. (2006). Remarks on the speech of Arabic-speaking children with cleft palate. *Journal of Multilingual Communication Disorders, 4,* 71–77.

Shriberg, L. & Kent, R.D. (2002). *Clinical phonetics* (3rd ed.). Boston, MA: Allyn and Bacon.

Shriberg, L. & Lof, G. (1991). Reliability studies in broad and narrow phonetic transcription. *Clinical Linguistics and Phonetics, 5,* 225–279.

Small, L. (2004). *Fundamentals of phonetics: A practical guide for students* (2nd ed.). Boston, MA: Allyn and Bacon.

PART IV

Instrumentation
Introduction

Part IV of the *Manual* is the longest, containing 20 chapters. These deal with the wide range of phonetic instrumentation that has been applied to the analysis of disordered speech. Due to the number of chapters, we have divided them into four subsections: preliminaries, instrumental analyses of articulatory phonetics, instrumental analyses of acoustic, auditory, and perceptual phonetics, and speech recognition and speech synthesis.

The Preliminaries subsection opens with a chapter by Nicola Bessell providing an overview of the instrumental approach to phonetics, in particular discussing what instrumentation can and cannot do. Adam Vogel then describes the recording of speech, and Yvan Rose and Gregory Hedlund look at speech databases, especially of disordered speech.

There then follow a series of chapters in the second subsection that describe techniques for measuring the different aspects of speech production. Muscle activity (electromyography, Cara Stepp & Jennifer Vojtech); aerodymanics (aerometry, David Zajac); larynx activity (laryngoscopy, Catherine Madill, Daniel Navakovic, Duong Duc Nguyen & Antonia Chacon); phonation and vocal fold activity (electroglottography, Chiara Celata & Irene Ricci); oral/nasal resonance (nasometry, Tim Bressmann); and articulation (electropalatography, Alice Lee).

These are then followed by 4 chapters that can be considered as imaging techniques that can cover more than one aspect of speech production. These are electromagnetic articulography (Pascal Van Lieshout), magnetic resonance imaging (Vikram Ramanarayanan and Christina Hagedorn), video tracking in speech (Christian Kroos) and ultrasound (Joanne Cleland).

The third subsection starts with a chapter concerned with speech acoustics: in particular, with sound spectrography (Chiara Meluzzi). The following four chapters deal with auditory and perceptual phonetics. Fei Zhao and Robert Mayr describe audiometry; Peter Howell and Liam Barrett give an account of time and frequency variated speech; Mária Gósy and Ruth Huntley Bahr cover dichotic listening; and Grant McGuire gives an overview of other perceptual phonetic techniques.

The final subsection consists of two chapters providing an overview of promising areas for clinical phonetics: automatic speech recognition, and speech synthesis. In the first of these, Loridana Buttigieg, Helen Grech, Simon Fabri, James Attard and Philip Farrugia describe initial versions of automatic speech recognition that could aid transcriptions of disordered speech. In the second chapter, Martine Smith and John Costello describe how speech synthesis can be used as part of augmentative and alternative communication systems.

Although we would like to think the coverage in Part 4 is comprehensive, there is one omission to the techniques covered, however; that is x-radiography. This is despite its long history in the investigation of both typical and disordered speech. The eventual decision to exclude it was based on two considerations. First, due to the inherent dangers of x-radiography, little work has been undertaken in recent times, especially since the development of safe imaging techniques such as magnetic resonance imaging, and ultrasound. Second, unlike the majority of techniques discussed in this part of the book, speech clinicians would not be able to undertake x-radiographic studies themselves. Nevertheless, a brief description of this type of imaging would be helpful. An overview of x-radiography and of the different types of imaging equipment is available in Ball and Gröne (1997). In speech research, low dosage systems such as x-ray microbeams, and video-fluorography were popular from the 1970s onwards, but other techniques, such as the relatively high dose xeroradiography, have also been used in the past. X-ray studies of disordered speech have covered craniofacial disorders, laryngeal disorders, fluency disorders, acquired speech disorders, articulation disorders, and speech disorders subsequent to hearing impairment (references to all these studies are in Ball & Gröne, 1997). Video-fluorography is still often employed today to study the swallowing action in clients with (suspected) dysphagia; however, this area, of course, does not fall under the remit of phonetics.

A video-fluorographic study of an unusual articulation can be briefly described here (Ball, Manuel & Müller, 2004). The imaging showed that the client (a 3;10 year-old boy) was often employing a velodorsal articulation in place of most consonants. This involved a raised but static tongue dorsum with the velum being used as the active articulator. The authors report that without the use of the imaging technique this atypical articulation type would not have been identified. In a similar case today, of course, techniques such as ultrasound or electromagnetic articulography would be safer ways of imaging this unusual articulation type.

References

Ball, M. J. & Gröne, B. (1997). Imaging techniques. In M.J. Ball & C. Code (Eds.), *Instrumental clinical phonetics* (pp. 194–227). London: Whurr.
Ball, M. J., Manuel, R. & Müller, N. (2004). Deapicalization and velodorsal articulation as learned behaviors: A videofluorographic study. *Child Language Teaching and Therapy*, 20, 153–162.

Preliminaries

17

THE NATURE OF PHONETIC INSTRUMENTATION

Nicola Bessell

Our earliest records of phonetic description come from Pāṇini's treatise on Vedic Sanskrit (5th century BCE). Pāṇini is mostly concerned with Sanskrit lexical and grammatical structure, but he does group Sanskrit segments into classes based on phonetic properties and morphophonological behavior (Cardona, 1976). From his descriptions, we would recognize the articulatory features of voicing, aspiration, place and manner of articulation. Pāṇini could have noted some of these properties from visual observation. Other features he may have inferred from cues at least one remove from their source, perhaps by feeling vibrations at the larynx, in addition to aural differences and sensory feedback from the vocal tract and respiratory system. However, there are limits to what one can directly observe or propriocept about speech sound production because most of the vocal tract is internal and views of it are increasingly obscured as sounds are made further back in the mouth. Early speech scientists were clearly frustrated by this limitation, particularly where both visual information and proprioceptive feedback are poor, as with vowel production. Erasmus Darwin (1731–1802) used a simple instrument to address this problem. He inserted a slim flexible tin cylinder into his mouth while producing vowels. For some vowels, the tongue gesture would indent the cylinder in a measurable place along its length (Jackson, 2005). This particular technique has its limitations: Darwin noted that the data he obtained using this method were somewhat crude.

Early speech scientists also recognized the limits of auditory perception to describe, record and categorize speech sounds. One limitation of auditory perception is that it does not provide direct information about how sounds are produced. A confounding difficulty is that sensitivity of auditory perception can vary from person to person and even from feature to feature. In addition, it is influenced by the language background of the perceiver. In reaction to this, Abbé Rousselot (1843–1897), who contributed to the development of early recording technology, remarked on the usefulness of speech records not limited to the "testimony" of the ear. In Abbé Rousselot's time records of speech, data were still being made in idiosyncratic and often insufficient orthographies used with varying perceptual sensitivity to the data. The development of audio speech recording has enabled significant advances in speech data storage, analysis and research.

These historical examples illustrate two general concerns that still inform the use and development of tools for investigating speech production and perception. On the one hand, we continue to seek access to data that are otherwise unobtainable due to the limits of our current observational techniques. Through instrumental techniques we can observe and measure aspects of anatomy and physiology, both typical and atypical, that are either inaccessible to unassisted observation or else inferred from existing technologies and in need of independent validation. The instrumental analysis of speech in the 20th century in particular has brought forth new data from which we have gained expansion and integration of knowledge about speech production and perception. The chapters in this volume bear clear witness to this fact. On the other hand, while impressionistic and perceptual analysis of both speech and voice is considered the gold standard within clinical linguistic practice, we encounter personal, language and culture-specific variation in perceptual responses that are reflected in description and evaluation of speech. While consistency in perceptual records improves with specialist training, there remains variance even among trained phoneticians and clinicians (see part 3 of this volume for discussion). To complicate matters further, there are some articulatory events that are not easily perceived with the degree of differentiation required for accurate linguistic or clinical description (nasality is an example, see Chapter 24). In addition, there can be non-linearities between auditory-acoustic cues and articulatory events. Gay, Lindblom, and Lubker (1981) demonstrated this experimentally for bite block vowels, where "super articulations" of the tongue and lips compensate for constraints on jaw movement in productions of /o, u/. A real-world example comes from dialects of English which produce/ɹ/-sounds with either a bunched/domal or an apical/retroflex articulation, with little auditory distinction (Ladefoged & Johnson, 2011). Given these factors, there is an obvious place for the use of objective instrumental data in speech description and analysis. Within clinical domains, such data is useful as a supplement to impressionistic analysis, to scaffold perceptual training and to inform therapy. For instance, some of the limits of impressionistic transcription can be ameliorated by the use of spectrography-assisted transcription, thus revealing details relevant to diagnosis and choice of treatment.

Chapters 20 to 34 in this volume outline the many contributions of instrumental techniques to clinical aspects of articulatory, acoustic, auditory and perceptual phonetics. Some techniques were developed with clinical linguistic practice in mind, and may even be developments of earlier non-clinical linguistic field techniques. Electropalatography (EPG) is an example of this developmental pathway (see Chapter 25). Other instruments now used for phonetic investigation were developed for medical or research use and then applied to typical speech production research before being applied to atypical speech production. Electromyography (Chapter 20) and magnetic resonance imaging (MRI) (Chapter 27) are examples. If we consider a cost-benefit analysis of the tools described in this volume, a number of common factors emerge. What follows is not necessarily exhaustive, but represents the type and range of factors that influence the use of instrumentation in clinical phonetics.

Equipment

The cost of equipment and associated software or other peripherals can determine access for research, inclusion in university teaching, and subsequent use in clinics. In addition to the initial outlay to acquire equipment, some tools require a high level of training and expertise to operate safely. Access to some procedures may be restricted to medical centers with technicians operating the equipment (e.g. MRI). Where there are different manufacturers of similar devices, differences in design or make of equipment can complicate the comparability of data, which in turn complicates the evaluation of research, which in turn informs arguments for clinical use.

Sometimes these costs reduce over time and portable units may be developed. An important example is the development of sound spectrography, which is now desktop accessible using freeware.

The first sound spectrographs were large, heavy and expensive pieces of specialist equipment originating in physics labs, and could not have been considered for clinical use. Nowadays, we can do spectrographic analysis on our laptops. Likewise, both EPG and ultrasound units have become more affordable and physically accessible. Clinicians can now use portable versions of this equipment. MRI on the other hand has yet to become readily accessible for speech production research or therapy, though it has enormous potential.

Procedures

Some techniques require invasive procedures, or are intrinsically risky because of the technology itself. X-ray imaging is no longer used for speech sound investigation because of exposure to dangerous radiation. Instead other imaging techniques are preferred, but few give as much useful information as MRI which is difficult to access for reasons of expense, restriction to medical centers and the expertise required to operate it. Some technologies are physically invasive and may not be well-tolerated, hence are not suitable for general clinical use. Direct laryngoscopy is an example. Its clinical use is generally confined to medical diagnosis, where other means of laryngeal examination such as flexible nasoendoscopy are not sufficient (see Chapter 22). Electroglottography (Chapter 23) is the most acceptable clinical procedure for therapeutic use with voice disorders since it is non-invasive and portable. The degree of client cooperation required by a technique can also limit use by age and client group, or require additional risks to overcome these limitations. For instance, very young children need to be anesthetized for automated brain stem response testing, while adults are able to remain quiet while being tested. Because of this, clinicians will exhaust other means of assessing children before resorting to this procedure (see Chapter 31 for standard behavioral audiological testing). Finally, variation in test procedures or protocols can affect the quality and interpretation of data from the same piece of equipment. Researchers and clinicians have to be aware of the context of data collection and interpret accordingly.

The data

Newly developed investigative techniques can contribute new types of data to the knowledge base of speech production and perception. This information has an uncontested basic research value. However, most data from new tools or new applications of existing tools has to be interpreted and possibly reformatted in order for it to be relatable to existing data and accessible to research or clinical communities. This process requires expert understanding and contextual analysis. The literature on cleft lip and palate illustrates this point since some patterns in speech production result from active gestures that compensate for compromised articulation (see Chapters 21 and 25). Poorly informed interpretation of any data can be misleading, but in clinical applications misinterpreted data can result in inappropriate diagnostic and treatment decisions.

It can take time for new techniques to be assessed for clinical value and if the data is produced in a format that is not easy to work with, this too can be a barrier to adoption. For instance, many SLTs/SLPs learn the basics of spectrography while in training. Spectrography requires an audio recording, which can be done on a smartphone nowadays, and familiarity with analysis software such as Praat, also readily available nowadays. But formant frequency data such as might be needed to assess vowel production is more useful converted into a vowel plot to compare with norms or as a form of visual feedback. An F1/F2 vowel plot presents the data in a format that is familiar, readily parsed, and can be used for evaluation and visual feedback during therapy. Unfortunately there are few affordable packages that facilitate automatic data manipulation of this sort in "one-stop shop," time efficient and clinically useful ways.

To be useful for comparative research and clinical application, the data produced by any tool or technique must be interpreted with reference to norms of some sort. Norming raises complex questions about the range of typical variation in performance both within and across individuals, registers and context, so it requires careful planning and execution. Norming typically requires subjects from statistically representative samples with careful attention to relevant variables. Norms are not available for all of the instrumental data that is of clinical linguistic interest. Depending on the technique and the type of data it generates, indices may be needed for useful clinical application. Data from a single assessment tool or any single measure may not be sufficient. Examples of clinical indices can be found in Chapter 21 (aerometry), Chapter 23 (electrolaryngography) and Chapter 25 (electropalatography).

Some tools produce readily accessible data that can be used in clinical contexts for feedback or monitoring, but are problematic for speech research without additional information that may be complex and inconvenient to acquire. Ultrasound is a non-invasive and safe technique that can be used to generate a real-time visual image of tongue movement within the mouth. Ultrasound can be used in the clinic for visual feedback by holding the probe under the chin without external stabilization. But research use of ultrasound data requires additional techniques to associate the ultrasound data with landmarks in the vocal tract. One solution is the use of head stabilizing gear that is challenging to wear.

Limitations of data

The type of stimuli used to elicit speech data can be a constraint on its transferability to clinical domains. In research contexts stimuli are often simplified or unnatural in the sense of not occurring in the real world, or being elicited in a formal environment (a speech laboratory). The use of /hVd/ stimuli to generate data on vowel quality has the virtue of maintaining an identical linguistic context for all vowels. But the paradigm requires the use of some words that don't exist for some speakers and the task is artificial and very formal even when the carrier phrase "I say /hVd/ again" is used. As a result /hVd/ data tells us nothing about coarticulation of vowels with consonants (other than alveolar /d/), and very little about vowel quality in natural speech, different registers or varying speech rates. Likewise, a great deal of basic information about consonant production, regardless of the investigative method, comes from single word production, yet we know that connected speech data can have different qualities from controlled single word data. This raises the problem of ecological validity of data, which has to be considered before the application of research data to clinical and therapeutic domains.

Uses of data

The emergence of data from new investigative techniques has immense primary research value, regardless of whether the data comes from clinical or non-clinical populations. Such data can develop our understanding of speech production and perception in general and may be part of assessment information that impacts diagnosis and treatment choices. Many of the techniques discussed in Part 4 are used for medical or clinical linguistic assessment and diagnosis, evaluation for intervention, treatment choice and monitoring. Despite the constraints noted, the recent wealth of different investigative tools for speech also presents opportunities for cross-correlation to validate existing and emerging data. Systematic correlation of data from different instrumental techniques may relieve a clinician of the need for a more invasive or less accessible procedure.

Instrumental data can be used in assessment, choice and design of therapy, for therapeutic tasks, for feedback, to measure outcomes and can boost client confidence. Therapeutic use may not require the rigorous methodology or protocols that accompany research work but norms or indices may be required. Where instruments have become relatively affordable, accessible and are reasonably easy for both client and therapist to use, therapeutic use can be considered providing it supports patient outcomes.

References

Cardona, G. (1976) *Pāṇini: A survey of research*. The Hague: Mouton.

Jackson, P. (2005). Mama and Papa: The ancestors of modern-day speech science. In C. Smith & R. Arnott (Eds). *The genius of Erasmus Darwin*. Aldershot, UK: Ashgate Publishing.

Gay, T., Lindblom, B., & Lubker, J. (1981). Production of bite-block vowels: Acoustic equivalence by selective compensation. *Journal of the Acoustical Society of America 69*(3), 802–10. doi: 10.1121/1.385591.

Ladefoged, P. & Johnson, K. (2011). *A course in phonetics* (6th ed.). Boston, MA: Wadsworth, Cengage Learning.

18

RECORDING SPEECH

Methods and formats

Adam P. Vogel and Hannah Reece

Hardware selection is an important and often overlooked component of speech research. All data are acquired using a microphone and a data capture and storage device. The precision, fidelity and utility of these configurations vary greatly between products and within manufacturers. There is evidence to suggest that differences between devices recorded simultaneously can sometimes be larger than differences between speakers (Vogel et al. 2014). If hardware is not harmonized from one study to the next within labs, between groups or across indications, the field will struggle to make concrete assumptions about the accuracy of studies and the features they describe. These limitations pose a significant logistical problem for groups looking to draw on historical recordings or combine data from other centers. However, these limitations are largely restricted to recordings made for the purpose of conducting acoustic analysis, and not necessarily for clinicians and scientists using speech recordings for listener based perceptual judgment. These assumptions raise important issues for hardware selection and the role different configurations play in research and the clinic. When deciding on the best tools to acquire speech, some key questions on purpose of recordings are helpful:

1. What is the post recording purpose of the speech samples? (e.g. listener-based judgment, language sampling, broad acoustic features or fine-grained analysis)
2. Where are the recordings taking place? (e.g. in the clinic, in the field, at home)
3. What is the budget? (e.g. does the team require individual devices, is testing conducted centrally requiring one set?)
4. What is the level of expertise of the user? (e.g. plug and play or bring your own device, versus complicated multi-component set ups)

There are no established criteria or standards to determine best practice in hardware selections. There are some practical constraints restricting access to the "best" hardware configuration like limited funding and access expertise necessary to purchase and operate complex hardware. However, expertise is available to many through collaboration and training and funding bodies recognize the value of high-fidelity instruments. With the advent of relatively affordable, high-quality recording devices that are designed for use by the general public, speech recordings are within the reach of most researchers. Key points around portability, software and microphone selection, recording environments, file formats and sampling rates remain. These points are discussed in this chapter with a focus on the strengths and weaknesses of each configuration and their utility in varying experimental contexts.

Recording devices

Hardware capable of capturing speech and voice are ubiquitous. We carry recording devices in our pockets, making access an issue of the past. Our review of recording devices in 2009 presented a different picture of speech research to what we experience today (Vogel & Morgan, 2009). Although remote voice capture was readily available before 2009 through interactive voice response technology and phone-based recording (Mundt, Perrine, Searles, & Walter, 1995), the quality of samples was considerably lower and the level of expertise required to set up the technology was more demanding. The variety of devices capable of recording sound now extends beyond traditional set ups using laptops, solid state recorders to smartphones, online portals and in-home voice activated technologies (e.g. Amazon's Alexa and Echo, Google Home) as well as in-car recordings.

The appeal of easy to use, relatively affordable recording devices, such as smartphones, is obvious. They carry the appearance of high-quality acquisition (irrespective of whether their fidelity actually matches purpose-built devices) and offer accessibility to users previously unable or unwilling to adopt new technologies. There are some caveats to their use, however, which limit their broader application in some speech science investigations. Microphone quality for example, often determines the overall quality of speech signals and these are discussed in the following section. File types (compression methods), (e.g. lossy compression), sampling rates, durability and storage capacity also play a part in their utility. The quality, portability, complexity, cost and limitations of prototypical hardware configurations are described in Table 18.1.

Users who want to have the option of analyzing any acoustic measure, are not restricted by budget, do not need the equipment to be portable and have access to user expertise, should continue to apply current gold standard configurations (Vogel & Morgan, 2009). Specifically, a configuration with a stand-alone hard disc recorder, an independent mixer to attenuate the incoming signal and insulated wiring combined with a high-quality microphone in an anechoic chamber or sound treated room has capacity to provide high-quality signals fit for any purpose.

Microphones

All speech samples are recorded using a microphone. The quality and reliability of recordings is strongly influenced by their specifications (See Table 18.2 for details). There are core features of the signal that need to be captured accurately for recordings to be truthfully acquired: fundamental frequency (f_0), timbre (sound spectrum) and the pressure amplitude measured via sound pressure level. For frequency, the range of the microphone response should be broad enough to capture the complete spectrum of sound, from the lowest to the highest frequency of interest. The low-frequency limit of the microphone should ideally be lower than the lowest frequency of voice (~50 Hz) and the upper frequency limit of the microphone should be above the highest frequency of interest (minimum 8,000 Hz). The frequency response of the microphone should be "flat" (variation of less than 2 dB) across the low-high frequency range (Švec, J. G., & Granqvist, S., 2010).

Directionality of the microphone is important. Omnidirectional microphones have the same sensitivity response to sound, regardless of where the sound is coming from and are well suited to recording conversations. Conversely, directional microphones respond differently to sound

Table 18.1 Features of commonly used speech recording devices

Hardware configuration (example)	Quality of acquired signal	Portability	Budget	Ease of use	Limitations	Overall utility
Hard disk recorder coupled with high quality microphone	Typically high.	Relatively low as specialized equipment required.	Relatively expensive.	Often complicated due to cabling additional equipment requirements.	Specialized equipment can be difficult to operationalize.	Good for specialized recording labs. Impractical for field work.
Solid State Recorder/flash recorder/MP3	Varying levels of quality depending on microphone input and compression options. Top of the range products provide high-quality recordings.	Medium-to-high portability; sizes range from shoe box to small MP3 player.	Costs have dropped over past decade; wide range from inexpensive to high end.	Can manually adjust pre-amplification; typically allow easy data transfer to data analysis systems.	Data needs to be transferred to alternative storage and analysis device. In-built microphones are typically unsuitable for fine grained acoustic analysis.	Good for field and clinical settings; suitable for dictation.
Personal computer	Medium (may not be appropriate for some measures of perturbation or timing) if using in built microphones.	Laptops: highly portable; likely part of the equipment taken in the field or in clinic. Desktop: not portable	Variable but typically included in any professional kit.	High, however some specialized recording equipment can require some expertise.	Noise of the computer can enter signal; quality of sound card needs to be considered; can be combined with specialized hardware.	Easy to use; potential for coupling with audio interfaces and high-quality microphones.

(Continued)

219

Table 18.1 (Continued)

Hardware configuration (example)	Quality of acquired signal	Portability	Budget	Ease of use	Limitations	Overall utility
Telephone (Landline)	For landline connections, low (frequency response is generally between 300 and 3 kHz).	Relies on user accessing their phone in the home; suitable for distance therapy and studies with participants living over a wide geographical area	Inexpensive; most participants and labs have access to a telephone.	Recording the signal requires specialized voice response technology software.	Limited frequency range restricting the type of acoustic variables that can be explored reliably.	Suitable for some acoustic analyses; however potential for fine grained analysis is likely limited.
Smartphone/ Tablet	Depends on microphone used; typically lower quality in-built microphones.	Extremely portable.	Can be expensive but often part of hardware kit.	Easy to use; many free and fee for service apps available to capture data.	Recording quality not as high as other options.	Suitable for language assessments and some acoustic analysis.
Internet browser/ Voice over Internet	Signal quality is dependent on Internet connection quality; typically inconsistent due to fluctuations in the Internet service.	Requires a computer or web-enabled device (e.g. smartphone).	Requires purpose-built webpages or software (e.g. Zoom or Skype). Data storage security needs to be considered.	Dependent on user interface; potentially straightforward Depends on hardware coupled with interface	Dependent on bandwidth of Internet connection; signal drop-outs can occur during recording.	Provides easy access to wide populations. Some control over hardware needs to be considered.

Table 18.2 Microphone features and configurations

Component	Features	Configurations
Power supply	Condenser, dynamic	Condenser: require external power (i.e. phantom power) and are typically able to pick up more subtle or fine-grained changes in sound. Dynamic: draw power from device they are attached to (do not require external power source), often have fewer moving parts, typically sturdy and less sensitive than condenser microphones.
Polar pattern[#]	Unidirectional (cardioid), omnidirectional, bidirectional	Cardioid (heart shaped) and unidirectional microphones are most sensitive to sound from a specific direction (i.e. mouth). They are designed to be sensitive to sound from one direction and therefore may pick up less ambient noise than omnidirectional options. Omnidirectional microphones are better suited to recording conversations or signals from multiple directions.
Sensitivity[*]	e.g. −38 dB	Lower the sensitivity the less responsive the microphone is to quieter sounds.
Frequency response[†]	e.g. 20 Hz–20 kHz	A wide flat frequency range is desirable, with a response curve that does not exaggerate or attenuate frequencies within the range of the human voice. Most microphones boost or dampen different frequencies to produce a more "natural" sounding voice. This may not be desirable for acoustic analysis.
Connection and wiring	XLR, 3.5 mm, USB, wireless	XLR connectors use a balanced wiring scheme, with two pins used to carry audio and the third as a ground connection. Wiring of 3.5 mm mini-plug connectors is typically not balanced as the components of the connection that provide grounding and carry the signal are in close proximity, potentially leading to interference. USB connectors bypass the sound card but may have other limitations such as lower frequency range. Wireless microphones require a transmitter and receiver. They use Bluetooth or radio waves to transmit the digital signal from the microphone to the receiver.
Positioning	Tabletop, handheld, head-mounted, lavaliere	Table-top options are suitable for recording conversations or in settings where the speaker does not want to have a device attached to them (e.g. behavioral disorders; avoiding physical contact with hardware to limit transferring viruses between users). Head-mounted options can limit the changes in mouth-to-microphone distances, ensuring amplitude remains relatively stable. Unidirectional microphones are influenced by the proximity effect which is an increase in lower frequencies as the microphone gets closer to the speaker. Lower frequencies can also pass through the microphone when the source is close, further distorting the signal. Some microphones cater for this phenomenon by providing a form of high pass filter to balance out the frequency.
Impedance[^]	Low (<600 Ω), medium (600–10,000 Ω), high (>10,000 Ω)	The higher the resistance/impedance the worse the signal.

[#] *Polar pattern (also known as directionality): the sensitivity of the microphone to sound from various directions.*
[*] *Sensitivity: reflects the amount of electrical output a microphone will produce at a certain sound pressure level (SPL).*
[†] *Frequency response: refers to the way microphones respond to different frequency levels.*
[^] *Impedance: denotes the way a microphone transfers the signal to the sound recorder or amplifier and is measured in Ohm (Ω; electrical resistance between two points of a conductor).*

depending on the direction of the sound source. The most common example of microphone directionality is the cardioid polar pattern, which optimizes the sound signal coming from directly in front of the microphone while minimizing the signal coming from other directions. Directional microphones are well suited for capturing speech/voice as they suppress any background or ambient noise. However, there are a number of frequency response issues that should be considered when using them. Directional microphones are sensitive to the pressure gradient, which is proportional to air particle velocity rather than the sound pressure itself. The *proximity effect*, where lower frequencies are disproportionally boosted when the microphone is close to the mouth, is one such effect. The proximity effect is important to consider when placing the microphone near the speakers' mouth: too close the signal will be distorted (especially lower frequencies and plosives from wind), too far and the signal will be weak.

The positioning and proximity of the microphone to the sound source (e.g. mouth) is important. Adhering to the manufacturers' requirements is recommended as they may provide information on optimal placement and direction of the microphone. Where manufacturers do not specify the microphone-to-mouth distance required for optimal sound signal a minimum distance of five centimetres (~2 inches) is recommended. If directional microphones are to be used for spectral measurements of voice and speech, the microphone specifications should contain information about the distance at which the frequency response is flat and the speech samples should be taken at that distance.

The noise level of a microphone is another notable component of their makeup. The noise level of the microphone (as well as environmental noise discussed late in the chapter) should be significantly lower than the level of the softest phonation expected in a recording. It is recommended that microphone noise levels be, at a minimum, 15 dB lower than the amplitude of the voice signal. Ideally the microphone should not be limited by distortion or clipping at high amplitudes (Švec & Granqvist, 2010).

The optimal type and configuration of a microphone is dictated by its intended use. Some microphones are highly calibrated and easily damaged and may not be suitable for use with young children or where the speaker is moving. Head-mounted microphones may not be ideal for populations with sensory needs. For acquisition of a single speaker, a set up that maintains a stable mouth to microphone distance can be achieved by using a head-mounted unidirectional or cardioid microphone or lavaliere microphone, positioned at a distance approximately 5–10 cm from the mouth (unless specifically specified by the manufacturer). The microphone itself should have a flat frequency response, an internal-noise level of at least 15 dB lower than the softest vocal sound and the highest level of the dynamic range should be above the sound levels of the loudest phonation (to avoid saturation or clipping) (Patel, Awan, Barkmeier-Kraemer, Courey, Deliyski, Eadie, … Hillman, 2018; Švec & Granqvist, 2010).

For readers interested in exploring the nature and fidelity of their own microphones, there are several steps that can be considered. Compare signals acquired simultaneously from known devices of high quality and new hardware at the same distance from the source using both electronic sounds and different voices. Trialing different voice types (e.g. non-periodic dysphonic male, female, pediatric) is important as signal quality itself varies from one speaker to the next, as does a microphone's capacity to accurately capture the signal. Testing hardware in different recording environments (e.g. soundproof booth, clinic testing room) will give data on the microphones' capacity to maintain an adequate signal-to-noise ratio. Other components of microphone performance can also be investigated by users including frequency response (by plotting estimate sound pressure level dB against frequency for an acquired signal), power spectral density and proximity effect. For examples where microphones have been compared empirically (see Parsa, Jamieson, & Pretty, 2001; Patel, Awan, Barkmeier-Kraemer, Courey,

Deliyski, Eadie, Hillman, 2018; Švec & Granqvist, 2010; Titze & Winholtz, 1993; Vogel & Maruff, 2008). Given the high variability in specifications and how microphones are used, it is desirable for clear reporting of each aspect of microphone use in study methods.

Analog-to-digital conversion and file formats

Sampling and quantization are integral parts of the analog-to-digital (A–D) conversion. The sampling rate (number of samples per second) and quantization level (the number of discrete levels of sound amplitude) of a recording determine how much of the signal is captured (Kellogg, 1967). It is often assumed that the higher values are better, however optimal sampling and quantization rates are dependent on minimum requirements.

The Nyquist Theorem (Nyquist, 2002) can be used as guiding principle for individuals determining an optimal sampling rate for their recording. The principle dictates that the sampling frequency should be at least double that of the frequencies of interest. If we consider that most of the *interesting* components of human speech fall within the first 10 kHz, a minimum sampling rate of 22.05 kHz is recommended. The most commonly available sampling rates include 44.1, 22.05, 11.025, 32, 24 and 16 kHz.

Practically speaking, analog-to-digital conversion occurs using a computer sound card, or preferably, an external analog-to-digital device (audio interface or external sound card) which connects to a computer via USB or other port (Patel, Awan, Barkmeier-Kraemer, Courey, Deliyski, Eadie, & Hillman, 2018). When choosing an appropriate external soundcard, minimum specifications include: a sampling rate of greater than 44.1 kHz, minimum resolution of 16 bits (24 bits preferred) and similarly to the microphone specifications—an internal noise level of at least 10 dB lower than the quietest phonation and an adjustable gain to ensure that the loudest phonation sounds are able to be captured without saturation or clipping (Patel, Awan, Barkmeier-Kraemer, Courey, Deliyski, Eadie, & Hillman, 2018).

How data are stored is steadily becoming a minor issue in speech research. We now have access to what seems like unlimited storage capacity, meaning we have little need for saving files in lossy compression formats (thus shrinking the size of each file). Ideally files should be stored in their uncompressed, pulse-code modulation (PCM) format which maintains the integrity of the captured signal. PCM is the standard audio file format used in CDs (sampling rate of 44.1 kHz and 16-bit quantization). Examples of the file types that store this uncompressed information are: RIFF (e.g. .avi, .wav) and AIFF (e.g. .aif). If files are compressed (e.g. MP3 compression format) the loss of signal quality will lead to changes in the robustness/validity/reliability of the results from acoustic analyses (Vogel & Morgan, 2009). While MP3 files use considerably less space to represent the audio recording than .wav files, some audio detail is lost in order to reduce the size of the file. Therefore, despite the audio sounding very similar to a .wav file, the quality of the signal has been significantly reduced. Thus, the current recommendation is that speech files be stored in PCM format to avoid problems associated with data analysis and signal quality.

Software

The range and scope of recording software has evolved over recent decades, offering the user a range of features including analysis. While hardware remains the most important component of speech recordings, software options are part of the process. For researchers using computers to collect data, software programs typically offer options for the specific hardware in terms of the sampling rate and quantization level, input (mono or stereo), file format and display options (spectrogram). In addition, some free and commercially available programs such as Praat (Boersma, 2001) provide both analysis and recording protocols.

Recording environments and how they influence recordings

Environmental or additive noise can compromise recordings. Background or environmental noise can significantly influence the quality of acquired signals and influence outcomes if fine grained acoustic features (e.g. perturbation) are targeted. To capture high-quality speech recordings, the following considerations are relevant:

1. The ambient/background noise level should be at least 10 dB weaker than the quietest phonation.
2. The signal-to-noise ratio (SNR) for vocal signal quality should be greater than 30 dB.
3. Reverberation should be kept to a minimum.

There are several practical modifications that can be deployed to ensure the environment meets the above specifications. For example, eliminating noise from talking, traffic and electrical equipment by closing doors, windows and switching-off appliances before commencing testing, avoiding recording in spaces with hard reflective surfaces, move recording devices with fans (e.g. laptops) away from the microphone. Access to sound-proof or sound-treated environments is ideal where possible (Patel, Awan, Barkmeier-Kraemer, Courey, Deliyski, Eadie, & Hillman, 2018).

Recordings outside of the lab

There is a significant and legitimate drive to extend speech recordings beyond traditional clinical and experimental environments to include remote, naturalistic settings that better represent habitual speech. In order to record speech in the home, we need to be assured that the devices used are not only accessible to individuals, appropriate for the researcher or clinician, but capable of capturing high-quality sound that is suitable for acoustic and perceptual analysis.

There have been mixed outcomes when validating alternative recording devices against the gold standard. A study comparing (a) a hard disc recorder, external mixer and table mounted microphone (b) landline telephone coupled with a computer to record the receiving end, (c) iPhone and a unidirectional head-mounted microphone and (d) laptop computer with USB unidirectional head-mounted microphone, revealed there were no statistically significant correlations between measures of voice quality across devices (Vogel et al., 2014). Yet, another study comparing (a) a laptop computer, audio interface and a unidirectional condenser microphone and (b) an iPhone/iPad and a unidirectional condenser microphone for smartphones/tablets (iRig) reported no statistically significant differences in acoustic analysis across any parameter or any speech task (Oliveira, Fava, Baglione, & Pimpinella, 2017). Both studies recorded speech of healthy control participants simultaneously with the above set ups. The divergent outcomes highlight the need for work in this space. They also show that statistical approaches and a priori hypotheses may influence interpretations of outcomes.

Taken together, these two example studies show that with the advent of new methods comes the need for evaluation of their fidelity and comparability to existing approaches. As technology continues to advance and the reliability and validity of these alternative recording devices is investigated further, speech recording outside the research or clinic environment is likely to increase. There are a number of benefits to recording speech outside the clinic environment including providing researchers with a unique opportunity to monitor change on a more frequent basis, and potentially provide a better indication of performance than one-off clinic-based assessments. If remote speech and voice diagnostics advance, individuals could attend specialist appointments remotely and costs to the patient and healthcare system may be reduced. Remote monitoring of speech could provide valuable information about disease progression or treatment response outside of traditional face-to-face visits.

There is promising evidence to suggest the use of at-home speech assessments to accurately monitor change in disease progression. One example, using an At Home Testing Device (AHTD) and a high-quality headset, participants with Parkinson's disease recorded their speech once a week for six months. Machine learning algorithms were used to map unique features of speech. Speech features significantly correlated with different aspects of disease severity (motor, speech, mood) as rated by the UPDRS (Tsanas, Little, McSharry, & Ramig, 2010). An example of more passive data collection method (i.e. recording naturalistic speech without specific tasks) of speech and language recording is LENA (Language ENvironment Analysis System) (Xu, Yapanel, & Gray, 2009). The system records and analyses a child's language and their surrounding language environment. LENA is a small wearable device that has capacity to record an auditory signal for up to 16 hours with potential for automatically labeling aspects of the input (e.g. amount of speech by target child, adults, background noise, etc.). While LENA does not automatically transcribe speech or acoustically analyze speech, it is able to collect data to investigate language acquisition in children, in a way that a single clinic visit would be unable to (Ganek & Eriks-Brophy, 2018).

Other options for long-format speech environment (LFSE) recordings (e.g. extended conversations, workplace, classroom or home-environments) are limited. It is challenging to set users up with the gold-standard hardware (computer, audio-interface, head-mounted microphone). However, similar specifications could be considered for portable devices including: the sampling frequency (higher sampling is better), bit rate (higher is better), compression (lower is better) and frequency response (as close to flat frequency is better) (Casillas & Cristia, 2019). Additionally, charging capabilities, user interface, method of securing the device on clothes and endurance to temperature/weather are also important considerations in some cases. USB audio recorders, iPods, wireless microphones and handheld recorders have been used effectively in some studies (Casillas & Cristia, 2019).

Speech is a promising non-invasive biomarker in several conditions including degenerative diseases, mental health conditions and cognitive abnormalities (Chan, Stout, & Vogel, 2019; Harel, Cannizzaro, Cohen, Reilly, & Snyder, 2004; Magee, Copland, & Vogel, 2019; Noffs, Perera, Kolbe, Shanahan, Boonstra, Evans, Vogel, 2018; Slavich, Taylor, & Picard, 2019; Voleti, Liss, & Berisha, 2020). With advancements in technology, many groups are investigating the role of more passive data collection methods including in-home monitoring. These approaches are appealing but come with risks relating to privacy and ethical concerns including how and where data are stored?; what happens if sensitive, health data is released without a users' consent?; what if the speech recording detects information about self-harm, suicide, or domestic violence? Discussion between privacy experts, developers, medical professionals and ethicists is needed before these opportunities are embraced (Cychosz, Romeo, Soderstrom, Scaff, Ganek, Cristia, & Weisleder, 2020; Slavich, Taylor, & Picard, 2019).

Conclusion

Technology, recording equipment and speech and voice analysis methods are advancing rapidly. While researchers and clinicians are faced with more options and inventive ways to record and measure speech, it is important to keep the research question, study population and target analysis at the forefront of decision making when choosing the best hardware, software and analysis methods for a study. Speech, voice and language analysis will continue to provide insight into human development, neurophysiology, health and daily life and therefore we must do our best to record it using the most appropriate methods available.

References

Boersma, P. & Weenink, D. (2001). PRAAT, a system for doing phonetics by computer. *Glot international.* 5. 341–345.

Casillas, M., & Cristia, A. (2019). A step-by-step guide to collecting and analyzing long-format speech environment (LFSE) recordings. In (Vol. 5).

Chan, J. C. S., Stout, J. C., & Vogel, A. P. (2019). Speech in prodromal and symptomatic Huntington's disease as a model of measuring onset and progression in dominantly inherited neurodegenerative diseases. *Neuroscience & Biobehavioral Reviews, 107*, 450–460. doi:https://doi.org/10.1016/j.neubiorev.2019.08.009

Cychosz, M., Romeo, R., Soderstrom, M., Scaff, C., Ganek, H., Cristia, A., Casillas, M., de Barbaro, K., Bang, J. Y., & Weisleder, A. (2020). Longform recordings of everyday life: Ethics for best practices. *Behavior research methods, 52*(5), 1951–1969. https://doi.org/10.3758/s13428-020-01365-9

Ganek, H., & Eriks-Brophy, A. (2018). Language ENvironment analysis (LENA) system investigation of day long recordings in children: A literature review. *Journal of Communication Disorders, 72*, 77–85. doi:10.1016/j.jcomdis.2017.12.005

Harel, B. T., Cannizzaro, M. S., Cohen, H., Reilly, N., & Snyder, P. J. (2004). Acoustic characteristics of Parkinsonian speech: a potential biomarker of early disease progression and treatment *(6)*, 439–453.

Kellogg, W. (1967). Information rates in sampling and quantization. *IEEE Transactions on Information Theory, 13*(3), 506–511. doi:10.1109/TIT.1967.1054019

Magee, M., Copland, D., & Vogel, A. P. (2019). Motor speech and non-motor language endophenotypes of Parkinson's disease. *Expert Review of Neurotherapeutics, 19*(12), 1191–1200. doi:10.1080/14737175.2019.1649142

Mundt, J. C., Perrine, M., Searles, J., & Walter, D. (1995). An application of interactive voice response (IVR) technology to longitudinal studies of daily behavior. *Behavior Research Methods, 27*(3), 351–357. doi:10.3758/bf03200429

Noffs, G., Perera, T., Kolbe, S. C., Shanahan, C. J., Boonstra, F. M. C., Evans, A., … Vogel, A. P. (2018). What speech can tell us: A systematic review of dysarthria characteristics in Multiple Sclerosis. *Autoimmunity Reviews, 17*(12), 1202–1209. doi:https://doi.org/10.1016/j.autrev.2018.06.010

Nyquist, H. (2002). Certain topics in telegraph transmission theory. *Proceedings of The IEEE, 90*(2), 280–305.

Oliveira, G., Fava, G., Baglione, M., & Pimpinella, M. (2017). Mobile digital recording: Adequacy of the iRig and iOS device for acoustic and perceptual analysis of normal voice. *Journal of Voice, 31*(2), 236.

Parsa, V., Jamieson, D. G., & Pretty, B. R. (2001). Effects of microphone type on acoustic measures of voice. *Journal of Voice, 15*(3), 331–343.

Patel, R. R., Awan, S. N., Barkmeier-Kraemer, J., Courey, M., Deliyski, D., Eadie, T., … Hillman, R. (2018). Recommended protocols for instrumental assessment of voice: American Speech-Language-Hearing Association Expert Panel to develop a protocol for instrumental assessment of vocal function. *American Journal of Speech-Language Pathology, 27*(3), 887–905. doi:10.1044/2018_AJSLP-17-0009

Slavich, G. M., Taylor, S., & Picard, R. W. (2019). Stress measurement using speech: Recent advancements, validation issues, and ethical and privacy considerations. *Stress (Amsterdam, Netherlands), 22*(4), 408–413. doi:10.1080/10253890.2019.1584180

Švec, J. G., & Granqvist, S. (2010). Guidelines for selecting microphones for human voice production research. *American Journal of Speech-Language Pathology, 19*(4), 356–368. doi:10.1044/1058-0360(2010/09-0091)

Titze, I. R., & Winholtz, W. S. (1993). Effect of microphone type and placement on voice perturbation measurements. *Journal of Speech & Hearing Research, 36*(6), 1177–1190.

Tsanas, A., Little, M. A., McSharry, P. E., & Ramig, L. O. (2010). Accurate telemonitoring of Parkinson's disease progression by noninvasive speech tests. *IEEE Transactions on Biomedical Engineering, 57*(4), 884–893. doi:10.1109/TBME.2009.2036000

Vogel, A. P., & Maruff, P. (2008). Comparison of voice acquisition methodologies in speech research. *Behavior Research Methods, 40*(4), 982–987

Vogel, A. P., & Morgan, A. T. (2009). Factors affecting the quality of sound recording for speech and voice analysis. *International Journal of Speech-Language Pathology, 11*(6), 431–437.

Vogel, A.P., Rosen, K.M., Morgan, A.T., & Reilly, S. (2014) Comparability of modern recording devices for speech analysis: smartphone, landline, laptop, and hard disc recorder. *Folia Phoniatrica et Logopaedica, 66*(*6*), 244–50. doi: 10.1159/000368227

Voleti, R., Liss, J. M., & Berisha, V. (2020). A review of automated speech and language features for assessment of cognitive and thought disorders. *IEEE Journal of Selected Topics in Signal Processing, 14*(2), 282–298. doi:10.1109/JSTSP.2019.2952087

Xu, D., Yapanel, U., & Gray, S. (2009). *Reliability of the LENA Language Environment Analysis System in young children's natural home environment* (Technical Report LTR-05-2). Boulder, CO: LENA Foundation.

19

THE PHONBANK DATABASE WITHIN TALKBANK, AND A PRACTICAL OVERVIEW OF THE PHON PROGRAM

Yvan Rose and Gregory J. Hedlund

Background

Clinical research in phonetics and phonology typically involves the analysis of significant sets of speech recordings. To engage in the analysis of these recordings, researchers and students must transcribe the samples both orthographically and phonetically, in order to extract patterns which relate to different factors such as word forms, syllable shapes or positions, phones, or phonological features, also in reference to stress or other prosodic contexts (e.g. Rose & Inkelas, 2011). Phonetic transcriptions can also serve as useful reference points toward acoustic analysis, given that each token to be measured must first be properly labeled. Given the complexity inherent to this type of research, and because of technical challenges posed by the representation of attributes such as syllable position or phonological features, each of which transcends basic means of phonetic transcription, research in clinical phonetics and phonology has traditionally suffered from a lack of useful software support or basic standards to enable corpus building across different computer platforms (MacWhinney, Spektor, Chen, & Rose, 2012; Rose & MacWhinney, 2014).

The situation began to change for the better with the creation of the PhonBank database (https://phonbank.talkbank.org; Rose & MacWhinney, 2014).[1] PhonBank initially began as an extension of the long-established CHILDES database (https://childes.talkbank.org; MacWhinney, 2000), a powerful resource for research on child language development and developmental language disorders, but with limited support for research in phonetics and phonology. In order to support this research, PhonBank needed a program for phonetic data transcription, annotation and analysis. It is in this context that we invented Phon (https://www.phon.ca; Hedlund & O'Brien, 2004; Hedlund & Rose, 2020; Rose, MacWhinney, Byrne, Hedlund, Maddocks, O'Brien, & Wareham, 2006) and, as of 2011, instituted PhonBank as a database separate from CHILDES, both of which are now standing alongside one another within the larger TalkBank system, described below.

In this chapter, we begin by situating PhonBank, CHILDES and TalkBank both in their historical context and also in light of current trends in open science, which aim at making scientific data and methods maximally transparent and readily accessible to everyone. With this communal setting as background, we then introduce Phon in more detail and describe how it can be used for developmental and clinical studies in phonetics and phonology. We contextualize our descriptions of Phon as part of two practical workflows commonly used in developmental and clinical research. We conclude with a brief summary, highlighting again the virtues of open science and its significance for current and future research in the field.

CHILDES and PhonBank within TalkBank

To study patterns of language production in any significant detail, either from typical or atypical learners or speakers, scholars must generally rely on large, maximally representative datasets documenting different languages and/or speaker populations. Likewise, longitudinal studies must document individual learners as frequently as possible throughout the duration of the observation period, a method which also generates significant amounts of data to transcribe and analyze. Working toward these goals, scholars must have access to computer-assisted methods for the systematic coding and analysis of these datasets, the size of which typically makes manual analyses impractical. The TalkBank project (https://talkbank.org; MacWhinney, 2016; MacWhinney, Fromm, Rose, & Bernstein Ratner, 2018) is currently the largest and most compelling linguistic database system worldwide. At present, TalkBank consists of 15 different databanks, each documenting different properties of language use, language acquisition and language disorders (e.g. AphasiaBank, BilingBank, CHILDES, FluencyBank, HomeBank, PhonBank, ...).

From a historical perspective, TalkBank is in fact one of the many extensions of the original CHILDES project (CHIld Language Data Exchange System), which began in 1983 through an initiative by Brian MacWhinney and Catherine Snow (MacWhinney & Snow, 1985). CHILDES was also a precursor to the more general open science movement, now a leading trend throughout the research world. Open science aims at the following four fundamental goals (http://openscience.org):

- Transparency in experimental methodology, observation and collection of data
- Public availability and reusability of scientific data
- Public accessibility and transparency of scientific communication
- Using web-based tools to facilitate scientific collaboration

Since its inception, CHILDES has made both child language datasets and the software programs required for the analysis of these data freely and openly accessible to the research community, thereby supporting and fostering a tremendous wealth of research on child language and developmental language disorders. This early model of open science then snowballed into different database projects related to the study of language and language disorders such as those listed above which, together, constitute the whole of TalkBank.

The datasets available through CHILDES as well as through most other TalkBank databases are primarily created and analyzed using the computer program CLAN (Computerized Language ANalysis), which offers a rich set of functions primarily geared toward the study of lexical, morpho-syntactic and conversational aspects of speech. However, in spite of its tremendous analytic power, CLAN has traditionally provided little support in the area of phonetics and phonology, primarily because of technical difficulties such as those mentioned above concerning the use of phonetic transcriptions in early computer programs. For example, just focusing on phonetic and phonological data representation, the word *crocodile* [ˈkɹɑkəˌdaɪɫ], as it is produced in many common dialects of English, includes three syllables with varying degrees of stress, an onset cluster, a diphthong and a dark [ɫ]. These phonological contexts each carry rich arrays of information about place and manner of articulation, voicing, also in relation to syllable stress and position within the word, many aspects of which can be quantified through acoustic analysis. The study of these and other phonological and phonetic properties of speech, especially in the context of language acquisition and phonological disorders, primarily motivated the invention of Phon, the free, open-source program that supports the needs of PhonBank.

More generally, and similar to every database within TalkBank, PhonBank and Phon are the outcomes of a community endeavor. The development of these open resources crucially relies both on public funding and on the commitment of active contributors within the scholarly and clinical communities, following a winning scenario for everyone involved: students, researchers and dedicated clinicians benefit from PhonBank data and Phon functions to do their work. In return, these people contribute to the building of PhonBank, through the open sharing of their corpus data and to the further development of Phon, through their provision of ideas and feedback. In turn, PhonBank and Phon have become true investments for all the funding institutions and corpus data contributors involved, in a number of concrete ways. From a financial standpoint, data sharing helps reduce the overall cost of research tremendously, as datasets built for individual projects can be reused in a virtually unlimited number of additional studies. Individuals who share their data also benefit from a unique platform to disseminate their work and strengthen their overall profile, through their active embrace of the tenets of open science listed above. Finally, data sharing levels the playing field for research, as open databases offer rich grounds to explore and compare different theories and ideas, from which everyone ultimately benefits, all the way to clinical applications emerging from cutting-edge research.

In sum, it is in the communal spirit of TalkBank, itself inspired by the original CHILDES system and the open science movement more generally, that we built the PhonBank database and developed the Phon program, to which we turn in the next section.

The Phon software program: a practical overview

Phon was invented in 2004, in the form of a proof of concept (Hedlund & O'Brien, 2004), and later introduced to the research community as a prototype (Rose, MacWhinney, Byrne, Hedlund, Maddocks, O'Brien, & Wareham, 2006). It has since evolved into a mature software platform with programs to segment, transcribe, annotate and analyze phonological and phonetic speech data (Hedlund and Rose, 2020). Phon supports phonological analyses at the level of segmental features, phones, clusters and diphthongs, word forms, tones and syllable stress, with each of these levels centrally relevant to mainstream research on phonetics and phonology (e.g. Ewen, Hume, Oostendorp, & Rice (Eds.), 2011; Goldsmith, 1996) and phonological disorders (e.g. Baker & Williams, 2010; Bernhardt, Stemberger, Ayyad, Ullrich, & Zhao, 2010; Ingram, 1981; see also contributions to McLeod (Ed.) 2007). Finally, Phon integrates Praat libraries (Boersma & Weenink, 2020) for the analysis of acoustic parameters such as duration, pitch, intensity, formant frequencies, spectral moments and voice onset time.

In the next section, we describe the process of building and analyzing a dataset using Phon, version 3.2, which we describe following two practical workflows. We take as our first example a semi-guided conversation between a participant and an interviewer. We then emphasize how to use Phon based on predetermined lists of stimuli (e.g. word or sentence repetition; picture naming; ...), which are frequently used toward assessments of speech productive abilities. In our discussion of each workflow, we assume the pre-existence of digital audio or video recorded data. We begin in the next section with the general setup relevant to both workflows.

General interface and corpus setup

Phon organizes corpus projects and transcripts following a hierarchical folder and file structure located on the user's computer hard drive, as listed in (1). Given this structure, a single transcript in Phon is nested within a corpus folder, itself part of a project folder, which for convenience can be located within a dedicated workspace folder.

1. Data structure in Phon

    a. Workspace: top organizing folder; contains at least one project
    b. Project: folder containing at least one corpus
    c. Corpus: folder containing at least one session
    d. Session: file containing all transcript and annotation data

Each project is listed within the Welcome window illustrated in Figure 19.1, which specifies the location of the workspace currently in use and also provides ready access to general user actions.

The basic steps to create a project, starting with the Welcome window, are as follows:

2. Creating a Phon project (step-by-step)

    a. Set the general user preferences

        i. Dictionary and syllabification languages
        ii. General (default) media folder location
        iii. (Other preferences as needed)

    b. Create project (from the Welcome window)
    c. Create corpus and session (using the Project Manager; see below)

The user can access the preferences directly from the actions panel located on the left of the Welcome window in Figure 19.1. Of the preference options, it is particularly important to assign a default dictionary language and syllabification algorithm, in Figure 19.2a, and a media folder, in Figure 19.2b, as these options might affect some of the automatized functions described below.

After the user preferences are set, we can create a new project by clicking on the "Create Project" action button in Figure 19.1. Phon then opens this new project within the Project Manager window, an interface designed to assist all tasks related to corpus and transcript

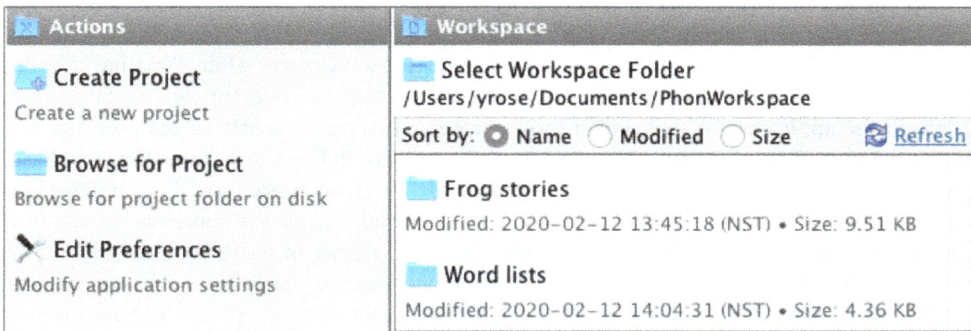

Figure 19.1   Welcome window: workspace, project list and general settings.

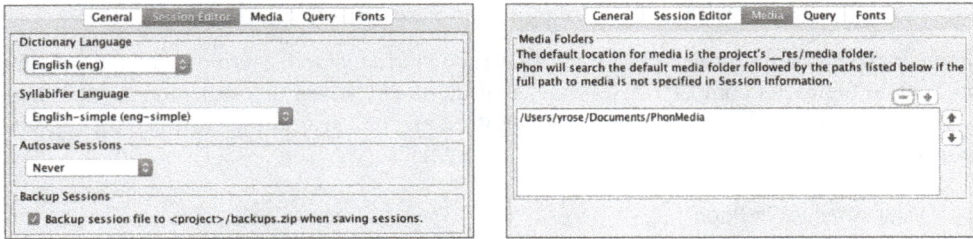

Figure 19.2 Language and general media folder location preferences. (a) Session Editor (b) Media folder.

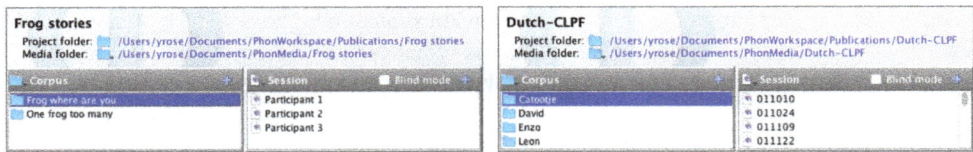

Figure 19.3 Project Manager. (a) Cross-sectional design (b) Longitudinal design.

management, including the assignment of specific media folders for either the whole project or each individual corpus contained in the project. What exactly we mean by "corpus" is entirely left to the user. For example, in Figure 19.3a, each corpus corresponds to a specific data elicitation task, as part of a cross-sectional design, with each session transcript corresponding to an individual participant. By contrast, in a longitudinal setting, illustrated in Figure 19.3b, a corpus typically documents an individual participant, with session transcripts each corresponding to a data recording session, where the six digits indicate the speaker's age (YYMMDD) at the time of recording, as illustrated here with the Dutch–CLPF corpus (Fikkert, 1994; Levelt, 1994). As we can also see in these illustrations, each of these projects is assigned a dedicated media folder, specified on top of the interface.

For each session transcript to be linked (time-aligned) to a media recording, the user must place a copy of the relevant media file within the dedicated media folder and create a new session for this media file. The user then opens this newly-created session within the Session Editor, whose default interface is illustrated in Figure 19.4.

The Session Editor consists of different view panels, each of which gives access to a specific set of functions within Phon. For example, in Figure 19.4, the Media Player, Session Information and Record Data panels are visible within the interface, while Timeline is hiding "behind" Session Information, but readily accessible through clicking on its tab button. Through the application's View menu (not represented in the screenshot), the user can load additional view panels, for example IPA Lookup, to access dictionary- or transliteration-based phonetic transcription systems for different languages, or Speech Analysis, for TextGrid generation, formatting and subsequent acoustic analysis. Besides adding or removing panels from the interface, the user can click and drag each panel's title bar to move the panel to another location within the interface, or use the buttons located on the right of the title bar for more configuration options.[1] User-defined layouts resulting from these operations can be saved or reset at will (still through the View menu), offering the user flexible computer environments to accomplish different tasks such as the ones described below.

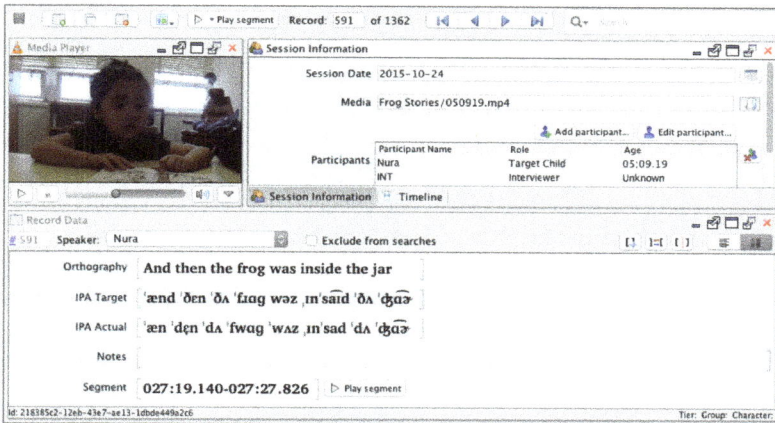

Figure 19.4   Session Editor.

Session and participant metadata

Returning to corpus building, the first step involved in filling a newly-created transcript is to enter the session and participant metadata. Before we detail this process, we urge every user to treat participant information with appropriate care. As long as the corpus remains private and is adequately protected on the researcher's or clinician's personal computer, using recording dates and birth dates can facilitate tasks around data management. For example, Phon relies on these dates to automatically compute participant age at the time of recording. However, in the context of open data sharing, such identifiers must be removed; Phon also provides functions to facilitate this operation. With this in mind, we can describe this task as follows:

3. Entering session and participant information (step-by-step)

    a. Enter session (recording) date
    b. Enter media filename
    c. Add participant(s)
    d. Assign participant role and enter participant name (or pseudonym)
    e. Enter participant age; alternatively enter participant birthdate (to compute age)

As soon as the filename is entered into the Media field in Figure 19.5a, Phon automatically opens the corresponding media file, assuming that this media file is correctly located within its dedicated folder, as discussed already. By clicking on the "Add participant" button, the user can then enter participant-specific information, as in Figure 19.5b.

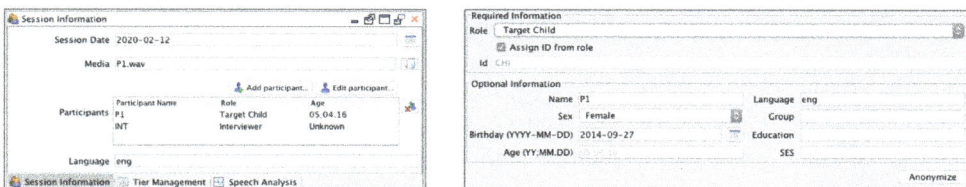

Figure 19.5   Session and participant information. (a) Session information (b) Participant information.

At this stage, the user is ready to begin the work in earnest, as we describe next, beginning with our general workflow. In case the corpus at hand does not involve media recordings, the user can proceed directly to data transcription and annotation, by manually inserting new records and filling them with the relevant data, as we describe in more detail below.

General workflow

The general workflow covers all cases where a speaker produces natural speech, whether unguided or semi-guided. Key to this workflow is that the speech targeted for analysis is not predetermined as part of a list of words or sentences. For example, frog stories, which consist of data elicitation through picture-only books such as *Frog, where are you?* (Mayer, 1969), are bound to elicit certain words (e.g. frog, boy, dog, ...), but the exact words used and the way these words are used may vary greatly across different participants or even versions of the same stories told by unique participants. Because of this, and similar to general interviews or unguided narrations, we must begin the work with an empty transcript, as per the steps in (4).

4. General workflow (step-by-step)

    a. Session creation
    b. Media segmentation
    c. Data transcription

        i. Orthography
        ii. IPA (using IPA Lookup when possible)

    d. Data annotation

        i. Syllabification and phone-by-phone alignment
        ii. Other annotations

    e. Data analysis

        i. Transcript-based analysis (textual and IPA data)
        ii. Acoustic analysis

After the user creates the new transcript within the relevant project and corpus, and enters the session and participant information, as described in the previous section, the first step is to engage with media segmentation.

Media segmentation

Media segmentation, also referred to as "time alignment" or "time stamping," is the task of identifying the parts of the recorded media which are relevant for analysis. For simplicity, we refer to these words or sentences as "utterances" in our discussion below. Media segmentation is achieved through the Timeline view panel. As illustrated in Figure 19.6a, Timeline displays a waveform of the media file, to which segments identifying the speech productions are aligned temporally on dedicated lines, for each speaker.

Media segmentation proceeds according to the following steps. The first three steps in (5a–c) are required to engage with the segmentation process. Concerning (5d), the number keys correspond to each speaker as they are ordered within Session Information. Alternatively, the user can press the space bar or the "0" number key to assign a speech segment to an unidentified speaker.

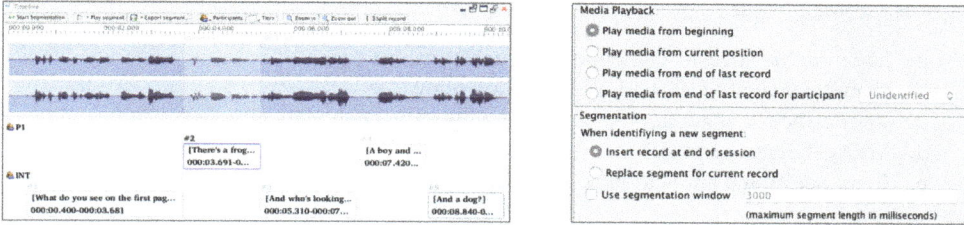

Figure 19.6   Timeline and general segmentation settings. (a) Timeline (b) Segmentation settings.

5. Segmenting a media recording (step-by-step)

   a. Click on the "Start Segmentation" button (top left of Figure 19.6a)
   b. Select relevant segmentation parameters (Figure 19.6b)
   c. Click on the "Start Segmentation" button on the bottom right corner of the segmentation parameter window
   d. After hearing an utterance, press the relevant number key or the space bar

After the initial segmentation is completed, each utterance is assigned to a participant and associated to its corresponding time interval on the recording within an otherwise empty (untranscribed) data record. It often happens, however, that some of the segments obtained through the process just described need to be further refined or, at times, assigned to a different speaker, split into multiple intervals and so on. Each of these operations can be done directly from the Timeline's interface. After completion of these adjustment tasks, the corpus is ready for transcription and annotation.

Data transcription and annotation

Data transcription and the addition of textual annotations to transcript records take place within the Record Data view panel, represented in Figure 19.7a. This screenshot contains the five default tiers in Phon as well as a user-defined tier, GrammCat, to which we return below.

   Because, under our current workflow, the content of the speech segments is largely unpredictable, transcription and annotation must be performed from scratch. For each data record, the general steps are as follows:

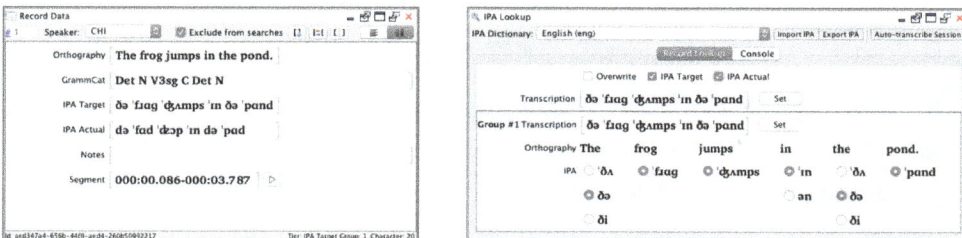

Figure 19.7   Transcription and Annotation (a) Record Data (b) IPA Lookup.

6. Transcribing record data (step-by-step)

   a. Listen to the speech segment of the current record
   b. Transcribe the speech segment in orthography
   c. Transcribe (or generate) the corresponding form(s) phonetically
   d. Verify the transcriptions
   e. Enter additional annotations (as needed)

The first two steps are self-explanatory. Concerning orthographic transcription, Phon supports different writing systems, as long as the relevant character sets are encoded in Unicode format. Moving to phonetic transcription, an unavoidably time-consuming task, Phon provides support for many languages in the form of dictionaries of citation forms and orthography-to-IPA transliteration systems, accessible through the IPA Lookup view panel in Figure 19.7b.[2] Both citation and transliterated forms obtained through IPA Lookup can be further modified by the user as needed. To enter phonetic transcriptions from scratch or to modify a form obtained through IPA Lookup, the user can use the IPA Map built into Phon, available from the Tools menu.

Finally, the user can enter additional annotations as needed, for example within user-defined tiers such as the GrammCat tier in Figure 19.7a. While this may not be obvious from this screenshot, Phon implicitly aligns each annotation between each record tiers on a word-by-word basis, based on the number of white spaces present between these words. One practical use of this implicit alignment is that the user can take advantage of it to look for words or phonological forms which correspond to particular grammatical categories. This is useful to analyze behaviors in different syntactic or morphological contexts, for example the omission of 3rd person singular "s" suffix of *jumps* in Figure 19.7a.

Syllabification and phone-by-phone alignment

Upon entering the phonetic transcriptions within the IPA Target and IPA Actual tiers, Phon automatically generates two additional levels of annotation, one for the labeling of each phone for position within the syllable, the other to obtain a systematic, phone-by-phone alignment of the corresponding target-actual pairs of IPA forms, as per the screenshot in Figure 19.8. These two annotations work together toward the systematic detection of segmental patterns (e.g. substitution, deletion, epenthesis) across different positions within the syllable or word.

Syllables are identified in Phon through visual groupings of phones, with syllable positions color-coded within each grouping (e.g. blue for syllable onsets; green for codas). Phone-by-phone alignments are represented through vertical alignments between target and actual phone pairs.

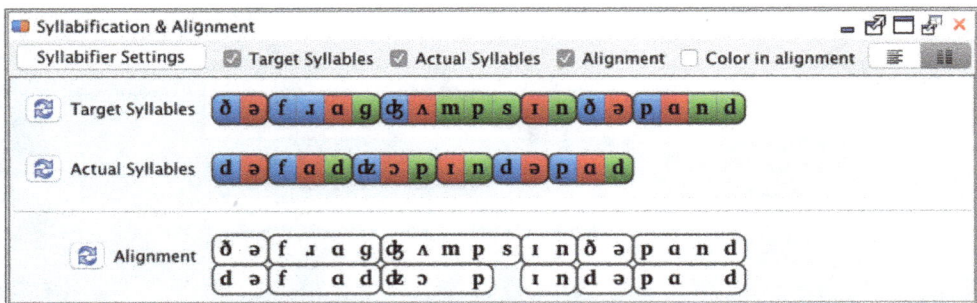

Figure 19.8   Syllabification and alignment.

Similar to textual transcriptions and annotations, all syllabification and alignment data encoded within this interface can also be modified at will by the user, whenever needed.

This completes our overview of the general workflow for data preparation. Before we turn to data analysis, we first discuss our second workflow, this time based on a pre-transcribed session template.

Template-based workflow

The template-based workflow best applies to contexts where the speech content relevant for analysis is (largely) predictable from a guided approach to speech elicitation. This includes picture naming and utterance repetition tasks, for example, which are commonly used in large-scale studies of speech sound productive abilities (e.g. Másdóttir, 2019; Mcleod & Baker, 2014; Skahan, Watson, & Lof, 2007; Smit, 1993). These and similar methods such as non-word repetition tasks (Coady & Evans, 2008), all of which can be used in clinical contexts, have in common the reliance on a predetermined list of stimuli, assuming that the stimuli are presented to the participants in a fixed order. This list will be our starting point for preparing the session template, the first step in the workflow in (7).

7. Template-based workflow (step-by-step, building on (4))

   a. Template preparation

      i. Create a session template (only once)
      ii. Copy a duplicate of the template into the relevant corpus (for each recording)

   b. Media segmentation (using the "replace segment" mode)
   c. Data transcription (based on template data)
   d. Data annotation (as needed)
   e. Data analysis (same as general workflow)

Following the step-by-step description in (7), the work begins with creating the session template, a one-time task. Once completed, the template becomes a significant time saver for the processing of the media recordings, something especially important in the context of both routine speech assessments and large-scale studies.

Template preparation

A template in Phon is, simply put, a maximally pre-filled session transcript which serves as a basis to derive individual transcripts. At the session level, the Session Date and Media fields of Figure 19.5a above should be left empty, as they are unique to individual recordings. Similarly, the key difference between the current workflow and that illustrated in Figure 19.5b is that only general attributes such as participant role or language(s) can be common to all participants; all other fields should also be left empty within the template, to be filled later, when the user derives individual transcripts from the template. Finally, concerning the list of participants, the user can decide to only include the target participant(s), or to include all speakers involved in the recording.

Turning now to Record Data, the simplest way is to manually enter the data to be included into the template (transcriptions and related annotations), with each data record corresponding to an utterance expected to be present in the recordings.[3] Each record should minimally consist of the form entered within the Orthography tier, alongside its phonetic transcription in the

IPA Target tier. For users adopting the transcription-by-modification approach (see below), the same phonetic form should be entered in the IPA Actual tier as well. Finally, template records may contain additional tiers and annotations, for example concerning the grammatical category, gloss and/or translation of each form present in Orthography.

Media segmentation

As indicated in the steps in (7), to begin segmentation of a new media recording, the user must first place a duplicate of the template file into the appropriate corpus folder and rename this duplicate appropriately.[4] The user then opens this new file to enter the details specific to this individual session transcript within Session Information, thereby linking it to its corresponding media file, and specifying the required information for each participant.

The user can now proceed with segmentation, as described for the general workflow above, with the difference that this time the segment times are assigned to already-existing records, instead of newly-inserted (blank) records, as per the segmentation settings in Figure 19.9.

At the beginning of segmentation, the current (visible) Phon record must correspond to the first utterance expected to be heard on the recording. Immediately after hearing the production of this form, the user presses the relevant key ("1" if only one participant is documented). Phon then assigns the segment time relative to this keypress, and automatically moves to the following record within the transcript file, indicating to the user the next utterance they must segment.

After this task is completed, the user can then refine the segment times as already described for the general workflow. In this regard, note that Figure 19.9 uses a specific segmentation window, which imposes a predefined limit on segment times (here, 2,000 milliseconds), as opposed to the open-ended segmentation window of Figure 19.6b. This setting is particularly useful for list-based elicitation, as it prevents the segmentation of overly lengthy time intervals covering portions of the recorded media which are irrelevant to the work at hand.[5] Using prespecified segmentation windows such as this also helps reduce the amount of time involved in refining the time interval of each segmented utterance.

Data transcription and annotation

As already mentioned, session templates are particularly useful for the time savings they provide in the areas of data transcription and annotation, given that much of the record data are readily available from the template. Concerning phonetic transcription, this is especially true if the user adopts the transcription-by-modification method, whereby the user arrives at the IPA Actual phonetic form through modifying the model form already present within the original

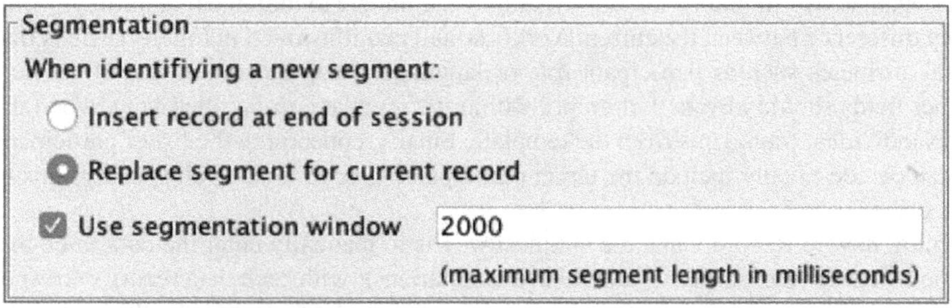

Figure 19.9 Template-based segmentation settings.

template file (McAllister Byun & Rose, 2016). For example, using this method, the elicited utterances produced accurately by the participant do not require any further work toward analysis. Likewise, deletion, modification or addition of a few phones or diacritics based on a pretranscribed form requires less work than entering the full IPA Actual form from scratch. Finally, in case the form produced by the participant differs significantly from the pretranscribed one, the user can simply transcribe this production from scratch.

In the same spirit, in case the participant produces a target form more than once, the user may decide to duplicate the relevant record for each repetition, duplicate the Orthography and IPA forms as many times as needed within a unique Phon record, or more simply consider only one of these productions toward analysis (and leave the other ones unsegmented). As well, if the participant produces an alternative form (e.g. a synonym or a regional variant of the target form), then adjustments to the corresponding data in other tiers (e.g. Orthography, IPA Target) are in order as well. Alternatively, the user can check the "Exclude from searches" option available for each record (see Figure 19.7a) to prevent the data contained in this record from unduly influencing data analysis.

Syllabification and phone-by-phone alignment

The final step toward data preparation is identical to both workflows described in this chapter: each time a form in the IPA Actual tier needs modification, the user should verify that syllabification and phone-by-phone alignments generated by Phon correspond to expectations, as we already described for the general workflow.

This completes our description of both the general and the template-based workflows for data preparation. Once the steps described above (for either workflow) are completed, the transcript is now ready for analysis. Within Phon, analyses can be conducted based on either transcript data (orthographic and/or IPA transcriptions and annotations) or speech acoustics, as we describe in turn in the next section.

Data analysis

Phon offers two main approaches to analyzing transcript data, namely a set of methods for data query and reporting as well as a series of built-in analyses, many of which are used standardly in clinical analyses of speech. Under either approach, Phon opens up a dedicated wizard designed to guide the user through each step in the process, also allowing them to backtrack to a previous step, for example to revise or rerun the current query or analysis.

Transcript data query and reporting

All transcript data (e.g. textual and phonetic) and associated metadata (e.g. participant role or age) can be used across the different Phon query methods listed in (8).

8. Query methods in Phon 3.2

   a. Data Tiers
   b. Deletions
   c. Epenthesis
   d. Phones
   e. Segmental Relations

Each one of these query methods is available from the Query menu, from which Phon opens an expandable query form, enabling the user to enter the relevant query criteria. Phon then combines these criteria within specialized algorithms designed to return the transcript data sought by the query. This form-based process makes accessible to the user query functions which would otherwise require advanced computing (scripting) skills.

Of the query types listed in (8), Data Tiers and Phones are the two most commonly used methods. The three other query methods follow the same logic, however in a more specific fashion, as the Deletions and Epenthesis queries consist of methods to detect exactly these phenomena, while Segmental Relations consists of a set of detectors for patterns such as phone or feature reduplication, migration, metathesis, or assimilation, among others, which are often encountered in developmental and disordered speech data. In the next paragraphs, we limit our focus to Data Tiers and Phones queries.

Data Tiers can be used to look for specific textual or phonological annotations present within data records. For example, in the Data Tiers form in Figure 19.10a, the user looks into the GrammCat tier for the expression "V3sg" (meaning Verb, 3rd pers. sing.), and returns, for each occurrence of such verbs, the orthography as well as the corresponding IPA forms and notes (if any); this query also applies specifically to the "Target Child" participant(s), as per the selection at the bottom of the form.

In addition to plain text expressions such as "V3sg" in Figure 19.10a, the user can select among other types of expressions, for example "regular" and "phonological" expressions. Regular expressions (or regex) combine textual strings with logical operators (e.g. "and" and "or" operators), wildcards, etc., to look for textual patterns. For example, the user can use the regex "p.nt" to find any textual string such as *pant*, *pent*, *pint*, *punt*, etc., where "." is a wildcard

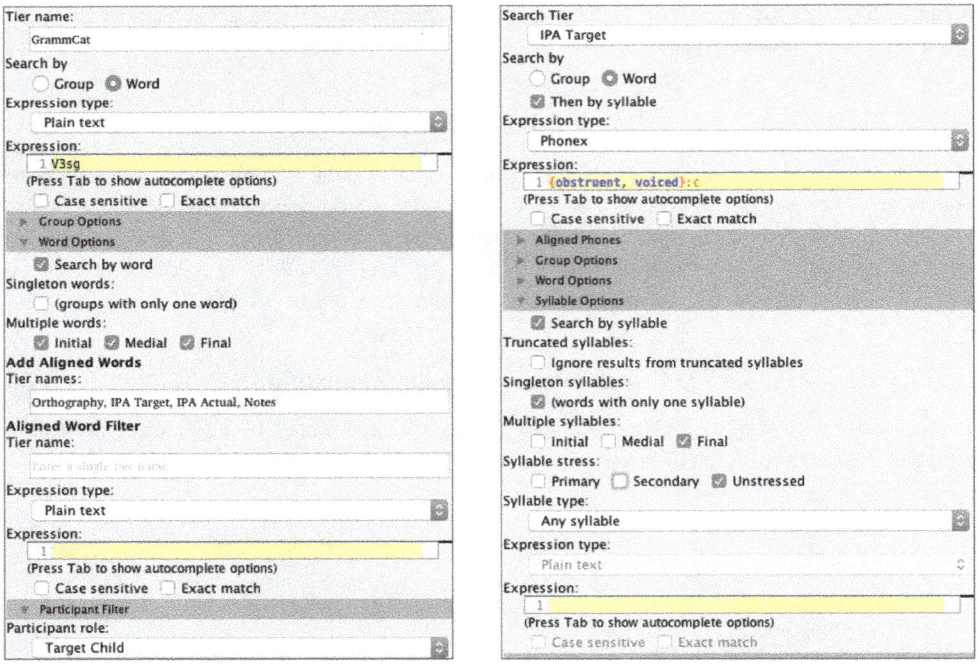

Figure 19.10 Example query forms. (a) Data Tiers (b) Phones.

for any unique character standing between "p" and "n," itself followed by "t." Phonological expressions (or phonex) consist of a special set of regular expressions with constructs built specifically for Phon to look for patterns represented in phonetic transcriptions, also in relation to syllabification. For example, the user can use the phonex "\c" to look for any consonant or "\v" to look for any vowel. Similarly, phone classes can be queried using their descriptive features; the phonex "{c, labial, continuant}" will return all labial continuant consonants (e.g. [f, v, β, w, …]) present in a given IPA tier. Just like regular expressions, phonological expressions can be much more elaborate, for example specifying positions within syllables (e.g. "\c:o" for any consonant in syllable onsets), or relative to syllable stress or word boundaries.

Phonological expressions are used most often within Phones queries, which also provide functions to perform comparisons between pairs of aligned phones, or to restrict the query to particular types of word or syllable forms. For example, in the Phones query in Figure 19.10b, the user looks for voiced obstruent consonants located in syllable codas in IPA Target forms; this query is also restricted to word-final, unstressed syllables, based on the selection of syllable-level criteria specified in the bottom section of the form displayed.[6]

After each query is completed, the user is then given options to either open individual session transcripts containing the results returned by the query or to generate data reports. In the former, Phon opens a Results Navigator window alongside the Session Editor, which the user can use to directly access each individual result returned by the query. In the latter, the user moves to the next step within the wizard, the Report Composer, an interface which allows the user to organize the query results as part of customizable reports. For example, the report composed in Figure 19.11 consists of an aggregate of the results obtained across all transcripts targeted by the query, followed by a listing of each individual result.

After the report is composed, Phon generates a report preview. Using this preview, the user can validate that the query results are organized as needed; the user can also directly open the relevant record of each individual result by clicking on this result. This is particularly useful to assess individual results within their contexts of occurrence. Finally, all reports can be saved as HTML files or exported in text-only (CSV) and Excel formats for further processing or use, for example within of spreadsheet, statistical analysis, text processing or presentation software.

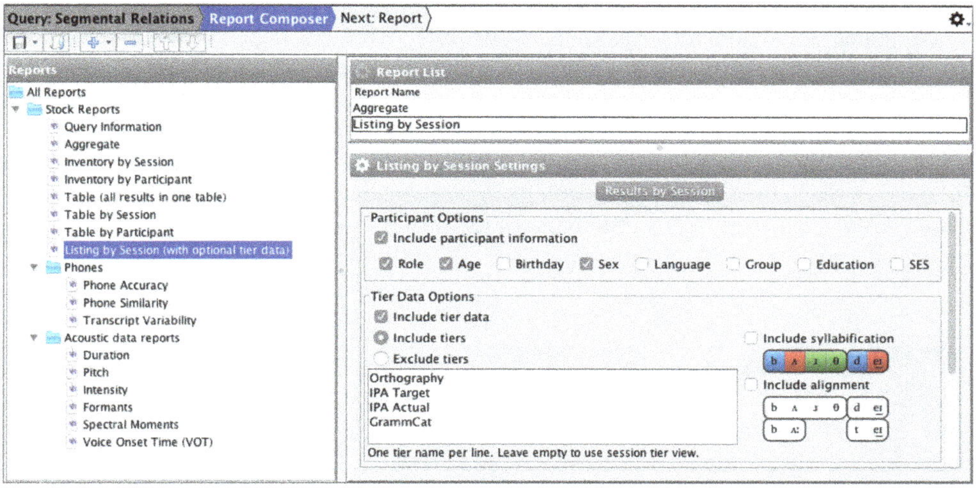

Figure 19.11   Report Composer.

Built-in analyses of transcript data

As mentioned above, the clinical user may be interested in particular types of measures of the session transcript data, many of which involve rather cumbersome, time-consuming computations if they are performed manually. To address this need, we built custom-purpose analyses directly into Phon, for example to obtain word and phone inventories (including their frequency counts) or extract general measures such as the PCC (Percentage of Consonants Correct; Shriberg, Austin, Lewis, McSweeny, & Wilson, 1997; Shriberg & Kwiatkowski, 1982) and the PMLU (Phonological Mean Length of Utterance; Arias & Lleó, 2013; Ingram, 2002). We also designed built-in analyses to detect commonly observed phonological processes such as velar fronting, fricative stopping, or consonant deletion. Finally, Phon offers implementations of more specialized analyses such as those developed by Mason (2015) and Masso (2016) for the analysis of multisyllabic word productions.

The key difference between the query and reporting methods described in the preceding section and built-in analyses discussed here is that the latter offer a more restricted set of predefined options, and are linked to preformatted reports, making the overall process of analysis maximally straightforward. Running a built-in analysis follows the logic illustrated in Figure 19.12, as Phon guides the user through the steps ordered on top of the interface.

As with query and reporting, the user can then save the reports as standalone HTML files or export them in text-only (CSV) and Excel formats.

In addition to queries, reports and built-in analyses, Phon incorporates functions for acoustic analysis from Praat (Boersma & Weenink, 2020), another open-source program for research in phonetics and phonology. In the next section, we describe how to obtain acoustic data measurements with Phon; this discussion assumes an understanding of speech acoustics and of how Praat works using TextGrids toward batch analyses of speech data.[7]

Acoustic analysis

To perform acoustic analyses, the user must go through a few more steps in data preparation. The relevant functions supporting this work in Phon are combined within the Speech Analysis view panel. After all the transcriptions and annotations are completed, as described above, the first additional step is to generate TextGrids from the data records, using the Praat menu located in the toolbar at the top of the Speech Analysis panel. After the TextGrids are generated, the user must align the TextGrid boundaries relevant to the phones to be measured. Starting with the "Open TextGrid in Praat" function located in the same Praat menu, the user opens the relevant portion of the media and associated TextGrid in Praat, and then adjusts the TextGrid alignments of the relevant phones. After these alignments are completed, the user updates the Phon data through the "Send back to calling program" function available from the File menu of Praat.[8] After completion of this task for all of the relevant records, everything is now in place for acoustic analysis.

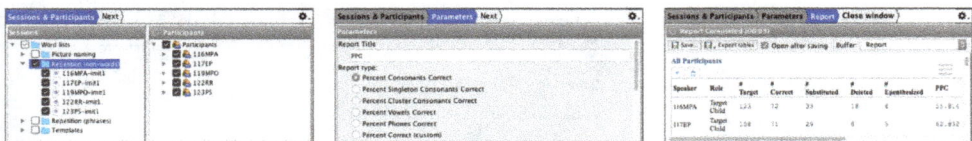

Figure 19.12 Example analysis: PPC. (a) Participant selection (b) Analysis selection (c) Analysis results.

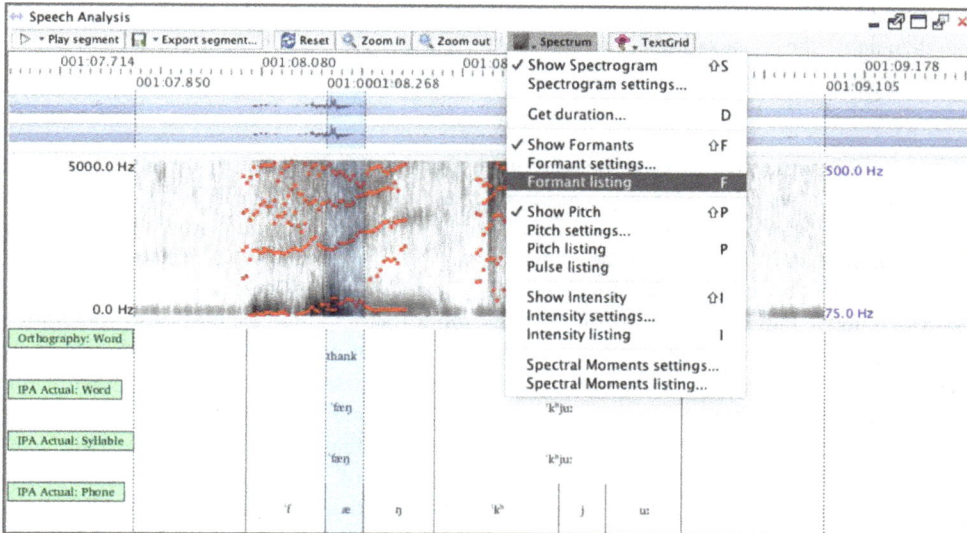

Figure 19.13 Speech Analysis.

To obtain individual measurements, the user can browse to the relevant record, select the relevant TextGrid interval to be measured from the Speech Analysis panel, and call up the required measurement from the Spectrum menu in the toolbar, as illustrated in Figure 19.13.

For batch analyses of multiple tokens within a session transcript, corpus, or project, the user first performs a Phones query, to identify the individual phones or phone classes to be measured acoustically. The phones returned by the query are then measured acoustically, based on the acoustic data reports set by the user within the Report Composer, which also incorporate all of the parameters for acoustic analysis supported by Praat.

Similar to the reports obtained from queries and analyses described above, acoustic measurements obtained through this method can be visualized in report previews within Phon or saved as part of HTML, CSV and Excel report formats.

Saving and combining queries, reports and built-in analyses

Returning to the topic of open science, recall that data and research methods are only truly useful to the extent that they can be reused as part of further analyses and/or shared transparently between different users. Addressing this need, Phon offers functions to save and later access user-specified queries, reports and analyses. Each of these analytic resources can then be used repeatedly (as needed) and also shared with colleagues or students.

When these resources are saved within a Phon project or the user's Phon library, they also become potential ingredients for the Analysis Composer, an advanced function to build analytic routines that combine different queries, reports and built-in analyses which can then be run at once. For example, the user can compose a custom analysis to extract transcript data relative to the production of the vowel [i] in stressed syllables, acoustically measure the duration and formant structure of these vowels, and interpret these results in light of general data on lexical or phonological productivity (e.g. the Percentage of Vowels Correct measure, one of the options in Figure 19.12b). In line with the system for data analysis described above, each custom analysis composed by the user can be saved internally for later uses and shared with other people, who can then apply the exact same set of analyses to their own datasets.

Conclusion

Through this chapter, we covered the essential aspects of PhonBank and of the Phon software program, which we situated within the larger context of CHILDES and TalkBank. Through practical descriptions of the main workflows supported by Phon, we also covered essential aspects of data transcription, annotation and formatting, the logic of which can be generalized to any study of phonological development and speech disorders. While some of the resources described above can be at times difficult to use on a routine basis, especially within clinical settings, primarily because of time constraints, they are central to much current research. These free and open resources are indeed supporting students and researchers worldwide, all of whom are working toward a better understanding of phonological development and speech disorders.

It is in this context that we want to emphasize once more that none of the resources discussed in this chapter would exist without the active participation of researchers and students in open science, most concretely through the sharing of their corpus data through PhonBank, CHILDES, or other TalkBank databases more generally. In light of this, we invite everyone engaging in corpus building to embrace this communal effort through their own work, present and future.

Notes

* The early development of Phon has benefited from funding from the Social Sciences and Humanities Research Council of Canada between 2004 and 2007 (grant #410-2004-1836) as well as from a 2006 Petro-Canada Young Innovator Award. The PhonBank Project has received funding from the National Institutes of Health since 2006 (R01 HD051698, R01 HD051698-06A1, R01 HD051698-11). We are grateful to all students, researchers and clinicians who are supporting PhonBank through data sharing, and indebted to every person and organization who has contributed resources and feedback toward the development of Phon.
1 Moving, hiding or closing view panels has no impact whatsoever on the contents of the session transcript.
2 All of the IPA dictionaries and transliteration systems built into Phon represent additional examples of open science.
3 Phon also offers methods to import pre-transcribed lists from CSV (comma-separated value) files, as documented within the Phon online manual (accessible through the Help menu of the application).
4 Within the Project Manager, the user can simply click on the template file and drag it to the relevant corpus folder, where Phon will generate a copy of this file, which can then be renamed as needed.
5 While the 2,000 ms suggested here is generally useful for word elicitation in languages like English, this limit may be adjusted based on the user's particular needs; for example, a larger window is likely to be needed for utterance (e.g. phrase or sentence) elicitation.
6 Participant selection is not included in this screenshot but is available in all query forms.
7 The skeptical reader might wonder why we are not sending the user directly to Praat. Our short answer is that this move would take the user away from all of the functions for database management, transcription and annotation that Phon provides (see Hernandez & Rose, to appear, for a more detailed discussion).
8 The user can also open and edit the TextGrids generated by Phon directly in Praat. By default, Phon saves TextGrid files alongside their corresponding audio files within the relevant media folder.

References

Arias, J., & Lleó, C. (2013). Rethinking assessment measures of phonological development and their application in bilingual acquisition. *Clinical Linguistics & Phonetics*, *28*(3), 153–175. https://doi.org/10.3109/02699206.2013.840681

Baker, E., & Williams, A.L. (2010). Complexity approaches to intervention. In A.L. Williams, S. McLeod, & R.J. McCauley (Eds.), *Intervention for speech sound disorders in children* (pp. 95–115). Baltimore, MD: Brookes Publishing.

Bernhardt, B.M., Stemberger, J.P., Ayyad, H., Ullrich, A., & Zhao, J. (2010). Nonlinear phonology: Clinical applications for Kuwaiti Arabic, German and Mandarin. In J.A. Guendouzi (Ed.), *Handbook of psycholinguistics and cognitive processing: Perspectives in communication disorders*. London, UK: Taylor and Francis.

Boersma, P., & Weenink, D. (2020). Praat: Doing phonetics by computer (Version 6.1.09). Retrieved from http://www.praat.org/

Coady, J.A., & Evans, J.L. (2008). Uses and interpretations of non-word repetition tasks in children with and without specific language impairments (SLI). *International Journal of Language & Communication Disorders, 43*(1), 1–40. https://doi.org/10.1080/13682820601116485

Ewen, C.J., Hume, E., Oostendorp, M. van, & Rice, K. (Eds.). (2011). *The Blackwell companion to phonology*. Malden, MA: Wiley-Blackwell.

Fikkert, P. (1994). *On the acquisition of prosodic structure*. The Hague: Holland Academic Graphics.

Goldsmith, J.A. (1996). *The handbook of phonological theory*. Cambridge, MA: Blackwell.

Hedlund, G.J., & O'Brien, P. (2004). *A software system for linguistic data capture and analysis*. B.Sc. Honours Thesis, Memorial University of Newfoundland.

Hedlund, G.J., & Rose, Y. (2020). *Phon 3* [Computer program]. Retrieved from https://www.phon.ca

Hernandez, A., & Rose, Y. (to appear). Introducing Phon to the sociophonetics community. In K. Martin (Ed.), *Proceedings of the 2019 Conference of the Canadian Linguistic Association | Actes du Congrès 2019 de l'Association canadienne de linguistique*. Retrieved from http://cla-acl.ca/congres-annuel-annual-conference-3/

Ingram, D. (1981). *Procedures for the phonological analysis of children's language*. Baltimore, MD: University Park Press.

Ingram, D. (2002). The measurement of whole-word productions. *Journal of Child Language, 29*(4), 713–733.

Levelt, C.C. (1994). *On the acquisition of place*. The Hague: Holland Academic Graphics.

MacWhinney, B. (2000). *The CHILDES project: Tools for analyzing talk* (3rd ed.). Mahwah, NJ: Lawrence Erlbaum.

MacWhinney, B. (2016). *The TalkBank Project: Tools for Analyzing Talk – Electronic Edition. Part 1: The CHAT Transcription Format*. Retrieved from https://talkbank.org/manuals/CHAT.pdf

MacWhinney, B., Fromm, D., Rose, Y., & Bernstein Ratner, N. (2018). Fostering human rights through Talkbank. *International Journal of Speech-Language Pathology, 20*, 115–119. https://doi.org/10.1080/17549507.2018.1392609

MacWhinney, B., & Snow, C.E. (1985). The child language data exchange system. *Journal of Child Language, 12*, 271–295.

MacWhinney, B., Spektor, L., Chen, F., & Rose, Y. (2012). Best practices for speech corpora in linguistic research. In *Proceedings of Best Practices for Speech Corpora in Linguistic Research, 8th International Conference on Language Resources and Evaluation (LREC)* (pp. 57–60).

Másdóttir, Þ. (2019). Hljóðþróun íslenskra barna á aldrinum tveggja til átta ára. *Netla*. https://doi.org/10.24270/netla.2019.11

Mason, G.K. (2015). *Multisyllabic word production of school aged children with and without protracted phonological development*. Ph.D. dissertation, University of British Columbia.

Masso, S. (2016). *Polysyllable maturity of preschool children with speech sound disorders*. Ph.D. dissertation, Charles Sturt University.

Mayer, M. (1969). *Frog, where are you?* New York, NY: Dial Books for Young Readers.

McAllister Byun, T., & Rose, Y. (2016). Analyzing clinical phonological data using Phon. *Seminars in Speech and Language, 37*(2), 85–105.

McLeod, S. (Ed.). (2007). *The international guide to speech acquisition*. Clifton Park, NY: Thomson Delmar Learning.

Mcleod, S., & Baker, E. (2014). Speech-language pathologists' practices regarding assessment, analysis, target selection, intervention, and service delivery for children with speech sound disorders. *Clinical Linguistics & Phonetics, 28*(7–8), 508–531.

Rose, Y., & Inkelas, S. (2011). The interpretation of phonological patterns in first language acquisition. In C.J. Ewen, E. Hume, M. van Oostendorp, & K. Rice (Eds.), *The Blackwell Companion to Phonology* (pp. 2414–2438). Malden, MA: Wiley-Blackwell.

Rose, Y., & MacWhinney, B. (2014). The PhonBank Project: Data and software-assisted methods for the study of phonology and phonological development. In J. Durand, U. Gut, & G. Kristoffersen (Eds.), *The Oxford handbook of corpus phonology* (pp. 380–401). Oxford, UK: Oxford University Press.

Rose, Y., MacWhinney, B., Byrne, R., Hedlund, G.J., Maddocks, K., O'Brien, P., & Wareham, T. (2006). Introducing Phon: A software solution for the study of phonological acquisition. In D. Bamman, T. Magnitskaia, & C. Zaller (Eds.), *Proceedings of the 30th Annual Boston University Conference on Language Development* (pp. 489–500). Somerville, MA: Cascadilla Press.

Shriberg, L.D., Austin, D., Lewis, B.A., McSweeny, J.L., & Wilson, D.L. (1997). The percentage of consonants correct (PCC) metric: Extensions and reliability data. *Journal of Speech, Language, and Hearing Research, 40*(4), 708–722.

Shriberg, L.D., & Kwiatkowski, J. (1982). Phonological disorders III: A procedure for assessing severity of involvement. *The Journal of Speech and Hearing Disorders, 47*(3), 256–270.

Skahan, S.M., Watson, M., & Lof, G.L. (2007). Speech-language pathologists' assessment practices for children with suspected speech sound disorders: Results of a national survey. *American Journal of Speech – Language Pathology, 16*(3), 246–259.

Smit, A.B. (1993). Phonologic error distribution in the Iowa-Nebraska articulation norms project: Consonant singletons. *Journal of Speech and Hearing Research, 36*(3), 533–547.

Instrumental analysis of articulatory phonetics

20

ELECTROMYOGRAPHY

Jennifer M. Vojtech and Cara E. Stepp

Introduction to Electromyography

Historical background

The electrical properties of living organisms have been of interest to humans across time. The earliest records of bioelectricity date back to c. 2750 BC when ancient Egyptians depicted electric fish on tomb walls (Kellaway, 1946). Ancient Greeks also knew of the bioelectric properties of some eels, rays and catfish, and even described using these properties to induce numbness in the body (Finger, Boller, & Tyler, 2009). Emil du Bois-Reymond (1848) was the first to demonstrate that the electrical activity of human muscle could be detected during a voluntary contraction. The first recording of this activity was produced by French scientist, Étienne Marey, in 1890. Marey later coined the term *electromyography* or EMG.

Early EMG studies were conducted to examine the activity of muscles related to speech production, such as the intrinsic and extrinsic laryngeal muscles (Faaborg-Andersen, 1957; Faaborg-Andersen, & Buchthal, 1956; Moulonget, 1955) and respiratory muscles (Campbell, 1955; Draper, Ladefoged & Whitteridge, 1959; Jones, Beargie, & Pauley, 1953; Stetson, 1951). Researchers began to investigate the relationship between specific muscle groups and speech sounds, including that of the larynx (Faaborg-Andersen, Edfeldt, & Nykøbing, 1958; Hiroto, Hirano, Toyozumi, & Shin, 1967), pharynx (Minifie, Abbs, Tarlow, & Kwaterski, 1974), and various orofacial and mandibular (Alfonso & Baer, 1982); Sussman, MacNeilage, & Hanson, 1973; Sussman, MacNeilage, & Powers, 1977; Tuller, Kelso, & Harris, 1982) and respiratory (Eblen, 1963) muscles. The role of individual speech articulators such as the lips (Gay, Ushijima, Hiroset, & Cooper, 1974; Öhman, 1967; Sussman, MacNeilage, & Hanson, 1973) and tongue (MacNeilage & Sholes, 1964; Smith, & Hirano, 1968) have also been investigated. The physiological theory, recording techniques and analysis methods of EMG research in the field of speech disorders is discussed in detail below.

Physiological theory of electromyography

During a muscle contraction, movement information is carried from the motor cortex in the brain to the brainstem or spinal cord by the work of upper motor neurons. These upper motor neurons form connections with a class of lower motor neurons called alpha motor neurons (α-MNs) to then transfer movement-related impulses to standard skeletal muscle fibers. Upon entering a skeletal muscle, the axons of the α-MN branch out, with each axon terminal making synaptic contact with a single muscle fiber; nerve impulses generated from the α-MN cause the muscle fiber to contract. The term for an α-MN and all the muscle fibers that it innervates is called a motor unit (MU; Liddell and Sherrington, 1925).

The MU is considered the basic functional unit of skeletal muscle. The range, force and type of voluntary contraction is related to the number of MUs recruited, as well as their pattern and frequency of firing (Moritani, Stegeman, & Merletti, 2004). It has been well documented that the force of a muscle contraction increases with a greater number and higher firing rate of MUs. Additionally, movement precision is related to the number of muscle fibers present in a MU, wherein a lower ratio of muscle fibers to motor neuron leads to finer motor control. For instance, the intrinsic laryngeal muscles are estimated to contain anywhere from 3–21 muscle fibers per motor unit (Rüedi, 1959; Santo Neto & Marques, 2008), with a combined MU size of 30 for all intrinsic laryngeal muscles (English & Blevins, 1969). The gastrocnemius muscle of the leg, on the other hand, is estimated to have around 1,300 muscle fibers per MU (Feinstein, Lindegard, Nyman, & Wohlfart, 1955). The intrinsic laryngeal muscles perform the rapid, precise movements necessary to regulate voice production (i.e. to enable vocal fold vibration) and respiration, whereas the gastrocnemius generates comparably slower, stronger forces needed for changes in body position (Purves, Augustine, Fitzpatrick, Hall, LaMantia, McNamara, & Williams, 2001).

When the α-MN is activated, an action potential travels through the neuron toward the nerve endings. An insulating layer comprised of myelin sheaths allow this electrical signal to travel quickly down the axon via salutatory conduction until it reaches the axon terminals. The site where the axon terminal meets the muscle fiber is called the neuromuscular junction; this is where the electrical signal may be transferred from the α-MN to the muscle fibers of the MU. The axon terminal, or synaptic bulb, releases a neurotransmitter called acetylcholine to transverse the space between the α-MN and muscle fiber. In this way, the electrical signal that passed through the neuron has been converted into a chemical signal. Upon reaching the muscle fiber, acetylcholine binds to acetylcholine receptors on the motor end plate of the muscle fiber. The influx of acetylcholine depolarizes the membrane, and, if the amplitude of depolarization is sufficient, triggers a muscle action potential. The chemical signal is thus converted back into an electrical signal that may travel along the muscle fibers of the MU. Because all the muscle fibers of the MU are activated simultaneously, the muscle action potentials are collectively termed "motor unit action potential (MUAP)." The MUAP propagates away from the motor end plate and along the innervated muscle fibers toward the fiber terminals by depolarizing muscle fiber membranes as an amplified version of α-MN activity. The depolarization of the muscle fiber stimulates the release of calcium ions from inside the muscle fiber to initiate contraction.

The detection and recording of the MUAPs at some distance is referred to as electromyography (EMG). It is important to note that there is an inherent delay of approximately 30–100 ms between the onset of electrical activation detected via EMG and measurable muscle force (Cavanagh & Komi, 1979). Because of this delay, it is possible for myoelectric activity to return to baseline before any changes in muscle force can be measured. An example of electromechanical delay is shown in Figure 20.1, wherein electromyographic activity of the anterior neck muscles are detected leading up to the production of the nonsense word /ifi/. The majority of EMG activity is captured prior to the start of audible speech.

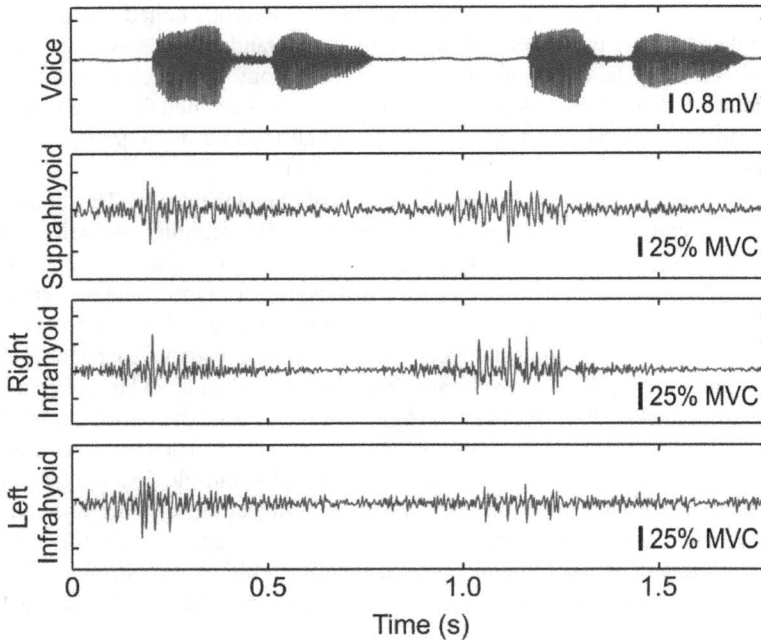

Figure 20.1 Example of acoustic signal and anterior neck myoactivity during the production of the nonsense word/ifi/. The raw acoustic signal (top panel) was captured via a headset microphone sampled at 30 kHz, whereas electromyographic signals of the suprahyoid and infrahyoid muscles (lower three panels) were captured at 2 kHz and normalized to speaker maximum voluntary contraction (MVC).

Electromyographic recording techniques

Electrode types

The myoelectric signal representing MUAP activity is detected using electrodes. There are two main types of EMG electrodes used in speech research: surface (skin) electrodes and intramuscular (wire, needle) electrodes. As their names imply, surface electrodes are placed on the surface of the skin, whereas intramuscular electrodes are inserted inside the muscle tissue. Choosing the appropriate electrode type and configuration depends on the nature of the desired information, as each type of electrode has advantages and limitations.

Surface electrodes

Surface electrodes provide a noninvasive means of capturing aggregated MU activity from muscles underlying the electrodes. Surface EMG (sEMG) leverages the chemical equilibrium between the surface of the skin and the detecting surface via electrolyte conduction (i.e. skin/electrolyte and electrolyte/electrode interfaces); in this way, current is able to flow from the body into the electrode as a representation of myoelectric activity. The electrodes used in sEMG are either passive or active.

Passive electrodes use conductive materials such as silver or silver-silver chloride to sense electrical current on the skin via the electrode-skin interface. These electrodes are often called "wet" electrodes because they require an electrolytic gel or paste act as a conductor between the skin and the electrode. Passive electrodes leverage a reversible chloride exchange interface between the electrode and the skin to reduce motion artifacts from skin potentials. Criticism of passive electrodes includes uncomfortable and/or irritating skin preparation (e.g. hair removal, skin abrasion, gel application), and a high sensitivity to perspiration and mechanical perturbations (Basmajian & De Luca, 1985; Roy, De Luca, Cheng, Johansson, Gilmore, & De Luca, 2007).

Active electrodes detect electrical current on the skin using signal amplification circuitry near the electrode-skin interface. Compared to their passive counterparts, active electrodes do not require conductive gel or paste to adhere to the skin; for this reason, active electrodes are often referred to as "dry" or "pasteless" electrodes. Although active electrodes provide online signal amplification and filtering, these electrodes often still require some degree of skin preparation (e.g. hair removal, skin abrasion) to reduce the skin-electrode impedance. Nevertheless, active electrodes remain preferable to passive counterparts due to higher signal fidelity and convenience of use.

Intramuscular electrodes

Intramuscular electrodes are inserted directly into the muscle of interest to detect MU activity. There are two types of intramuscular electrodes: needle and fine wire. Concentric needle electrodes are the most common type of needle electrode used in speech and swallowing research (e.g. see Ertekin & Aydogdu, 2003). In its most basic form, the concentric needle detects myoelectric activity as the differential between the tip of the center wire (at the tip of the needle) and the outer, uninsulated cannula. Hooked-wire electrodes are a lighter, flexible alternative to the needle electrode. These electrodes comprise two separate, insulated fine-wires that pass through a hypodermic needle. After the needle is inserted into the muscle, it is withdrawn. Hooks on the end of the fine-wires act as a barb to keep the wires inserted within the muscle. Myoelectric activity is detected between the two wires that remain in the muscle.

Hooked-wire electrodes are typically recommended over needle electrodes in speech research (Hirano & Ohala, 1969). The size and weight of the needle electrodes may increase patient pain and discomfort, while needle rigidity has been observed to increase the likelihood of electrode dislodgment and movement artifacts when producing speech behaviors (Gay & Harris, 1971). Despite observed improvements in patient comfort, however, Jaffe, Solomon, Robinson, Hoffman, and Luschei (1998) demonstrated that EMG waveform morphology, inflammatory response and hematoma formation do not significantly differ when using hooked-wire versus concentric needle electrodes.

Contrasting surface and intramuscular electrodes

Surface electrodes are a simple and noninvasive method of detecting the myoelectric signal. Because surface electrodes must be positioned on the surface of the skin, their use is limited to superficial muscles. Surface electrodes are also much larger than intramuscular electrodes, such that they cannot be used to acquire signals selectively from small muscles due to concerns of crosstalk from neighboring sources (Fuglevand, Winter, Patla, & Stashuk, 1992). The smaller detection volume available with intramuscular electrodes is more suitable for detecting myoelectric activity from small muscles; however, the small detection volume also lends itself to difficulties repositioning the electrode to detect the same MUs.

Electrode configurations

The segment of the electrode that contacts the recording site is referred to as the detection surface. The signal captured at the detection surface is typically collected relative to a reference signal, or ground, in order to minimize the amount of bioelectrical noise that can otherwise contaminate the desired signal. There are a wide variety of electrode configurations for use in recording myoelectric activity, each with its own advantages and limitations.

Monopolar electrode configurations rely on one detection surface to capture the myoelectric signal. This electrode configuration allows for a large detection volume, as one electrode is placed on the desired recording site and another electrode is placed away from the recording site to act as a ground. The signal between the electrodes is then amplified and recorded. The large detection volume is advantageous when aiming to provide a more global view of muscle activation, as a greater number of MUs can be detected with larger detection volumes. However, this configuration can suffer from poor spatial resolution due to the large detection volume sampling from fibers of neighboring muscles (i.e. crosstalk; De Luca, 2006; Gerdle, Karlsson, Day, & Djupsjöbacka, 1999).

As an alternative, differential electrode configurations rely on multiple detection surfaces to capture myoelectricity. In a differential configuration, electrodes are placed parallel to underlying muscle fibers to detect MUAPs as they propagate down the fiber. These configurations use linear combinations of different electrodes to amplify the difference between the electrodes when placed over the muscle of interest. Differential electrodes operate on the principle of common-mode rejection to eliminate bioelectrical noise that is common to the electrodes. This type of configuration is more spatially sensitive, as each electrode needs to be properly configured according to the direction of the muscle fibers to help isolate the electrical activity of interest. Electrode size and interelectrode distance should be taken into consideration when using differential electrodes, as electrode size determines the number of active MUs that can be detected and interelectrode distance determines the bandwidth of the electrode configuration. A larger interelectrode distance leads to a higher signal amplitude (i.e. from sampling a larger surface area), the resultant signal will be less spatially specific (Fuglevand, Winter, Patla, & Stashuk, 1992; Roeleveld, Stegeman, Vingerhoets, & Van Oosterom, 1997).

Electrode placement

Surface electrodes

In an effort to standardize sEMG methodology, the Surface Electromyography for the Noninvasive Assessment of Muscles (SENIAM) project set forth guidelines for electrode type, configuration, and placement. Yet there may be difficulties following SENIAM recommendations to detect myoelectric activity from speech musculature because the muscles of the face and neck are small, interdigitating and overlapping. Caution should be exercised when applying these recommendations to speech musculature.

The position and orientation of surface electrodes play a crucial role in detecting myoelectric activity from the muscle of interest. The size and shape of the electrode characterize the detection surface from which active MU activity may be collected, and—as mentioned previously—the interelectrode distance determines the bandwidth of the electrode configuration. SENIAM recommends a maximum electrode size of 10 mm and maximum interelectrode distance of either 20 mm or 25% of the length of the muscle fiber (whichever is smaller; Hermens, Biomedical, C.o.t.E.C., & Programme, 1999).

Prior to placing a surface electrode, the skin must be properly prepared to obtain a good quality EMG signal. This requires reducing the skin-electrode impedance by removing hair, dead cells and oils from the surface of the skin. SENIAM recommends the intended sensor site be shaved if it is covered with hair, then cleaned with alcohol to remove any moisture on the skin (Hermens, Biomedical, C.o.t.E.C., & Programme, 1999). Rubbing a medical abrasive paste on the skin has been shown to reduce the skin-electrode impedance by nearly 90% (Merletti & Hermens, 2004), but is often considered messy and uncomfortable. Instead, combining shaving and alcohol skin preparation steps with skin "peeling" using hypoallergenic tape has been adopted as a more tolerable alternative, effectively reducing the skin-electrode impedance from 40% (shaving + alcohol) to 70% (shaving + alcohol + skin peel; Merletti, & Hermens, 2004). The skin peeling technique involves repeated placement and removal of the hypoallergenic tape to peel off the layer of dead cells on the surface of the skin.

After preparing the skin, the surface electrode should be placed parallel to the orientation of the muscle fibers to maximize the measured conduction velocity of MUAPs, and thus, the amplitude and frequency content of the detected signal (De Luca, 1997). Care should be exercised to avoid excessive skin, fatty tissue and bony obstructions that could reduce the amplitude and frequency content of the signal. The shape and size of the muscle should be regarded to minimize crosstalk from neighboring muscles, and the electrode should not be placed over the edge of the muscle or over a myotendinous junction (tendinous insertion of the muscle). Past work from De Luca (2002) recommends placement over the muscle belly since target muscle fiber density is the highest at this location. The ground electrode should be placed at a nearby yet distinct location, such as the spinous process of the C7, acromion process, glabella (forehead), nose, or earlobe (Stepp, 2012). In cases where monopolar electrodes are used, avoid placing the ground electrode below the head to minimize contamination from cardiac activity (Willigenburg, Daffertshofer, Kingma, & van Dieën, 2012).

Figure 20.2 shows an example of electrode placements over the neck musculature that may be used to capture sEMG from speech and swallowing anatomy. Surface recordings of the submental surface via single differential electrodes may detect activations of the anterior belly of the digastric and mylohyoid during gestures such as lowering the jaw under resistance and swallowing, respectively (O'Dwyer, Quinn, Guitar, Andrews, & Neilson, 1981). Infrahyoid muscle activity may be captured using single or double differential

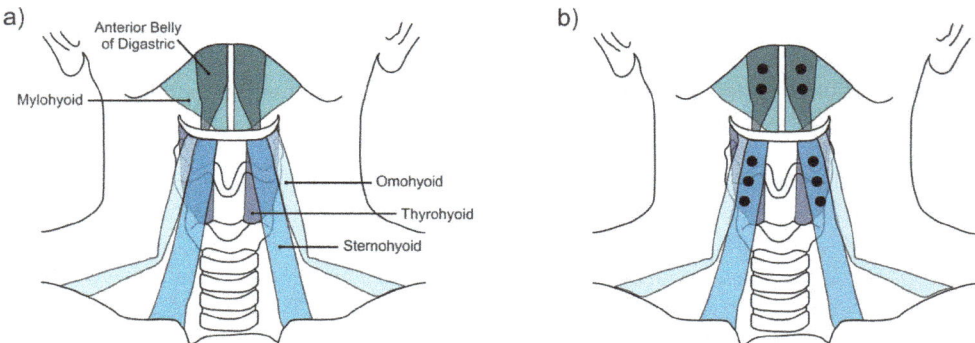

Figure 20.2 Diagram of anterior neck muscles illustrating (a) suprahyoid (green) and infrahyoid (blue) muscles that may contribute to surface recordings, and (b) suggested sensor placements, with electrodes placed parallel to the longitudinal axis of the muscle body (in line with the fibers of the muscle).

electrodes; the choice of double differential electrodes (as illustrated in Figure 20.2b) are recommended to reduce conduction volume by minimizing crosstalk from surface musculature common to all electrode contacts (Rutkove, 2007).

Depending on sensor placements, single or double differential electrodes may detect activations primarily of the sternohyoid and omohyoid. Although the thyrohyoid is within the same region as these muscles, it is unlikely that the thyrohyoid substantially contributes to surface recordings due to its depth relative to the sternohyoid (Stepp, 2012). When positioning electrodes over the anterior neck muscles, it must be noted that the resulting signal may be contaminated by activity of the platysma, a thin, superficial sheet of muscle thought to activate during swallow (Palmer, Luschei, Jaffe, & McCulloch, 1999) as well as act as an antagonist to the orbicularis oris inferior muscle during speech (McClean & Sapir, 1980).

Intramuscular electrodes

Intramuscular electrodes are a popular choice for performing laryngeal EMG. This is because the relatively deep location of the intrinsic laryngeal muscles is unlikely to contribute to the detected signal when using surface electrodes. As with surface electrodes, the skin must first be prepared prior to inserting the electrode. Local anesthetics may be used to reduce patient discomfort during needle insertion. Investigators must use anatomical landmarks as a reference for needle insertion (see Heman-Ackah, Mandel, Manon-Espaillat, Abaza, & Sataloff, 2007; O'Dwyer, Quinn, Guitar, Andrews, & Neilson, 1981). Surface electrodes may be used as reference electrodes when applicable. During intramuscular electrode insertion, electrode placement may be validated by examining EMG signal activity during specific participant gestures (e.g. phonating the sound /i/, swallowing, smiling).

Electromyographic signal acquisition

Signal conditioning

Since the myoelectric signal is relatively weak, proper EMG equipment should be used to condition and amplify the signal prior to acquisition. These steps may involve a pre-amplification module, as well as hardware or software filters, additional amplification steps, and analog-to-digital (A/D) conversion.

The myoelectric signal is highly influenced by noise (e.g. electromagnetic radiation from power line interference or fluorescent lights). Differential amplification is one method of noise reduction. This technique amplifies the difference in potential between two electrodes and amplifies the difference. In addition to applying differential amplification to reduce noise, the EMG signal should be filtered to measure the effective bandwidth of the EMG signal. The International Society of Electrophysiology and Kinesiology reports that the majority of the power of the EMG signal is between 5 and 450 Hz for sEMG and between 5 and 1500 Hz for intramuscular EMG. Movement artifacts may create signals in the range of 0–20 Hz, and as such, should be minimized by use of a high-pass filter with a cut-off frequency between 10 and 20 Hz (De Luca, Gilmore, Kuznetsov, & Roy, 2010). Filtering may be applied using hardware (prior to digitization) or software (post-digitization). Hardware filtering is preferred to avoid aliasing (i.e. when the analog signal is undersampled). From here, the analog EMG signal should be digitized via A/D conversion for visualization and analysis purposes.

Visualization

When sampled from multiple MUs, the detected EMG signal is the result of the asynchronous summation of MUAPs. As such, the EMG signal may be referred to as an interference pattern or recruitment pattern. MUs are visualized as spikes that vary in amplitude, duration, phase, rise time and firing rate according to the number of muscle fibers within a MU and their degree of synchronicity. This activity may be assessed by examining signal amplitude and frequency.

The amplitude of the EMG signal is related to the degree of muscle activation and force, but is affected by factors such as muscle length and fatigue. The raw EMG signal is useful to determine the activation timing of a muscle but should not be used to generalize the degree of muscle activation or estimate the force produced by a muscle. This is because peak amplitudes from the raw signal are not necessarily representative of overall activity. Instead, the root-mean-square or average rectified value should be used to more reliably represent this activity.

The frequency of the EMG signal is related to individual characteristics of the MUAPs (e.g. size) and their distance from the recording electrode. Frequency information can be extracted to monitor muscle fatigue rates and assess levels of muscle recruitment (e.g. Boucher, Ahmarani, & Ayad, 2006; Koutsos, & Georgiou, 2014; Walker, Davis, Avela, & Häkkinen, 2012). Muscle fatigue occurs as lactic acid builds up in the muscle from continuous activation. Accumulated lactic acid reduces the pH of extracellular fluid, thereby increasing action potential duration. This, in turn, leads to a decline in conduction velocity and an overall larger spread of contraction potentials in time. Mean and median frequency can capture this change in conduction velocity by decreasing as MUAP asynchronicity increases. The degree of muscle recruitment, on the other hand, is modulated by the number of MUAPs of active MUs. Higher levels of recruitment can be assessed using mean and median frequency, as MUAP pulse trains tend to fire at higher frequencies.

Electromyographic analysis of speech disorders

EMG is used to evaluate neuromuscular health for the assessment and rehabilitation of speech and language disorders. The use of sEMG to study voice, speech and swallowing is becoming increasingly popular due to its less invasive and simple-to-use nature. However, intramuscular EMG is still regarded as an important technique for assessing oropharyngeal and laryngeal function via providing spatially sensitive and precise timings of myoelectric activity. The use of these techniques in the assessment and treatment of speech disorders is discussed in detail below.

Disorders of the voice

Laryngeal dystonia

Laryngeal dystonia, previously called "spasmodic dysphonia," is a neurological voice disorder that affects the muscles of the vocal folds. It is a task-specific focal dystonia that causes irregular and uncontrollable vocal fold movements (spasms) that interfere with voice production. There are two main types of laryngeal dystonia: adductor laryngeal dystonia (AdLD) and abductor laryngeal dystonia (AbLD). AdLD is described by spasms that force the vocal folds to involuntarily stiffen and close, making it difficult to vibrate for voice

production. AbLD is characterized by spasms that force the vocal folds open, which ceases vocal fold vibration during voice production. Rarely, individuals can exhibit symptoms of both AbLD and AdLD; such cases are appropriately referred to as mixed laryngeal dystonia (MLD).

LEMG offers a useful application in cases of laryngeal dystonia for guiding botulinum toxin (Botox) injections into targeted musculature and assessing the myoelectric activity of the muscles that are affected by this disorder. Prior to injecting the Botox, confirmation of needle localization is done by observing EMG activity during a sustained phonation of "eee" for AdLD, and by sniffing for AbLD (Tisch, Brake, Law, Cole, & Darveniza, 2003). Upon successful injection, Botox blocks acetylcholine release from the neuromuscular junction to prevent the muscle from contracting.

In addition to guiding Botox injections, LEMG has also been used to assess the different laryngeal dystonia types. For instance, Rodriquez, Ford, Bless, and Harmon (1994) showed that LEMG differentiate muscle activity of the thyroarytenoid and cricothyroid muscles between AdLD and AbLD, but could not distinguish MLD from AbLD or AbLD. The authors further used LEMG to characterize this muscle activity: AbLD was described predominantly by spasms in the cricothyroid, whereas AdLD was found to result in spasms in both the thyroarytenoid and cricothyroid muscles.

Vocal hyperfunction

Vocal hyperfunction is a common accompaniment of voice disorders (Roy, 2003). It is defined as "conditions of abuse and/or misuse of the vocal mechanism due to excessive and/or "imbalanced" muscular forces" (Hillman, Holmberg, Perkell, Walsh, & Vaughan, 1989, p. 373) and is characterized as excessive laryngeal and/or paralaryngeal muscle tension associated with phonation. There has been no objective evidence to demonstrate increased tension of the intrinsic laryngeal system, as perturbing these muscles and structures via intramuscular EMG may alter typical muscle function. Yet it is known that tension in the extrinsic laryngeal musculature modifies the height and stability of the larynx, which, in turn, disturbs the cartilages of the larynx to alter intrinsic laryngeal muscle tension. As such, EMG is a useful tool that can serve as an indicator of laryngeal muscle tension.[1]

Surface EMG-based biofeedback has been used to treat vocal hyperfunction with the goal of assisting the patient in reducing excessive tension associated with phonation. Andrews, Warner, and Stewart (1986) examined the effectiveness of two voice treatments to relax the laryngeal musculature: progressive relaxation and sEMG biofeedback. For the participants assigned to the sEMG biofeedback group, a continuous visual stimulus was provided to demonstrate muscle activity. The authors had targeted the cricothyroid; however, the deep location of the muscle suggests that the biofeedback signal was likely composed of activations of the sternohyoid and possibly omohyoid (Loucks, Poletto, Saxon, & Ludlow, 2005). Regardless, the authors found that sEMG biofeedback significantly reduced laryngeal muscle tension and improved self-rated voice quality. In a similar study, Allen, Bernstein, and Chait (1991) provided visual sEMG biofeedback to a 9-year-old individual with vocal nodules. Surface electrodes were positioned over the thyrohyoid membrane to capture extrinsic laryngeal muscle activity. The child was instructed to attempt to reduce tension below an established threshold, which would lower when met during at least 80% of recorded trials for three consecutive sessions. The authors saw marked reductions in muscle tension and vocal nodules that were maintained at a 6-month follow-up.

Disorders of speech

Stuttering

Stuttering is a fluency disorder marked by interruptions in the smooth flow of speech. These interruptions can include repetitions, prolongations and blocks. Early studies into adults who stutter report increased muscle activity (e.g. Freeman & Ushijima, 1978; van Lieshout, Peters, Starkweather, & Hulstijn, 1993); however, additional conducted in adults who stutter found relatively equal or smaller EMG amplitudes in orofacial and laryngeal muscles during phonation (McClean, Goldsmith, & Cerf, 1984; McLean & Cooper, 1978; Smith, Denny, Shaffer, Kelly, & Hirano, 1996). It has also been shown that stuttering can also present with abnormal peaks (Denny & Smith, 1992; McClean, Goldsmith & Cerf, 1984) or tremor-like oscillations (Denny & Smith, 1992; Smith, 1989) or in orofacial EMG activity within the range of 5–15 Hz following a disfluency. Taken together, these studies describe the extreme heterogeneity in the muscle activation patterns that underlie stuttering. Self-reports of stuttering note that these disfluencies are often accompanied by the presence of physical tension (Bloodstein & Bernstein Ratner, 2008), which may be increased under various external stressors (e.g. speaking in front of a crowd).

EMG biofeedback has been explored as a treatment for stuttering in both adults and children. Employing EMG biofeedback to manage stuttering has showed relatively consistent results across different investigations. In particular, muscle activity has been shown to decrease in orofacial (Block, Onslow, Roberts, & White, 2004; Craig, Hancock, Chang, McCready, Shepley, McCaul, Costello, Harding, Kehren, Masel, & Reilly, 1996; Craig & Cleary, 1982; Guitar, 1975; Lanyon, 1977) and extrinsic laryngeal (Cross, 1977; Guitar, 1975; Hanna, Wilfling, & McNeill, 1975) muscles following the presentation of an auditory or visual feedback signal. Despite these promising results, investigations examining the effects of EMG biofeedback were conducted in small samples (<15 individuals). Thus, even though the use of EMG feedback has been shown to be an effective strategy in the treatment of stuttering, future investigations should be conducted in a larger group of individuals to comprehensively assess the effects of EMG feedback.

Apraxia of speech

Apraxia of speech (AOS) is a motor speech disorder relating to problems in motor planning and programming. AOS is characterized by understanding others but having difficulty in coordinating the muscle movements necessary to produce speech. Current AOS research involving EMG is limited and has largely set out to characterize the neuromuscular pathophysiology of the disorder rather than to apply biofeedback as treatment. Fromm, Abbs, McNeil, and Rosenbek (1982) examined lip, jaw and chin muscle activity in three apraxic and three normative speakers, ultimately finding substantially distinct coordination abilities between the two groups. The authors reported antagonistic co-contraction, tone, movement without producing voice, discoordination, additive movements and groping patterns that were not exhibited in normative speakers. This work confirmed the difficulties in distinguishing the underlying myoelectric physiopathology of AOS without controlling for those physiological variables (e.g. abnormal patterns may be perceived as normal because the speaker is compensating). Investigations into AOS vowel acoustics report slow and inaccurate articulator movements and long vowel durations (Caligiuri & Till, 1983; Collins, Rosenbek, & Wertz, 1983; Kent & Rosenbek, 1983; Seddoh, Robin, Sim, Hageman, Moon, & Folkins, 1996; Ziegler, 2002), which were speculated to be associated with reduced muscle activity. Yet upon directly examining timing patterns, Strauss and Klich (2001) demonstrated that the timing of lip muscle activity was relatively similar between normative and apraxic speakers. However, this study was limited to two normative speakers and two speakers with AOS, and as a result, these findings may not be generalizable. In a study on the viability of EMG biofeedback on AOS, McNeil, Prescott, and Lemme (1976) provided feedback from the frontalis as a treatment in four individuals with AOS. Participants were provided two types (auditory and visual) of feedback. The authors saw a decrease in frontalis muscle activity as compared to baseline conditions. These findings suggest that external muscle feedback could be beneficial in AOS; but, a comprehensive analysis in a large sample size is needed to confirm generalizability.

Dysarthria

Dysarthria is a motor speech disorder that affects the timing, strength and tonicity of the muscles involved in speech. The application of EMG biofeedback to dysarthric speech has been investigated since the late 1960s. Case studies involving dysarthric participants with unilateral facial paralysis (Booker, Rubow, & Coleman, 1969; Daniel & Guitar, 1978) demonstrated that visual and auditory feedback were effective mechanisms for relaying myoelectric activity between normal and paralyzed sides of the face. Similar case studies used EMG biofeedback to increase patient awareness of hypertonia in the lip (Netsell & Cleeland, 1973), mandible (Nemec & Cohen, 1984) and forehead (Rubow, Rosenbek, Collins, & Celesia, 1984). Participants retained this ability even after biofeedback was removed.

EMG has also been most extensively applied to investigate dysarthria in Parkinson's disease (PD), a neurodegenerative disease known for primary motor symptoms of body tremor and rigidity. Approximately 90% of individuals with PD develop hypokinetic dysarthria, characterized by imprecise articulation, reduced loudness and flat prosody (Moya-Galé & Levy, 2019). A study by Netsell, Daniel, and Celesia Gastone (1975) suggests that Parkinsonian dysarthria extends past the primary motor symptoms of tremor and rigidity, encompassing additional neuromuscular bases of impaired articulatory acceleration and weakness.

Levadopa is a popular drug treatment to manage PD; however, the effects of the drug on dysarthric symptoms have not been fully characterized. Gallena, Smith, Zeffiro, and Ludlow (2001) used LEMG to examine laryngeal movement control during speech in individuals with idiopathic PD. Increased laryngeal muscle activity was associated with impaired speech in the absence of medication. Similarly, Moore and Scudder (1989) examined jaw muscle activity of individuals with PD, and found impaired muscle coordination. When examining the effects of levodopa treatment on dysarthric symptoms, it has been shown that levodopa treatment may affect muscle activity at the laryngeal and supralarygeal levels in speakers with PD (Leanderson, Meyerson, & Persson, 1971; Leanderson, Meyerson, & Persson, 1972; Nakano, Zubick, & Tyler, 1973).

Additional EMG studies have been performed in non-Parkinsonian dysarthria. Hirose, Kiritani, Ushijima, & Sawashima (1978) analyzed articulatory muscles in an individual with cerebellar degeneration and an individual with amyotrophic lateral sclerosis (ALS). The speaker with cerebellar degeneration produced abnormal and inconsistent articulatory patterns, varying in both range and velocity of movement. The speaker with ALS produced articulatory movements that were slow and reduced in range. In a separate study, Neilson and O'Dwyer (1981) found no evidence of tonic hyperactivity of articulatory musculature in cerebral palsy. Although these participants varied in their articulatory patterns, the authors noted that exploring the dynamic aspects of articulation via EMG was a promising technique for characterizing the physiopathology of the dysarthrias.

Conclusion

There is great potential for EMG to investigate the neuromuscular aspects of speech production. EMG is an objective and quantitative means of assessing pathophysiology of irregular motor patterns of speech-language disorders such as dysarthria, as well as for applying biofeedback to treat abnormal speech production. Although there has been much research in the realm of speech-language disorders, further work must be done to develop controlled and standardized methods of biofeedback treatments. The clinical use of EMG shows promise for elucidating the physiological mechanisms of speech production; however, further development must be taken to reduce cost and clarify measurement protocols for simple, easy-to-interpret, and effective data collection techniques.

Note

1 Although these studies support sEMG as an effective mechanism of biofeedback, it is difficult to compare this tool to other interventions due to the limited number of studies on EMG-based biofeedback for vocal hyperfunction. It is important to note that these regard a reduction in muscle activity as a reduction in muscle tension. However, muscle tension is dependent on muscle length and velocity, such that sEMG activity (asynchronous summation of myoelectric activity near the electrode site) does not provide a direct measure of muscle tension.

References

Alfonso, P.J., & Baer, T. (1982). Dynamics of vowel articulation. *Lang Speech*, *25*(2), 151–173.

Allen, K.D., Bernstein, B., & Chait, D.H. (1991). EMG biofeedback treatment of pediatric hyperfunctional dysphonia. *J Behav Ther Exp Psy*, *22*(2), 97–101.

Andrews, S., Warner, J., & Stewart, R. (1986). EMG biofeedback and relaxation in the treatment of hyperfunctional dysphonia. *Int J Lang Comm Dis*, *21*(3), 353–369.

Basmajian, J.V., & De Luca, C.J. (1985). *Muscles Alive: Their Functions Revealed by Electromyography*. Baltimore, MD: Williams & Wilkins.

Block, S., Onslow, M., Roberts, R., & White, S. (2004). Control of stuttering with EMG feedback. *Adv Speech Lang Pathol*, *6*(2), 100–106.

Bloodstein, O., & Bernstein Ratner, N. (2008). *A Handbook on Stuttering* (6th ed.). Clifton Park, NY: Thomson-Delmar.

Booker, H.E., Rubow, R.T., & Coleman, P.J. (1969). Simplified feedback in neuromuscular retraining: An automated approach using electromyographic signals. *Arch Phys Med Rehabil*, *50*(11), 621–625.

Boucher, V.J., Ahmarani, C., & Ayad, T. (2006). Physiologic features of vocal fatigue: Electromyographic spectral-compression in laryngeal muscles. *Laryngoscope*, *116*(6), 959–965.

Caligiuri, M.P., & Till, J.A. (1983). Acoustical analysis of vowel duration in apraxia of speech: A case study. *Folia Phoniatr (Basel)*, *35*(5), 226–234.

Campbell, E.J. (1955). An electromyographic examination of the role of the intercostal muscles in breathing in man. *J Physiol*, *129*(1), 12–26.

Cavanagh, P.R., & Komi, P.V. (1979). Electromechanical delay in human skeletal muscle under concentric and eccentric contractions. *Eur J Appl Physiol Occup Physiol*, *42*(3), 159–163.

Collins, M., Rosenbek, J.C., & Wertz, R.T. (1983). Spectrographic analysis of vowel and word duration in apraxia of speech. *J Speech Hear Res*, *26*(2), 224–230.

Craig, A., Hancock, K., Chang, E., McCready, C., Shepley, A., McCaul, A., Costello, D., Harding, S., Kehren, R., Masel, C., & Reilly, K. (1996). A controlled clinical trial for stuttering in persons aged 9 to 14 years. *J Speech Hear Res, 39*(4), 808–826.

Craig, A.R., & Cleary, P.J. (1982). Reduction of stuttering by young male stutterers using EMG feedback. *Biofeedback Self Regul, 7*(3), 241–255.

Cross, D.E. (1977). Effects of false increasing, decreasing, and true electromyographic biofeedback on the frequency of stuttering. *J Fluency Disord, 2*(2), 109–116.

Daniel, B., & Guitar, B. (1978). EMG feedback and recovery of facial and speech gestures following neural anastomosis. *J Speech Hear Disord, 43*(1), 9–20.

De Luca, C.J. (1997). The use of surface electromyography in biomechanics. *J Appl Biomech, 13*, 135–163.

De Luca, C.J. (2002). Surface Electromyography: Detection and Recording. Retrieved from https://www. delsys.com/downloads/TUTORIAL/semg-detection-and-recording.pdf

De Luca, C.J. (2006). Electromyography. In J.G. Webster (Ed.), *Encyclopedia of Medical Devices and Instrumentation*, (pp. 98–109). Hoboken, NJ: Wiley-Interscience.

De Luca, C.J., Gilmore, L.D., Kuznetsov, M., & Roy, S.H. (2010). Filtering the surface EMG signal: Movement artifact and baseline noise contamination. *J Biomech, 43*(8), 1573–1579.

Denny, M., & Smith, A. (1992). Gradations in a pattern of neuromuscular activity associated with stuttering. *J Speech Hear Res, 35*(6), 1216–1229.

Draper, M.H., Ladefoged, P., & Whitteridge, D. (1959). Respiratory muscles in speech. *J Speech Hear Disord, 2*(1), 16–27.

Du Bois-Reymond, E. (1848). *Untersuchungen über thierische Elektricität*. Berlin: Reimer.

Eblen, R.E. (1963). Limitations on use of surface electromyography in studies of speech breathing. *J Speech Hear Disord, 6*(1), 3–18.

English, D.T., & Blevins, C.E. (1969). Motor units of laryngeal muscles. *Arch Otolaryngol, 89*(5), 778–784.

Ertekin, C., & Aydogdu, I. (2003). Neurophysiology of swallowing. *Clin Neurophysiol, 114*(12), 2226–2244.

Faaborg-Andersen, K. (1957). Electromyographic investigation of intrinsic laryngeal muscles in humans. *Acta Physiol Scand, 41*(Suppl. 140), 1–150.

Faaborg-Andersen, K., & Buchthal, F. (1956). Action potentials from internal laryngeal muscles during dhonation. *Nature, 177*(4503), 340–341.

Faaborg-Andersen, K., Edfeldt, Å.W., & Nykøbing, F. (1958). Electromyography of intrinsic and extrinsic laryngeal muscles during silent speech: Correlation with reading activity: Preliminary report. *Acta Otolaryngol, 49*(1), 478–482.

Feinstein, B., Lindegard, B., Nyman, E., & Wohlfart, G. (1955). Morphologic studies of motor units in normal human muscles. *Acta Anat (Basel), 23*(2), 127–142.

Finger, S., Boller, F., & Tyler, K.L. (2009). *History of Neurology*. Amsterdam, Netherlands: Elsevier Science.

Freeman, F.J., & Ushijima, T. (1978). Laryngeal muscle activity during stuttering. *J Speech Hear Res, 21*(3), 538–562.

Fromm, D., Abbs, J.H., McNeil, M.R., & Rosenbek, J.C. (1976). Simultaneous perceptual-physiological method for studying apraxia of speech. In R.H. Brookshire (Ed.), *Clinical Aphasiology: Conference Proceedings, Oshkosh, WI (pp. 251–262)*. Minneapolis, MN: BRK Publishers.

Fuglevand, A.J., Winter, D.A., Patla, A.E., & Stashuk, D. (1992). Detection of motor unit action potentials with surface electrodes: Influence of electrode size and spacing. *Biol Cybern, 67*(2), 143–153.

Gallena, S., Smith, P.J., Zeffiro, T., & Ludlow, C.L. (2001). Effects of levodopa on laryngeal muscle activity for voice onset and offset in Parkinson disease. *J Speech Hear Res, 44*(6), 1284–1299.

Gay, T., & Harris, K.S. (1971). Some recent developments in the use of electromyography in speech research. *J Speech Hear Disord, 14*(2), 241–246.

Gay, T., Ushijima, T., Hiroset, H., & Cooper, F.S. (1974). Effect of speaking rate on labial consonant-vowel articulation. *J Phon, 2*(1), 47–63.

Gerdle, B., Karlsson, S., Day, S., & Djupsjöbacka, M. (1999). Acquisition, processing and analysis of the surface electromyogram. In U. Windhorst & H. Johansson (Eds.), *Modern Techniques in Neuroscience Research*. Berlin, Heidelberg: Springer-Verlag.

Guitar, B. (1975). Reduction of stuttering frequency using analog electromyographic feedback. *J Speech Hear Disord, 18*(4), 672–685.

Hanna, R., Wilfling, F., & McNeill, B. (1975). A biofeedback treatment for stuttering. *J Speech Hear Disord, 40*(2), 270–273.

Heman-Ackah, Y.D., Mandel, S., Manon-Espaillat, R., Abaza, M.M., & Sataloff, R.T. (2007). Laryngeal electromyography. *Otolaryngol Clin North Am, 40*(5), 1003–1023.

Hermens, H.J., Biomedical, C.o.t.E.C., & Programme, H.R. (1999). *European Recommendations for Surface Electromyography: Results of the SENIAM Project.* Enschede, Netherlands: Roessingh Research and Development.

Hillman, R.E., Holmberg, E.B., Perkell, J.S., Walsh, M., & Vaughan, C. (1989). Objective assessment of vocal hyperfunction: An experimental framework and initial results. *J Speech Hear Res, 32*(2), 373–392.

Hirano, M., & Ohala, J. (1969). Use of hooked-wire electrodes for electromyography of the intrinsic laryngeal muscles. *J Speech Hear Disord, 12*(2), 362–373.

Hirose, H. (1974). The activity of the lip in articulation of a Japanese vowel/O/: A simultaneous EMG and stroboscopic study. *Auris Nasus Larynx, 1*(1), 33–41.

Hirose, H., Kiritani, S., Ushijima, T., & Sawashima, M. (1978). Analysis of abnormal articulatory dynamics in two dysarthric patients. *J Speech Hear Disord, 43*(1), 96–105.

Hiroto, I., Hirano, M., Toyozumi, Y., & Shin, T. (1967). Electromyographic investigation of the intrinsic laryngeal muscles related to speech sounds. *Ann Otol Rhinol Laryngol, 76*(4), 861–872.

Jaffe, D.M., Solomon, N.P., Robinson, R.A., Hoffman, H.T., & Luschei, E.S. (1998). Comparison of concentric needle versus hooked-wire electrodes in the canine larynx. *Otolaryngol Head Neck Surg, 118*(5), 655–662.

Jones, D.S., Beargie, R.J., & Pauley, J.E. (1953). An electromyographic study of some muscles on costal respiration in man. *Anat Rec, 117*(1), 17–24.

Kellaway, P. (1946). The part played by electric fish in the early history of bioelectricity and electrotherapy. *Bull Hist Med, 20*(2), 112–137.

Kent, R.D., & Rosenbek, J.C. (1983). Acoustic patterns of apraxia of speech. *J Speech Hear Res, 26*(2), 231–249.

Koutsos, E., & Georgiou, P. (June, 2014). An analogue instantaneous median frequency tracker for EMG fatigue monitoring. In *2014 IEEE International Symposium on Circuits and Systems (ISCAS)*, Melbourne VIC, Australia, (pp. 1388–1391). Piscataway, NJ: IEEE.

Lanyon, R.I. (1977). Effect of biofeedback-based relaxation on stuttering during reading and spontaneous speech. *J Consult Clin Psychol, 45*(5), 860–866.

Leanderson, R., Meyerson, B.A., & Persson, A. (1971). Effect of L-dopa on speech in Parkinsonism. An EMG study of labial articulatory function. *J Neurol Neurosurg Psychiatry, 34*(6), 679–681.

Leanderson, R., Meyerson, B.A., & Persson, A. (1972). Lip muscle function in Parkinsonian dysarthria. *Acta Otolaryngol, 74*(5), 350–357.

Liddell, E.G.T., & Sherrington, C.S. (1925). Recruitment and some other features of reflex inhibition. *Proc R Soc B, 97*(686), 488–518.

Loucks, T.M., Poletto, C.J., Saxon, K.G., & Ludlow, C.L. (2005). Laryngeal muscle responses to mechanical displacement of the thyroid cartilage in humans. *J Appl Physiol, 99*(3), 922–930.

MacNeilage, P.F., & Sholes, G.N. (1964). An electromyographic study of the tongue during vowel production. *J Speech Hear Disord, 7*, 209–232.

McClean, M., Goldsmith, H., & Cerf, A. (1984). Lower-lip EMG and displacement during bilabial disfluencies in adult stutterers. *J Speech Hear Res, 27*(3), 342–349.

McClean, M., & Sapir, S. (1980). Surface electrode recording of platysma single motor units during speech. *J Phon, 8*(2), 169–173.

McLean, A.E., & Cooper, E.B. (1978). Electromyographic indications of laryngeal-area activity during stuttering expectancy. *J Fluency Disord, 3*(3), 205–219.

McNeil, M.R., Prescott, T.E., & Lemme, M.L. (1976). An application of electromyographic biofeedback to aphasia/apraxia treatment. In R.H. Brookshire (Ed.), *Clinical Aphasiology: Conference Proceedings, Wemme, OR (pp. 151–171)*. Minneapolis, MN: BRK Publishers.

Merletti, R., & Hermens, H.J. (2004). Detection and conditioning of the surface EMG signal. In R. Merletti & P. Parker (Eds.), *Electromyography* (pp. 107–131). Hoboken, NJ: John Wiley & Sons, Inc.

Minifie, F.D., Abbs, J.H., Tarlow, A., & Kwaterski, M. (1974). EMG activity within the pharynx during speech production. *J Speech Hear Disord, 17*(3), 497–504.

Moore, C., & Scudder, R. (1989). Coordination of jaw muscle activity in parkinsonian movement: Description and response to traditional treatment. In K. Yorkston & D. Beukelman (Eds.), *Recent Advances in Clinical Dysarthria*. Boston, MA: College-Hill.

Moritani, T., Stegeman, D., & Merletti, R. (2004). Basic physiology and biophysics of EMG signal generation. In R. Merletti & P. Parker (Eds.), *Electromyography*, (pp. 1–25). Hoboken, NJ: John Wiley & Sons, Inc.

Moulonget, A. (1955). Notions nouvelles concernant la physiologie de la phonation. *Exposes annuelles d'oto-rhino-laryngologie*, *44*(2), 169–180.

Moya-Galé, G., & Levy, E. (2019). Parkinson's disease-associated dysarthria: Prevalence, impact and management strategies. *Res Rev Parkinsonism*, *9*, 9–16.

Nakano, K.K., Zubick, H., & Tyler, H.R. (1973). Speech defects of Parkinsonian patients: Effects of levodopa therapy on speech intelligibility. *Neurology*, *23*(8), 865–870.

Neilson, P.D., & O'Dwyer, N.J. (1981). Pathophysiology of dysarthria in cerebral palsy. *J Neurol Neurosurg Psychiatry*, *44*(11), 1013.

Nemec, R.E., & Cohen, K. (1984). EMG biofeedback in the modification of hypertonia in spastic dysarthria: Case report. *Arch Phys Med Rehabil*, *65*(2), 103–104.

Netsell, R., & Cleeland, C.S. (1973). Modification of lip hypertonia in dysarthria using EMG feedback. *J Speech Hear Disord*, *38*(1), 131–140.

Netsell, R., Daniel, B., & Celesia Gastone, G. (1975). Acceleration and weakness in Parkinsonian dysarthria. *J Speech Hear Disord*, *40*(2), 170–178.

O'Dwyer, N.J., Quinn, P.T., Guitar, B.E., Andrews, G., & Neilson, P.D. (1981). Procedures for verification of electrode placement in EMG studies of orofacial and mandibular muscles. *J Speech Hear Res*, *24*(2), 273–288.

Öhman, S. (1967). *Peripheral motor commands in labial articulation*. (STL-QPSR 4/1967) Stockholm, Sweden: Royal Institute of Technology. http://www.speech.kth.se/prod/publications/files/qpsr/1967/1967_8_4_030-063.pdf

Palmer, P.M., Luschei, E.S., Jaffe, D., & McCulloch, T.M. (1999). Contributions of individual muscles to the submental surface electromyogram during swallowing. *J Speech Lang Hear Res*, *42*(6), 1378–1391.

Purves, D., Augustine, G.J., Fitzpatrick, D., Hall, W.C., LaMantia, A., McNamara, J.O., & Williams, S.M. (2001). The motor unit. In *Neuroscience*. Sunderland, MA: Sinauer Associates.

Rodriquez, A.A., Ford, C.N., Bless, D.M., & Harmon, R.L. (1994). Electromyographic assessment of spasmodic dysphonia patients prior to botulinum toxin injection. *Electromyogr Clin Neurophysiol*, *34*(7), 403–407.

Roeleveld, K., Stegeman, D.F., Vingerhoets, H.M., & Van Oosterom, A. (1997). The motor unit potential distribution over the skin surface and its use in estimating the motor unit location. *Acta Physiol Scand*, *161*(4), 465–472.

Roy, N. (2003). Functional dysphonia. *Curr Opin Otolaryngol Head Neck Surg*, *11*(3), 144–148.

Roy, S.H., De Luca, G., Cheng, M.S., Johansson, A., Gilmore, L.D., & De Luca, C.J. (2007). Electromechanical stability of surface EMG sensors. *Med Bio Eng Comput*, *45*(5), 447–457.

Rubow, R.T., Rosenbek, J.C., Collins, M.J., & Celesia, G.G. (1984). Reduction of hemifacial spasm and dysarthria following EMG biofeedback. *J Speech Hear Disord*, *49*(1), 26–33.

Rüedi, L. (1959). Some observations on the histology and function of the larynx. *J Laryngol Otol*, *73*(1), 1–20.

Rutkove, S.B. (2007). Introduction to volume conduction. In A.S. Blum & S.B. Rutkove (Eds.), *The Clinical Neurophysiology Primer* (pp. 43–53). Totowa, NJ: Humana Press.

Santo Neto, H., & Marques, M.J. (2008). Estimation of the number and size of motor units in intrinsic laryngeal muscles using morphometric methods. *Clin Anat*, *21*(4), 301–306.

Seddoh, S.A., Robin, D.A., Sim, H.S., Hageman, C., Moon, J.B., & Folkins, J.W. (1996). Speech timing in apraxia of speech versus conduction aphasia. *J Speech Hear Res*, *39*(3), 590–603.

Smith, A. (1989). Neural drive to muscles in stuttering. *J Speech Hear Res*, *32*(2), 252–264.

Smith, A., Denny, M., Shaffer, L.A., Kelly, E.M., & Hirano, M. (1996). Activity of intrinsic laryngeal muscles in fluent and disfluent speech. *J Speech Hear Res*, *39*(2), 329–348.

Smith, T.S., & Hirano, M. (1968). Experimental investigations of the muscular control of the tongue in speech. *J Acoust Soc Am*, *44*(1), 354–354.

Stepp, C.E. (2012). Surface electromyography for speech and swallowing systems: measurement, analysis, and interpretation. *J Speech Hear Res*, *55*(4), 1232–1246.

Stetson, R.H. (1951). *Motor Phonetics: A Study of Speech Movements in Action*. Amsterdam, The Netherlands: North Holland Publishers.

Strauss, M., & Klich, R.J. (2001). Word length effects on EMG/vowel duration relationships in apraxic speakers. *Folia Phoniatr Logop, 53*(1), 58–65.

Sussman, H.M., MacNeilage, P.F., & Hanson, R.J. (1973). Labial and mandibular dynamics during the production of bilabial consonants: preliminary observations. *J Speech Hear Disord, 16*(3), 397–420.

Sussman, H.M., MacNeilage, P.F., & Powers, R.K. (1977). Recruitment and discharge patterns of single motor units during speech production. *J Speech Hear Disord, 20*(4), 613–630.

Tisch, S.H., Brake, H.M., Law, M., Cole, I.E., & Darveniza, P. (2003). Spasmodic dysphonia: Clinical features and effects of botulinum toxin therapy in 169 patients - An Australian experience. *J Clin Neurosci, 10*(4), 434–438.

Tuller, B., Kelso, J.S., & Harris, K.S. (1982). Interarticulator phasing as an index of temporal regularity in speech. *J Exp Psychol Hum Percept Perform, 8*(3), 460–472.

van Lieshout, P.H.H.M., Peters, H.F.M., Starkweather, C.W., & Hulstijn, W. (1993). Physiological differences between stutterers and nonstutterers in perceptually fluent speech. *J Speech Hear Res, 36*(1), 55–63.

Walker, S., Davis, L., Avela, J., & Häkkinen, K. (2012). Neuromuscular fatigue during dynamic maximal strength and hypertrophic resistance loadings. *J Electromyogr Kinesiol, 22*(3), 356–362.

Willigenburg, N.W., Daffertshofer, A., Kingma, I., & van Dieën, J.H. (2012). Removing ECG contamination from EMG recordings: A comparison of ICA-based and other filtering procedures. *J Electromyogr Kinesiol, 22*(3), 485–493.

Ziegler, W. (2002). Psycholinguistic and motor theories of apraxia of speech. *Semin Speech Lang, 23*(4), 231–244.

21

SPEECH AEROMETRY

David J. Zajac

Introduction

Speech is essentially an overlaid function on respiration, with the pulmonic system initiating a pressurized air stream that is modified (regulated) by laryngeal (phonatory) and supralaryngeal (articulatory) activities, respectively. The production of the stop-plosive /p/, for example, is characterized by the momentary stoppage of the air stream by the lips that results in the build-up of intraoral air pressure followed by release of the occlusion resulting in a burst of oral airflow. These aerodynamic events—which give rise to the acoustic and perceptual aspects of speech—can be detected and recorded using modern instrumentation. Some speech disorders, however, fundamentally disrupt aerodynamic processes. Individuals with velopharyngeal dysfunction (VPD), for example, are likely to have difficulty producing speech with normal aerodynamic, and thus, acoustic-perceptual, characteristics. VPD can occur congenitally from structural defects such as cleft palate or it can occur from acquired neurogenic disorders such as traumatic brain injury and amyotrophic lateral sclerosis (ALS). There is a need, therefore, for specialized instrumentation to describe the speech aerodynamics of these and other disorders.

As reviewed in Chapter 6 of this volume, individuals with VPD experience two major types of aerodynamic problems. The first is the loss of oral air pressure through the velopharyngeal port during attempts to occlude and/or constrict the oral cavity. This occurs during production of stops and fricatives that require adequate levels of air pressure to generate stop bursts and frication noise, respectively. Perceptually, the loss of oral air pressure reduces overall intensity of these sounds, often referred to as "weak pressure consonants" by clinicians. The second, and related, problem is nasal air escape through the velopharyngeal port. Under certain conditions, this air escape can become audible, adding noise to the intended speech signal. Although this noise typically does not reduce intelligibility (except in severe cases), it is perceptually distracting to the listener. Often, individuals with VPD also exhibit hypernasality. This is primarily an acoustic-resonance phenomenon that occurs during production of vowels and voiced consonants. Although it is associated with some nasal airflow, the airflow itself is typically not audible. Chapter 24 in this volume covers instrumental approaches to describe hypernasal resonance.

Passive (obligatory) versus active (learned) nasal air emission

The clinical literature is filled with many different terms used to describe nasal air escape. This is not surprising given (a) the complex anatomy of the nasal passages, (b) individual variations in nasal anatomy, often exacerbated due to surgical intervention in cases of cleft lip and palate and (c) individual variations in speech production (e.g. respiratory effort levels). As indicated in Chapter 6 of this volume, however, there is general consensus regarding two broad etiological categories of nasal air emission—passive (or obligatory) and active (or learned). Obligatory nasal air escape occurs due to some degree of VPD. Perceptually, it has been described as occurring across a continuum from inaudible (visible only) to audible to turbulent (Peterson-Falzone, Hardin-Jones & Karnell, 2001; Zajac & Vallino, 2017). Inaudible nasal air escape can only be detected by instrumental means. A common clinical technique is to hold a small mirror under the nostrils of the speaker to detect fogging during production of oral pressure consonants. The lack of accompanying noise indicates that the nasal air stream is moving in a laminar (relatively straight-line) flow pattern. Peterson-Falzone et al. (2001) describe "audible" nasal air escape as the sound that one can make by forcefully exhaling through the nose. Under this condition, the velum is relaxed and the air stream becomes turbulent (nonlaminar) as it passes through and exits the nasal cavity. Audible nasal air emission has a hissing-like quality that may be relatively low in intensity. This type of nasal air emission typically occurs in speakers with relatively large velopharyngeal gaps and accompanying hypernasality. In these cases, the hypernasality is usually the most perceptually salient symptom. Finally, Peterson-Falzone et al. (2001) describe "turbulent" nasal air escape as a more perceptually severe form of audible nasal air escape. By this they mean that the noise is relatively louder, has extra components and draws more listener attention than audible nasal air escape. Peterson-Falzone et al. (2001) attributed the extra components of "turbulent" nasal air emission to either tissue vibration and/or displacement of mucous in the velopharyngeal port or nasal passages. Various terms have been used to clinically describe this type of nasal air escape including nasal rustle. Turbulent nasal air escape is typically associated with relatively small velopharyngeal gaps (Kummer, Curtis, Wiggs, Lee, & Strife, 1992). Of importance, Zajac and Preisser (2016) showed that "turbulent" nasal air emission was actually associated with a relatively strong (intense) quasi-periodic noise in spectrographic analyses. This finding is consistent with both a small velopharyngeal port and tissue vibration as the primary source of the "turbulent" noise quality.

Active (or learned) nasal air escape occurs during articulation of nasal fricatives. Harding and Grunwell (1998) described active nasal fricatives as articulations with simultaneous oral stopping and all airflow directed through the nose. The location of the oral stopping gesture can be bilabial, lingual-alveolar or lingual-velar. These articulations, typically used by young children with and without palatal anomalies, can replace any or all of the oral fricatives and affricates. Of clinical importance (and concern), these articulations can sound similar to either audible or turbulent types of obligatory nasal air emission. Zajac (2015) used spectrographic analyses of separately recorded oral and nasal acoustic signals to show spectral distinctions between two types of active nasal fricatives that he referred to as anterior and posterior, respectively. Both types showed silent intervals on the oral signal indicating oral occlusion. Nasal spectrograms of anterior nasal fricatives were characterized solely by aperiodic hissing noise, similar to obligatory audible nasal air emission. Conversely, nasal spectrograms of posterior nasal fricatives were characterized primarily by relatively intense quasi-periodic noise, similar to obligatory "turbulent" nasal air emission. As described later in this chapter, aerometric techniques can also identify the oral stopping component of active nasal fricatives.

It is an axiom of clinical phonetics that auditory-perceptual analysis is the gold standard for describing speech disorders and, indeed, this is true. As the above review of VPD has shown, however, some perceptually similar (even identical) symptoms can occur with diametrically opposite underlying causes and treatment needs. The rest of this chapter, therefore, focuses on instrumental aerodynamic techniques that not only can quantify the primary symptoms of VPD—weak pressure consonants and audible/turbulent nasal air escape—but also provide essential information to aid in differential diagnosis of obligatory versus learned behaviors.

Brief background to aerometric techniques

Technological advances in the middle part of the last century stimulated considerable research on normal speech aerodynamics. Indeed, during the 1960s and 1970s, numerous studies appeared using electronic pressure gauges and transducers to describe intraoral air pressure and oral/nasal airflow of various consonants (see Baken & Orlikoff, 2000, for a review). Also during this time, Warren and colleagues pioneered the application of fluid dynamic principles to study VPD of individuals with palatal clefts (Warren, 1964a, 1964b; Warren & DuBois, 1964). Warren's approach—which uses measures of oral-nasal air pressure and nasal airflow to estimate velopharyngeal port size—has come to be known as the pressure-flow method.

Basic principles of the pressure-flow method

Warren and DuBois (1964) used a model of the upper vocal tract to show that the cross-sectional area of a constriction (or orifice) can be calculated if the differential pressure across the orifice and rate of airflow are measured simultaneously. Figure 21.1 shows fluid flow (water in this example) through a pipe with a constriction. The static pressures (i.e. pressure associated with the moving stream) are detected before and after the constriction. The difference between these pressures is the pressure loss, shown by a drop in the height of the water column downstream of the constriction. Assuming a similar pipe with airflow that is steady (or nonturbulent), the area of the constriction can be calculated using the pressure loss and a modification of Bernoulli's equation as follows:

$$A = V/[2(p_1 - p_2)/D]^{1/2}$$

where A is area in cm^2, V is airflow in ml/s, p_1 is static pressure in dynes/cm before the constriction, p_2 is static pressure in dynes/cm after the constriction and D is the density of air (.001 gm/cm).

The above equation assumes ideal (i.e. nonturbulent) flow conditions. As indicated by Warren and DuBois (1964), however, ideal conditions do not exist in the human anatomy.

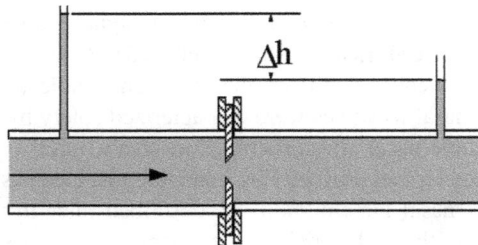

Figure 21.1   Water flow in a pipe with a constriction.

Given that turbulent airflow would likely occur downstream of the constriction, they introduced a "correction factor k." This was a dimensionless coefficient, 0.65, derived from model tests using known orifice openings. Based on these model tests, Warren and DuBois (1964) modified the equation as follows:

$$A = V/k[2(p_1 - p_2)/D]^{\frac{1}{2}}$$

where k is 0.65. Although Warren and DuBois (1964) referred to this as a working equation, it has subsequently become known as the "orifice equation."

Accuracy of the orifice equation

As reported by Warren and DuBois (1964), accuracy of area estimates decreases with increasing size of orifice openings, especially at very large openings (e.g. greater than 100 mm^2). This occurs due to difficulty detecting relatively low levels of air pressure associated with large openings. This concern, however, has limited impact on clinical decisions because, as reviewed later in the chapter, VPD typically occurs once velopharyngeal area exceeds 20 mm^2. The accuracy of area estimates for smaller orifices is actually quite good. Zajac and Yates (1991), for example, reported an approximately 7% error between known and estimated orifice area when a short tube with a cross-sectional area of 18.1 mm^2 was placed in the oropharynx of a normal speaker. A related concern is that accuracy of area estimates depends on the value of the coefficient k used in the orifice equation to correct for turbulent flow. Warren and DuBois (1964) used a value of 0.65 based on model studies that used short tubes and thin orifice plates with sharp entrances. As indicated by Yates, McWilliams, and Vallino (1990), the entrance geometry of the velopharyngeal port is likely tapered and rounded. This geometry will result in less turbulent flow and a higher value for the coefficient. This means that calculated velopharyngeal area using a k value of 0.65 is larger (by up to 35%) compared to using a value of 0.99, which may be more representative of actual port geometry. As described later in the chapter, the use of a new speaker-centered aerometric index negates the concern regarding the value of k.

Clinical application

Figure 21.2 shows the clinical application of the pressure-flow method. To obtain differential pressure across the velopharyngeal port, an open-tip catheter is placed in the oral cavity and another catheter is placed in one nostril of the speaker.[1] The nasal catheter is secured with a foam plug that also occludes the nostril and creates a stagnation pressure. The oral and nasal catheters are connected to separate differential pressure transducers. Nasal airflow is obtained by fitting a plastic tube into the other nostril of the speaker. This is connected in series to a pneumo-tachograph (flowmeter) and another differential pressure transducer. Specific procedures for placement of the catheters/flow tube and calibration of transducers are described below.

How to do aerometric testing

Obtaining oral-nasal air pressures

Air pressure of consonants can be associated with a moving airstream during production of fricatives or a nonmoving air volume during production of stops. To detect these pressures, small-bore catheters must be positioned *behind* the articulators of interest. The detection of

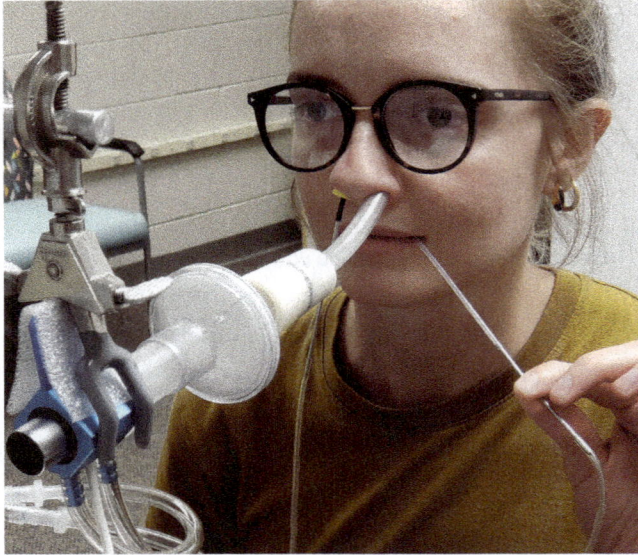

Figure 21.2   Clinical application of the pressure-flow method.

peak air pressure associated with stops is relatively easy, at least for bilabials. For these stops, the open end of the catheter is simply placed behind the lips. The orientation of the catheter is inconsequential—as long as it is behind the lips—due to equal pressure being exerted in all directions. To detect air pressure associated with alveolar stops, the catheter should be inserted from the corner of the mouth. This will usually ensure placement behind the alveolar ridge. This may interfere with articulation, however, in some speakers. Placement for velar stops is most difficult. To detect these pressures, the catheter either must be placed along the buccal sulcus of the oral cavity and angled to the midline behind the last molar or inserted through the nose as initially done by Warren and DuBois (1964). Neither of these approaches, especially the latter, is practical with young children in a clinical setting. To detect pressures associated with fricative sounds, care must be taken to ensure that the open end of the catheter is positioned perpendicular to the direction of airflow. [2] Inserting the catheter from the corner of the mouth will usually achieve this requirement, at least for fricatives produced at the alveolar ridge. Because of practical concerns for oral catheter placement, clinical speech samples are typically limited to bilabial stops, especially for young children. Nasal air pressure associated with either nasal consonants or oral consonants in the presence of VPD can be detected by securing a catheter in the vestibule of the nose (described in detail below).

The oral and nasal catheters need to be attached to calibrated differential pressure transducers referenced to atmosphere. Various types of transducers are available. In the author's lab, variable capacitance transducers are used (Setra, model 239). This transducer has a diaphragm and an insulated electrode that forms a variable capacitor. As pressure is applied to the high (center) port relative to the low (or atmospheric) port, capacitance increases in proportion. The transducers used for oral and nasal air pressure are bidirectional with a pressure range of ±0–15 inches of water (approximately ±0–38 cm H_2O), useful for recording pressures associated with most speech activities. The upper limit of these transducers, for example, is approximately twice as high as pressures associated with even loud speech.

The pressure transducers are calibrated by applying a known pressure using a manometer. Traditionally, a U-tube manometer was used. This is a water-filled U-shaped glass tube with an adjustable centimeter scale. Zero on the scale is positioned at the level of the water in the two columns. A syringe is attached to one end of the U-tube and the pressure transducer to be calibrated to the other end. When a pressure is applied via the syringe, the water column in that arm will be depressed below zero on the scale (e.g. down 3 centimeters) while the water column in the other arm will be elevated above zero (e.g. up 3 centimeters). The total pressure applied is the sum of water displacement in both arms (e.g. 6 centimeters of water in this example). Digital manometers have largely replaced U-tube and other types of fluid-filled manometers making calibration easier. A digital manometer is simply connected to the transducer, a pressure is selected (e.g. 6 centimeters of water) and the pressure is directly applied. Calibration is completed following directions of any commercially available software programs (e.g. PERCI-SARS, TF32 Lab Automation).[3] These programs will compute a scale factor that relates the electrical output of the transducer to a pressure value. Once calibrated, air pressure transducers, at least the variable capacitance kind used by the author, are stable and do not require frequent recalibration. Calibration checks (i.e. applying a known pressure and observing the software output), however, should be done periodically to ensure fidelity of the system.

Obtaining nasal airflow

The recording of nasal (or oral) airflow is typically done using a heated pneumotachograph (Figure 21.3). This device provides a constant resistance to airflow by means of a small screen or a bundle of small diameter tubes housed within a larger conduit. The rate of airflow is determined by measuring the differential pressure drop across the resistance. Higher rates of airflow will produce a proportionally greater pressure drop for a given resistance. As shown in Figure 21.3, the pneumotachograph has two pressure taps that are connected to the high and low ports of a differential pressure transducer. The pressure transducer is the same as that used for oral/nasal air pressure but has a smaller range, typically ±0–0.5 or ±0–1.0 inches of water. The smaller range is used because the pressure drops associated with airflow during speech are relatively low compared to vocal tract air pressure. Pneumotachographs are available in different sizes for different applications. As indicated by Baken and Orlikoff (2000), the Fleisch #1 pneumotachograph (shown in Figure 21.3) is appropriate for many speech applications.[4] It has a maximum useful flow rate of 1.0 L/s, a resistance of 1.5 cm H_2O/L/s and a dead space of 15 ml. The pneumotachograph is heated by a low-voltage direct current. This is done to eliminate condensation from the breath stream on the resistive element.

The pneumotachograph is typically calibrated by applying a known flow rate from a compressed air cylinder that is routed through a rotameter. A float or ball in the rotameter rises in proportion to the applied rate of airflow. Calibration is completed using software to compute a scale factor that relates the electrical output of the transducer to a flow value. A large syringe (e.g. 1–3 liters) may also be used to apply a known volume of air across the pneumotachograph in a given period of time for calibration purposes. The advantage of this approach is that it eliminates the need for a compressed air supply that may not be available in a clinical setting. Once the pneumotachograph is calibrated, nasal airflow can be obtained by means of a flow tube inserted into one nostril or a small mask placed over the nose (described in detail below).

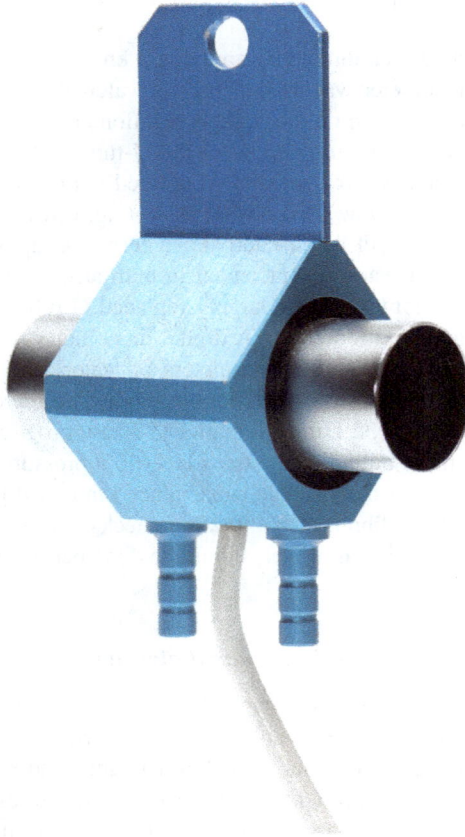

Figure 21.3   Fleisch #1 pneumotachograph.

Step-by-Step clinical procedures

The pressure-flow technique as shown in Figure 21.2 is minimally invasive to the patient. It does require, however, a certain level of cooperation. Thus, children under the ages of 5–6 years may not be good candidates. The procedure also requires that both nasal passages of the patient be open. Specific procedures for obtaining nasal air pressure, nasal airflow and oral air pressure are as follows:

1. A foam plug/catheter assembly is first inserted in one nostril of the patient to obtain nasal air pressure. The least patent (open) nostril should be selected. This can be determined by asking the patient to pinch each nostril closed while breathing to subjectively determine the least/most patent nostril. The end of the catheter is connected to the high port of the bidirectional differential pressure transducer (±0–15 inches of water). To ensure a comfortable but snug fit, the author uses foam ear inserts that are used in audiometric testing. These inserts come in various sizes that fit most patients. After the plug/catheter is secured in the nostril, the clinician should confirm patency by asking the patient to breathe quietly with the mouth closed while monitoring the nasal air pressure signal on the computer software. If nasal pressure does not consistently rise and fall during the respiratory cycle,

then the nostril is not patent and the procedure cannot be done. In this case, the nasal mask approach described in the next section may be used.

2. Next, a plastic tube is inserted into the patient's other nostril to obtain nasal airflow. [5] The tube is connected in series to the heated pneumotachograph and bidirectional differential pressure transducer (±0–1 inches of water) (see Figure 21.2). The upstream pressure tap on the pneumotachograph is connected to the high port on the transducer; the downstream pressure tap is connected to the low port.

3. To obtain oral air pressure, the clinician places a catheter behind the patient's lips. Although older patients can hold the catheter, it is recommended that the clinician do this if phonemes other than /p/ or /b/ are tested to ensure appropriate placement. The catheter is connected to the high port of another bidirectional differential pressure transducer (±0–15 inches of water).

4. A small electret microphone is either clipped to the patient's shirt collar or attached to the tubing that holds the oral catheter.

5. Once the pressure catheters and flow tube are in place, the clinician instructs the patient to repeat a series of speech samples. The author uses the syllables /pi/, /pa/, /bi/, /ba/, /si/ and /mi/, the word *hamper* and the sentence *Peep into the hamper*. Each sample is produced three to five times on a single breath and repeated at least twice.

As previously indicated, placement of the oral catheter must be behind the articulator of interest in order to record a valid pressure. For the /si/ sample, the oral catheter should be placed from the corner of the mouth so that the open end approximates the midline of the oral cavity.

Nasal mask approach

The pressure-flow method can be adapted for children as young as three years of age who may not tolerate the insertion of plugs and tubing into the nostrils. As illustrated in Figure 21.4,

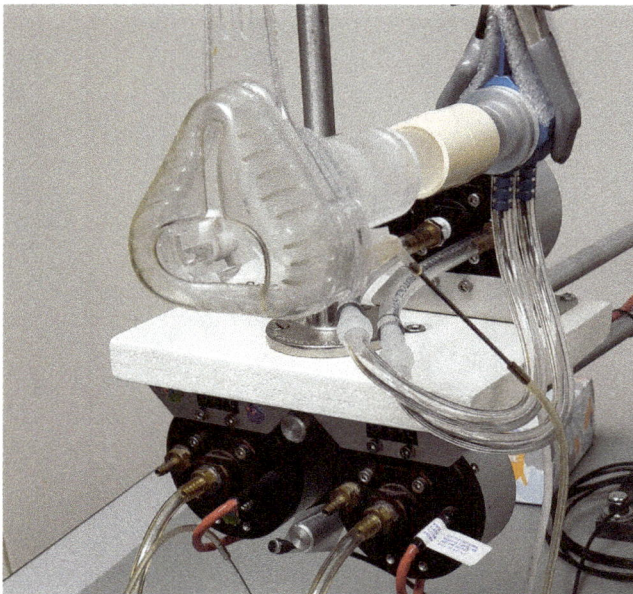

Figure 21.4   Nasal mask approach to pressure-flow testing.

a small nasal mask is used to eliminate the need for the flow tube and catheter plug. The open end of the mask is attached to the pneumotachograph; the nasal pressure catheter is attached to a tap on the mask. Because nasal mask pressure is detected rather than pressure within the nasal cavity, the differential pressure includes drops across both the velopharyngeal port and the nasal cavity. Estimated area, therefore, should be considered an effective velopharyngeal-nasal area. [6] As discussed later in the chapter, this actually may be an advantage relative to improving correspondence between area estimates and perceptual characteristics of speech.

Oral-nasal mask approach

The pressure-flow method as described above does not provide measures of oral airflow. Oral airflow can be obtained, however, by using a divided circumferentially-vented mask (Figure 21.5). The mask is partitioned into nasal and oral chambers. Each chamber has fine mesh, wire screens that serve as flow-resistive pneumotachographs. Catheters are inserted into each chamber to detect pressure variations associated with airflow. A microphone is positioned outside of the mask to record the audio signal. Because the resistive elements are located on the periphery of the mask, not centrally in the air stream, condensation is largely eliminated. Thus, heating of the wire mesh can also be eliminated.

Each chamber of the divided mask must be calibrated separately using a known flow rate as described above for the pneumotachograph. The catheters inside the chambers are connected to the high ports of separate differential pressure-transducers; low range transducers are used as with the pneumotachograph. Scale factors are obtained via software for each chamber. Calibration can be problematic due to the shape of the mask chambers. The author uses thermoforming plastic that is cut to the shape of each chamber to ensure a seal during calibration.

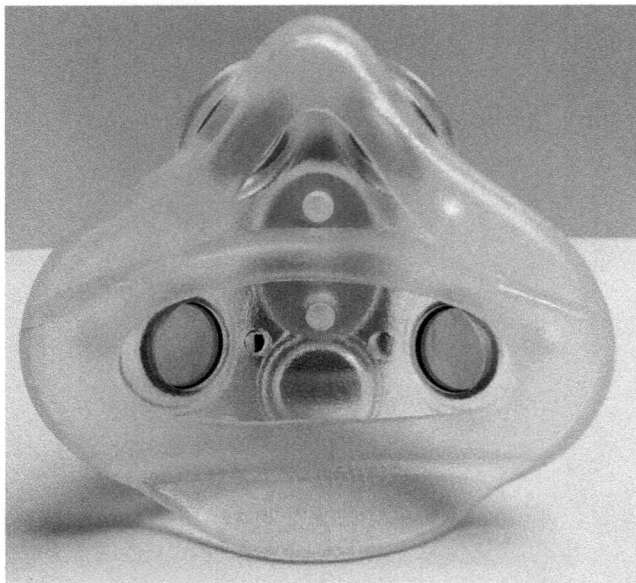

Figure 21.5   Divided oral-nasal circumferentially-vented mask.

Examples of aerometric outputs

The following three examples were obtained using the pressure-flow method as shown in Figure 21.2. Each output shows intraoral air pressure, nasal airflow and audio of the speaker; nasal air pressure was obtained but is not shown. Figure 21.6 shows output of an adult speaker with normal velopharyngeal function saying a series of five /pa/ syllables on a single breath. As shown in the figure, oral air pressure approximates 6 to 7 centimeters of water for the /p/ segments, typical of adult males (Zajac, 2000). Nasal airflow during breathing is evident before and especially after the utterance; positive airflow reflects exhalation and negative airflow reflects inhalation. The positive nasal airflow peak immediately prior to the first syllable is due to the transition of the velopharyngeal port from open during respiration to closed during speech. As shown in the figure, nasal airflow during the utterance is essentially zero reflecting complete velopharyngeal closure.

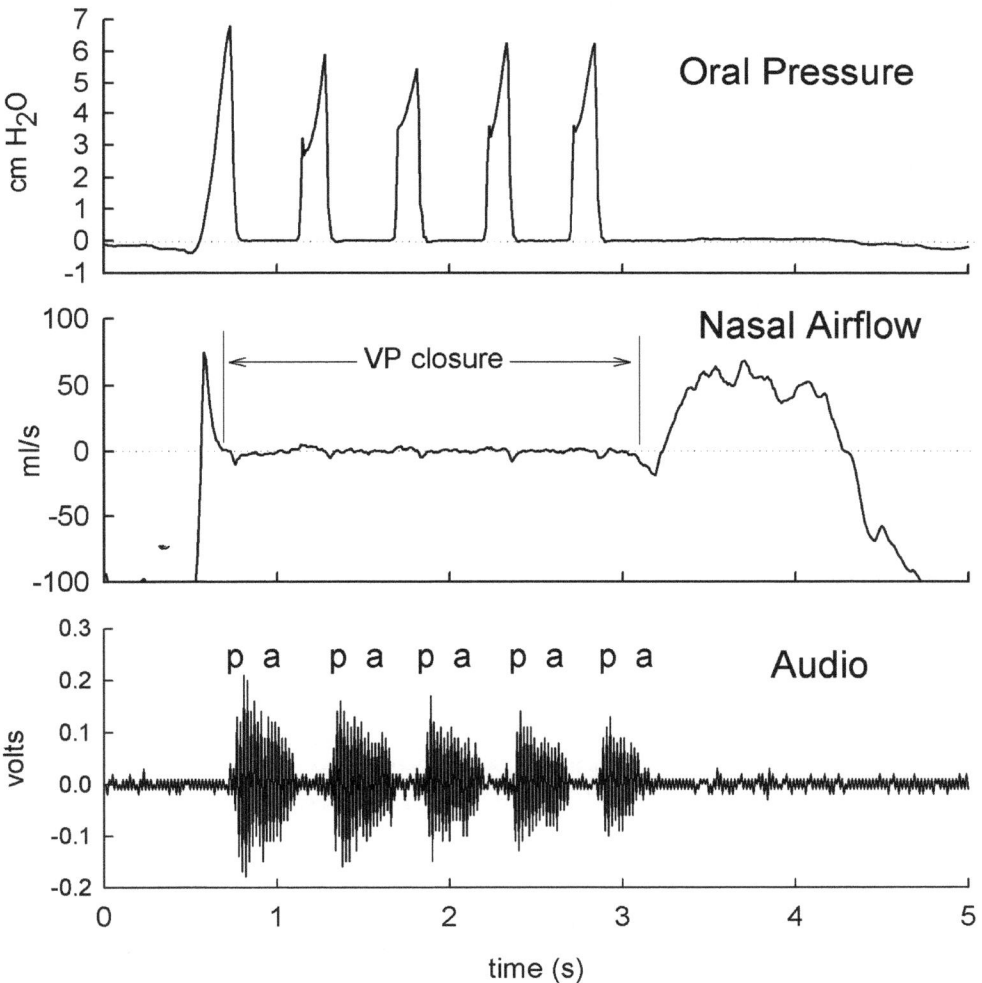

Figure 21.6 Pressure-flow output of a typical speaker saying /pa /syllables.

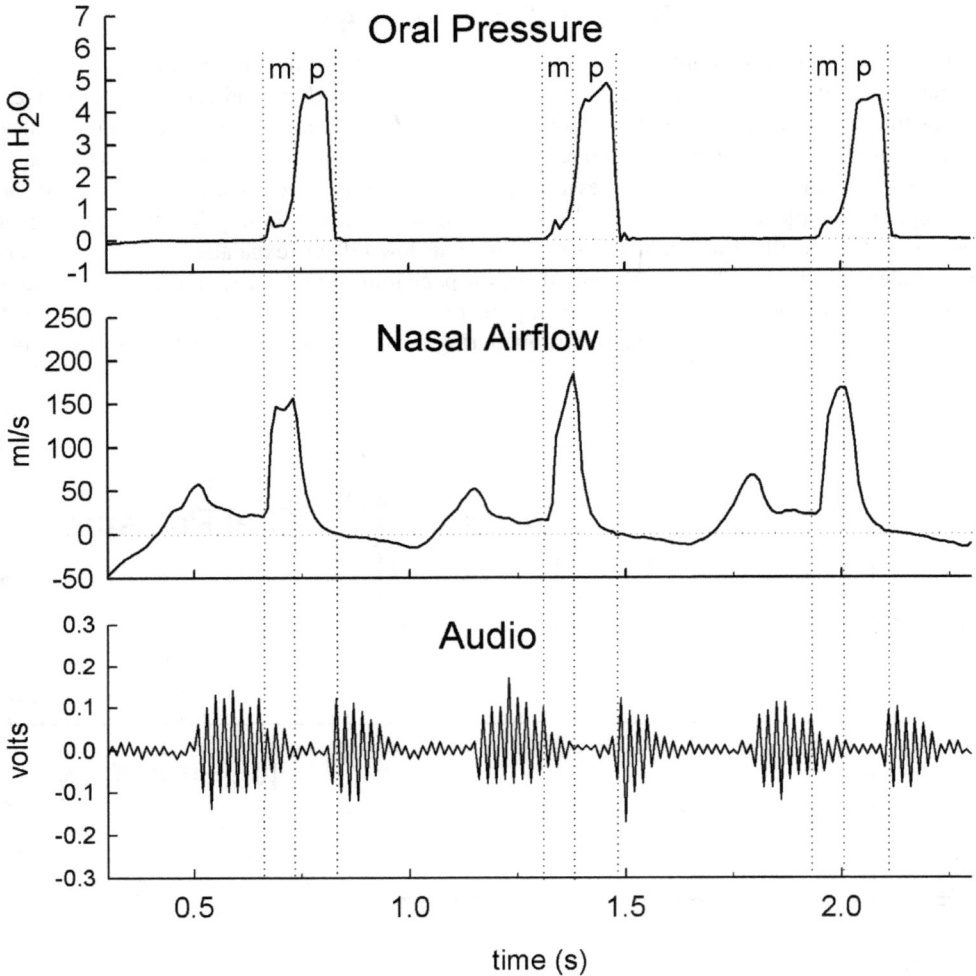

Figure 21.7 Pressure-flow output of a typical speaker saying *hamper* three times.

Figure 21.7 shows the same speaker as in the previous figure saying the word *hamper* three times on a single breath. Oral air pressure approximates 5 centimeters of water for each /p/ segment, slightly less than the speaker's production of /pa/. Nasal airflow peaks between 150 and 200 mL/s for each /m/ segment followed by a rapid decline toward zero for each /p/ segment. Estimated velopharyngeal areas during /m/ and /p/ segments were approximately 24 and less than 1 mm², respectively. These values are consistent with typical adult males (Zajac, 2000). Anticipatory nasal airflow prior to each /m/ segment is also evident in the figure. Although the phonetic segments are not labeled, nasal airflow begins with the /h/ segment and continues through the vowel of each word. Of note, nasal airflow is reduced during the vowel compared to the voiceless /h/ due to voicing.

Pressure-flow outputs from a speaker with repaired cleft palate saying *hamper* three times are shown in Figure 21.8. The speaker was a 13-year-old female who exhibited hypernasality, weak pressure consonants and audible nasal air emission (hissing type). The most striking

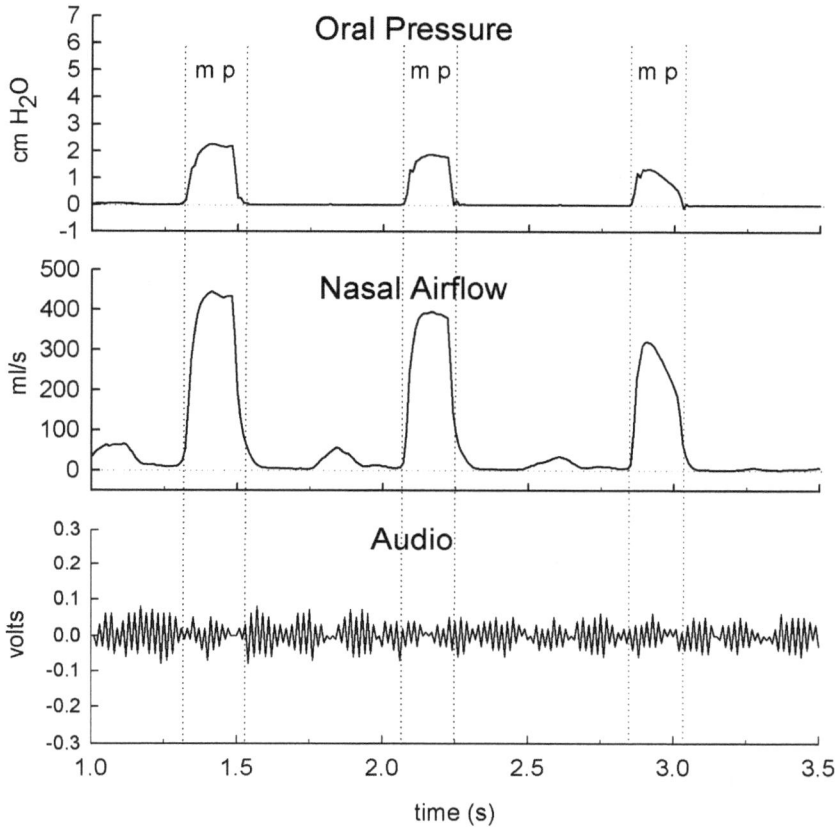

Figure 21.8 Pressure-flow output of a speaker with velopharyngeal dysfunction saying *hamper* three times.

feature of the output is the reduced oral air pressure associated with /p/ segments, only 2–3 cm of water. Although the speaker's nasal air pressure is not shown in the figure, it almost equaled oral air pressure. Thus, differential pressure was close to zero indicating an extremely large velopharyngeal opening, estimated at greater than 100 mm^2. Another striking feature of the output is the complete temporal overlap of the nasal airflow and oral air pressure pulses of the /m/ and /p/ segments. In essence, the speaker's VPD was so severe that she was not able to aero-dynamically separate the segments.

As previously noted, auditory-perceptual discrimination of obligatory versus learned nasal air emission may be difficult, even for experienced clinicians. Although the defining characteristic of a learned nasal fricative is an oral stopping gesture, this articulation is not always perceptually salient.[7] The following two examples illustrate oral-nasal airflow recordings obtained with a divided circumferentially-vented mask. The first is from a speaker who exhibited obligatory nasal air emission during production of both /p/ and /s/ phonemes. The second is from a speaker who produced /p/ normally but used a posterior nasal fricative to replace /s/.

Figure 21.9 shows nasal airflow, oral airflow and audio from a 6-year-old male who exhibited hypernasality and obligatory nasal air emission (hissing type) due to VPD. Although the child

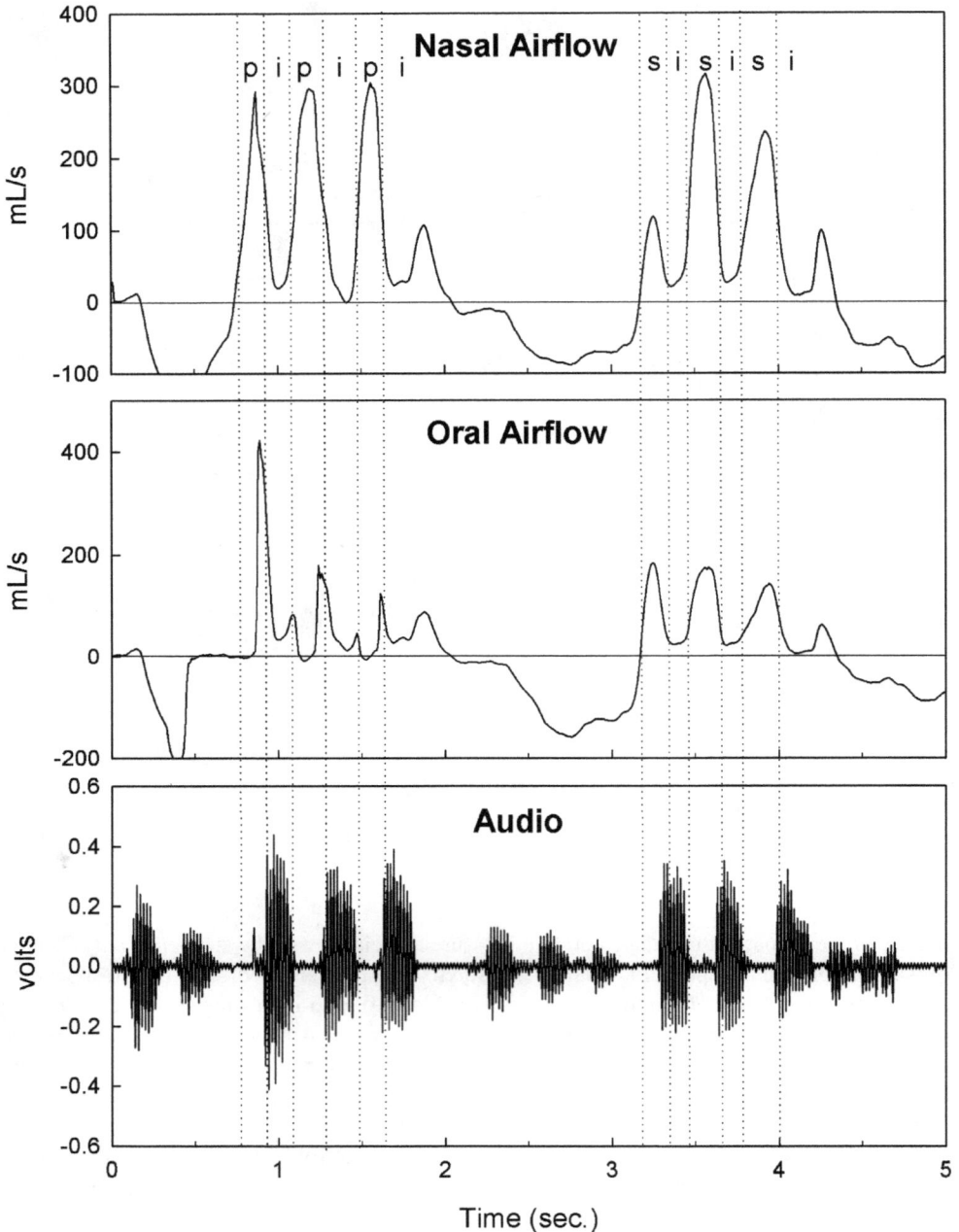

Figure 21.9 Nasal and oral airflow output of a speaker with obligatory nasal air emission.

did not have cleft palate, video nasoendoscopy showed a deep pharyngeal cavity that precluded velopharyngeal closure. The figure shows the child saying a series of three /pi/ syllables followed by a series of three /si/ syllables, each on separate breath groups. It should be noted that the fourth airflow peak in each series reflects end-of-utterance nasal and oral airflow, respectively. The extra audio signals preceding the child's productions are those of the examiner who prompted the responses. As shown in the figure, the child exhibited excessive nasal airflow on all /p/ and /s/ segments, often approaching 300 mL/s except for the first /s/ segment. This pattern of consistent nasal airflow during production of both stops and fricatives is a reliable indicator of obligatory audible nasal air emission due to a structural anomaly, a deep nasopharynx in this case.

Figure 21.10 shows nasal airflow, oral airflow and audio from a 9-year-old female who used posterior nasal fricatives to replace /s/. The child did not have cleft palate or VPD. The figure shows the child saying the same syllables as in the previous example. As shown in the figure, the child had complete velopharyngeal closure during production of /pi/ syllables as evidenced by the lack of nasal airflow.[8] Production of /si/ syllables, however, is accompanied by nasal airflow that approach rates of 200 mL/s and the absence of oral airflow, except during the vowel segments. In essence, the child produced /s/ as an oral stop, similar to the oral airflow of her /p/ productions. This pattern of (a) stops produced normally without nasal airflow and (b) fricatives produced abnormally with nasal airflow but without oral airflow is consistent with the use of nasal fricatives as a learned maladaptive articulation. It should be noted that a child who has VPD might also use nasal fricatives. In this case, there may be some obligatory nasal airflow during stops. The production of a nasal fricative, however, will still show the oral stopping component.

Some clinical studies

Dalston, Warren, Morr, and Smith (1988) used the pressure-flow method to study oral air pressure levels in 267 speakers with varying degrees of VPD. The speakers ranged in age from 4 to 58 years, most (93%) had repaired cleft palate. They produced the word *hamper* and were categorized into five groups based on velopharyngeal area during the /p/ segment: (1) "adequate" if area was less than 5 mm^2, (2) "adequate-borderline" if area was between 5 and 9 mm^2, (3) "borderline-inadequate" if area was between 10 and 19 mm^2, (4) "inadequate" if area was between 20 and 80 mm^2, and (5) "grossly inadequate" if oral and nasal air pressures were essentially equal that precluded accurate area estimates. Dalston et al. reported that peak oral air pressure associated with the /p/ segment decreased systematically across the five groups: 6.7 (SD = 2.4), 4.5 (SD = 1.9), 4.1 (SD = 1.7), 3.5 (SD = 2.0) and 3.0 (SD = 1.3) centimeters of water, respectively.

Warren, Dalston, Morr, and Hairfield (1989) used the pressure-flow method to investigate rate of nasal airflow in 107 speakers with repaired cleft palate. They ranged in age from 5 to 58 years. The speakers were categorized into four groups based on velopharyngeal area during the /p/ segment of *hamper*: (1) adequate, (2) adequate-borderline, (3) borderline-inadequate and (4) inadequate. Area criteria were the same as used by Dalston et al. (1988). Warren et al. (1989) reported that mean nasal airflow during production of /p/ increased systematically across the four groups: 32 (SD = 25), 102 (SD = 34), 149 (SD = 51) and 313 (SD = 188) mL/s, respectively.[9]

Speech aerometric techniques have also been used to investigate velopharyngeal function of individuals with various neurologic disorders. Rong et al. (2016) obtained nasal airflow along with kinematic (movement), acoustic and perceptual speech measures of 66 individuals with ALS. The patients were studied longitudinally to document progression of the disease and accompanying decline in overall speech intelligibility. Rong et al. (2016) obtained nasal airflow using a small nasal mask during production of syllables including /pi/ and the

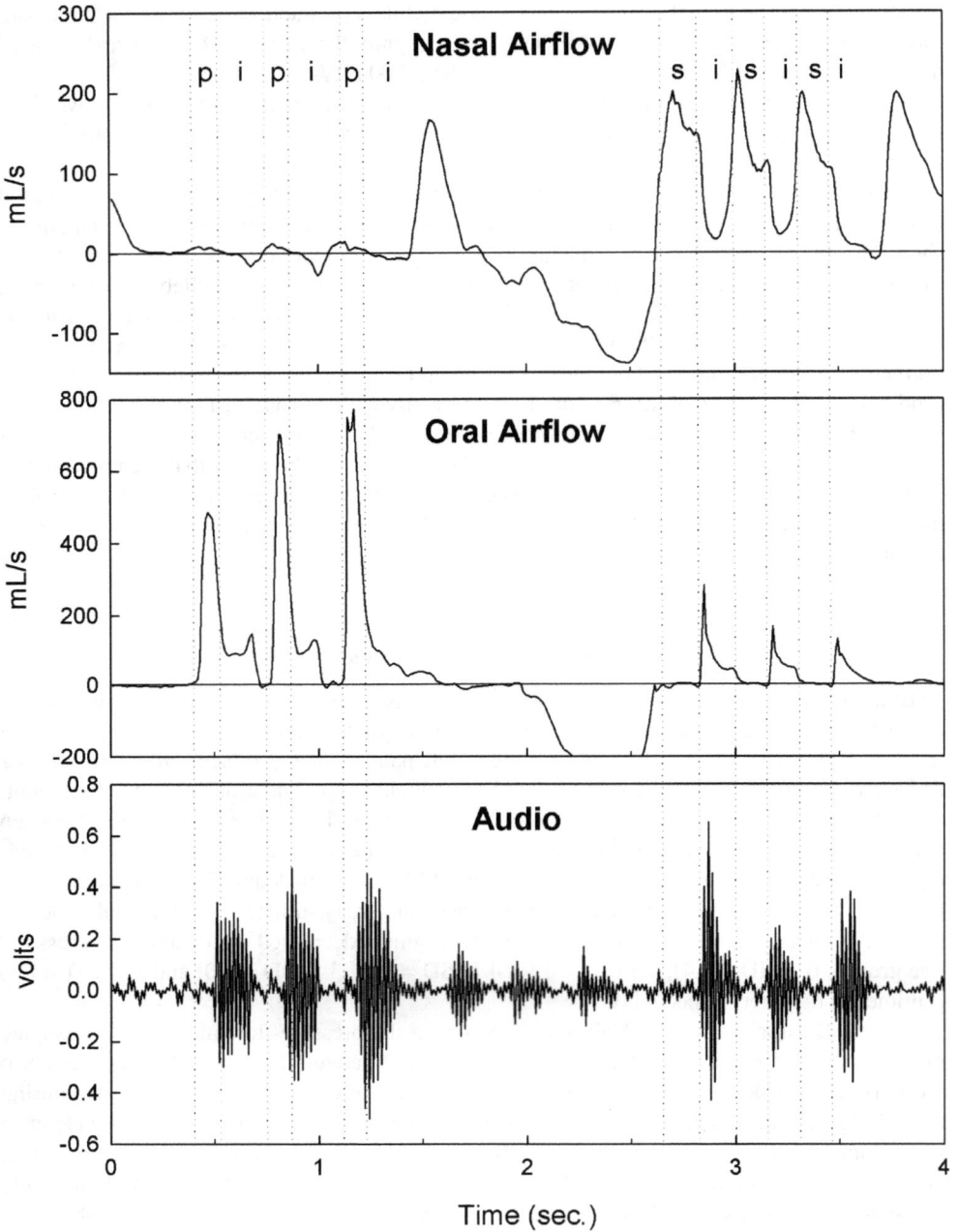

Figure 21.10 Nasal and oral airflow output of a speaker with active (learned) nasal air emission as part of a posterior nasal fricative.

word *hamper*. They reported that slowed lip and jaw movements accounted for the most variance (57.7%) followed by increased nasal airflow during /pi/ (22.7%) in predicting decline in speech intelligibility.

The PaCE index

Perrotta and Zajac (2019) introduced a new aerodynamic metric to describe velopharyngeal function using a speaker-centered approach. It involves calculation of a palatal closure efficiency (PaCE) index based on a speaker's production of the syllables /mi/ and /bi/, a nasal-stop minimal pair. Essentially, PaCE reflects the extent that a speaker achieves closure relative to his/her own velopharyngeal opening during production of the nasal consonant /m/. As reported by Zajac (2000), estimated velopharyngeal areas for /m/ are age dependent, with younger children typically having smaller areas than adults. The PaCE index is calculated as: $100 - ((bi \text{ area} \div mi \text{ area}) \times 100)$, expressed as a percentage.

To explain the index and highlight interpretation, consider the following clinical case of a three-year-old male with repaired unilateral cleft lip and palate. He exhibited moderate hypernasality and audible nasal air escape (hissing type), at times with a nasal grimace. Using the nasal mask approach (Figure 21.4), his estimated velopharyngeal-nasal areas during production of /mi/ and /bi/ were 9.8 and 7.3 mm², respectively. His calculated PaCE index was 26%, meaning that he was able to close the velopharyngeal port only 26% during /bi/ as compared to his opening during /mi/. Of interest, his estimated area for /bi/ would be considered "adequate-borderline" based on traditional area criteria (i.e. 5–9 mm²). Obviously, in this case, the PaCE index is more consistent with the child's moderate, at least, perceptual symptoms than traditional area categories. [10]

Perrotta and Zajac (2019) reported PaCE measures for 23 children and adolescents with repaired cleft palate between 6 and 18 years of age. Based on clinical assessments, most of the children had varying degrees of VPD, from mild to severe. A few of the children were judged to have adequate velopharyngeal function. The calculated PaCE indices, based on production of /mi/ and /bi/, ranged from 0 to 100% (mean = 60%, standard deviation = 36). These preliminary findings suggest that the PaCE index may have clinical utility. Major advantages of PaCE are that it is speaker-centered and expresses area estimates as part of a ratio, thus negating concerns regarding age differences and accuracy of area estimates, respectively. One potential disadvantage of PaCE is that two of the children studied by Perrotta and Zajac (2019) had larger estimated areas during /bi/ than /mi/, resulting in a negative PaCE. These cases were reported as zero. Obviously, additional research is needed to determine the overall clinical utility of PaCE, especially how it corresponds to perceptual symptoms such as weak pressure consonants and audible/turbulent nasal air emission.

Notes

1   Warren and DuBois (1964) initially used a single balloon-tipped catheter placed in the posterior oropharynx to detect pressure before the velopharyngeal port. The catheter was passed through a nostril and secured by a cork at a level just below the resting velum. The balloon was used to eliminate the possibility of saliva occluding the catheter. Because the balloon-tipped catheter was positioned behind the tongue, air pressures associated with the place of articulation of all stops (bilabial, alveolar and velar) could easily be detected without interfering with tongue movement. This approach, however, had two distinct disadvantages. First, the differential pressure also included a nasal pressure loss when the velopharyngeal port was open. This occurred because the pressure transducer was referenced to atmosphere. Calculated velopharyngeal area, therefore, was reduced, to some extent, due to the

additional nasal pressure drop. Although this could be corrected by obtaining nasal resistance of the speaker while breathing, the additional procedures were time consuming. Second, as discussed in the text, transnasal passage of a catheter is not practical in a clinical setting, especially with young children.

2 Orientation of the open end of the catheter perpendicular to the air stream avoids a spurious increase in pressure due to kinetic impact of air particles. Another way to avoid this is to plug the open end of the catheter and drill multiple side holes along the catheter wall. This will allow static pressure of the moving air stream to be detected without the influence of impact pressure.

3 PERCI-SARS is a hardware and software system marketed by MicroTronics Corp. (Chapel Hill, NC). It is specifically designed to obtain oral air pressure, nasal air pressure, nasal airflow and audio (voice) to calculate velopharyngeal area based on the orifice equation. The company, however, no longer sells new units of the system. TF32 is a commercially available software program developed by Paul Milenkovic at the University of Wisconsin (http://userpages.chorus.net/cspeech/). Although designed to obtain intraoral air pressure, oral airflow and audio to calculate laryngeal resistance, it can easily be modified to obtain nasal air pressure and nasal airflow. No hardware (e.g. pressure transducers, A/D converter), however, is provided with the program and the user must obtain these separately.

4 Fleisch pneumotachographs are no longer commercially available. Hans Rudolph, Inc., however, carries similar screen-type pneumotachographs (https://www.rudolphkc.com/).

5 Plastic tubing with various diameters can be obtained from sources such as Fischer Scientific (https://www.fishersci.com/us/en/home.html). These should be cut to lengths of approximately 5–6 inches. It is always better to use a flow tube with a slightly larger diameter than the patient's nostril to ensure a snug fit and prevent the escape of air.

6 As indicated in Note 1, the nasal pressure component due to the mask can be determined during quiet breathing and removed from the differential pressure. In the author's experience, this correction only marginally changes the area estimation except in cases of relatively increased nasal airway resistance.

7 Many clinicians who suspect a nasal fricative will occlude the speaker's nose while sustaining /s/. If a nasal fricative is produced, all airflow will abruptly stop due to oral occlusion. If oral airflow continues, then obligatory nasal air emission is indicated. This procedure, however, is not foolproof as the act of occluding the nose may facilitate oral airflow in some cases when nasal fricatives are present.

8 As shown in Figure 21.10, there are small positive and negative peaks of nasal airflow associated with each /pi/ syllable. These peaks reflect upward and downward movement of the elevated velum against the posterior pharyngeal wall due to active muscle contractions during each syllable. Upward movement will displace some volume of air out of the nose; downward movement will draw some air into the nose. The author refers to this phenomenon as "velar bounce."

9 Warren (1967) reported a strong linear relationship between velopharyngeal area and rate of nasal airflow in speakers with gaps up to 20 mm². When port size exceeded this value, especially 40 mm², the relationship plateaued. Warren attributed this to the nasal cavity becoming the flow-limiting factor when velopharyngeal area is large.

10 Even with a correction for the nasal pressure drop due to the mask, the child's estimated velopharyngeal area during /pi/ would be less than 10 mm², still in the adequate-borderline category.

References

Baken, R.J. & Orlikoff, R.F. (2000). *Clinical Measurement of Speech and Voice*, (*2nd Ed.*). San Diego, CA: Singular.

Dalston, R.D., Warren, D.W., Morr, K.E. & Smith, L.R. (1988). Intraoral pressure and its relationship to velopharyngeal inadequacy. *Cleft Palate Journal*, 25, 210–219.

Harding, A. & Grunwell, P. (1998). Active versus passive cleft-type speech characteristics. *International Journal of Language and Communication Disorders*, 33(3), 329–352.

Kummer, A. W., Curtis, C., Wiggs, M., Lee, L. & Strife, J.L. (1992). Comparison of velopharyngeal gap size in patients with hypernasality, hypernasality and audible nasal emission, or nasal turbulence (rustle) as the primary speech characteristic. *Cleft Palate Journal*, 29, 152–156.

Perrotta, L. & Zajac, D.J. (November, 2019). The PaCE index: A new pressure-flow metric to evaluate velopharyngneal function. Poster presented at the Annual Convention of the American Speech-Language-Hearing Association, Orlando, FL.

Peterson-Falzone, S., Hardin-Jones, M. & Karnell, M. (2001). *Cleft Palate Speech, (3rd ed.)*. St. Louis, MO: Mosby, Inc.

Rong, P., Yunusova, Y., Wang, J., Zinman, L., Pattee, G.L., Berry, J.D., Perry, B. & Green, J.R. (2016). Predicting speech intelligibility decline in amyotrophic lateral sclerosis based on the deterioration of individual speech subsystems. *PLoS One*, 11(5):e0154971. Published 2016 May 5.

Warren, D.W. (1964a). Velopharyngeal orifice size and upper pharyngeal pressure-flow patterns in normal speech. *Plastic and Reconstructive Surgery*, 33, 148–161.

Warren, D.W. (1964b). Velopharyngeal orifice size and upper pharyngeal pressure-flow patterns in cleft palate speech: A preliminary study. *Plastic and Reconstructive Surgery*, 34, 15–26.

Warren, D.W. (1967). Nasal emission of air and velopharyngeal function. *Cleft Palate Journal*, 16, 279–285.

Warren, D.W. & DuBois, A. (1964). A pressure-flow technique for measuring velopharyngeal orifice area during continuous speech. *Cleft Palate Journal*, 1, 52–71.

Warren, D.W., Dalston, R.M., Morr, K. & Hairfield, W. (1989). The speech regulating system: Temporal and aerodynamic responses to velopharyngeal inadequacy. *Journal of Speech and Hearing Research*, 32, 566–575.

Yates, C.C, McWilliams, B.J. & Vallino, L.D. (1990). The pressure-flow method: Some fundamental concepts. *Cleft Palate Journal*, 27, 193–198.

Zajac, D.J. (2000). Pressure-flow characteristics of /m/ and /p/ production in speakers without cleft palate: Developmental findings. *The Cleft Palate-Craniofacial Journal*, 37(5), 468–477.

Zajac, D.J. (2015). The nature of nasal fricatives: Articulatory-perceptual characteristics and etiologic considerations. *Perspectives in Speech Science and Orofacial Disorders*, 25, 17–28.

Zajac, D.J. & Preisser, J. (2016). Age and phonetic influences on velar flutter as a component of nasal turbulence in children with repaired cleft palate. *The Cleft Palate-Craniofacial Journal*, 53(6), 649–656.

Zajac, D.J. & Vallino, L.D. (2017). *Evaluation and management of cleft lip and palate: A developmental perspective*. San Diego, CA: Plural.

Zajac, D.J. & Yates, C. (1991). Accuracy of the pressure-flow method in estimating induced velopharyngeal orifice area: effects of the flow coefficient. *Journal of Speech and Hearing Research*, 34, 1073–1078.

22

LARYNGOSCOPY AND STROBOSCOPY

Duy Duong Nguyen, Catherine Madill, Antonia Chacon, and Daniel Novakovic

Historical overview of laryngeal visualization

Laryngoscopy originated as a technique for visualization of the larynx in the mid-1700s (Pantano, 2015). The first documentation of indirect laryngoscopy reported French surgeon André Leveret's use of a bent reflective spatula surface in 1743 to facilitate removal of antrochoanal polyps (Lapeña, 2013). Philipp Bozzini first described the principles of laryngoscopy in 1806, comprising of two metal tubes positioned parallel to one another, with either sun or candlelight used for illumination (Lapeña, 2013).

Laryngoscopy continued to develop in the ensuing century, with Charles Cagniard de la Tour developing a method of 'autolaryngoscopy' with the use of two mirrors; however, was limited in his ability to only visualize the epiglottis through this method (Lapeña, 2013). Devices developed thereafter, such as Benjamin Guy Babington's 'glottiscope' in 1829 and Francesco Bennati's tubular device in 1832 highlighted various challenges in laryngeal visualization, including the need for an appropriate light source and the likelihood of gagging from an inappropriately-sized apparatus (Bailey, 1996). Surgeon Robert Liston in 1840 recorded the first instance of using a dental mirror in laryngeal examination (Thomson, 1905), at a time where various surgeons began seeking to address the challenge of poor illumination through various light sources; culminating in Antoine Jean Desormeaux's projection of a directed light beam down the larynx through use of a gaslight lamp (Stell, 1990).

The first attempt at laryngeal photography occurred with Czermak's approach of using a refined mirror with a concentrated source of light in 1860 (Moore, 1937; Sircus, 2003), prior to Manuel Garcia's production of a laryngoscope using two mirrors and the sun as an external light source to view the glottis in 1881 (García, 1881). By 1895, Alfred Kirkstein developed an autoscope to perform the first documented instance of direct laryngoscopy. He is later described as adding an electric light source to the handle of the autoscope, enabling the epiglottis to be moved and the vocal folds visualized (Hirsch, Smith, & Hirsch, 1986).

Direct laryngoscopy

Introduction

Direct laryngoscopy (DL) is a procedure used to visualize the larynx via direct line of sight.

Indications and technique

DL is most widely used in the field of anesthesia for patients requiring endotracheal intubation. It is always performed in hospital with the administration of anesthesia and the primary equipment required is a laryngoscope with an integrated or attached light source. Absolute contraindications include patients with impeding airway obstruction due to glottic or supraglottic pathology.

In the field of Otolaryngology Head and Neck Surgery, DL is routinely used as the first part of a microlaryngoscopy procedure to gain access to the larynx for diagnostic or therapeutic purposes. The patient is anesthetized to optimize access and minimize upper airway reactivity and placed in a supine position; either flat or on a head ring. An appropriate laryngoscope with illumination is introduced transorally until the distal end of the scope is engaged in the vallecula or underneath the epiglottis, at which point the endoscope is lifted to expose the laryngeal structures. A laryngoscope holder can then be attached to the handle to secure the device externally.

Diagnostic use

Securing the laryngoscope places the patient into suspension, allowing hands-free line of sight access to the laryngeal structures for further diagnostic or therapeutic procedures. Direct visualization of the larynx has been superseded by the routine adjunct use of the surgical microscope or rigid endoscopes, which offer a greatly magnified view of laryngeal structures for diagnostic purposes once access has been established using DL.

Rigid endoscopes coupled to a remote camera head can be introduced to allow detailed videoendoscopy of laryngeal structures. With distal viewing angles ranging from 0 to 70 degrees, rigid videoendoscopy has the advantage of being able to closely inspect areas which are not in the DL line of sight, such as the laryngeal ventricle and the under surface of the vocal folds. When coupled with optical imaging technologies, rigid videolaryngoscopy can reveal hidden detail in conditions with vascular abnormalities.

The surgical microscope allows for detailed stereoscopic evaluation of the larynx at magnifications typically up to 400:1. Arguably the greatest diagnostic benefit of microlaryngoscopy is that it affords hands-free visualization, allowing the surgeon to introduce laryngeal instruments with both hands in order to palpate and manipulate laryngeal structures. This is especially important when assessing arytenoid mobility and examining the vocal folds for subepithelial pathology such as scar tissue or sulcus vocalis. When coupled with subepithelial saline infusion into the superficial layer of the lamina propria, microlaryngoscopy and palpation is a powerful exploratory diagnostic tool.

Indirect laryngoscopy

Introduction

Laryngoscopy is currently an indispensable examination method for visualizing and documenting anatomical, functional and pathological characteristics of the vocal folds and other pharyngeal and laryngeal structures. The term 'indirect laryngoscopy' refers to laryngeal examination procedures that allow the examiner to observe the larynx indirectly via an instrument which is either a laryngeal mirror (mirror indirect laryngoscopy) (Lapeña, 2013) or an endoscope (rigid or flexible indirect laryngoscopy). Indirect mirror laryngoscopy dates back to the nineteenth century when García introduced his laryngeal mirror for laryngoscopy in 1855 (Goldman & Roffman, 1975). With the development of advanced endoscopic technology, mirror laryngoscopy has been gradually replaced by indirect laryngoscopy using rigid and flexible endoscopes.

Indications and contraindications

Indirect laryngoscopy is used to visually assess laryngeal structures, subglottic areas, lower pharyngeal walls and piriform sinuses. The technique is indicated in patients with vocal symptoms, dysphagia, airway problems suspected of pharyngeal or laryngeal origin, pre- and post-thyroid surgery, a pharyngeal issue and suspected presence of a foreign body.

There is no absolute contraindication of indirect laryngoscopy. However, care must be taken in patients with dyspnea, stridor, a known history of laryngospasm and/or a suspected laryngeal or pharyngeal foreign body; especially in the child or elderly patient. A rarely occurring complication related to laryngoscopy is vasovagal syncope, which results in no health risk to most people but can be fatal for some patients with congenital cardiac conditions. It is essential that a careful history be taken in light of these factors, and that the patient is informed of all necessary details of the procedure.

Equipment

Mirror laryngoscopy

- Headlight
- Laryngeal or dental mirrors
- Gauze sponge
- Alcohol lamp, or an alternate heat source to warm the mirror
- Anesthetic spray (e.g. Xylocaine 10% spray)
- Ear Nose Throat (ENT) examination chair
- Personal protective equipment for the examiner: Facemask, examination gloves and eye goggles.

Rigid telescopic laryngoscopy

- 70-degree endoscope
- Light source and light cable
- Charge-coupled device (CCD) camera head and processor
- Liquid-crystal display (LCD) monitor
- Gauze sponge
- Local anesthetic spray (e.g. Xylocaine 10%)
- ENT examination chair
- Personal protective equipment for the examiner as mentioned above.

Technique

Mirror laryngoscopy

In performing a mirror laryngoscopy, the patient should be informed of both the indications for the procedure and associated risks. One or two sprays of Xylocaine 10% into the mouth is sufficient to anesthetize the pharynx for mirror laryngoscopy. This procedure should be undertaken in a well-lit room (Ponka & Baddar, 2013) with the patient seated upright in an examination chair facing the clinician. The patient is asked to lean forward with their chin directed upward, while relaxing their shoulders and arms. The clinician sits opposite the patient throughout the examination.

The mirror is warmed above an alcohol lamp to prevent fogging before its temperature is tested on the examiner's palm to ensure it is not hot. The patient is asked to open their mouth and protrude their tongue for the examiner to grasp with a gauze sponge. The patient is advised to relax and breathe regularly. The mirror is inserted gently into the mouth toward the rear of the tongue with the glass surface pointing downward. Care is taken to ensure the mirror does not contact the tongue base and posterior pharyngeal wall to avoid stimulating the gag reflex and blurring the mirror. Once the mirror is at the rear of the oropharynx, the examiner is to adjust its position and angle to visualize the target structures (pharyngeal walls, epiglottis, vocal folds). The patient is advised to continue breathing through his/her nose during the procedure. When examining the vocal folds, the patient is asked to phonate a prolonged /i:/ sound. This will help open the laryngeal inlet and the two vocal folds can be seen. The fogged mirror should be re-heated.

Rigid telescopic laryngoscopy

The clinician should provide an explanation to the patient regarding the procedure and possible risks, before answering any questions the patients may have. One to two sprays of Xylocaine 10% are administered into the pharynx. The patient is required to sit in the examination chair, lean forward and position their chin upward (sniffing position), gazing at a fixed point (e.g. picture) on the window or wall. This positioning must be maintained throughout the procedure. The patient's legs are to remain uncrossed and should be placed firmly on the footrest of the examination chair. The telescope is connected to the light cable and the camera head and is adjusted for accurate focus. The camera should be tested for white balance before scoping.

The patient is required to open the mouth and protrude his/her tongue for the clinician to grasp with a gauze sponge. He or she is advised to breathe gently and regularly through the nose during the procedure. The telescope with the 70°-viewing angle, directed downward, is inserted and directed to the back of the mouth to visualize the larynx. Care is taken not to contact the posterior pharyngeal wall with the tip of the scope. When the scope is in position, the patient is asked to take a deep breath and produce a prolonged /i:/ sound. The angle and position of the scope should be adjusted by the examiner while looking at the monitor to optimize their view of the larynx. Structures in view during scoping include the tongue base, epiglottis, vocal folds, arytenoids, anterior and posterior commissure, aryepiglottic folds, inter-arytenoid space, piriform sinuses and lower pharyngeal walls. Depending on diagnostic requirements, specific vocal tasks will be performed by the patient as directed by the examiner. Typical tasks usable in rigid laryngoscopy include prolonged /i:/ phonation and upward and downward pitch gliding on /i:/.

Interpretation of examination

In mirror laryngoscopy, the structures visible include the epiglottis in the upper margin of the mirror, the arytenoids in the lower margin and the aryepiglottic folds on either side. Note that the presenting image is contralateral to the clinician, so that the right vocal fold is visible on the left-hand side, and the anterior commissure at the top. In rigid laryngoscopy, the anterior commissure is presented at the bottom of the monitor screen, with the side still being contralateral to the examiner.

Anatomical landmarks and functional movements should be checked carefully for signs of malformation and abnormality related to airway, phonation and swallowing. Although mirror laryngoscopy can provide the view of the larynx in real color, it is challenging to evaluate small lesions such as varices or small vocal fold masses. It is therefore recommended to perform laryngoscopy using a rigid scope connected to a camera system or flexible videolaryngoscope for videolaryngoscopy as this enables review and close inspection of the recorded images. The epiglottis should have a slightly curved shape and smooth surface without any swelling, ulcerative, or corrosive lesions. The vocal fold mucosa should present with a translucent white color and smooth surface, with its medial edge being regular and straight. The glottis should close completely during phonation and open completely in respiration. The two arytenoids should move medially and laterally in synchronization with the movement of the vocal folds. The mucosa of the arytenoid should be smooth and not erythematous. The first few tracheal rings can also be observed in the subglottic area during abduction. The mucosa of the lower pharyngeal walls should be smooth and pink in color. Piriform sinuses should be clear and free of saliva (Figure 22.1).

Perceptual errors in indirect laryngoscopy have been documented by Brewer (1966), inclusive of technical errors (insufficient illumination, position of the patient, inadequate laryngeal mirror size, position of the laryngeal mirror) and recognition errors (e.g. lack of established routine, inability to visualize the anterior commissure due to epiglottic contraction, error in perception of mucus and mucosal changes). Caution must be taken to avoid these errors to ensure this serves as an accurate examination method for both clinical and research purposes.

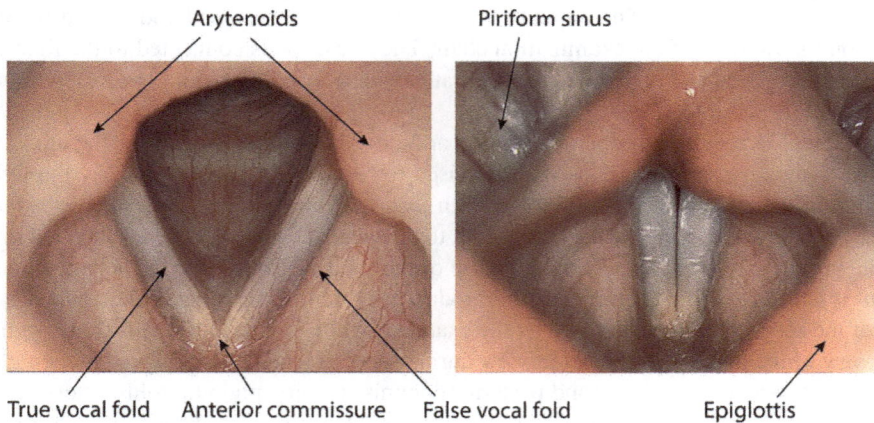

Figure 22.1 View of a normal larynx under rigid telescopic laryngoscopy. Left panel: Breathing/abduction position. Right panel: Phonation/adduction position.

Advantages and disadvantages

Mirror laryngoscopy

The advantage of mirror laryngoscopy is that it only requires simple equipment including a laryngeal mirror and a light source. In addition, with sufficient illumination, the target structures can be viewed in real color and size. Disadvantages include the dependence on an external light source, the inability to record images for review or future assessment and the lack of magnification. Compared with rigid videolaryngoscopy, mirror laryngeal examination is also considered inferior as it results in significant patient discomfort and gag reflex (Dunklebarger, Rhee, Kim, & Ferguson, 2009).

Rigid telescopic laryngoscopy

Rigid telescopic laryngoscopy, especially when coupled with a digital camera for video recording, is superior to mirror laryngoscopy in terms of patient comfort, laryngeal visualization extent and patient preference (Dunklebarger et al., 2009). A magnified, detailed and well-illuminated view of the vocal folds is the most advantageous feature of rigid laryngoscopy (Heman-Ackah, 2004) allowing the clinician to evaluate anatomical and pathological characteristics of the larynx, and for close-up examination of the vocal fold mucosa (Yanagisawa, Owens, Strothers, & Honda, 1983). These features make rigid laryngoscopy more accurate than flexible laryngoscopy in the assessment of mucosal lesions (Eller et al., 2009).

However, in rigid laryngoscopy, only limited, non-speech vocal tasks can be performed (mainly phonation of the prolonged vowel /i:/). This does not allow for examination of speech-related articulatory features of the larynx. Neck extension and tongue protrusion create an unnatural phonation position, resulting in laryngeal images that do not reflect the laryngeal postures present in normal physiologic states (Heman-Ackah, 2004), and can provoke supraglottic muscle tension patterns and preclude a clear view of the vocal folds. The determination of laryngeal features such as a glottal gap can be affected by rigid laryngoscopy (Chandran, Hanna, Lurie, & Sataloff, 2011). The assessment of abnormal muscle tension patterns is also not necessarily accurate through rigid laryngoscopy.

Transnasal flexible laryngoscopy

Introduction

Transnasal flexible laryngoscopy (TFL) using a constant light source is the most commonly used technique for visualization of the larynx. It is employed for both diagnostic and therapeutic purposes by most otolaryngologists and many speech language pathologists (SLPs). Also commonly known as fiberoptic nasendoscopy (FNE), it can be used to visualize the upper aero-digestive tract including the nasal cavity, nasopharynx and post-nasal space, oropharynx, hypopharynx, larynx and upper trachea in a simple and well-tolerated fashion in an office-based setting. Flexible endoscopes became commercially available in medicine in the 1960s (Campbell, Howell, & Evans, 2016) and were initially fiberoptic in design. There have been major technological advances in this field over time resulting in improved image quality and diagnostic/therapeutic capabilities. There are very few contraindications for TFL, the main being impeding airway obstruction from pathology such as supraglottitis where there is risk of laryngospasm. In such cases, TFL must be performed by an experienced operator in a controlled setting such as the operating room.

Equipment

Transnasal laryngoscopy requires a flexible endoscope of a diameter small enough to pass through the nasal cavity whilst retaining adequate resolution. A diameter of approximately 4 mm seems to be the optimal balance between image quality and patient comfort. Smaller diameter endoscopes (down to 2.6 mm) are useful for the pediatric population or difficult access patients, with some compromise on image quality and resolution. Larger diameter endoscopes (up to 5.1 mm) can be variably accommodated by most patients and may include a working channel for procedural intervention. A working length of 300 mm is standard. Endoscopes generally have a proximal control lever which can flex the end of the endoscope uni-dimensionally using wires integrated into the endoscope sheath.

There are two types of transnasal endoscopes:

- Fiberoptic laryngoscope (Analog) – the image is delivered to a proximal eyepiece using optical fibers integrated into the endoscope sheath. The image is viewed through the eyepiece or on a screen via an attached remote video camera head.

- Videolaryngoscope (Digital) – the image is captured on a small sensor at the tip of the endoscope and transmitted digitally to a processor for viewing on a screen. The sensor can be a CCD or complementary metal oxide semiconductor (CMOS).

In each endoscope, a light source is required to illuminate the region of interest. Light is usually delivered from an external source down the flexible endoscope by an optic fiber system, although more recent developments in technology have seen an LED light source integrated into the tip of some digital flexible endoscopes, including single-use disposable flexible endoscopes.

An LCD or LED screen with a video/image capture device is desirable for review and archiving purposes.

Topical anesthesia with nasal decongestant may be administered to the nasal cavity (either atomized or on cotton pledgets) to reduce patient discomfort (Sahin, Kokoglu, Gulec, Ketenci, & Unlu, 2017); however, the clinician must be aware of potential drug reactions and side effects. Lubrication gel, alcohol wipes and tissues are also useful to have on hand.

Technique

As with other forms of laryngoscopy, indications and risks are first discussed with the patient. Prior to endoscopy, the clinician briefly examines the anterior nasal cavity for any obvious anatomical factors (e.g. nasal septal deviation) which may impede passage of the scope. Topical anesthesia and decongestant (if used) is administered at this stage. The patient is seated comfortably in an examination chair and instructed to lean forward at the hips and extend the head whilst flexing their neck (sniffing position) (Figure 22.2).

The clinician passes the endoscope (usually via the more patent nares) into the nasal cavity. Generally, this is done along the floor of the nose between the septum and inferior turbinate, or just above the inferior turbinate until the scope reaches the post-nasal space. At this point, velopharyngeal competence can be assessed prior to proceeding further to the larynx by downward vertical deflection of the endoscope tip (Figure 22.3).

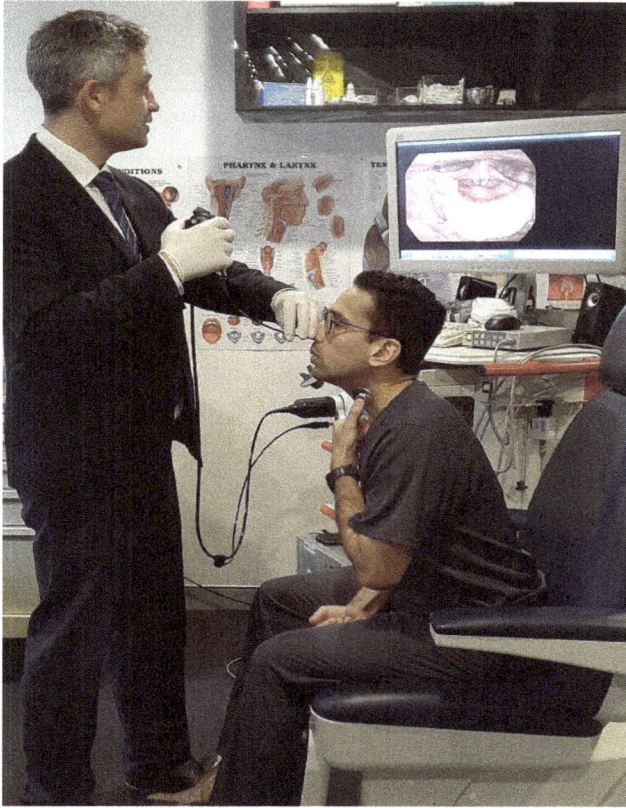

Figure 22.2   Position of the clinician and patient during flexible transnasal laryngoscopy.

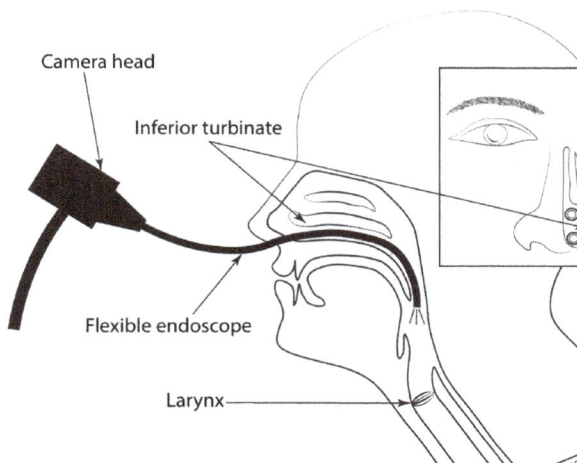

Figure 22.3   Transnasal flexible laryngoscopy. Inset: Coronal view showing the position of the flexible scope in the nasal cavity (circles).

Source: © Duy Duong Nguyen, used with permission.

Table 22.1 Vocal tasks for transnasal flexible laryngoscopy and stroboscopy evaluation

Instructions for a standardized assessment for visual evaluation of the larynx

Evaluating anatomical structures and nonvibratory movements of the larynx:

1 Breathing:

"Breathe normally for three complete breath cycles (inhalation and exhalation)."

2 Laryngeal diadochokinetic tasks:

"say /ʔiʔiʔiʔiʔiʔi/"

3 Maximum range of adduction and abduction with sniffing.

"Say /i/ then sniff as quickly as you can six times- /i/-sniff, /i/-sniff…"

Evaluating supraglottic movement on phonation:

4 Voice onset in connected speech:

"Count from 80-90 in your normal voice at a steady rate"
"Read the CAPE-V phrases as written here"
"Tell me what you will do after you leave here"

5 For singers:

"Can you please sing Happy Birthday"
"Can you please sing a verse and chorus from a song of your choice (that demonstrates the problem you are having with your voice)?"

Evaluating vocal fold vibratory characteristics (using videostrobsocopy) in addition to the above:

6 Production of a sustained vowel /i/:

"Say /i/ for as long as you can keeping the volume and pitch constant."

7 Production of a prolonged vowel with varying pitch and loudness:

"Say /i/ and go as high / low in pitch as you can"
"Say /i/ as quietly / loudly as you can"

Interpretation of examination

Once in view, the larynx and its surrounds are observed carefully during quiet breathing before the patient is asked to perform tasks to allow assessment of laryngeal function appropriate to the presenting complaint. These may include connected speech, sustained phonation, phonatory repetitive tasks, singing, laughing and even a trial of voice therapy tasks to provide biofeedback (see Table 22.1). A detailed description of features for evaluation of TFL examination is provided below (see Table 22.2).

Advantages and disadvantages

Advantages of TFL compared with other methods of laryngeal examination:

- Can be performed in an office-based setting with minimal or no anesthesia
- Well-tolerated by the majority of people with less propensity to trigger a gag reflex by stimulation of the oral cavity and oropharynx

Table 22.2 Specific features for evaluation of transnasal flexible laryngoscopy /stroboscopy parameters. Tasks listed refer to Table 22.1

Movement	Mucosa	Muscle tension	Mucosal wave
Constant light	Constant light	Constant light	Stroboscopic light
Assessed on breathing, tasks of sustained phonation or connected speech (Tasks 1–7)	Assessed during quiet breathing (Task 1)	Assessed on tasks of sustained phonation or connected speech (Tasks 4 - 7)	Assessed in sustained phonation at various frequencies and levels of loudness (Tasks 6 and 7)
Global appearance	Appearance/global structure of larynx	Any extraneous movement beyond the arytenoid/vocal fold	Amplitude
Asymmetry	Edema	Lateral supraglottic constriction obscuring vocal folds partially or completely	Progression
Axis	Erythema	Unilateral false vocal fold hyperfunction	Closure pattern – open vs. closed vs. normal range
Abnormal movement: – Abduction / adduction – Rotation – Sluggish movement – Abduction lag on repetitive tasks	Mucous lesions – location, nature, appearance	Anteroposterior supraglottal movements obscuring view of vocal folds	Phase symmetry
Paradoxical vocal fold movement during breathing	Vascular patterns (e.g. varix, herald vessel)	Vertical movement of the larynx	Periodicity
Arytenoid asymmetry Glottal closure Axis rotation on pitch glide			Inspiratory maneuver

- Allows for assessment of the entire upper aerodigestive tract; i.e. it is not just limited to visualization of the larynx
- Allows for an accurate assessment of laryngeal functions in an awake patient with the larynx in a physiologically natural state
- Addition of stroboscopic assessment can take place during the same examination
- Incorporation of working channels into flexible scopes allows for an extended range of therapeutic capabilities such as delivery of injectable agents, biopsy via flexible forceps and treatment of lesions using flexible laser fibers

Disadvantages of TFL:

- Resolution and color accuracy of flexible laryngoscopy has historically been inferior compared with transoral rigid endoscopy. Progressive technologies such as CCD and CMOS video chips have significantly closed the gap between rigid and flexible laryngoscopy, especially in recent years

- Topical nasal decongestant and anesthesia is generally required prior to examination
- Anatomical factors, especially structural abnormalities of the nose, may restrict the ability of the endoscope to pass comfortably in a small proportion of people

Strobolaryngoscopy

Historical background

The principle of stroboscopy was first discovered by Simon von Stamfer of Vienna in 1833, when it was identified as a means of studying periodic oscillation of objects (Tarafder, Chowdhury, & Tariq, 2012). The first laryngeal stroboscope was created by Öertel in 1878, comprising of a bright light shone upon a perforated rotating disk which reflected off a laryngeal mirror (Rajput & Poriya, 2017). Despite its clinical utility, the widespread use of stroboscopes in laryngeal examination was limited by the impact of background noise in altering the rate of image capture, decreased illumination with increasing disk rotation speed, poor image quality and the need for frequent disc-changing, amongst other factors (Hoffmann, Mehnert, & Dietzel, 2013; Tarafder et al., 2012).

In 1913, the first motion picture of the larynx was created by Chevronton and Vles, with the first laryngostroboscopic film being developed in the same year by Hegener and Panconcelli-Calzia (Moore, 1937). Hegener advanced strobolaryngoscopy further through the development of a disk stroboscope, involving a series of lenses that enabled the light source to focus upon the vocal folds without distortion. At the same time, Wethlo is reported to have developed a strobolaryngoscopic instrument renowned for its practicality and compact form (Moore, 1937). The principle of a flash tube was later introduced by Leo Kallen in 1932, which involved a gas-filled lamp emitting a sharp flash using transformers and induction coils once its voltage reached a particular valve (Kallen, 1932). The functionality and value of strobolaryngoscopy in aiding laryngeal diagnosis was endorsed widely by Stern, Weiss, Maljutin and Heymann, as they recognized that where a laryngoscope fails to identify an abnormality in vocal fold structure or function, a stroboscope holds the potential to reveal it (Moore, 1937).

How stroboscopy works

Two important visual phenomena underlie the principle of stroboscopy; the flicker-free perception of light and the perception of apparent motion (Mehta, Deliyski, & Hillman, 2010). In photographing moving objects, using a camera exposure time that is shorter than the time needed for an action/movement to take place leads to an image that is sharp in quality. In contrast, if a photo is taken using a long exposure time on a moving object, the resultant image will be blurred. If a fast-exposed image is taken continuously of quickly moving objects, the view in sequence will provide a slow-motion image of the object. Similarly, stroboscopy generates an apparent slow-motion view of vocal fold vibration by selectively capturing consecutive phases across successive vibratory cycles (Mehta et al., 2010).

In phonation, the human vocal folds vibrate at a fundamental frequency of hundreds of cycles per second (hertz). The human eye cannot capture this fast vibration under constant light. Stroboscopy technology uses flashing, short-lasting light instead of constant light to illuminate the vocal folds at varied time points across different cycles of mucosal vibration. If the frequency of the flashing light is exactly the same as that of vocal fold vibration, assumed to be perfectly periodic, the lights will illuminate the vocal folds at the *same* time point in the vibratory cycle and the observer will have the impression that the vocal folds are not moving.

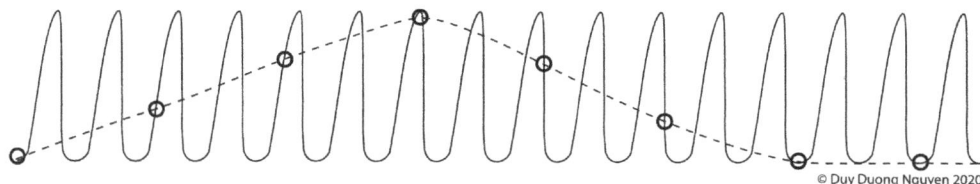

© Duy Duong Nguyen 2020

Figure 22.4 Principle of stroboscopy. The continuous line represents the vibratory waveform of the vocal folds. The black circles represent the moments in the vibratory cycle when the flashing light illuminates the vocal folds. The dashed line represents the reconstructed vibration pattern provided by stroboscopic images, which has a much lower frequency than the actual waveform.

If the time that the flash illuminates the vocal fold is adjusted, so that there is a phase difference between flashing/stroboscopic frequency and the vibratory frequency of the vocal folds, the light will *illuminate* different vocal fold positions across the successive cycles and the subsequent video image will be that of vibrating vocal folds in slow motion. The images provided by the stroboscopic light do not reflect the true vibration of the vocal folds, but rather, different moments across different vibratory cycles. If the flashing frequency is lower than vibration frequency (fundamental frequency) of the vocal folds, by capturing different vocal fold positions across successive vibratory cycles and reconstructing the image sequence in a certain frame rate, the visual effect is that the vocal folds appear to vibrate *more slowly* than they do in actuality. The continuous flow of images provided by the stroboscope results in a visual representation of a waveform pattern with a significantly lower frequency than the actual waveform (Figure 22.4). The frequency of the reconstructed wave (Δf) is equal to the difference between the original fundamental frequency of the vocal folds and the flashing/stroboscopic light frequency.

If the flashing frequency is slightly higher than fundamental frequency, there will be a reversal of the reconstructed waveform so that the mucosal waves seem to propagate toward the glottis (rather than away from the glottis), creating an artifact. In addition, there are circumstances where the image by stroboscopy will be affected. If the light exposure time is too long, then the image will be blurred. Furthermore, if there is irregularity in either the frequency of the vocal folds (for example, in voice disorders) or the frequency of the flashing light, the stroboscopic image sequence will be distorted.

The rate at which the stroboscopic light flashes is therefore dependent on the fundamental frequency of vocal fold vibration. For stroboscopy to function correctly, a microphone or electroglottograph that can detect the fundamental frequency of phonation must be attached to the computer; regulating the stroboscopic light source to enable the flashing rate to be adjusted as fundamental frequency changes during phonation.

Equipment

Stroboscopy can be performed using either a rigid transoral endoscope coupled to a camera, or a flexible videolaryngoscope; both of which are detailed above. Fiberoptic laryngoscopy is generally of insufficient image quality to provide useful additional information during the stroboscopic examination. A laryngeal microphone (often surface mounted to the neck) or electroglottograph receives real-time phonation frequency information. This is transmitted to the stroboscopy processor, which adjusts and controls the frequency of light delivered by the endoscope based upon the real-time phonation information received. The processor and light control system are generally integrated into the stroboscopic light source as a single unit.

Stroboscopic light systems are implemented in different ways according to the manufacturer. In some, a Xenon or LED light source is emitted in an extremely short burst (5 ms). Other systems rely upon a constant LED light source which electronically shutters the image sensor of the camera (Mehta & Hillman, 2012). In addition to the incoming frequency signal, the stroboscopic unit must also synchronize the recording camera unit to ensure that frame dropouts do not occur. A recording system that integrates the audio and video data collected during the examination is imperative for archiving, review and longitudinal tracking. This should also record data about vibration frequency in a readable fashion.

Strobolaryngoscopy technique

Techniques for stroboscopic examination of the vocal folds can be considered an extension of those described above for flexible and rigid laryngoscopy. Stroboscopy is performed as part of that same examination, giving supplemental information to that obtained during white light endoscopy. The operator must first instruct the light control system to switch from continuous to stroboscopic light source mode. This is usually done by way of foot pedal control but can also be performed manually if independent light sources are being used. The patient is instructed to perform sustained phonation at multiple frequencies and intensities relevant to the presenting symptoms. The focus of the examination at this point should be on the vocal folds themselves, with the operator adjusting the position of the camera to give an optimal view of both vocal folds during entrained mucosal wave vibration. The camera should be positioned as close as possible to the vocal folds while remaining comfortable for the patient. Supplemental techniques can be employed here, such as the inspiratory maneuver (asking the patient to breathe in whilst phonating) to gain extra information about vibratory characteristics, or supraglottic deconstriction maneuvers, which improve the view of vocal fold vibration in case of obstruction by specific patterns of supraglottic muscle tension. It is always recommended that the stroboscopic exam is recorded along with audio, frequency and intensity data. This allows for slow motion playback and assessment of potentially important findings which may not have been appreciated during the initial examination. Table 22.1 shows common tasks that are used in stroboscopy examination.

Interpretation of strobolaryngoscopic assessment

Interpretation of visual images of the larynx requires subjective evaluation of what is seen by the clinician. As in any subjective evaluation of a perceptual phenomenon, identification and quantification of specific features can be influenced by a range of factors. Image quality, clinician experience and training, clear understanding and definitions of the features of interest, evaluation of single versus multiple features at a time and use of comparison or anchor stimuli to which features can be compared all impact the reliability of rating visual and auditory perceptual phenomena (Hapner & Johns, 2007; Iwarsson & Reinholt Petersen, 2012). Subsequently, it is recommended that clinicians use a rating system to guide their evaluation and interpretation of laryngoscopic images. A number of laryngoscopic and stroboscopic rating tools have been developed over the last 25 years. These include The Australian Fiberscopic Profile (AFP) (Pemberton et al., 1993), The University of Wisconsin Videostroboscopic rating form (Bless, 1991), the Stroboscopy Research Instrument (Rosen, 2005) and the Voice-Vibratory Assessment with Laryngeal Imaging (VALI) (Poburka, Patel, & Bless, 2017).

All of these rating tools include a range of common features for the clinician to identify and evaluate upon inspection of laryngoscopic footage, with some listing a large range of features requiring detailed analysis. A simplified system for evaluating TFL and stroboscopy of the larynx is to systematically consider four main categories; movement, mucosa/mucosal lesions, muscle tension and mucosal wave.

Movement

Movement within the larynx includes those of the arytenoid complex and the vocal folds, changes in laryngeal posture around its axis (rotation), and changes in vertical position. In the ideal, nonpathological larynx, movement of both vocal folds should be equal and symmetrical with respect to range and speed of motion. Movement is assessed at rest (during quiet breathing), on sustained phonation and during a range of vocal tasks. These tasks are designed to unmask subtle asymmetry, such as abduction lag or sluggish movement, which may be a sign of neurological dysfunction of the larynx. The examiner should also look for evidence of inappropriate vocal fold abduction during inspiration and any abnormal movements such as laryngeal tremor at rest or during phonation.

Mucosa/Mucosal lesions

Mucosal features of the larynx related to color, erythema, edema and vascular pattern should be systematically evaluated. Organic lesions of the vocal fold or elsewhere in the larynx may be identified and characterized. The contour of the vocal fold medial edge (straightness, smoothness and superior mucosal surface) should be assessed. The presence of accumulative mucus can affect rating, so the patient should be asked to perform a throat clear followed by a swallow to facilitate visualization. The addition of spectroscopy where available can enhance the identification of vascular markings, which may be relevant for some pathologies such as carcinoma.

Muscle tension

Muscle tension patterns refers to global movements of laryngeal structures during phonation and are best evaluated using flexible transnasal laryngoscopy. Supraglottic muscle tension constriction patterns can be seen in both vocally-healthy phonation as laryngeal articulation in certain phonemes (e.g. glottal stops) (Stager, Bielamowicz, Regnell, Gupta, & Barkmeier, 2000), and muscle tension voice disorders (muscle tension dysphonia with or without vocal fold mucosal lesions) (Koufman & Blalock, 1991; Morrison & Rammage, 1993). Antero-posterior (AP) constriction is the appearance of movement of the epiglottis toward the arytenoids such that the endoscopic view of the vocal folds is precluded in part or in whole. Several rating scales of AP constriction exist to classify degree of this tension pattern. Lateral constriction is the medial compression of the false vocal folds toward the midline, which may partially or completely obscure the endoscopic view of the vocal folds during phonation. Similar rating scales exist for this muscle tension pattern (Morrison & Rammage, 1993). Asymmetry in muscle tension patterns, such as unilateral false vocal fold hyperfunction or unilateral arytenoid prolapse, should raise suspicion regarding a possible underlying nonfunctional cause of dysphonia.

Mucosal wave

The mucosal wave is an important component which distinguishes the diagnostic capabilities of stroboscopic examination above and beyond those of white light endoscopy alone. It gives critical information about the functional aspects of vocal fold mucosal vibration throughout the glottal cycle.

There are several important measures to be considered within this category that reflect the function of the vocal fold mucosa:

- *Phase symmetry* is evaluated by comparing the direction and amplitude of the mucosal wave between the left and right vocal folds. Symmetry can be assessed as *in phase, 90° out of phase*, or *180° out of phase*.
- *Phase closure* is the rating of the relative duration of each of the stages in a vibrating cycle. The outcome can be normal closure, predominating open phase (e.g. in breathy voice), or predominating closed phase (in strained voice/hyperfunctional state). Phase closure is an important stroboscopy criterion to evaluate whether there exists a glottic insufficiency, which can vary greatly from subtle to an extensive degree.
- *Amplitude* refers to the lateral displacement of the vocal fold free edge during the glottal vibratory cycle.
- *Regularity* relates to the periodicity of the vocal fold vibratory pattern over successive cycles. On the rating form this can be any degree between *always regular* and *always irregular*, or *regularly regular* and *irregularly regular*.
- *Vertical plane* is the height difference between the vocal fold medial edges in the closed phase.
- *Nonvibrating portion* refers to the presence of a mucosal area that does not vibrate in phase with the vocal fold mucosa.
- *Glottal shape* is determined during the closed phase and may indicate complete closure, incomplete closure, an hour-glass glottal shape, anterior glottal gap, posterior glottal gap, spindle gap, irregular glottal gap, or variable gap (Figure 22.5). The assessment of glottal shape necessitates using a flexible endoscope as rigid strobolaryngoscopy images do not reflect the view normally seen in natural phonation.

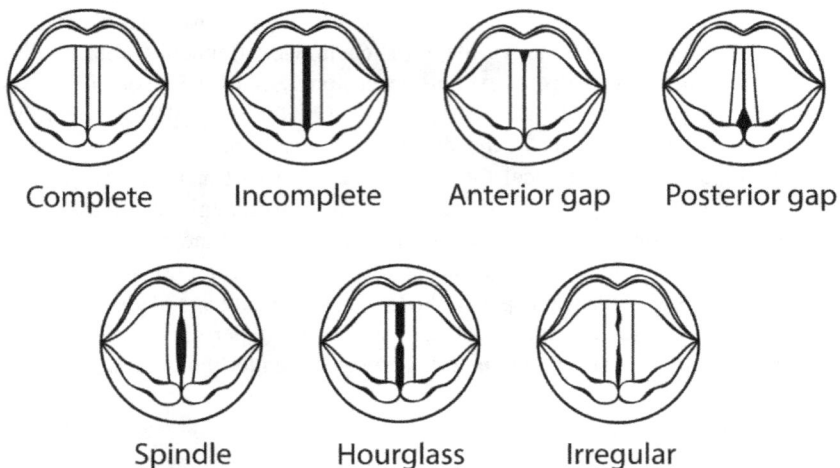

© Duy Duong Nguyen 2020

Figure 22.5 Glottal closure patterns observed during flexible laryngoscopy.

A standardized battery of vocal tasks is recommended for comprehensive assessment of laryngeal function during laryngoscopy with stroboscopy (Table 22.2). Key features of the exam should be systematically identified and documented as necessary across the four main categories discussed above. Of these, movement, mucosa and muscle tension can be examined using white light endoscopy. Evaluation of the mucosal wave requires supplemental stroboscopy.

Strobolaryngoscopy rating form

Strobolaryngoscopy allows the examiner to assess dynamic aspects of laryngeal function (Poburka, 1999) which provide critical information for diagnosis, treatment planning, and outcome assessment. Findings from strobolaryngoscopy can be assessed both quantitatively and qualitatively. With advanced personal computers and image analysis programs, strobo-scopic images can be processed to quantify the glottal area waveform and obtain information regarding the vibratory patterns of the vocal folds (Noordzij & Woo, 2000). Although such ana-lyses are useful for understanding vocal fold physiology, in daily clinical practice, quantitative analyses of stroboscopic images are time-consuming and impractical. Therefore, stroboscopy assessment mainly depends upon the examiner's perception of visual information, which is subjective and prone to reliability issues. A number of studies have shown low to moderate intra- and inter-rater reliability of stroboscopic rating. Some authors have found that inter-rater reliability for some parameters (vertical level, glottal closure, phase closure, phase symmetry and regularity) is too low to be rated in stroboscopy (Nawka & Konerding, 2012). The design and use of stroboscopy rating forms is one of the factors that influences the reliability of strobo-scopic assessment.

There are a range of stroboscopy rating forms to be found in the literature. However, it is worth summarizing four major categories that need to be included in any rating system.

Vocal fold movement

An example of measures to be assessed for vocal fold movement is shown in Table 22.3, which is part of an online stroboscopy rating form used in Bridge2practice.com (Madill, Corcoran & So, 2019), which the authors designed for clinical assessment and clinician training. Movement evaluation involves identification of normal and abnormal vocal fold position, adduction, abduction, length and axis rotation during phonation and requires the patient to perform spe-cific tasks (Tables 22.1 and 22.2).

Table 22.3 Ratings of vocal fold movement

Movement			
Gross vocal fold movement (Right)	☐ Normal	☐ Decreased	☐ Absent
Gross vocal fold movement (Left)	☐ Normal	☐ Decreased	☐ Absent
Abduction lag	☐ None	☐ Left	☐ Right
Axis rotation at rest	☐ None/NA	☐ Clockwise	☐ Anticlockwise
Axis rotation on pitch glide	☐ None/NA	☐ Clockwise	☐ Anticlockwise
Vocal fold length	☐ Equal	☐ Left shorter	☐ Right shorter

Table 22.4 Ratings of muscle tension

Muscle tension				
Unilateral false vocal fold hyperfunction	☐ None	☐ Left	☐ Right	
Lateral supraglottic constriction	☐ Absent	☐ Mild	☐ Moderate	☐ Severe
Antero-posterior supraglottic constriction	☐ Absent	☐ Mild	☐ Moderate	☐ Severe

Muscle tension

Table 22.4 shows three important abnormal muscle tension patterns that need to be judged during strobolaryngoscopy. The rating and documentation of these patterns are implemented most accurately using flexible scoping, as this allows for natural phonation. Judgment of muscle tension patterns during rigid laryngoscopy is not recommended. The ratings of AP constriction are based on the visibility of the vocal fold length from the anterior commissure to the vocal process of the arytenoid. If more than three-quarters of the vocal fold can be visible, the AP constriction is mild. If half of the vocal fold length is visible, AP constriction is moderate. If less than one quarter of the vocal fold length is visible, AP constriction is severe. Lateral constriction is rated based on the degree of medial compression of the false vocal folds toward the midline that precludes visibility of vocal fold width at the mid-point of the membranous portion. Mild, moderate and severe lateral constriction corresponds to visibility of more than two-thirds, half and less than half of the vocal fold width, respectively.

Mucosal wave

An example of the stroboscopy form for assessing the mucosal wave is shown in Table 22.5. Documenting the mucosal wave is the most challenging task in stroboscopy rating and is associated with considerable intra- and inter-rater inconsistency. The judgment of phase closure is difficult as the rater/clinician must estimate the relative duration of the open and closed phases and essentially transform the visual images into a mental representation of a glottal waveform (Poburka, 1999). Phase symmetry is a parameter used to evaluate whether the two vocal folds are vibrating as a mirror image of each other (in phase) or whether they are in different phases by 90° or 180° (out of phase) (Woo, 2009). Periodicity is another parameter associated with low reliability (Nawka & Konerding, 2012) and will require different tasks in different pitch ranges to be identified (Poburka, 1999). It is not possible to judge irregularity

Table 22.5 Ratings of mucosal wave

Mucosal wave				
Glottic closure	☐ Complete	☐ Irregular	☐ Incomplete	☐ Hourglass
	☐ Anterior gap	☐ Posterior gap	☐ Spindle gap	
Vertical level on phonation	☐ On-plane	☐ Left lower	☐ Right lower	
Phase symmetry	☐ In-phase	☐ 90° out-of-phase	☐ 180° out-of-phase	
Phase closure (modal voice)	☐ Normal	☐ Predominating open phase	☐ Predominating closed phase	
Amplitude/progression (R)	☐ Normal	☐ Decreased	☐ Increased	
Amplitude/progression (L)	☐ Normal	☐ Decreased	☐ Increased	
Periodicity	☐ Regular	☐ Regularly irregular	☐ Irregularly irregular	

Table 22.6 Ratings of mucosal lesions

Mucosa/Mass lesions			
VF edge/contour (Right) □ Normal/smooth	□ Bowed/concave □ Convex		□ Irregular
VF edge/contour (Left) □ Normal/smooth	□ Bowed/concave □ Convex		□ Irregular
VF lesion present □ None	□ Unilateral	□ Left	□ Right
VF lesion position □ Anterior commissure	□ Anterior VF	□ Mid VF	□ Posterior VF
□ Superior surface	□ Free edge	□ Inferior surface	
Other mucosal lesions □ VF erythema	□ VF edema	□ VF varices	□ Thick mucus
Mucosal lesions noted □ Polyp	□ Cyst	□ Nodules	□ Sulcus
□ Scar	□ Neoplasm	□ Pseudocyst	□ Hemorrhage

in vocal fold vibration when the stroboscopy device fails to accurately track the fundamental frequency of the mucosal wave, leading to temporary changes in stroboscopic images, such as quivering (Poburka, 1999).

Apart from gross mucosal wave patterns, it is important to identify and describe nonvibrating portions with regard to size, location and color.

Mucosal characteristics

The stroboscopy rating form should include fields to judge the vocal fold mucosa in terms of contour, color and the presence/absence of pathologies (Table 22.6). The vibrating/medial edge should be evaluated during breathing, normal phonation and inhalation phonation for features such as smoothness and straightness. It is more difficult to judge medial edge straightness when it is irregular/not smooth. Therefore, checking during both respiration and phonation with specific tasks is necessary for accurate assessment.

Advantages and disadvantages of strobolaryngoscopy

Stroboscopy allows for visualization of vocal fold mucosa vibration and provides a clinical visual record of vocal function (Bless, Hirano, & Feder, 1987; Hirano, Yoshida, Yoshida, & Tateishi, 1985; Mehta & Hillman, 2012; Poburka & Bless, 1998). It enables more accurate diagnosis (Sataloff, Spiegel, & Hawkshaw, 1991) and is particularly useful in the diagnosis of patients with functional dysphonia (Casiano, Zaveri, & Lundy, 1992), vocal fold paralysis (Estes, Sadoughi, Mauer, Christos, & Sulica, 2017) and in the detection of subtle vocal fold lesions. Strobolaryngoscopy can impact intervention planning and treatment outcome (Casiano et al., 1992). The use of stroboscopy in a multidisciplinary model of care has been shown to result in changes in diagnosis and treatment (Cohen et al., 2015). Stroboscopy is also useful in planning voice therapy (Brockmann, 2006) and making surgical decisions (Mehta & Hillman, 2012).

There are, however, disadvantages associated with stroboscopic examination. It is a reconstruction of a sequence of images captured from different successive vibratory cycles as a slow-motion view, rather than a real-time image (Wittenberg, Tigges, Mergell, & Eysholdt, 2000). Given its dependence upon vocal fundamental frequency tracking, stroboscopy only works reliably for periodic vocal fold vibration (Mehta & Hillman, 2012) and stroboscopic data may not be interpretable for vibratory function in severe dysphonia (Patel, Dailey, & Bless, 2008). It cannot investigate irregular vibrations (Švec & Schutte, 1996) nor the onset and offset of phonation (Cutler & Cleveland, 2002). It also requires complicated and expensive equipment associated with extensive clinical training and clinician experience (Poburka & Bless, 1998). The documentation of stroboscopy findings requires dedicated rating forms, which is impractical to use in clinical settings as a result of complicated rating scales (Poburka et al., 2017). It is also difficult and time-consuming to quantify stroboscopy parameters (Woo, 1996). The reliability in stroboscopy ratings is low especially for phase closure and regularity (Nawka & Konerding, 2012; Poburka & Bless, 1998). Finally, the stroboscopic assessment in pediatric patients is more challenging than in adults (Hartnick & Zeitels, 2005; Mortensen, Schaberg, & Woo, 2010).

Enhanced optimal imaging of the larynx

Introduction

Several recently developed technologies have been introduced by various manufacturers to help improve sensitivity and diagnostic accuracy during flexible endoscopy procedures, including laryngoscopy. Known by various names including virtual chromoendoscopy, optical imaging and digital chromoendoscopy, these are designed to provide detailed contrast enhancement of the mucosa and blood vessels as an alternative to more traditional dye-based chromoendoscopy techniques, with an aim to help highlight and identify pathologies in a manner that is superior to white light endoscopy alone (Manfredi et al., 2015). Some systems rely on post-image processing to enhance color and contrast. In laryngoscopy, the most widely studied optical image enhancing technology is Narrow Band Imaging (NBI), proprietary of the Olympus Corporation. It works on the principal of filtering light delivered from a xenon lamp to allow only two narrow bands to pass through to the tissue of interest (415 nm and 540 nm), which correspond to the absorption light peaks of hemoglobin. The result of this is a strong emphasis upon blood vessel visualization in the resulting endoscopic image.

Classification and application

By enhancing our ability to view the microvascular network of the vocal fold and larynx, enhanced optical imaging appears to be evolving as a useful adjunct tool to routine laryngoscopy. For the diagnosis of laryngeal malignancy, it demonstrates higher sensitivity and accuracy compared with white light imaging alone (Davaris, Voigt-Zimmermann, Kropf, & Arens, 2019). A classification system for suspected cancerous or precancerous vocal fold lesions has been developed (Ni et al., 2011), which is based upon vascular features identified in vivo using narrow band imaging. This demonstrates the ability to differentiate malignant from nonmalignant laryngeal lesions with high accuracy using capillary morphology.

Furthermore, there is growing evidence for the use of enhanced optical imaging during microlaryngoscopy. This aims to improve detection of neoplastic laryngeal lesions intraoperatively (Klimza, Jackowska, Piazza, Banaszewski, & Wierzbicka, 2019) and subsequently reduce the incidence of positive surgical margins during the treatment of glottic cancer, leading to improved clinical outcomes (Campo, D'Aguanno, Greco, Ralli, & de Vincentiis, 2020).

Laryngeal high-speed videoendoscopy

Introduction

Ultra-high speed photography was first documented in the 1930s (Farnsworth, 1940). Since then, development of increased frame rate and camera technology has resulted in high-speed imaging of the vocal folds in clinical and research settings. During laryngeal high-speed videoendoscopy (LHSV) examination, a constant light source is used with camera frame rates of between 4,000 and 10,000 frames per second (fps) to capture a short segment (usually two seconds) of vocal fold vibratory activity. Playback of the images provides a slow-motion view of vocal fold vibration with high resolution.

LHSV allows imaging of the vibratory movement of the true vocal folds at the onset and offset of phonation, and is considered to be the only imaging technique that can capture the actual intracycle vibration of the true vocal folds (Deliyski et al., 2008). Unlike videostroboscopy, LHSV is not dependent on a predominantly periodic vibration pattern and acoustic signal to view the vibratory pattern of the vocal folds. Video images captured using LHSV can also be processed to produce a videokymogram (Figure 22.6); a single image of aggregated custom-selected line images produced from each frame (Švec & Schutte, 1996).

Equipment

LHSV units are comprised of four primary elements; a 70-degree or 90-degree rigid laryngeal endoscope, a digital high-speed camera (color or monochrome) with trigger button; a powerful light source (usually 300 watts constant xenon) and digital processor with specialized software for image acquisition and real-time video feedback. A computer monitor and endoscopic lens adaptor are also required. Given the high frame rate of LHSV, a high volume of data is collected during the examination, which requires longer timeframes to process and save.

Technique

Collection of LHSV images is similar to that of videostrobosocopy. A rigid scope is inserted in the mouth (or nose if flexible nasendoscopy is available). LHSV utilizes a continuous recording

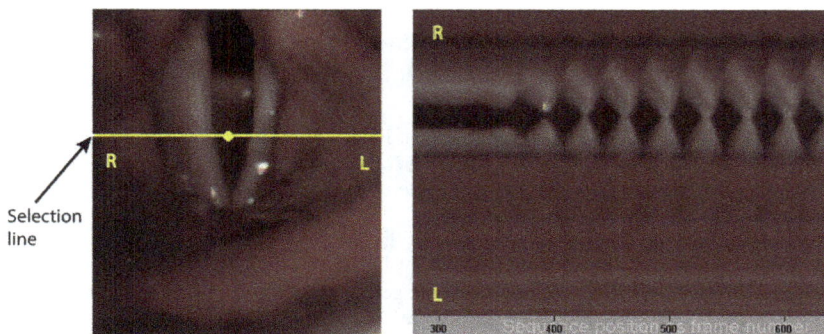

Figure 22.6 Videokymogram obtained from high-speed videoendoscopy. Normal mode is shown in the left panel with a horizontal line indicating the position of the selection line. This results in the high-speed line-imaging mode present in the right panel.

format with capture of required images achieved by pressing the trigger button. The images captured prior to stopping capture are retained for a set period of time (commonly two seconds).

Interpretation of examination

The slow-motion replay of the film can be visually inspected, or further computer analysis may be undertaken. Visual assessment of LHSV images should involve rating the same parameters of the mucosal wave as are rated in videostroboscopy. LHSV images can be analyzed further via the use of videokymography (frequency, amplitude of the vocal fold vibration, left-right asymmetries, open and closed phases of the glottal cycle (open and closed quotient) and propagation of mucosal waves) (Švec & Schutte, 1996); phonovibrograms (Unger, Schuster, Hecker, Schick, & Lohscheller, 2016), phonovibrographic wavegrams (Unger et al., 2013) and glottal area waveform analysis (Maryn et al., 2019).

Advantages and disadvantages

LHSV has a number of advantages over videostroboscopy. The image is continuously illuminated so that no visual data is lost as it is in videostroboscopy. LSHV can capture onset and offset of vocal fold vibration and aperiodic vibratory movements; a feature not available in videostroboscopy where stable frequency detection is needed for stroboscopic light production. The LHSV footage can be processed into a single still image or videokymogram, providing an overview of the pattern of vibration, and enabling closer inspection of specific vibratory features over time.

LHSV judgments have been shown to be more sensitive than videostroboscopy for evaluating vocal fold phase asymmetry (Mehta & Hillman, 2012) and to provide more reliable assessment of mucosal wave vibratory activity compared to stroboscopy (Zacharias et al., 2016). LHSV has not, however, been proven to be of greater clinical value than videostroboscopy in improving diagnostic accuracy (Mendelsohn, Remacle, Courey, Gerhard, & Postma, 2013).

Disadvantages of LHSV over other imaging techniques are few. However, processing of the digital file can take many minutes due to the high frame rate and large amount of data collected. Currently, increased cost and lack of commercial availability has prevented LHSV from being widely adopted in the clinical setting.

References

Bailey, B. (1996). Laryngoscopy and laryngoscopes-Who's first?: The forefathers/four fathers of laryngology. *Laryngoscope*, *106*(8), 939–943.

Bless, D.M. (1991). Assessment of laryngeal function. In C.N. Ford & D.M. Bless (Eds.), *Phonosurgery: Assessment and Surgical Management of Voice Disorders*. New York, NY: Raven Press.

Bless, D.M., Hirano, M., & Feder, R.J. (1987). Videostroboscopic evaluation of the larynx. *Ear Nose Throat J*, *66*(7), 289–296.

Brewer, D.W. (1966). Perceptual errors in indirect laryngoscopy. *Laryngoscope*, *76*(8), 1373–1379. doi:10.1288/00005537-196608000-00007

Brockmann, M. (2006). Advantages and disadvantages of the videolaryngostroboscopic examination when planning voice therapy. *Forum Logopadie*, *20*(1), 14–19.

Campbell, I.S., Howell, J.D., & Evans, H.H. (2016). Visceral vistas: Basil Hirschowitz and the birth of fiberoptic endoscopy. *Ann Intern Med*, *165*(3), 214–218. doi:10.7326/M16-0025

Campo, F., D'Aguanno, V., Greco, A., Ralli, M., & de Vincentiis, M. (2020). The prognostic value of adding narrow-band imaging in transoral laser microsurgery for early glottic cancer: A review. *Lasers Surg Med*, *52*(4), 301–306. doi:10.1002/lsm.23142

Casiano, R.R., Zaveri, V., & Lundy, D.S. (1992). Efficacy of videostroboscopy in the diagnosis of voice disorders. *Otolaryngol Head Neck Surg*, *107*(1), 95–100. doi:10.1177/019459989210700115

Chandran, S., Hanna, J., Lurie, D., & Sataloff, R. T. (2011). Differences between flexible and rigid endoscopy in assessing the posterior glottic chink. *J Voice*, *25*(5), 591–595. doi:10.1016/j.jvoice.2010.06.006

Cohen, S.M., Kim, J., Roy, N., Wilk, A., Thomas, S., & Courey, M. (2015). Change in diagnosis and treatment following specialty voice evaluation: A national database analysis. *Laryngoscope*, *125*(7), 1660–1666. doi:10.1002/lary.25192

Cutler, J.L., & Cleveland, T. (2002). The clinical usefulness of laryngeal videostroboscopy and the role of high-speed cinematography in laryngeal evaluation. *Curr Opin Otolaryngol Head Neck Surg*, *10*(6), 462–466. doi:10.1097/00020840-200212000-00009

Davaris, N., Voigt-Zimmermann, S., Kropf, S., & Arens, C. (2019). Flexible transnasal endoscopy with white light or narrow band imaging for the diagnosis of laryngeal malignancy: Diagnostic value, observer variability and influence of previous laryngeal surgery. *Eur Arch Otorhinolaryngol*, *276*(2), 459–466. doi:10.1007/s00405-018-5256-1

Deliyski, D.D., Petrushev, P.P., Bonilha, H.S., Gerlach, T.T., Martin-Harris, B., & Hillman, R.E. (2008). Clinical implementation of laryngeal high-speed videoendoscopy: Challenges and evolution. *Folia Phoniatr Logop*, *60*(1), 33–44. doi:10.1159/000111802

Dunklebarger, J., Rhee, D., Kim, S., & Ferguson, B. (2009). Video rigid laryngeal endoscopy compared to laryngeal mirror examination: An assessment of patient comfort and clinical visualization. *Laryngoscope*, *119*(2), 269–271. doi:10.1002/lary.20020

Eller, R., Ginsburg, M., Lurie, D., Heman-Ackah, Y., Lyons, K., & Sataloff, R. (2009). Flexible laryngoscopy: A comparison of fiber optic and distal chip technologies-part 2: Laryngopharyngeal reflux. *J Voice*, *23*(3), 389–395. doi:10.1016/j.jvoice.2007.10.007

Estes, C., Sadoughi, B., Mauer, E., Christos, P., & Sulica, L. (2017). Laryngoscopic and stroboscopic signs in the diagnosis of vocal fold paresis. *Laryngoscope*, *127*(9), 2100–2105. doi:10.1002/lary.26570

Farnsworth, D.W. (1940). High-speed motion pictures of human vocal cords. *Bell Laboratories Record*, *18*, 203–208.

García, M. (1881). On the invention of the laryngoscope. *Transactions of the international medical congress, seventh session* (pp. 197–199). London, UK: International Medical Congress.

Goldman, J.L., & Roffman, J.D. (1975). Indirect laryngoscopy. *Laryngoscope*, *85*(3), 530–533. doi:10.1288/00005537-197503000-00010

Hapner, E.R., & Johns, M.M. (2007). Recognizing and understanding the limitations of laryngeal videostroboscopy. *Perspect Voice Voice Disord*, *17*(1), 3–7. doi:doi:10.1044/vvd17.1.3

Hartnick, C.J., & Zeitels, S.M. (2005). Pediatric video laryngo-stroboscopy. *Int J Pediatr Otorhinolaryngol*, *69*(2), 215–219. doi:10.1016/j.ijporl.2004.08.021

Heman-Ackah, Y.D. (2004). Diagnostic tools in laryngology. *Curr Opin Otolaryngol Head Neck Surg*, *12*(6), 549–552.

Hirano, M., Yoshida, T., Yoshida, Y., & Tateishi, O. (1985). Strobofiberscopic video recording of vocal fold vibration. *Ann Otolaryngol*, *94*(6), 588–590. doi:10.1177/000348948509400613

Hirsch, N., Smith, G., & Hirsch, P. (1986). Alfred Kirstein: Pioneer of direct laryngoscopy. *Anaesthesia*, *41*(1), 42–45.

Hoffmann, R., Mehnert, D., & Dietzel, R. (2013). How did it work? Historic phonetic devices explained by coeval photographs. In INTERSPEECH-2013, 14th Annual Conference of the International Speech Communication Association, Lyon, France. August 25-29, 2013; 558–562.

Iwarsson, J., & Reinholt Petersen, N. (2012). Effects of consensus training on the reliability of auditory perceptual ratings of voice quality. *J Voice*, *26*(3), 304–312. doi:10.1016/j.jvoice.2011.06.003

Kallen, L.A. (1932). Laryngostroboscopy in the practice of otolaryngology. *Arch Otolaryngol*, *16*(6), 791–807.

Klimza, H., Jackowska, J., Piazza, C., Banaszewski, J., & Wierzbicka, M. (2019). The role of intraoperative narrow-band imaging in transoral laser microsurgery for early and moderately advanced glottic cancer. *Braz J Otorhinolaryngol*, *85*, 228–236.

Koufman, J.A., & Blalock, P.D. (1991). Functional voice disorders. *Otolaryngol Clin North Am*, *24*(5), 1059–1073.

Lapeña, J.F. (2013). Mirrors and reflections: The evolution of indirect laryngoscopy. *Ann Saudi Med*, *33*(2), 177–181.

Madill C, Corcoran S & So T. (2019). Bridge2practice: Translating theory into practice. https:// bridge2practice.com/. Accessed 8 March, 2019.

Manfredi, M.A., Abu Dayyeh, B.K., Bhat, Y.M., Chauhan, S.S., Gottlieb, K.T., … Banerjee, S. (2015). Electronic chromoendoscopy. *Gastrointest Endosc, 81*(2), 249–261. doi:10.1016/j.gie.2014.06.020

Maryn, Y., Verguts, M., Demarsin, H., van Dinther, J., Gomez, P., Schlegel, P., & Dollinger, M. (2019). Intersegmenter variability in high-speed laryngoscopy-based glottal area waveform measures. *Laryngoscope, 130*(11), e654–e661.. doi:10.1002/lary.28475

Mehta, D.D., Deliyski, D.D., & Hillman, R.E. (2010). Commentary on why laryngeal stroboscopy really works: Clarifying misconceptions surrounding Talbot's law and the persistence of vision. (Letter to the Editor)(Report). *J Speech Lang Hear Res, 53*(5), 1263. doi:10.1044/1092-4388(2010/09-0241)

Mehta, D.D., & Hillman, R.E. (2012). Current role of stroboscopy in laryngeal imaging. *Curr Opin Otolaryngol Head Neck Surg, 20*(6), 429–436. doi:10.1097/MOO.0b013e3283585f04

Mendelsohn, A.H., Remacle, M., Courey, M.S., Gerhard, F., & Postma, G.N. (2013). The diagnostic role of high-speed vocal fold vibratory imaging. *J Voice, 27*(5), 627–631. doi:10.1016/j.jvoice.2013.04.011

Moore, P. (1937). A short history of laryngeal investigation. *Q J Speech, 23*(4), 531–564.

Morrison, M.D., & Rammage, L.A. (1993). Muscle misuse voice disorders: Description and classification. *Acta Otolaryngol, 113*(3), 428–434.

Mortensen, M., Schaberg, M., & Woo, P. (2010). Diagnostic contributions of videolaryngostroboscopy in the pediatric population. *Arch Otolaryngol Head Neck Surg, 136*(1), 75–79. doi:10.1001/archoto.2009.209

Nawka, T., & Konerding, U. (2012). The interrater reliability of stroboscopy evaluations. *J Voice, 26*(6), 812 e811–e810. doi:10.1016/j.jvoice.2011.09.009

Ni, X.G., He, S., Xu, Z.G., Gao, L., Lu, N., Yuan, Z., … Wang, G.Q. (2011). Endoscopic diagnosis of laryngeal cancer and precancerous lesions by narrow band imaging. *J Laryngol Otol, 125*(3), 288–296. doi:10.1017/s0022215110002033

Noordzij, J.P., & Woo, P. (2000). Glottal area waveform analysis of benign vocal fold lesions before and after surgery. *Ann Otollaryngol, 109*(5), 441–446. doi:10.1177/000348940010900501

Pantano, K. (2015). History of the laryngoscope. *The Triological Society: ENTtoday.*

Patel, R., Dailey, S., & Bless, D. (2008). Comparison of high-speed digital imaging with stroboscopy for laryngeal imaging of glottal disorders. *Ann Otolaryngol, 117*(6), 413–424. doi:10.1177/000348940811700603

Pemberton, C., Russell, A., Priestley, J., Havas, T., Hooper, J., & Clark, P. (1993). Characteristics of normal larynges under flexible fiberscopic and stroboscopic examination: an Australian perspective. *J Voice, 7*(4), 382–389. doi:10.1016/s0892-1997(05)80262-0

Poburka, B.J. (1999). A new stroboscopy rating form. *J Voice, 13*(3), 403–413.

Poburka, B.J., & Bless, D.M. (1998). A multi-media, computer-based method for stroboscopy rating training. *J Voice, 12*(4), 513–526. doi:10.1016/s0892-1997(98)80060-x

Poburka, B.J., Patel, R.R., & Bless, D.M. (2017). Voice-vibratory assessment with laryngeal imaging (VALI) form: Reliability of rating stroboscopy and high-speed videoendoscopy. *J Voice, 31*(4), 513. e1–513.e14. doi:10.1016/j.jvoice.2016.12.003

Ponka, D., & Baddar, F. (2013). Indirect laryngoscopy. *Can Fam Physician, 59*(11), 1201.

Rajput, S.D., & Poriya, M.J. (2017). Stroboscopy: An evolving tool for voice analysis in vocal cord pathologies. *Int J Otorhinolaryngol Head Neck Surg, 3*(4), 927–931.

Rosen, C.A. (2005). Stroboscopy as a research instrument: Development of a perceptual evaluation tool. *Laryngoscope, 115*(3), 423–428. doi:10.1097/01.mlg.0000157830.38627.85

Sahin, M.I., Kokoglu, K., Gulec, S., Ketenci, I., & Unlu, Y. (2017). Premedication methods in nasal endoscopy: A prospective, randomized, double-blind study. *Clin Exp Otorhinolaryngol, 10*(2), 158–163. doi:10.21053/ceo.2016.00563

Sataloff, R.T., Spiegel, J.R., & Hawkshaw, M.J. (1991). Strobovideolaryngoscopy: Results and clinical value. *Ann Otolaryngol, 100*(9 Pt 1), 725–727. doi:10.1177/000348949110000907

Sircus, W. (2003). Milestones in the evolution of endoscopy: A short history. *J R Coll Physicians Edinb, 33*(2), 124–134.

Stager, S.V., Bielamowicz, S.A., Regnell, J.R., Gupta, A., & Barkmeier, J.M. (2000). Supraglottic activity: Evidence of vocal hyperfunction or laryngeal articulation? *J Speech Language Hear Res, 43*(1), 229–238. doi:10.1044/jslhr.4301.229

Stell, P. (1990). Give light to them that sit in darkness. *Med Hist, 3*, 3–12.

Švec, J.G., & Schutte, H.K. (1996). Videokymography: High-speed line scanning of vocal fold vibration. *J Voice, 10*(2), 201–205. doi:10.1016/S0892-1997(96)80047-6

Tarafder, K.H., Chowdhury, M.A., & Tariq, A. (2012). Video laryngostroboscopy. *Bangladesh J Otorhinolaryngol, 18*(2), 171–178.

Thomson, C. (1905). The history of the laryngoscope. *Laryngoscope, 15*(3), 181–184.

Unger, J., Meyer, T., Herbst, C.T., Fitch, W.T., Dollinger, M., & Lohscheller, J. (2013). Phonovibrographic wavegrams: Visualizing vocal fold kinematics. *J Acoust Soc Am, 133*(2), 1055–1064. doi:10.1121/1.4774378

Unger, J., Schuster, M., Hecker, D.J., Schick, B., & Lohscheller, J. (2016). A generalized procedure for analyzing sustained and dynamic vocal fold vibrations from laryngeal high-speed videos using phonovibrograms. *Artifi Intell Med, 66*, 15–28. doi:10.1016/j.artmed.2015.10.002

Wittenberg, T., Tigges, M., Mergell, P., & Eysholdt, U. (2000). Functional imaging of vocal fold vibration: Digital multislice high-speed kymography. *J Voice, 14*(3), 422–442. doi:10.1016/S0892-1997(00)80087-9

Woo, P. (1996). Quantification of videostrobolaryngoscopic findings–measurements of the normal glottal cycle. *Laryngoscope, 106*(3), 1–27.

Woo, P. (2009). *Stroboscopy*. San Diego, CA: Plural Publishing.

Yanagisawa, E., Owens, T.W., Strothers, G., & Honda, K. (1983). Videolaryngoscopy. A comparison of fiberscopic and telescopic documentation. *Ann Otolaryngol, 92*(5), 430–436. doi:10.1177/000348948309200504

Zacharias, S. R. C., Brehm, S. B., Weinrich, B., Kelchner, L., Tabangin, M., & Alarcon, A. d. (2016). Feasibility of clinical endoscopy and stroboscopy in children with bilateral vocal fold lesions. (Research Article)(Report). *American journal of speech-language pathology, 25*(4): 598. doi:10.1044/2016_AJSLP-15-0071

23

ELECTROLARYNGOGRAPHY/ ELECTROGLOTTOGRAPHY[1]

Chiara Celata and Irene Ricci

Basic information about the functioning of the vocal folds

Voiced speech is the loudest and most frequent form of speaking. It has the physical form of a quasi-periodic sound and is produced by the vibration of the vocal folds in the larynx. Phonation is the process of producing voiced speech at the larynx level, whereas articulation is the process of producing resonances by changing the configuration of the vocal tract through articulator movement.

Vocal fold movements may be analyzed through direct imaging (as in laryngeal stroboscopy; see Chapter 22) or indirect visualization, as in electrolaryngography (ELG), also known as electroglottography (EGG). Basically, an electrolaryngograph is an instrument that provides a reasonably good approximation to changes in the medial contact area between the vocal folds during phonation. The highest values in the electrolaryngographic signal correspond to maximum contact, whereas the lowest values correspond to absence of contact between the vocal folds, that is, to the opening of the glottis (Figure 23.1).

The voiced excitation of the vocal tract is very complex. According to the myoelastic aerodynamic theory of phonation (Van den Berg, 1958), the vocal folds are put into motion as a consequence of the airflow generated by the lungs and passing through the glottis. At the glottis level, the channel is narrower than below and above the glottis; the constriction produces an increase of the airflow velocity and a decrease of the pressure perpendicular to the flow (the so-called Bernoulli–Venturi effect, from the names of the two physicists who, as early as in the eighteenth century, demonstrated the inverse relationship between velocity and pressure that holds when a fluid flows through a constriction in a tube). When the subglottal pressure is high enough to overcome the myoelastic resistance of the vocal folds, the folds are pulled apart and the airflow goes through the glottis. In so doing, the airflow increases its velocity and the lateral pressure on the vocal folds decreases; the pressure exerted on the vocal folds is therefore lower than the pressure exerted on the tissues immediately above and below the folds. This temporary vacuum condition automatically results in the vocal folds being pulled together, thus generating the basic vibratory movement of the two membranes.

In addition to this general aerodynamic principle, the vocal fold oscillatory behavior during phonation is also sustained by the fact that each fold is not a uniform mass of muscle but, rather, shows a very complex internal structure: there are two different covering membranes, plus an

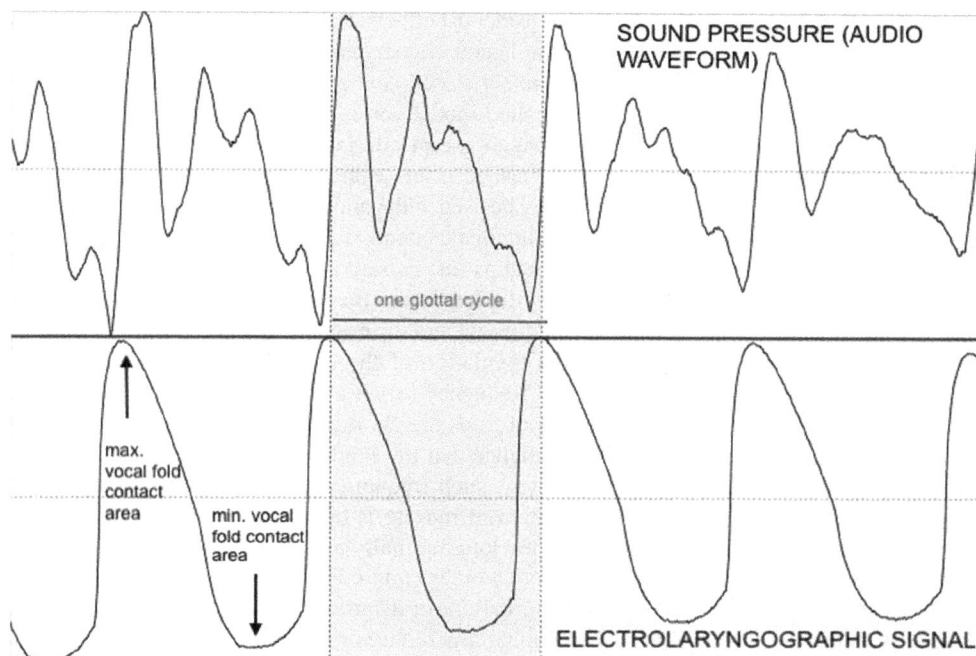

Figure 23.1 Time-aligned sound pressure waveform (audio signal; upper part) and vibratory vocal fold cycles (lower part).

intermediate layer and an internal muscle fiber (Hirano, 1974). This layered structure generates multiple masses, which independently contribute to the vibration pattern (Titze, 1973). The film of mucous covering the vocal folds further adds to the complexity of the process (Broad, 1979) and, consequently, to the acoustic complexity of the voice signal. As an example, we can consider people with laryngitis; they are not as easily understood as when their larynx is fully functioning and lubricated.

This short review of the basic functioning of phonation has thus shown how complex the mechanism of vocal fold adduction and abduction is. Before looking at how the electrolaryngographic signal may help in decoding and analyzing the many facets of this complex mechanism, it is essential to emphasize that vocal fold vibration is a three-dimensional movement, to which temporal constraints apply.

The first and most obvious dimension refers to the horizontal opening and closing of the glottis, which occurs from the back forward. The second dimension is the vertical one, to the extent that, as explained above, the combined effect of the Bernoulli–Venturi principle and the elasticity of the tissues implies that the vocal folds are rapidly sucked together from the bottom upward and then peeled apart again from the bottom upward. A third fundamental dimension is vocal fold length, which can also be considered in terms of muscle tension. The length of the vocal folds derives from the contraction of a specific set of muscles of the intrinsic anatomy of the larynx, i.e. the lateral cricoarytenoid muscles. The contraction of the lateral cricoarytenoid muscles is essential for the correct positioning and tensing of the vocal folds, which must be close enough to one another but not too tightly pressed together. The importance of this parameter, which also impacts on both the vertical and the horizontal dimensions of vibration, can be appreciated when we consider the effects of some deviant contacting patterns on voice production. For instance, when the lateral cricoarytenoid muscles are not sufficiently contracted, the glottis cannot reach a completely closed configuration, as required by the most common and "bright" type of phonation (called modal voice); this means that the vocal folds stay open for a relatively long time and more air escapes during voice production. This pattern produces a quieter phonation, sometimes described as an "aspirated" type of voice that is specifically called breathy voice. Breathy voice may be used with paralinguistic functions (e.g. to sound more gentle or sexy) but also to implement linguistic contrasts (like in Hindi, a language which contrasts modally and breathy voiced stops and nasals; Esposito, Khan & Hurst (2007).

Another muscle that directly impacts on the tension of the vocal folds is the cricothyroid, which determines the distance between the thyroid and the cricoid cartilages. The cricothyroid muscle has a primary importance for the regulation of the overall rate of vibration of the vocal folds, that linguists call fundamental frequency (often indicated with f_0) or pitch. When the cricothyroid muscle is relaxed, the vocal folds are shortened and thicker (i.e. their mass per unit length increases), with the consequence that the fundamental frequency of vibration decreases; form the perceptual point of view, such frequency decrease is associated with a lower pitch. By contrast, when the cricothyroid muscle is contracted, the thyroid cartilage tilts forward and the vocal folds are stretched longitudinally and thinned, which facilitates an increase in vocal fold vibration and therefore a higher pitch. In falsetto voice, a type of phonation that correlates with several voice perturbations or disorders (see below), the cricothyroid muscle stretches the vocal folds to their limits; this reduces the variation of vocal fold vibration along the vertical component and results in the perceptual effect of a voice sounding "like the string of a guitar."

Time is a fourth, very important variable to look at in analyzing voice production and voice pathologies. The number of contacting-decontacting (i.e. separating) cycles per time unit determines the overall frequency of vibration that is characteristics of an individual voice. The fundamental frequency thus depends on the mass of the vocal folds (the smaller or thinner the vocal fold, the faster its vibration pattern and thus the higher its f_0). Moreover, as mentioned above, vibration rate also depends on how much the vocal folds are stretched or in tension. Finally, there may also be linguistic choices (e.g. related to tonal or intonational variations) to determine pitch changes with specific communicative functions.

Time is also important as the duration ratio between the two basic phases of vocal fold vibration, that are the contacting and the decontacting phase. In normal conditions, the process by which the vocal folds are pulled together is much quicker and more abrupt than the process by which they are pulled apart. With respect to the duration of the entire cycle, the contacting phase is shorter than the decontacting phase. The reasons for this are related to the aerodynamic and myoelastic conditions reviewed above. Measuring deviations from this general pattern may be useful to characterize some pathological phonation dynamics. For instance, if contact is incomplete (possibly because of incorrect activity of the cricoarytenoid muscle) or shorter than normal, the egressive airflow is produced at a higher rate and the voice shows overall reduced amplitude, due to the presence of a continuous open passage between the trachea and the vocal tract. By contrast, if the vocal folds stay contacted for a longer time interval (because of slack vocal folds, which increases their mass per length unit) and the opening phase is slower, only a small amount of air escapes from the glottis. In this condition, the cycles turn out to be more irregular in both duration (what linguists and clinicians call acoustic "jitter") and intensity ("shimmer"); the resulting voice quality is usually referred to as creaky voice (or vocal fry) and is typical of a type of speech produced by people with physiological or pathological weariness who need to conserve energy while speaking.

In sum, the myoelastic aerodynamic theory coupled with the principles of the multiple-mass theory and the details about the physiology of the vocal folds provide a global model of phonation that has proven extremely powerful at explaining a variety of patterns in voice production. Since the development of this knowledge, a large body of modeling studies (e.g. Rothenberg M., 1981) has corroborated the theory through parameterization of laryngeal functions such as the glottal area, the vocal fold contact area and the glottal airflow. The power of the theory is also demonstrated by the fact that the same basic principles apply to a wide variety of sounds produced by mammals of a large range of body sizes, including elephants and their infrasonic (< 20 Hz) sounds (Herbst, Stoeger, Frey, Lohscheller, Titze, Gumpenberger, Fitch, 2012).

As already anticipated, each individual speaker is characterized by a specific type of vocal fold vibration, to which a specific fundamental frequency range can be associated. The type and the rate of vibrations together contribute largely to perceived personal features such as age, sex or accent; and this has been shown to happen even in the absence of supraglottal information (Abberton & Fourcin, 1978). Besides the linguistic uses of voice parameter variations (such as the intonational variations commonly used by the speakers of any language to index different sentence modalities in dialogues), variations in the overall rate of vibration or perturbations from the modal voice model may have a paralinguistic motivation, e.g. to signal the emotional state of the speaker, or his/her social patterning with specific speech communities. For instance, it is common knowledge that French women tend to speak with a higher fundamental frequency than women of other speech communities such as Italian or Spanish; sometimes, deviant uses of vocal parameters such as global f_0 patterns contribute to the perception of so-called foreign accent in non-native speakers. However, variations and perturbations of model patterns may also be due to pathological conditions, as the rest of this chapter will show. Given that the use of voice pattern variation by humans is so widespread and multifunctional, intervening voice or hearing pathologies may represent strong limitations to someone's social and communicative activities, sometimes biasing negatively their overall quality of life. In tone languages like Chinese, perturbations of fundamental frequency (or disabilities to perceive pitch distinctions) change the lexical identity of words and are therefore particularly disruptive (Yiu, van Hasslet, Williams, Woo, 1994).

How the electrolaryngograph works

General characteristics

Although phonation as produced at the glottal level and resonances as added at the supraglottal level (from epilaryngeal to oral structures) strongly interact in speech production (e.g. Esling & Harris, 2003), the experimental analysis of each can be separated and one or the other may be selectively impaired.

Electrolaryngography is a widely used method of indirect visualization of vocal fold vibration, based on principles of electrical impedance first discovered by Fabre (1957). Early descriptions of the functioning of electrolaryngographs as well as of their outputs may be found in Baken (1992), Fourcin (1974, 1981), Fourcin and Abberton (1971), Fourcin et al. (1975).

The literature shows that the term "electroglottography" is also used besides electrolaryngography. To some extent, the two terms can be seen as synonyms. Electroglottography makes more direct reference to the glottis, which strictly speaking is the volume between the vocal folds. However, as will be explained below, the instrument does not provide information about the size of the glottal aperture. Rather, it provides information about the contact phase of the vocal fold vibration, from the beginning of the contacting phase to the rapid achievement of maximum contact and up to the gradual decontacting phase. Therefore, in this respect, the term electrolaryngography should be seen as more correct and less ambiguous. In spite of this, EGG seems to be more frequently used as an acronym than ELG. In this chapter, we have opted for using the terms electrolaryngograph (and electrolaryngography) and avoiding acronyms.

A particularly interesting feature of electrolaryngographic analysis is that the laryngographic signal allows inspection of period-by-period vocal fold contact patterns. When calculated from the acoustic signal, f_0 is an average measurement that implies uniformity of vocal fold vibration and hides cross-cycle differences in glottal opening patterns. By contrast, in both normal and pathological voices, significant variations can occur from one vibratory cycle to the next, as will be shown in more detail below. This makes electrolaryngography very useful in the clinical domain.

Most often, the laryngographic signal is recorded during the comfortable sustained production of vowels, which allows gathering clear data about the prototypical phonation of the subject in the absence of intervening articulation or laryngeal mechanisms. The supraglottal activity that is needed to articulate voiced consonants may be a major source of perturbation of the laryngographic signal and, more generally, of glottal activity itself. One such example is the production of the apical trill [r], which requires an aerodynamically sustained oscillatory movement of the tongue tip against the alveolar ridge at a frequency of approximately 18–33 Hz (Lindau, 1985). Although phonological descriptions tend to classify this sound as voiced, there is an apparent conflict between maintenance of voicing and tongue tip trilling (Celata, Ricci, Nacci, & Romeo, 2016), that is clearly visible in terms of discontinuities at the level of the laryngographic signal (Figure 23.2).

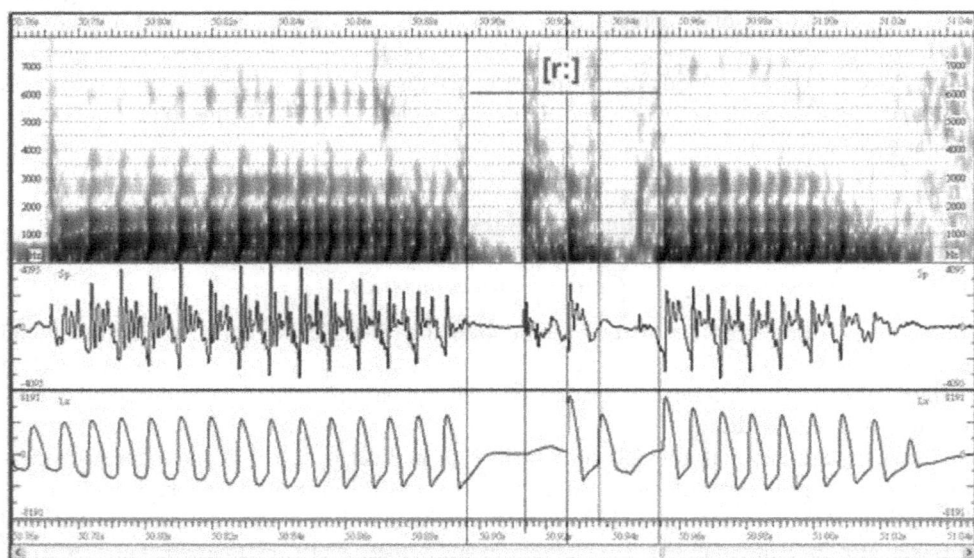

Figure 23.2 Time-aligned sound spectrogram, sound waveform and laryngographic signal. The portion of speech that is represented in the figure is [ar:a]. Alternations of tongue tip closures and openings for the production of the apical trill are detectable from the spectrogram and the waveform. The laryngographic signal shows glottal opening during most of the tongue tip closure and irregular vibrations as an effect of the aerodynamic conflict between phonation and articulation.

Instrumental components

The electrolaryngograph measures electric impedance between two gold-plated electrodes that are placed externally on the neck, on either side of the thyroid notch. Between the electrodes flows a low-voltage (0.5 V) and high-frequency current (usually between 300 kHz and 5 MHz), whose impedance changes with contacting and decontacting movements of the vocal folds. Due to the weakness of the electrical signal and the absence of any stimulation of nerves or muscles, the method is noninvasive and does not impact on phonation or speaking.

Electrodes have the form of rings or rectangles covering an area ranging from 3 to 9 cm^2. Sometimes a third electrode is used as a reference for impedance measurements; in this case, it may be designed as a separate electrode or as a ring electrode encircling each of the two other electrodes. The electrodes are usually mounted on a flexible band whose length may be adjusted to hold the electrodes in a steady position and yet to allow the subject to speak comfortably and breath naturally. In certain cases, the electrodes are mounted on a small holder that is pressed against the throat by hand.

The correct placement of the electrodes and good contact between their surface and the neck is essential to obtain a good electrolaryngographic signal.

It is usually assumed that the greater the contact area between the vocal folds, the more electricity is conducted between the electrodes; consequently, the electrolaryngographic signal provides rather detailed information on the degree of closure of the glottis. For the same reason, information about glottal opening (i.e. the size of the space between completely abducted vocal folds) is not provided. The contacting phase includes maximum contact but also the phase of progressively increasing contact, from the lower to the upper margins (which amounts to approximately 25% of the entire contact phase, Orlikoff (1991), and the decontacting phase, which is more gradual. Rigorous empirical tests (e.g. via stroboscopy) have demonstrated that there is a strong relationship between vocal fold contact area and the electrolaryngographic voltage values (Scherer, Druker, & Titze (1988); Hampala, Garcia, Švec, Scherer, & Herbst (2016)). However, authors also suggest caution in the interpretation of quantitative and statistical data derived from the electrolaryngographic signal, because of potentially intervening factors (such as subcutaneous tissue conductance) that may introduce small amounts of non-random variation (Hampala, Garcia, Švec, Scherer, & Herbst (2016)).

Experimental sessions with electrolaryngography require careful preparation and setup. Signal quality may be influenced or degraded by external factors such as background noise (which can be reduced by using gel to increase the contact between neck and the electrodes), the choice of an incorrect high-pass filter cutoff frequency, improper size of the electrodes or even their incorrect placement (e.g. Colton & Conture (1990)). Moreover, the larynx is subject to vertical displacements not only in processes such as swallowing, in which vertical displacement is large and essential, but also in singing and speaking, where vertical displacement may be small and auxiliary. Therefore, systems have been developed that provide multi-electrode arrays on each side of the neck, basically to capture the vertical dimension in addition to the default horizontal dimension. An early and famous example is the TMEGG - Tracking Multichannel Electrolaryngograph developed by Rothenberg (1992), equipped with an upper and a lower electrode on each side of the neck. Increasingly sophisticated systems (with up to 12 electrodes disposed in two 2 × 3 arrays, thus producing 36 electricity paths) are being developed currently; these include software tools that are able to decode and visualize the larynx displacements along the coronal plane (e.g. Tronchin, Kob & Guarnaccia (2018)).

Types of analysis

A first and very basic use that can be made of the laryngographic signal is the calculation of the fundamental frequency of vocal fold vibration. However, considering that the acoustic signal already allows a precise estimation of f_0, this is currently not the most widespread use. Laryngographic analyses rather tend to focus on the possibility of estimating the relative duration of selected subparts of the vibratory cycle and characterizing cycle-to-cycle variability.

As explained above, the electrical impedance varies with the area of contact between the vocal folds during the glottal vibratory cycle. However, since the percentage variation in the impedance caused by vocal fold contact can be extremely small and may vary considerably among subjects, no absolute measure of contact area can be obtained through electrolaryngography; rather, the electrolaryngographic signal represents a pattern of variation. Its analysis is therefore focused on landmarks on the waveform that are judged to correspond to essential moments of the vibratory cycle.

The most important and useful landmarks are those that are assumed to correspond to the instants of contacting and decontacting of the vocal folds, i.e. the glottal closing and glottal opening instants. These two instants are generally defined on the basis of the first mathematical derivative of the laryngographic signal (e.g. Henrich, Alessandro, Doval, & Castellengo, 2004), whose positive and negative peaks should correspond to the instants of maximum rate of change of the vocal fold contact area. Several studies have questioned the mathematical precision of this correspondence, particularly with respect to the opening instant (see e.g. Herbst, 2020). However, qualitative and quantitative analyses required for linguistic research and clinical assessments may rely on either the laryngographic signal or its first derivative to establish relevant cross-cycle changes and overall patterns of voice production, based on well-established laryngographic indices.

One such index, called the Contact Quotient, is used to calculate the ratio of the contacting phase duration to the duration of the total laryngeal cycle. There are different methods to calculate the Contact Quotient (see Herbst & Ternström (2006) for a review), either based on purposely established thresholds (after normalization of the amplitude of the signal) or—as mentioned above—based on the peaks of the first derivative of the signal.

Other indices that can be found in the literature target the "speed" or the "abruptness" of the vocal fold contact increase, under the assumption that a sudden increase of contact correspond to an abrupt cessation of the glottal airflow. An early example is the ratio of rise-time to fall-time within one vibratory cycle proposed by Esling (1984). Sometimes, these indices are calculated on the first derivative of the laryngographic waveform.

Systems currently in use

One of the first electrolaryngographs was produced by Glottal Enterprises, a company with over 30 years of professional experience and innovative research in voice measurement. Glottal Enterprises products were based on M. Rothenberg's original research in speech, voice and language, mostly developed at the Speech Research Laboratory of Syracuse University. Rothenberg's patented designs have provided researchers with an impressive amount of airflow and pressure measurement tools. The Glottal Enterprises electrolaryngograph produces a very low-noise laryngographic waveform that can even be used with children (provided that they are older than 4 years of age), and develops a series of features according to the specific requests of researchers and clinicians.

The most recent version is the EG2-PCX (first produced by Glottal Enterprise in 2015), a patented dual-channel configuration that is able to indicate proper electrode placement thanks to an LED electrode placement indicator. It also provides a quantitative indication of the vertical displacements of the larynx; by checking a signal produced by a DC voltage that changes with movements of the electrodes on the neck, along with the laryngographic signal, it is possible to control for the desired position while the data are being recorded. Moreover, the system offers easy connection to a personal computer and is capable of interacting with the most popular speech software packages; it is also possible to connect the system with any other data acquisition system through an analogue line-level output. The gold-plated electrodes provided by Glottal Enterprise are 34 mm diameter large, but 27 mm electrodes may be provided as an additional option. It is possible to select waveform polarity to measure either vocal fold contact area or inverse vocal fold contact area. Moreover, it is possible to set the signal strength manually, which is useful for a preliminarily verification that the waveform has a sufficiently high amplitude to reliably indicate vocal fold contact variation; also, the system is equipped with an optional calibration procedure (larynx simulator) that allows a verification of the laryngographic signal amplitude in terms of percentage variation in neck resistance. Finally, the system comes with a dual rechargeable battery that assures that recordings will not be interrupted in the event of a discharged battery.

Another system that is widely used is the one produced by Laryngograph Ltd. This company has produced since 1973 display and assessment systems that provide accurate, relevant and representative measures of the most important constituents of speech. It boasts wide collaboration activity with speech therapists, hearing clinicians, speech scientists and singing teachers throughout the world.

As early as 1995, researchers from University College London demonstrated the Laryngograph Ltd software in combination with the acoustic signal derived from a microphone, for the real-time analysis of speech and voice (Fourcin, Abberton, Miller & Howells (1995)). In that environment, time-aligned waveform and laryngographic signals were available so that vocal fold contact corresponded to the acoustic period of excitation and the system provided the duration of the contact phase of vocal fold movement. This in turn allowed the estimation of airflow through the vocal folds. The system was conceived of for both quantitative analysis and qualitative displays for teaching and interactive therapy. Fourcin, Abberton, Miller, & Howells (1995)) also described a clinical workstation combining acoustic signal recording and laryngography with other articulatory facilities such as nasality sensors or endoscopes for the visualization of vocal fold vibration.

Currently, the Digital Laryngograph® is a portable system providing clear laryngographic outputs via a USB connection with a personal computer. It features four analogue inputs that are useful for the acquisition of additional signals from other devices (such as electropalatography; see Chapter 25) and a digital image acquisition channel for quality precision stroboscopy, which can be used to synchronize the laryngographic signal with the images from an endoscope. The sampling rate may vary (either 24, 16 or 12 kHz) according to the specific needs of the experimenter. The electrodes also come in small, medium and large sizes.

The Laryngograph software package, called SpeechStudio, has been especially designed for phoneticians and speech scientists as well as for quantitative work by clinicians and speech and language therapists (Fourcin, McGlashan & Blowes (2002). It is Windows-based and can be used for analysis of data already recorded and stored on a hard disk, for real-time display and instantaneous quantitative analysis, and in the pattern target mode that is useful for speech training. The basic visualization can be customized by the individual user by adding or suppressing individual displays; the software is able to display real-time sound

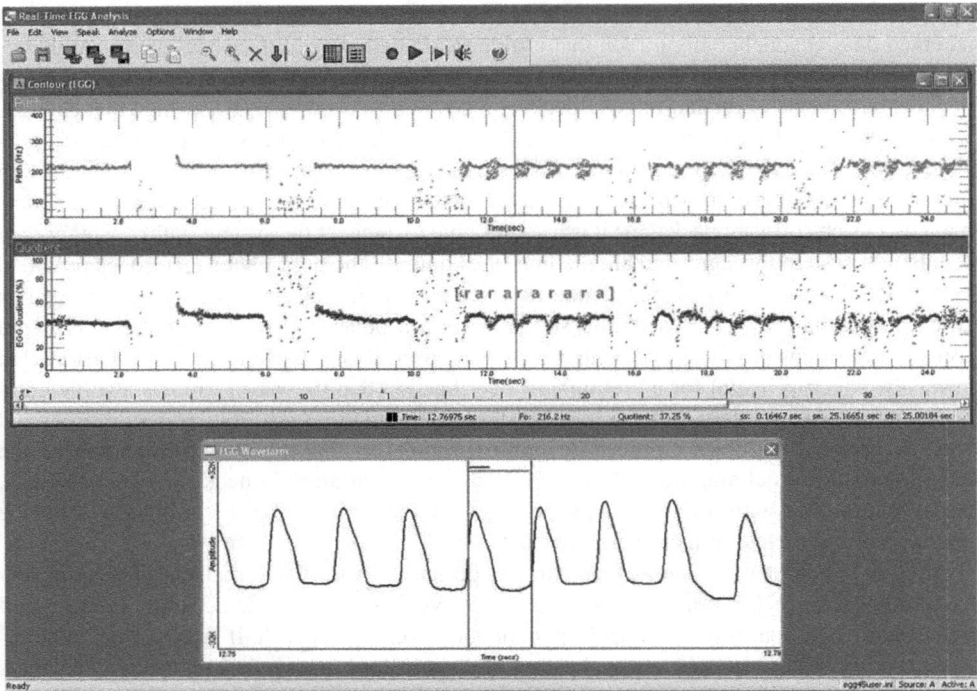

Figure 23.3 Example of time-aligned f_0 (upper box) and contact index (middle box) visualization within SpeechStudio. The boxes show sustained vowels (first three intervals) and rhotic-vowel sequences (intervals four to six) as produced by a female Italian speaker with no speech or hearing disabilities. The fourth interval, in particular, correspond to the production of [r:ar:ar:ar:ar:a]; the cursor is placed at the onset of the second intervocalic apical trill and shows variable and irregular f_0 and contact index values during trill production, as opposed to canonical vowel production. The lower box is a magnification of the laryngographic signal during trill production and shows the comparatively longer duration of the open glottis phase over the total duration of the glottal cycle.

pressure waveforms, fundamental frequency (Fx), amplitude (Ax), contact quotient (Qx), sound spectrogram and Linear predictive coding (LPC) spectrum.

SpeechStudio has been conceived of to perform a large number of analyses of both sustained vowels and connected speech (Figure 23.3). Most often, speech scientists and clinicians rely on fundamental frequency contours, signal amplitude (including its minimum, maximum, average and standard deviation) and contact quotient. It is however also possible to measure jitter and shimmer by simply selecting a voiced segment of the recorded signal and visualize relative f_0 variations. Also estimates of nasality and frication are available.

Currently, new software packages are being developed around the world to provide clinicians with easy and fast ways to calculate and—crucially—visualize voice parameters. This circumstance attests the increasing diffusion of electrolaryngography across the scientific and medical communities. There is an increasing demand for smart tools to assist scientists working with voice physiology and pathology, but also to support patients who may benefit from interactive training (see below). Many software packages for voice analysis are nowadays based on the analysis of the acoustic signal, whereas others are designed to decode and analyze the laryngographic signal, and in this case they can be coupled with existing systems of laryngographic data acquisition.

Electrolaryngographic characteristics of speech and voice pathologies

According to the American Speech-Language-Hearing Association (ASHA; www.asha.org), voice disorders may be grossly divided into two groups. Organic disorders have an origin in the physiology and particularly in the breathing mechanism, the larynx or the vocal tract. By contrast, functional disorders have no anatomical or physiological origin but rather derive from a misuse or abuse of the voice production mechanism. Vocal abuse arises as a consequence of the hyperfunctioning of the laryngeal mechanism. When repeated or habitual, vocally abusive behaviors may induce pain, strain or even damage to the laryngeal tissues and muscles. For instance, factory workers or teachers forced to shout to overcome environmental noise may encounter vocal fatigue; incessant and non-productive throat clearing or coughing, whatever their etiology, can also count as hyperfunctional voice disorders.

However, there may be overlap between the two categories, inasmuch as repeated misuse of the voice may lead to organic damage at some level of the physiological apparatus, and vice-versa.

Organic voice dysfunctions may be associated with difficulties and impairments of central or peripheral origin.

In the first case, structural voice dysfunctions may be caused by either physical abnormalities, lesions of the larynx (such as ulcers, polyps, nodules, cysts) or previous surgical interventions (such as intubation in premature children). Polyps or carcinomas may increase the mass of one fold, giving rise to asymmetric conditions in vibration velocity, which are reflected in irregular adduction-abduction dynamics. Excessive dryness of the vocal folds may arise from laryngitis or other reasons and may have a negative impact on the regularity of vibration because of lack of the necessary lubrication.

Neurogenic disorders affecting voice production may be monolateral or bilateral vocal fold paralysis and laryngeal dystonia; other neurogenic disorders such as Parkinson's disease or multiple sclerosis may also indirectly cause voice problems. Paralysis of one fold generally causes an asymmetry in the stiffness of the vocal folds, which impacts on the regularity of the vibration. Voice disorders related to abnormal muscular tension especially in children may occur as a consequence of other speech disorders such as dyspraxia and velopharyngeal insufficiency associated with cleft palate.

Finally, dysphonia may also reflect the existence of unsolved psychological conflicts. These dysfunctions are rare and cannot be classified as either organic or functional. Psychogenic voice disorders may happen for different reasons (chronic stress, anxiety, depression etc.), for instance during adolescence and post-pubertal development, but also children or adults may be affected. In these cases, voice disorders are unrelated to specific physical or neural problems. Electrolaryngographic measurements may not only highlight the laryngeal correlates of these pathological conditions, but also help to quantitatively distinguish the vibratory correlates of pathologies with auditorily similar voice qualities (Leff & Abberton (1981)).

The relationship between irregular laryngographic waveforms and anatomical or physiological conditions is not biunique, to the extent that a given perturbation of vocal fold periodicity as reflected in the electrolaryngographic signal may originate from different conditions of the organs or different patterns of laryngeal (dys)function. Pitch and amplitude (or voice loudness), in addition to the regularity of vibration, may also be affected in the case of dysphonia. Therefore, pathological voices change simultaneously with respect to different parameters and the electrolaryngographic signal includes relevant information from different anatomical and physiological sources. Starting from this observation, "holistic" approaches have been developed that show that a global variability index summing both amplitude and velocity variations may significantly characterize pathological voices of different origins

315

from non-pathological voices, particularly at the level of the final phase of vocal fold contact (Nacci, Romeo, Cavaliere, Macerata, Bastiani, Paludetti, Galli, Marchese, Barillari, Barillari, Berrettini, Laschi, Cianchetti, Manti, Ursino, & Fattori (2019)).

Abnormal voice conditions that are easily detected through laryngographic inspection are irregular (i.e. non-periodic) vibration, shorter than normal contact phases and anomalies in f_0 contour shape and range. For instance, deaf adults are known to have difficulties in maintaining modal voice parameters (e.g. Fourcin & Abberton, 1971). Sometimes, monotonous voice and insufficient variation of intonational contours (that is, a reduced f_0 range) are reported as indices of pathological voice (e.g. Abberton et al., 1991), whereas smokers are reported to have a comparatively lower f_0 than non-smokers (Guimaraes & Abberton, 2005). Interestingly, this may have consequences at the level of phonemic contrasts as well. As a matter of fact, we know that in the production of the voicing distinction (i.e. voiced vs. voiceless consonants), voiced consonants exhibit a physiological lowering of f_0 compared to the surrounding vowels. In pathological speech, where f_0 patterns are already compromised and f_0 ranges of variation are reduced, there may be cessation of vibration during voiced consonants (e.g. Fourcin, 1981), with the consequence of decreasing the degree of distinctiveness.

Electroglottography can be extremely useful in differential diagnosis of functional dysphonia. For instance, the open quotient is a parameter allowing the differentiation of hypofunctional from hyperfunctional dysphonia (Szkiełkowska, Krasnodębska, Miaśkiewicz, & Skarżyński, 2018): patients with hyperfunctional dysphonia were found to be not statistically different from the control group, whereas in patients with hypofunctional dysphonia, significantly higher values of open quotient were observed.

Spasmodic dysphonia is a neurologic voice disorder that gives rise to a severely hyperfunctional voice, sounding "strained-strangled" with frequent pitch or voicing breaks that interrupt the continuity of phonation. The auditory and perceptual quality of "strain" in this pathology can be measured by electrolaryngography (and particularly in terms of the decontacting slope quotient and peak skewness), thus indicating that laryngographic parameters may serve as markers for an improved characterization of the disturbance and for the quantification of the response to clinical treatments (Somanath & Mau, 2016).

A large amount of laryngographic work has been devoted to the analysis and treatment of abnormal voice patterns in hearing-impaired speakers. Deaf and poorly hearing speakers lack an adequate auditory monitoring of their own speech and therefore may develop irregular or hypo-differentiated f_0 patterns, tendencies to falsetto or creaky voice qualities and insufficient control of distinctive intonation (e.g. Fourcin & Abberton, 1971, 1991; Abberton, Fourcin, Rosen, Howard, Douek, & Moore, 1985).

Reduced vocal fold adduction, together with disturbance of the respiratory functioning, is also considered to be at the origin of low vocal intensity, monotonicity and hoarseness typical of speakers affected by Parkinson's disease (e.g. Ramig & Dromey, 1996).

There are many other fields in which electrolaryngography has proved useful in characterizing clinical work on voice production, and they appear to be increasing in most recent times; among them are chronic cough (Vertigan, Theodoros, & Winkworth, et al., 2008), laryngopharyngeal reflux (Ramirez, Jimenez, & Lopez, et al., 2017), multiple sclerosis (Putzer, Barry & Moringlane, 2007) and *sulcus vocalis* (Lim, Kim, & Choi et al., 2009).

In Figures 23.4–23.6, we illustrate electrolaryngraph patterns, aligned with the acoustic waveform for modal voice, creaky voice and murmur (or whispery voice, perceptually very close to breathy voice). These last two can occur in vocal pathologies, as well as in typical speech. The larynx traces at the foot of each figure clearly demonstrate the difference in vocal fold activity between the three voice qualities.

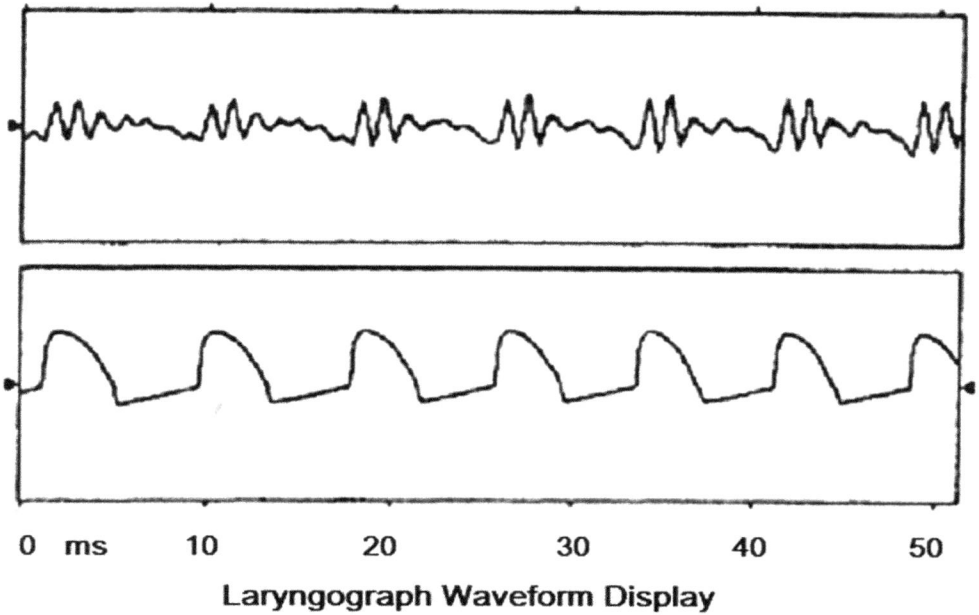

Figure 23.4 Acoustic waveform and laryngographic trace of modal voice for the vowel in "are." (With permission of Adrian Fourcin.)

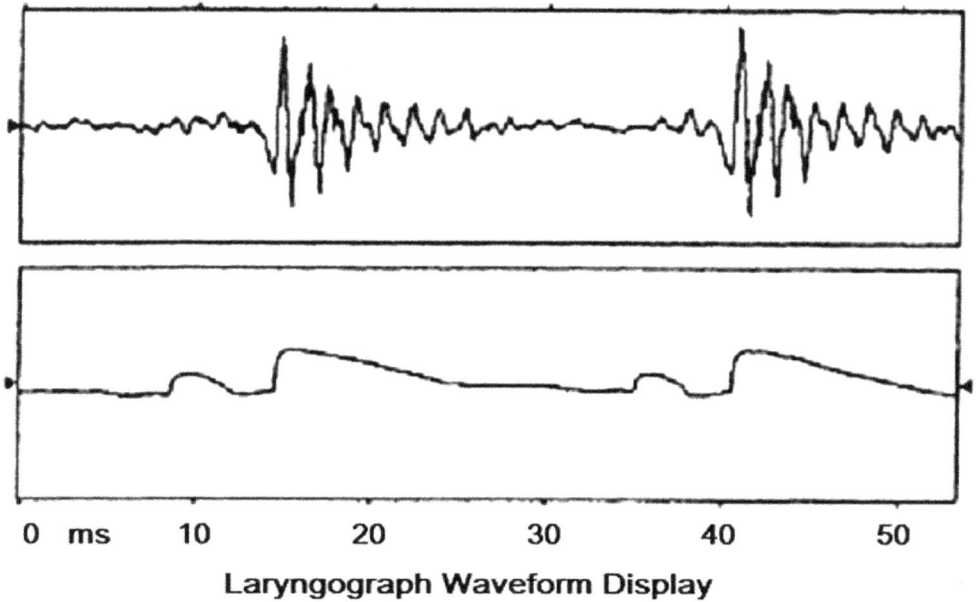

Figure 23.5 Acoustic waveform and laryngographic trace of creaky voice for the vowel in "are." (With permission of Adrian Fourcin.)

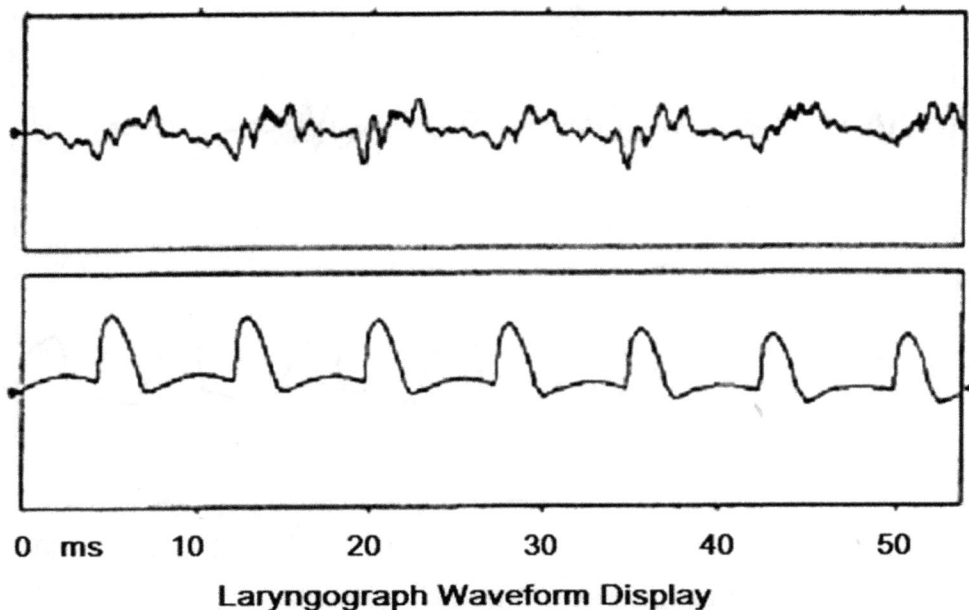

Laryngograph Waveform Display

Figure 23.6 Acoustic waveform and laryngographic trace of murmur for the vowel in "are." (With permission of Adrian Fourcin.)

Speech and voice therapy using electrolaryngography

Electrolaryngography may be a useful tool for interactive therapy through visual biofeedback. Dynamic displays give a clear visual indication of the smooth vocal fold vibration signal associated with clear modal voice and of any departure from the reference pattern associated with laryngeal problems or incorrect f_0 modulations. The software usually allows the simultaneous visualization of the client's voice and the reference model on the computer screen, which facilitates the comparison and the intuitive evaluation of the (mis)match.

Compared to raw speech pressure waveforms or spectrograms, laryngographic signals show less acoustic detail but, crucially, such detail is entirely functional to the specific purpose of the rehabilitation and requires much less effort in interpretation.

Moreover, not only the glottal wave with its shape and frequency pattern, but also the interactive displays of various measures associated with f_0 patterns that are produced by the software, such as larynx frequency distribution, distribution of speech intensity etc., may be of great usefulness in allowing the speaker and the clinician to visualize features of the phonation that are otherwise difficult to observe.

As emphasized by Abberton and Fourcin (1997), concomitant auditory evaluation is always necessary: since the correspondence between the laryngographic detail and the perceptual impact of voice perturbations is indirect, it is important that the clinician and the patient develop sensitivity to the global auditory output of voice pattern variations.

Another advantage of laryngographic-based rehabilitation paradigms, compared to other instrumental technique, is that the recordings can be made in quiet as well as in noisy environments with the same accuracy.

According to Cavalli & Hartley (2010), electrolaryngography is very well tolerated by children as young as three years of age, thus allowing wide sampling from all types of populations.

For instance, the live mode recording feature of the SpeechStudio software allowed children with either vocal fold palsy, mutational falsetto (puberphonia) or supraglottal voice production (following intubation associated with a history of prematurity) to successfully recover not only from their speech disorders but also from their inefficient swallowing dynamics (Cavalli, L. & Hartley, B.E.J., 2010). In a different study, inspection of the laryngographic signal could highlight the presence of diplophonia (that is, a bimodal distribution of fundamental frequency) in a subset of patients with mutational dysphonia, and the identification of this characteristic improved the success of the voice therapy, leading to a ready recovery of these patients (Lim J, Choi, Kim, 2007; see also Carlson, 1995; Chernobelsky, 2002).

Various voice quality parameters in adults with non-organic dysphonias may benefit from laryngographic feedback during treatment (Carding, Horsley, & Docherty, 1999). Speakers with habitually breathy voice may learn to better activate the cricoarythenoid muscles controlling vocal fold adduction (see above) after a training that includes real-time feedback provided by electrolaryngography (Herbst, Howard & Schlömicher-Their, 2010). It has also been shown that interactive training based on electrolaryngography can improve the control of fundamental frequency variations in hearing impaired children (Wirz & Anthony, 1979, Chernobelsky, 2002).

Note

1 This chapter has been jointly developed by two authors. The following sections were written by C. Celata: *Basic information about the functioning of the vocal folds, How the electrolaryngograph works: General characteristics, Electrolaryngographic characteristics of speech and voice pathologies, Speech and voice therapy using electrolaryngography.* The following sections were written by I. Ricci: *Instrumental components, Types of analysis, Systems currently in use.*

References

Abberton, E., & Fourcin, A. J. (1978). Intonation and speaker identification. *Language and Speech, 21,* 305–318.

Abberton, E., & Fourcin, A. J. (1997). Electrolaryngography. In M. J. Ball & C. Code (Eds.), *Instrumental clinical phonetics* (pp.119–148). London, United Kingdom: Whurr.

Abberton, E., Fourcin, A. J., & Hazan, V. (1991). Fundamental frequency range and the development of intonation in a group of profoundly deaf children. In *Actes du XIIème Congrès International des Sciences Phonétiques/Proceedings of the XII International Congress of Phonetic Sciences, Vol. 5* (pp. 142–145). Aix-en-Provence, France: Université de Provence, Service de Publications.

Abberton, E., Fourcin, A. J., Rosen, S.M., Howard, D. M., Douek, E. E., & Moore, B. C. J. (1985). Speech perceptual and productive rehabilitation. In R. A. Schindler & M. M. Merzenich (Eds.), *Cochlear Implants* (pp. 527–538). New York, NY: Raven Press.

Baken, R. J. (1992). Electroglottography. *Journal of Voice, 6*(2), 98–110.

Baken, R. J. (1987). *Clinical measurement of speech and voice.* Boston, MA: College Hill Press.

Broad, D. (1979). The new theories of vocal fold vibration. In N. Lass (Ed.), *Speech and Language: Advances in Basic Research and Practice* (pp. 203–256). New York, NY: Academic Press.

Carding, P., Horsley, I., Docherty, G. (1999). A study of the effectiveness of voice therapy in the treatment of 45 patients with nonorganic dysphonia. *Journal of Voice, 13*(1), 72–104.

Carlson, E. (1995). Electrolaryngography in the assessment and treatment of incomplete mutation (puberphonia) in adults. *European Journal of Disorders of Communication, 30*(2), 140–148.

Carlson, E., & Miller, D. (1998). Aspects of voice quality: display, measurement and therapy. *International Journal of Language & Communication Disorders, 33* Suppl, 304–309.

Cavalli, L., & Hartley, B. E. J. (2010). The clinical application of electrolaryngography in a tertiary children's hospital. *Logopedics Phoniatrics Vocology, 35*(2), 60–67.

Celata, C., Ricci, I., Nacci, A., & Romeo, S. (2016). Voiced apical trills: glottal, supraglottal and tongue root activity. Paper presented at XII Convegno Nazionale Associazione Italiana Scienze della Voce, Salerno, Italy, 27-29 January, 2016. Retrieved from https://www.researchgate.net/profile/Chiara_Celata/research

Chernobelsky, S. (2002). The use of electroglottography in the treatment of deaf adolescents with puberphonia. *Logopedics Phoniatrics Vocology*, 27(2), 63–65.

Colton, R., & Conture, E. (1990). Problems and pitfalls of electroglottography. *Journal of Voice, 4*(1), 10–24.

Esling, J. (2005). There are no back vowels. The Laryngeal Articulator Model. *The Canadian Journal of Linguistics/La revue canadienne de linguistique, 50*, 13–44.

Esling, J., & Harris, J. (2003). An Expanded Taxonomy of States of the Glottis. In M. J. Solé, D. Recasens, & J. Romero (Eds.), *ICPhS-15, Proceeding of the XV International Conference of Phonetic Sciences* (pp. 1049–1052), Barcelona, Spain. Retrieved from https://www.internationalphoneticassociation.org/icphs-proceedings/ICPhS2003/index.html

Esposito, C., Khan, S. D., & Hurst, A. (2007). Breathy Nasals and/Nh/Clusters in Bengali, Hindi, and Marathi. *Indian Linguistics, 68*(1–2), 275–299.

Fabre, P. (1957). Un procédé électrique percutané d'inscription de l'accolement glottique au cours de la phonation: glottographie de haute fréquence, premiers résultats. *Bulletin de l'Académie Nationale de Médécine, 141*(3–4), 69–99.

Fourcin, A. J. (1974). Laryngographic examination of vocal fold vibration. In B. Wyke (Ed.), *Ventilatory and phonatory control mechanisms* (pp. 315–333). London, United Kingdom: Oxford University Press.

Fourcin, A. J. (1981). Laryngographic assessment of phonatory function. In C. K. Ludlow & M. O'Connel Hart (Eds.), *Proceedings of the Conference on the Assessment of Vocal Pathology* (pp. 116–127). Rockville, MD: American Speech-Language-Hearing Association.

Fourcin, A. J., & Abberton, E. (1971). First applications of a new laryngograph. *Medical and Biological Illustration, 21*, 172–182.

Fourcin, A. J., Abberton, E., Miller, D., & Howells, D. (1995). Laryngograph: speech pattern element tools for therapy, training and assessment. *European Journal of Disorders of Communication, 30*, 101–115.

Fourcin, A. J., McGlashan, J., & Blowes, R. (2002). Measuring voice in the clinic - Laryngograph Speech Studio analyses. Retrieved from http://www.laryngograph.com/pdfdocs/paper7.pdf

Guimaraes, I., & Abberton, E. (2005). Health and voice quality in smokers: an exploratory investigation. *Logopedics Phoniatrics Vocology, 30*(3), 85–191.

Hacki, T. (1996). Electroglottographic quasi-open quotient and amplitude in crescendo phonation. *Journal of Voice, 10*(4), 342–347.

Hampala, V., Garcia, M., Švec, J. G., Scherer, R.C., & Herbst, C.T. (2016). Relationship Between the Electroglottographic Signal and Vocal Fold Contact Area. *Journal of Voice, 30*(2), 161–171.

Henrich, N., d'Alessandro, C., Doval, B., & Castellengo, M. (2004). On the use of the derivative of electroglottographic signals for characterization of nonpathological phonation. *The Journal of the Acoustical Society of America, 115*(3), 1321–1332.

Herbst, C. T. (2020). Electroglottography - An Update. *Journal of Voice, 34*(4), 503–526.

Herbst, C. T., Howard, D. M., & Schlömicher-Thier, J. (2010). Using electroglottographic real-time feedback to control posterior glottal adduction during phonation. *Journal of Voice, 24*(1), 72–85.

Herbst, C. T., Stoeger, A. S., Frey, R., Lohscheller, J., Titze, I. R., Gumpenberger, M., & Fitch, W. T. (2012) How Low Can You Go? Physical Production Mechanism of Elephant Infrasonic Vocalizations. *Science, 337*(6094), 595–599.

Herbst, C. T., Ternström, S. (2006). A comparison of different methods to measure the EGG contact quotient. *Logopedics Phoniatrics Vocology, 31*(3), 126–138.

Hirano, M. (1974). Morphological structure of the vocal cord as a vibrator and its variations. *Folia Phoniatrica et Logopaedica, 26*: 89–94.

Jilek, C., Marienhagen, J., & Hacki, T. (2004). Vocal stability in functional dysphonic versus healthy voices at different times of voice loading. *Journal of Voice, 18*(4), 443–453.

Lecluse, F. L. E., Brocaar, M. P., & Verschurre, J. (1975). The electroglottography and its relation to glottal activity. *Folia Phoniatrica et Logopaedica, 27*, 215–224.

Leff, J., & Abberton, E. (1981). Voice pitch measurements in schizophrenia and depression. *Psychological Medicine, 11*(4), 849–852.

Lim, J. Y., Lim, S. E., Choi, S. H., Kim, J. H., Kim, K. M., & Choi, H. S. (2007). Clinical characteristics and voice analysis of patients with mutational dysphonia: clinical significance of diplophonia and closed quotients. *Journal of Voice*, *21*(1), 12–19.

Lim, J. Y., Kim, J., Choi, S. H., Kim, K. M., Kim, Y. H., Kim, H. S., & Choi, H. S. (2009). Sulcus configurations of vocal folds during phonation. *Acta Oto-Laryngologica*, *129*(10), 1127–1135.

Lindau, M. (1985), The story of r. In V. A. Fromkin (Ed.), *Phonetic Linguistics* (pp. 157–168). Orlando, FL: Academic Press.

Nacci, A., Romeo, S. O., Cavaliere, M. D., Macerata, A., Bastiani, L., Paludetti, G., Galli, J., Marchese, M. R., Barillari, M. R., Barillari, U., Berrettini, S., Laschi, C., Cianchetti, M., Manti, M., Ursino, F., Fattori, B. (2019). Comparison of electroglottographic variability index in euphonic and pathological voice. *Acta Otorhinolaringologica Italica*, *39*(6), 381–388.

Orlikoff, R. F. (1991). Assessment of the dynamics of vocal fold contact from the electroglottogram: data from normal male subjects. *Journal of Speech and Hearing Research*, *34*(5), 1066–1072.

Pützer, M., Barry, W., & Moringlane, J. (2007). Effect of deep brain stimulation on different speech subsystems in patients with multiple sclerosis. *Journal of Voice*, *21*(6), 741–753.

Ramig, L., & Dromey, C. (1996). Aerodynamic mechanisms underlying treatment-related changes in vocal intensity in patients with Parkinson disease. *Journal of Speech Language and Hearing Research*, *39*(4), 798–807.

Ramírez, D., Jiménez, V., López, X. H., & Ysunza, P. A. (2018). Acoustic Analysis of Voice and Electroglottography in Patients With Laryngopharyngeal Reflux. *Journal of Voice*, *32*(3), 281–284.

Rothenberg, M. (1981). Some Relations Between Glottal Air Flow and Vocal Fold Contact Area. In C. K. Ludlow & M. O'Connel Hart (Eds.), *Proceedings of the Conference on the Assessment of Vocal Pathology* (pp. 88–96). Rockville, MD: American Speech-Language-Hearing Association.

Rothenberg, M. (1992). A Multichannel Electroglottograph. *Journal of Voice, 6*(1), 36–43.

Scherer, R. C., Druker, D. G., & Titze, I. R. (1988). Electroglottography and direct measurement of vocal fold contact area. In O. Fujimura (Ed.), *Vocal Fold Physiology, Vol. 2: Voice Production, Mechanisms and Functions* (279–290). New York, NY: Raven Press.

Somanath, K., & Mau, T. (2016). A Measure of the Auditory-perceptual Quality of Strain from Electroglottographic Analysis of Continuous Dysphonic Speech: Application to Adductor Spasmodic Dysphonia. *Journal of Voice*, *30*(6), 770.e9–770.e21.

Szkiełkowska, A., Krasnodębska, P., Miaśkiewicz, B., & Skarżyński, H. (2018). Electroglottography in the diagnosis of functional dysphonia. *European Archives of Oto-Rhino-Laryngology*, *275*(10), 2523–2528.

Titze I. R. (1973). The human vocal cords: a mathematical model, part I. *Phonetica*, *28*, 129–170.

Titze I. R. (1974). The human vocal cords: a mathematical model, part II. *Phonetica*, *29*, 1–21.

Titze I. R. (1984). Parameterization of the glottal area, glottal flow, and vocal fold contact area. *The Journal of the Acoustical Society of America*, *75*(2), 570–580.

Tronchin L., Kob, M., & Guarnaccia, C. (2018). Spatial information on voice generation from a multichannel electroglottograph. *Applied Sciences*, *8*(9), 1560.

van den Berg, J. W. (1958). Myoelastic-aerodynamic theory of voice production. *Journal of Speech and Hearing Research*, *1*(3), 227–244.

Vertigan, A. E., Theodoros, D. G., Winkworth, A. L., & Gibson, P. G. (2008). A comparison of two approaches to the treatment of chronic cough: Perceptual, acoustic, and electroglottographic outcomes. *Journal of Voice*, *22*(5), 581–589.

Wirz, S. L., & Anthony, J. (1979). The use of the voiscope in improving the speech of profoundly deaf children. *British Journal of Disorders of Communication*, *14*(2), 137–151.

Yiu, E. M., van Hasselt, C. A., Williams, S. R., & Woo, J. K. (1994). Speech intelligibility in tone language (Chinese) laryngectomy speakers. *European Journal of Disorders of Communication*, *29*(4), 339–347.

24
NASOMETRY

Tim Bressmann

Introduction

Nasality is an important and perceptually salient feature of speech production. To produce nasal or nasalized speech sounds, the soft palate is lowered and the velopharyngeal sphincter opens so that sound resonates in the nasal cavities (Bressmann, 2019; Kummer, 2008). The nasal cavities are mostly static anatomical structures (Amino & Arai, 2009). However, the nasal contribution to the spectral content of the speech signal can be frustratingly difficult to measure (Curtis, 1970).

Nasometry is an acoustic method to quantify the relative contribution of the sound pressure level (SPL) of the sound emanating from the nose to the total SPL, added from the oral and nasal speech signals. The SPL measures are made in Pascals to facilitate the calculations. The resulting measure is called nasalance (Fletcher, Sooudi, & Frost, 1974). Nasalance is reported as a percentage based on the formula:

$$\% \text{ Nasalance} = \frac{\text{Nasal SPL}}{\text{Nasal SPL} + \text{Oral SPL}} \times 100$$

Disorders of oral-nasal balance can affect the intelligibility and acceptability of speech (Kummer, 2008). The main types of oral-nasal balance disorders can be subsumed under three categories: Hypernasality, hyponasality and mixed nasality (de Boer & Bressmann, 2015). Hypernasality is characterized by too much sound emission from the nose, resulting in the nasalization of oral speech sounds. It is caused by velopharyngeal dysfunction, which Trost-Cardamone (1989) differentiates further into structurally related *velopharyngeal insufficiency* (related to conditions such as cleft palate or tumor resections), *velopharyngeal incompetence* (related to neuromotor or other physiological causes) and *velopharyngeal mislearning*. In hypernasality, nasalance scores for a non-nasal speech stimulus are higher than normal. In hyponasality, too little sound emanates from the nose, resulting in de-nasalization of nasal sounds. Hyponasality is caused by structural blockage of the nasal air passage because of conditions like septum deviation or hypertrophic nasal turbinates. Nasalance scores for a speech stimulus loaded with nasal sounds are lower than normal. Both hyper- and hyponasality may occur at the same time, resulting in mixed nasality. In this case, oral sounds are too nasal and nasal sounds are not nasal enough, which is reflected in higher nasalance scores for non-nasal speech stimuli and lower nasalance scores for stimuli loaded with nasal sounds (Bressmann et al., 2000; Kummer, 2008). Hypernasality, hyponasality and mixed nasality all result in a changed loudness balance between the oral and nasal cavity in speech, so they can be assessed with nasometry (de Boer & Bressmann, 2015).

History of the Nasometer

It has long been observed that clinicians struggle to make reliable and reproducible auditory-perceptual assessments of oral-nasal balance disorders (Fletcher, 1970; Keuning, Wieneke, Van Wijngaarden, & Dejonckere, 2002). Beginning in the 1950s, researchers attempted to make separate recordings of the oral and nasal speech signals, using separator plates, "nasal sound traps" (i.e. enclosures around the nose), or cannulas inserted into the nares (Shelton, Knox, Arndt, & Elbert, 1967). The idea that oral-nasal balance disorders could be measured and quantified was not uncontroversial even then. When Weatherley-White, Dersch, and Anderson (1964) proposed a design for a machine to automatically measure hypernasality from the acoustic signal, Moll (1964) responded that the auditory-perceptual assessment by a trained clinician should always be considered the gold standard and that acoustic measures could only be adjuncts. Moll's position is still a guiding principle for speech-language pathologists' clinical assessment of patients with oral-nasal balance disorders (Kuehn & Moller, 2000).

For recordings of a measure called The Oral Nasal Acoustic Ratio (TONAR; Fletcher, 1970), the participant pressed his or her prolabium against a contoured separator plate in a box with oral and nasal sound chambers. The signals from the oral and nasal microphones were bandpass-filtered with a center frequency of 500 Hz and a range of 350–650 Hz because this frequency was expected to correspond best to the perception of nasality. The intensity measurements for the band-pass filtered signals were displayed as oscillograph readouts, averaged over one second intervals. Fletcher and Bishop (1970) demonstrated that the ratio of the nasal divided by the oral SPL corresponded well to auditory-perceptual ratings of hypernasality. Fletcher (1972) suggested that the oscillographic readouts of the TONAR could be used to provide biofeedback in speech therapy. Fletcher et al. (1974) introduced the term "nasalance," calculated according to the formula given in the first paragraph of this chapter. Fletcher (1976) investigated the association between nasalance and listener judgments with an upgraded TONAR II. Stimuli used were the Zoo Passage, a short text without nasal consonants (Fletcher, 1972), the Nasal Sentences (Fletcher, 1978) and the phonetically balanced Rainbow Passage (Fairbanks, 1960). These stimuli are still used today for nasometric assessments. Weinberg, Noll and Donohue (1979) found that the frequency response characteristics of the TONAR II microphones were imbalanced, and they suspected that the sound separator chambers distorted the measurements further. Fletcher (1979) refuted these criticisms but also embarked on improvements.

The successor instrument to the TONAR II was called the Nasometer 6200[1] (Dalston, 1989). Marketed by Kay Elemetrics (now Pentax Medical, Montvale NJ), the Nasometer 6200 interfaced with a personal computer and ran with software in the Microsoft Disk Operating System (MS DOS). The new wearable headset used a metal separator plate that rested on the speaker's prolabium, perpendicular to the face (Figure 24.1). The signal was bandpass-filtered with a center frequency of 500 Hz and converted into direct current for the nasalance measurements. Because of the direct current conversion, it was not possible to play back the audio signals from the nasalance recordings. The nasalance trace ("nasogram") could be observed in real-time or stored for later review (Figure 24.2). The Nasometer software also included games for biofeedback exercises.

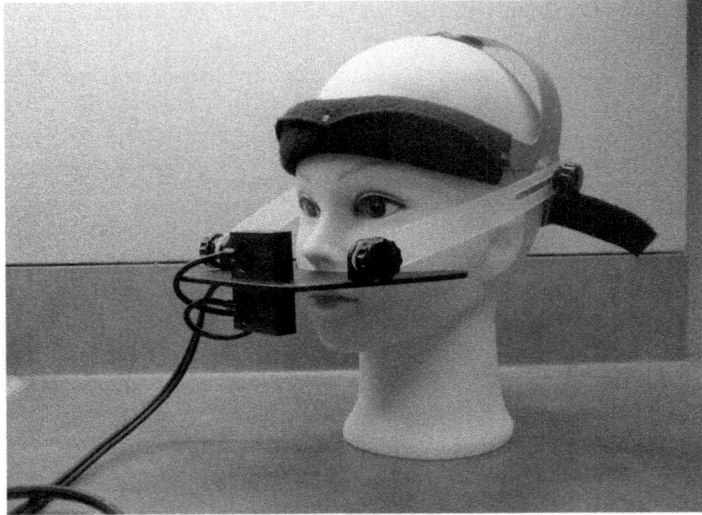

Figure 24.1 Nasometer headset.

The overall design and operation of the Nasometer hardware and software has remained remarkably unchanged. In the years since its introduction, the Nasometer was updated to work with a computer sound card (Nasometer II 6400) and the Microsoft Windows operating system. The current version (Nasometer II 6450) uses a proprietary universal serial bus sound converter, and the headset holder can be replaced with handles attached to the separator plate. The metal separation plate of the Nasometer is very effective for separating the nasal and oral channels but the headset has a certain weight as a consequence. Moisture from the nasal airflow

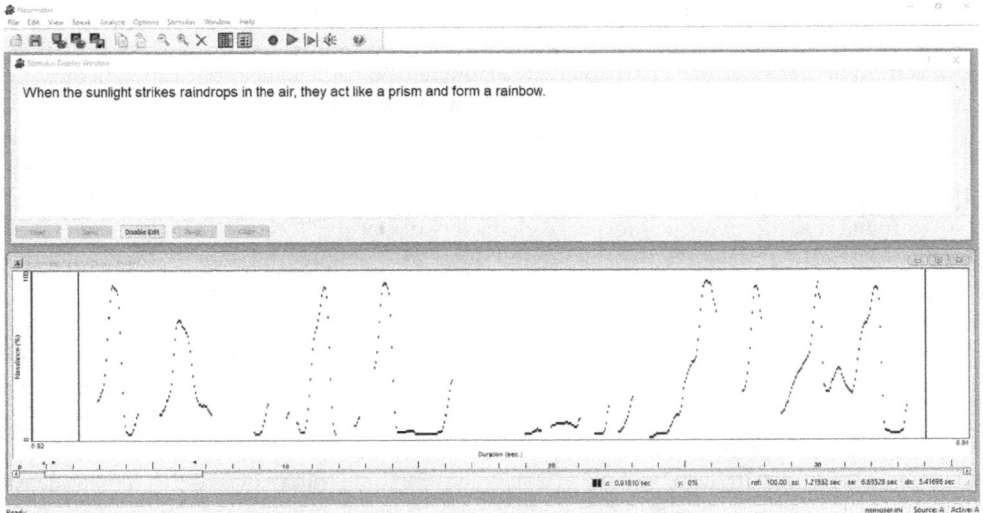

Figure 24.2 Nasometer software, showing a nasalance trace for the sentence "When sunlight strikes raindrops in the air, they act like a prism and form a rainbow," spoken by a typical speaker. The nasal segments are visible as peaks in the nasalance contour.

can condensate and accumulate on the nasal side of the separation plate during longer sessions. Ever since the Nasometer 6400 started using analog-to-digital sound conversion (rather than the direct current conversion used in the original Nasometer 6200), it has also become possible to record and play back the audio. The software uses a proprietary file format with a low sampling rate that cuts off frequencies above 4,000 Hz. For the purpose of obtaining nasalance recordings, this is more than enough signal resolution since only band-pass filtered low frequency bands around the center frequency of 500 Hz are used to obtain nasalance scores. However, the recordings sound rather muffled and would not be sufficient for detailed auditory-perceptual analyses.

Watterson, Lewis, and Brancamp (2005) found significant differences between scores obtained with the Nasometers 6200 and 6400. The authors attributed the differences mostly to intra-subject variability and headgear changes, and less to actual differences between the machines. Awan and Virani (2013) reported considerable differences of 7% for non-nasal stimuli between the Nasometers 6200 and 6400. In contrast, de Boer and Bressmann (2014) found only small differences of 1–2% between nasalance scores obtained with the Nasometers 6200 and 6450.

Speech materials and norms for nasalance scores

Soon after the introduction of the Nasometer 6200, a number of studies developed cut-off scores that mark the transition from normal oral-nasal balance to pathological hypernasality and hyponasality. To summarize these findings, for non-nasal stimuli such as the Zoo Passage (Fletcher, 1978), nasalance scores under 20% are considered normal. Nasalance scores above 20% are considered elevated but not clearly pathological. Using calculations of sensitivity (i.e. the percentage of individuals correctly found to have a trait of interest) and specificity (i.e. the percentage of individuals correctly found not to have the trait of interest), Dalston, Warren, and Dalston (1991a) proposed 32% as the cut-off score for hypernasality in American English. In a second study, Dalston, Neiman, and Gonzalez-Landa (1993) determined 28% as the cut-off score for hypernasality in American English while Hardin et al. (1992) arrived at 26%. Based on clinical experience, Watterson (2020) argued for a more conservative cut-off of 30% for normal or borderline hypernasal speech, 31–35% as the range of mild hypernasality, 36–45% for moderate hypernasality and more than 45% for severe hypernasality. Dalston, Warren, and Dalston (1991b) and Hardin, Van Demark, Morris, and Payne (1992) found that nasalance scores lower than 50% for the Nasal Sentences corresponded to an auditory-perceptual impression of hyponasality.

Fletcher's (1978) Zoo Passage and Nasal Sentences may be difficult for younger speakers. The alternative Simplified Nasometric Assessment Procedure (SNAP test, Kummer, 2008) consists of consonant repetitions and short phrases. Illustrations for target words have been incorporated into the Nasometer software. Watterson, Hinton, and McFarlane (1996) introduced the Turtle Passage as a simpler alternative to the Zoo Passage and showed that numerically identical nasalance scores could be obtained.

Longer nasometric assessment procedures do not necessarily produce more accurate results. Watterson, Lewis, and Foley-Homan (1999) evaluated the effect of stimulus length on nasalance scores and concluded that sentences needed to be at least six syllables in order to obtain reliable and reproducible nasalance scores. Bressmann et al. (2000) demonstrated that comparable diagnostic accuracy could be attained with short, individual sentences and longer stimuli.

Nasometric testing stimuli and cut-off scores for hypernasality have been developed for many different languages around the world, including North American English (Seaver, Dalston, Leeper, & Adams, 1991), Irish English (Lee & Browne, 2013; Sweeney, Sell, & O'Regan, 2004), Spanish (Anderson, 1996), German (Küttner et al., 2003; Stellzig, Heppt, & Komposch, 1994), Japanese (Tachimura et al., 2000), Dutch (Van Lierde et al., 2001), Cantonese (Whitehill, 2001), Malaysian (Mohd Ibrahim, Reilly, & Kilpatrick, 2012), Vietnamese (Nguyen, Lehes, Truong, Hoang, & Jagomägi, 2019), Swedish (Brunnegård & van Doorn, 2009), Greek (Okalidou, Karathanasi, & Grigoraki, 2011), Turkish (Karakoc, Akcam, Birkent, Arslan, & Gerek., 2013); Egyptian Arabic (Abou-Elsaad, Quriba, Baz, & Elkassaby, 2013), Korean (Park et al., 2014), Brazilian Portuguese (Marino et al., 2016, 2018) and Estonian (Lehes et al., 2018). Clinical cut-off scores for hypernasality have also been developed for different languages (Mayo & Mayo, 2011).

Clinical application of the Nasometer

The Nasometer has been used extensively in clinical research to investigate a diverse range of conditions and interventions, as demonstrated by the following, admittedly incomplete, overview.

Nasalance scores have been used to document surgical outcomes in different populations. To give but a few examples, there has been research on the outcomes of cleft palate surgery (Ekin et al., 2017; Nellis, Neiman, & Lehman, 1992; Reddy et al., 2016; Van Lierde, Claeys, De Bodt, & Van Cauwenberge, 2004; Van Lierde, Bonte, Baudonck, Van Cauwenberge, & De Leenheer, 2008), orthognathic surgery (Alaluusua et al., 2019; Kudo et al., 2014; Zemann, Feichtinger, Santler, & Kärcher, 2006), head and neck cancer surgery (Al-Qahtani et al., 2015; Browne, Butler, & Rees, 2011; Kim et al., 2017; Rieger, Wolfaardt, Seikaly, & Jha, 2002), adenoidectomy surgery (Tuzuner et al., 2014) and sleep apnea surgery (Karakoc et al., 2015; Li, Lee, Fang, Lin, & Lin, 2010; Van Lierde, Van Borsel, Moerman, & Van Cauwenberge, 2002). Nasalance has also been used to show the effectiveness of prosthodontic treatment and speech bulb prostheses (Ayliffe, Bressmann, Al Mardini, & Jokstad, 2014; Pinborough-Zimmerman, Canady, Yamashiro, & Morales, 1998; Tachimura, Kotani, & Wada, 2004). Nasalance scores have been used to document the success of therapy exercises to remediate hypernasality (Cahill et al., 2004; Ferreira et al., 2020; Van Lierde et al., 2004).

While the Nasometer is probably most frequently used to assess oral-nasal balance disorders in speakers with cleft palate, individuals with deafness and profound hearing loss have also been studied, starting with some of the earliest work with the TONAR (Fletcher & Daly, 1976; Kim et al., 2012). Most nasometry research, such as the studies cited above, has focused on hypernasality, but the Nasometer has also been used to assess nasal obstruction. Williams, Eccles, and Hutchings (1990) showed a good correlation of nasalance scores and nasal airway resistance in speakers with colds and matched controls. Since then, the Nasometer has often been used to document improvement after endonasal surgery (Amer, Elaassar, Anany, & Quriba, 2017; Jiang & Huang, 2006; Kim, Lee, Park, & Cho, 2013; Kim et al., 2017; Soneghet et al., 2002).

Sources of variation of nasalance scores

Nasalance scores are used to make clinical decisions about interventions such as surgery, prosthodontic devices or speech therapy, all of which may have a considerable impact on the patient's life. Therefore, it is important that the nasalance scores are as accurate as possible.

However, speech production is characterized by considerable variability, and this is often reflected in variable nasalance scores. In the initial assessments of immediate test-retest reliability of Nasometer scores, between 94% and 100% of recordings were within 3 points (Litzaw and Dalston, 1992; Seaver et al., 1991). Watterson and Lewis (2006) assessed test-retest variability of nasalance scores in hypernasal speakers and found that most repetitions were within a range of 5%. However, they also pointed out that changing the headgear increased the variability between measurements. In longer-term testing of typical speakers over several weeks, de Boer and Bressmann (2014) found that a 6–8-point interval was needed to capture 90% of the participants' data. It has been noted that variability of nasalance scores increases with the proportion of nasal consonants in the sentence (Whitehill, 2001). If nasal sounds are present, there will be corresponding peaks in the nasalance trace, which may skew the mean nasalance score (de Boer & Bressmann, 2014).

It can be difficult to pinpoint the sources of the variability. Factors of speech production such as speaking volume (Watterson, York, & McFarlane, 1994), air pressure of consonants (Watterson, Lewis, & Deutsch, 1998), speaking rate (Gauster, Yunusova, & Zajac, 2010) and fundamental frequency (Mandulak & Zajac, 2009) were all found to have limited effects on nasalance scores. Higher levels of nasal congestion were found to result in lower nasalance scores (Williams, Eccles, & Hutchings, 1990). Pegoraro-Krook et al. (2006) suggested that nasal decongestion should be applied routinely before nasometric recordings but Watterson, Lewis, Ludlow, and Ludlow (2008) reasoned that it is usually not necessary to go such lengths.

Nasalance scores are usually lower in young children and increase with age (Van Lierde, Wuyts, De Bodt, & Van Cauwenberge, 2003; Marino et al., 2016). Further increases in nasalance have been reported for elderly speakers (Hutchinson, Robinson, and Nerbonne, 1978; Marino et al., 2018). There are divergent reports in the literature whether nasalance scores differ by speaker sex. Some studies found no differences between male and female speakers (Brunnegård and van Doorn, 2009; D'haeseleer, Bettens, de Mets, de Moor, & Van Lierde, 2015; Lee & Browne, 2013; Sweeney, Sell, & O'Regan, 2004). Where studies did find sex differences, the nasalance scores for female speakers were higher (Awan et al., 2015; Marino et al., 2016; Rochet, Rochet, Sovis, & Mielke, 1998; Van Lierde et al., 2003). However, nasalance differences related to age and speaker sex are usually quite small and will have little clinical or diagnostic impact (Marino et al., 2018; Watterson, 2020).

Nasalance scores can be influenced by the vowel content of the speech stimuli. The bandpass filter of the Nasometer focuses the measurement on voiced segments in lower frequency bands. Lewis, Watterson, and Quint (2000) demonstrated that nasalance scores were highest for high front vowels. These differences also affect retest reliability, which is poorer for high vowels (Ha, Jung, & Koh, 2018). Since vowels and other features of speech differ across dialects of a language, a speaker's particular local dialect can also have a bearing on nasalance scores (Awan et al., 2015; Bae, et al., 2020; Dalston et al., 1993; D'haeseleer et al., 2015).

Mayo, Floyd, Warren, Dalston, and Mayo (1996) investigated possible differences between the nasalance scores and nasal cross-sectional areas for typical Black and Caucasian speakers of American English. No differences were found, with the exception of higher nasalance scores for the Nasal Sentences spoken by the Caucasian participants. Craniofacial growth trajectories are largely similar between different ethnic groups (Durtschi, Chung, Gentry, Chung, & Voperian, 2009), so few differences are to be expected. However, some researchers have not hesitated to attribute otherwise seemingly inexplicable group effects to supposed morphological differences between different ethnic groups (e.g. Shin, Kim, and Kim, 2017).

Gildersleeve-Neumann and Dalston (2001) investigated why typical nasalance scores on oral sounds are often low but never zero. The authors concluded that some acoustic energy may be transmitted through the palate. Scarsellone, Rochet, and Wolfaardt (1999) found slightly higher nasalance scores when speakers were wearing their complete maxillary dentures. Blanton, Watterson, and Lewis (2015) assessed the effect of covering only the hard or both the hard and soft palate in typical speakers. They concluded that most acoustic energy was transferred at the soft palate but that this effect was limited to high front vowels.

Even microphones of the same type may differ slightly in their frequency responses. Zajac, Lutz, and Mayo (1996) compared microphone sensitivities in different Nasometer headsets and found small differences in nasalance scores. Such hardware differences might affect the comparison of nasalance scores from different centers. Typically, nasalance scores are reported as mean values for a longer linguistic stimulus such as a sentence or a text passage. The Nasometer software only shows a nasalance trace but no accompanying speech oscillograms, so it does not lend itself to more fine-grained research on phonetic segments. Kummer (2008) described how some phonetic details can be observed in nasalance traces. Zajac and Preisser (2016) used a Nasometer headset to investigate mechanisms of nasal turbulence.

Alternative instruments for the acoustic assessment of oral-nasal balance

The Nasometer is the most widely used instrument for the assessment of oral-nasal balance but it is expensive. The quality of the audio recordings is poor, and the recordings are saved in a proprietary format that must be exported and converted file-by-file to be used with different software. Over the years, a number of alternative devices for the assessment of oral-nasal balance have been developed.

The NasalView (Awan, 1997) used a styrene sound separator plate with a headset holder similar to the Nasometer (Figure 24.3). To improve sound separation, a mass-loaded rubber layer was attached to the top- and undersides of the styrene plate. The device was marketed by TigerDRS (Seattle, WA). Sound separation was not as effective as that achieved by the

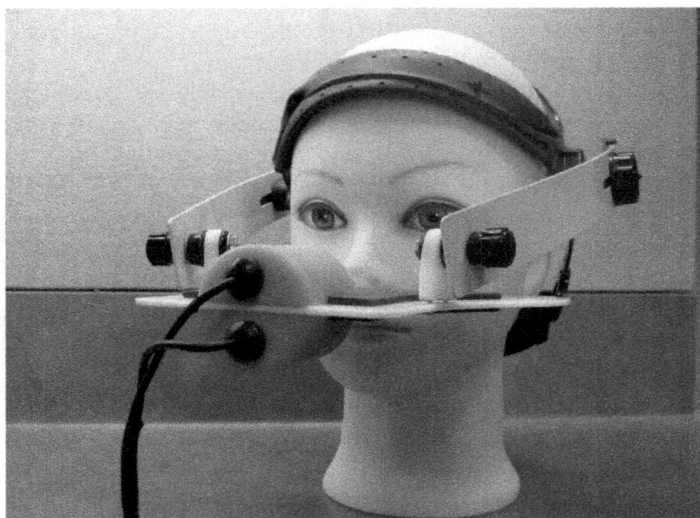

Figure 24.3   NasalView headset.

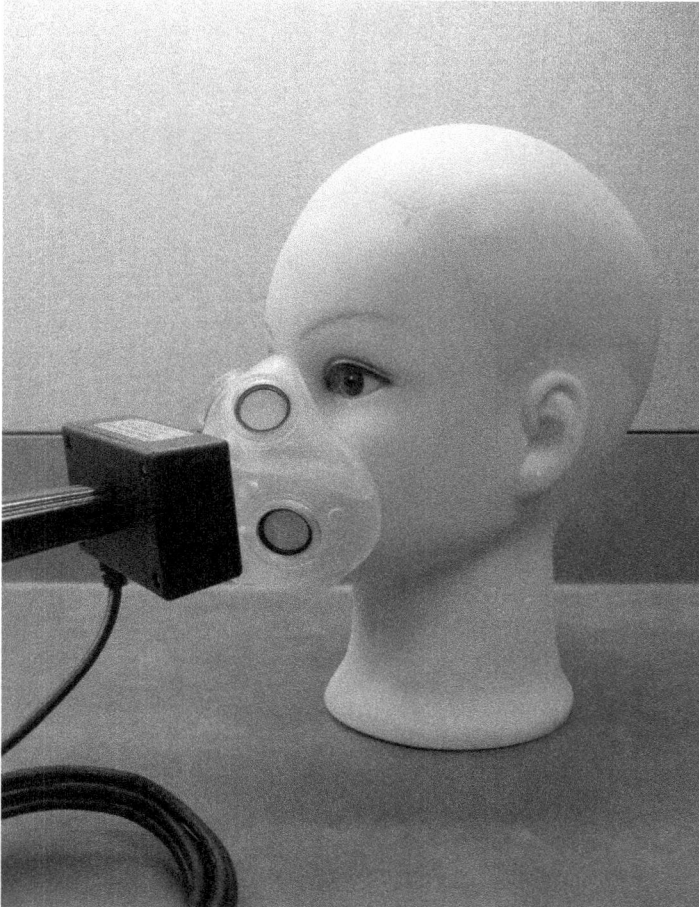

Figure 24.4 Nasalance System with face mask.

metal baffle plate of the Nasometer (Bressmann, 2005). Lewis and Watterson (2003) compared nasalance scores from the Nasometer 6200 and the NasalView and concluded that these were qualitatively and quantitatively different because of differences in signal processing.

The Nasalance System (formerly called the OralNasal System) by Glottal Enterprises (Syracuse, NY) comes with either a circumvented face mask (Figure 24.4) or with a plastic separator plate (Figure 24.5). The sound separation of the mask is better than that of the plate (Woo, Park, Oh, and Ha, 2019). To compensate for acoustic spillover between the oral and nasal channels, a proprietary algorithm calculates a corrected nasalance score. The software also calculates the inverse, termed "oralance". The device is marketed primarily as a biofeed-back instrument, and the manufacturer cautions against using nasalance scores for diagnostic purposes.

The lingWAVES Nasality is distributed by WEVOSYS (Braunach, Germany). It uses a nasal Continuous Positive Airway Pressure (CPAP) mask to isolate the nasal signal and measures sound pressure level with a microphone at the end of an attached air hose. The software calculates a nasalance score and provides different kinds of visual biofeedback for speech therapy.

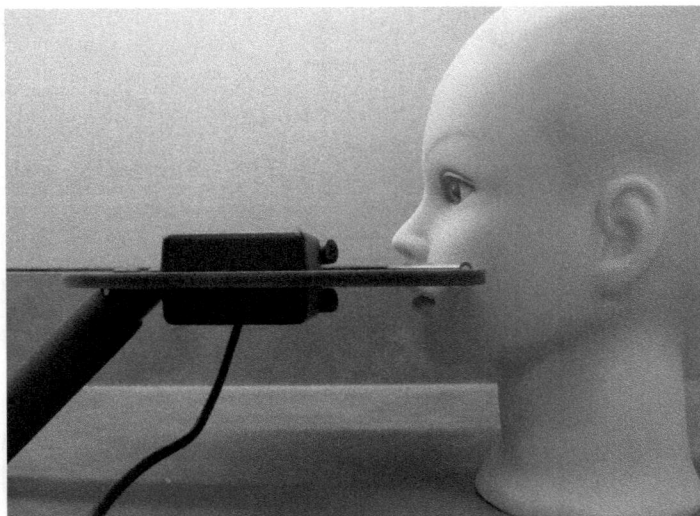

Figure 24.5   Nasalance System with separator plate.

Derrick, Duerr, and Kerr's (2019) Rivener brings the separation plate close to the participant's face but does not touch the prolabium. To maintain a constant distance, the separation plate is held by a headgear. While the contact-free approach may seem unusual at first, it should be noted that little gaps between the separation plate and the speaker's face can also often be observed with the standard Nasometer headset. Individuals' faces do not always fit the contour of the separation plate perfectly. If these gaps are small enough, they probably do not affect the nasalance score. However, with bigger gaps or an increasing distance between the prolabium and the baffle plate, the degree of acoustic spillover between the oral and nasal signals will increase.

Instead of microphones and a separation plate, Horii (1980) used accelerometers attached to the side of the nose and the larynx to calculate the ratio of the nasal SPL to the laryngeal source signal. The resulting measure was called the Horii Oral-Nasal Coupling (HONC) Index. A similar system from Sweden was the Nasal Oral Ratio Meter (NORAM; Karling, Larson, Leanderson, Galyas, & De Serpa-Leitao, 1993). A number of studies reported HONC scores for typical speakers as well as speakers with simulated or clinical hypernasality (Horii and Lang, 1981; Laczi, Sussman, Stathopoulos, & Huber, 2005; Mra, Sussman, & Fenwick, 1998; Sussman, 1995). The use of the technique for biofeedback was explored again by Heller-Murray, Mendoza, Gill, Perkell, and Stepp, (2016). Cler et al. (2016) used accelerometry to identify nasal emission. Despite their apparent promise, these accelerometer-based systems are not commonly used in clinical practice, yet.

Stewart and Kohlberger (2017) used small handheld earbud headphones to record separate oral and nasal signals for linguistic fieldwork. Ha, Sim, Zhi and Kuehn (2004) used a microphone headset with one microphone trained toward the nose and the other toward the mouth to investigate the timing characteristics of transitions from nasal to oral sounds. These methods worked well to detect when nasality was present. They would not be reliable enough to measure an accurate nasalance score.

The task of separating oral and nasal speech signals and deriving separate intensity measurements may seem simple enough but has a few challenges in practice. One problem is achieving sufficient sound separation of the nasal and oral signals. The Nasometer's metal baffle plate separates the sound more effectively than the alternative instruments. Achieving reliable and reproducible loudness measurements is not a trivial task, either. Švec and Granqvist (2018) explained how small changes in microphone position can make a big difference when measuring sound intensity at close range from the sound source. This may cause considerable variability in recordings with accelerometers or microphones positioned right by or on the nose and mouth, which could affect nasalance scores calculated from these measurements. For intensity measurements for voice research, Švec and Granqvist (2018) recommend a 30 cm distance between sound source and measurement microphone to obtain reproducible decibel readings. For nasalance recordings, this would require an impractically large and wide baffle plate to keep the oral and nasal sound sufficiently separated. Devices such as the Nasometer, the NasalView, or the OralNasal System place the microphones about 5 cm away from nose and mouth. This relatively close placement means that small variations in headset placement and angle may affect nasalance scores (Watterson & Lewis, 2006).

Future perspectives for nasometry

The Nasometer continues to be a popular instrument in clinical practice and research. However, the problem of variable agreement between nasalance scores and auditory-perceptual assessments remains. Studies have run the gamut from strong to weak agreement (Nellis, Neiman, & Lehman, 1992; Watterson, McFarlane, & Wright, 1993; Sweeney & Sell, 2008), irrespective of the rating scales used (Brancamp, Lewis, & Watterson, 2010). Watterson (2020) concluded that "some of the poor correspondence between nasalance scores and nasality ratings may be due to the instability of nasality ratings" (p. 157).

Clinicians find it unsettling if nasalance scores do not reflect what they think they hear. As a result, researchers have explored alternative measures. Vallino-Napoli and Montgomery (1997) investigated the diagnostic use of the nasalance standard deviation but concluded that the mean value was the better measure. Bressmann et al. (2000, 2006) tested nasalance distance and ratio measures to characterize the relationship between speakers' maximum nasalance for nasal stimuli and minimum nasalance for non-nasal stimuli. Keuning et al. (2004) found these measures only moderately correlated with auditory-perceptual ratings.

Van Lierde et al. (2006) developed a composite measure named the Nasal Severity Index. This measure was calculated as a weighted score of nasalance and a nasal mirror-fogging test, and the authors found high values of sensitivity and specificity. Bettens, Van Lierde, Corthals, Luyten, and Wuyts (2016) developed a new Nasality Severity Index 2.0 based on nasalance scores and a spectrographic measure. The final measure was calculated as NSI 2.0 = 13.20 – (.0824 * nasalance score /u:/) – (.260 * nasalance score oral text) – (.242 * voice low tone to high tone ratio of /i:/ 4.47* intensity of the fundamental frequency in decibels). Bettens et al. (2016) demonstrated good test-retest validity of the Nasality Severity Index 2.0 and a moderate association with auditory-perceptual ratings of hypernasality. Bettens, Wuyts, Jonckheere, Platbrood, and Van Lierde (2017) reported reference values for children and adults.

De Boer and Bressmann (2015) argued that the term "resonance disorders," which is commonly used by Speech-Language Pathologists to describe disorders of oral-nasal balance, may add unnecessary complexity to the diagnostic process. For example, a condition called cul-de-sac resonance is characterized by a muffled quality because sound is trapped in a blind pouch in the speaker's vocal tract. However, cul-de-sac may be observed as a nasal, oral or pharyngeal phenomenon, i.e. it may be independent from oral-nasal balance (Kummer, 2011). De Boer and Bressmann (2015) suggested that diagnoses of oral-nasal balance with the Nasometer should be limited to the categories of normal, hypernasal, hyponasal and mixed (concurrent hyper- and hypernasality), which can be reasonably quantified with nasalance scores. Other qualitative features such as audible nasal air emission, nasal frication sounds, or cul-de-sac are best assessed by auditory-perceptual analysis and should be documented separately. The authors also observed that nasometry has traditionally mainly been used to quantify hypernasality. However, many patients with cleft palate also have deviations of the nasal septum and other obstructions of the nose that may result in hyponasal or mixed oral-nasal balance. With a group of typical speakers simulating the four oral-nasal balance conditions, the authors demonstrated that a linear discriminant analysis of the nasalance scores for one oral and one nasal sentence separated accurately between the conditions. When Bettens, de Boer, Bressmann, Bruneel, and Van Lierde (2019) applied the original discriminant functions from de Boer and Bressmann (2015) to data of Dutch-speaking children, they found good accuracy after the functions were re-derived for the different population and language. De Boer et al. (2020) demonstrated how the agreement between experienced listeners' assessments improved when they made their diagnoses *after* reviewing nasalance-based pre-classifications of the type and severity of the oral-nasal balance disorders.

Conclusion

Nasometry provides a simple and seemingly straightforward measure of the nasal contribution to the speech produced. The nasalance score is one of the most widely used acoustic measures in Speech-Language Pathology but the received wisdom in the profession is that auditory-perceptual assessment must always supersede quantitative acoustic measures (Moll, 1964). An overly strict adherence to this tenet may be problematic because clinicians' auditory-perceptual assessments can be quite variable (Counihan & Cullinan, 1970; Fletcher, 1970; Galek & Watterson, 2017; Keuning et al., 2002, 2004). However, while clinicians should not rely unthinkingly on nasalance scores as the sole source of information for their diagnosis, acoustic measures do not have to detract from the clinician's authority. For example, de Boer at al. (2020) demonstrated how nasalance-based pre-classifications of the quality and severity of oral-nasal balance disorders resulted in improved agreement between trained listeners. This way, nasalance scores could be used to scaffold auditory-perceptual assessments, while still leaving the final say to the clinician.

Notes

1 The first occurrence of the term "Nasometer" in the literature describes an instrument for the assessment of nasal patency (Seltzer, 1957), which does not seem to have stood the test of time.

References

Abou-Elsaad, T., Quriba, A., Baz, H., & Elkassaby, R. (2013). Standardization of nasometry for normal Egyptian Arabic speakers. *Folia Phoniatrica et Logopaedica*, 64(6), 271–277.

Alaluusua, S., Turunen, L., Saarikko, A., Geneid, A., Leikola, J., & Heliövaara, A. (2019). The effects of Le Fort I osteotomy on velopharyngeal function in cleft patients. *Journal of Cranio-Maxillofacial Surgery*, 47(2), 239–244.

Al-Qahtani, K., Rieger, J., Harris, J.R., Mlynarek, A., Williams, D., Islam, T., & Seikaly, H (2015). Treatment of base of tongue cancer, stage III and stage IV with primary surgery: survival and functional outcomes. *European Archives of Oto-Rhino-Laryngology*, 272(8), 2027–2033.

Amer, H.S., Elaassar, A.S., Anany, A.M., & Quriba, A.S. (2017). Nasalance changes following various endonasal surgeries. *International Archives of Otorhinolaryngology*, 21(2), 110–114.

Amino, K., & Arai, T. (2009). Speaker-dependent characteristics of the nasals. *Forensic Science International*, 185(1–3), 21–28.

Anderson, R.T. (1996). Nasometric values for normal Spanish-speaking females: A preliminary report. *Cleft Palate-Craniofacial Journal*, 33(4), 333–336.

Awan, S.N. (1997). Analysis of nasalance: Nasalview. In: W. Ziegler & K. Deger. (Eds.) *Clinical Phonetics and Linguistics* (pp. 518–525). London: Whurr-Publishers.

Awan, S.N., & Virani, A. (2013). Nasometer 6200 versus Nasometer II 6400: Effect on measures of nasalance. *Cleft Palate-Craniofacial Journal*, 50(3), 268–274.

Awan, S.N., Bressmann, T., Poburka, B., Roy, N., Sharp, H., & Watts, C. (2015). Dialectical effects on nasalance: A multicenter, cross-continental study. *Journal of Speech, Language, and Hearing Research*, 58(1), 69–77.

Ayliffe, B.W., Bressmann, T., Al Mardini, M., & Jokstad, A. (2014). Evaluation of a modular palatal lift prosthesis with a silicone velar lamina for hypernasal patients. *Journal of Prosthetic Dentistry*, 112(3), 663–671.

Bae, Y., Lee, S.A.S., Velik, K., Liu, Y., Beck, C., & Fox, R.A. (2020). Differences in nasalance and nasality perception between Texas South and Midland dialects. *Journal of the Acoustical Society of America*, 147(1), 568–578.

Bettens, K., de Boer, G., Bressmann, T., Bruneel, L., & Van Lierde, K. (2019). Clinical application of a new approach to identify oral–nasal balance disorders based on nasalance scores. *Cleft Palate-Craniofacial Journal*, 56(5), 628–638.

Bettens, K., Van Lierde, K.M., Corthals, P., Luyten, A., & Wuyts, F.L. (2016) The nasality severity index 2.0: Revision of an objective multiparametric approach to hypernasality. *Cleft Palate-Craniofacial Journal*, 53(3), e60–e70.

Bettens, K., Wuyts, F.L., D'haeseleer, E., Luyten, A., Meerschman, I., Van Crayelynghe, C., & Van Lierde, K.M. (2016). Short-term and long-term test-retest reliability of the Nasality Severity Index 2.0. *Journal of Communication Disorders*, 62, 1–11.

Bettens, K., Wuyts, F.L., Jonckheere, L., Platbrood, S., & Van Lierde, K. (2017). Influence of gender and age on the Nasality Severity Index 2.0 in Dutch-speaking Flemish children and adults. *Logopedics Phoniatrics Vocology*, 42(3), 133–140.

Blanton, A., Watterson, T., & Lewis, K. (2015). The differential influence of vowels and palatal covering on nasalance scores. *Cleft Palate-Craniofacial Journal*, 52(1), 82–87.

Brancamp, T.U., Lewis, K.E., & Watterson, T. (2010). The relationship between nasalance scores and nasality ratings obtained with equal appearing interval and direct magnitude estimation scaling methods. *Cleft Palate-Craniofacial Journal*, 47(6), 631–637.

Bressmann, T. (2005). Comparison of nasalance scores obtained with the Nasometer, the NasalView, and the OroNasal System. *Cleft Palate-Craniofacial Journal*, 42 (4), 423–433.

Bressmann T. (2019). Nasality. In: M.J. Ball, J. Damico (Eds.), *Encyclopedia of Human Communication Sciences and Disorders* (pp. 1220–1223). Thousand Oaks, CA: Sage.

Bressmann, T., Klaiman, P., & Fischbach, S. (2006). Same noses, different nasalance scores: Data from normal subjects and cleft palate speakers for three systems for nasalance analysis. (2006) *Clinical Linguistics and Phonetics*, 20(2-3), 163–170.

Bressmann, T., Sader, R., Whitehill, T.L., Awan, S.N., Zeilhofer, H.-F., & Horch, H.-H. (2000). Nasalance distance and ratio: Two new measures. *Cleft Palate-Craniofacial Journal*, 37(3), 248–256.

Browne, J.D., Butler, S., & Rees, C. (2011). Functional outcomes and suitability of the temporalis myofascial flap for palatal and maxillary reconstruction after oncologic resection. *Laryngoscope*, 121(6), 1149–1159.

Brunnegård, K., & van Doorn, J. (2009). Normative data on nasalance scores for Swedish as measured on the Nasometer: Influence of dialect, gender, and age. *Clinical Linguistics and Phonetics*, 23(1), 58–69.

Cahill, L.M., Turner, A.B., Stabler, P.A., Addis, P.E., Theodoros, D.G., & Murdoch, B.E. (2004). An evaluation of continuous positive airway pressure (CPAP) therapy in the treatment of hypernasality following traumatic brain injury: A report of 3 cases. *Journal of Head Trauma Rehabilitation*, 19(3), 241–253.

Cler, M.J., Lien, Y.-A.S., Braden, M.N., Mittelman, T., Downing, K., & Stepp, C.E. (2016). Objective measure of nasal air emission using nasal accelerometry. *Journal of Speech, Language, and Hearing Research*, 59(5), 1018–1024.

Counihan, D., & Cullinan, W. (1970). Reliability and dispersion of nasality ratings. *Cleft Palate Journal*, 7, 261–270.

Curtis, J.F. (1970). The acoustics of nasalized speech. *Cleft Palate Journal*, 7, 480–496.

Dalston, R.M. (1989). Using simultaneous photodetection and nasometry to monitor velopharyngeal behavior during speech. *Journal of Speech and Hearing Research*, 32(1), 195–202

Dalston, R.M., Neiman, N.S., & Gonzalez-Landa, G. (1993). Nasometric sensitivity and specificity: A cross-dialect and cross-culture study. *Cleft Palate-Craniofacial Journal*, 30(3), 285–291.

Dalston, R.M., Warren, D.W., & Dalston, E.T. (1991a). Use of nasometry as a diagnostic tool for identifying patients with velopharyngeal impairment. *Cleft Palate-Craniofacial Journal*, 28(2), 184–188.

Dalston, R.M., Warren, D.W., & Dalston, E.T. (1991b). A preliminary investigation concerning the use of nasometry in identifying patients with hyponasality and/or nasal airway impairment. *Journal of Speech and Hearing Research*, 34(1), 11–18.

De Boer, G., & Bressmann, T. (2014). Comparison of nasalance scores obtained with the nasometers 6200 and 6450. *Cleft Palate-Craniofacial Journal*, 51(1), 90–97.

De Boer, G., & Bressmann, T. (2015). Application of linear discriminant analysis to the nasometric assessment of resonance disorders: A pilot study. *Cleft Palate-Craniofacial Journal*, 52(2), 173–182.

De Boer, G., Marino, V.C.C., Dutka, J.C.R., Pegoraro-Krook, M.I., & Bressmann, T. (2020). Nasalance-based preclassification of oral-nasal balance disorders results in higher agreement of expert listeners' auditory-perceptual assessments: Results of a retrospective listening study. *Cleft Palate-Craniofacial Journal*, 57, 448–457.

Derrick, D., Duerr, J., & Kerr, R.G. (2019). Mask-less oral and nasal audio recording and air flow estimation for speech analysis. *Electronics Letters*, 55(1), 12–14.

D'haeseleer, E., Bettens, K., de Mets, S., de Moor, V., & Van Lierde, K. (2015). Normative data and dialectical effects on nasalance in Flemish adults. *Folia Phoniatrica et Logopaedica*, 67, 42–48.

Durtschi, R.B., Chung, D., Gentry, L.R., Chung, M.K., & Voperian, H.K. (2009). Developmental craniofacial anthropometry: Assessment of race effects. *Clinical Anatomy*, 22(7), 800–808.

Ekin, O., Calis, M., Kayikci, M.E.K., Icen, M., Gunaydin, R.O., & Ozgur, F. (2017). Modified superior-based pharyngeal flap is effective in treatment of velopharyngeal insufficiency regardless of the preoperative closure pattern. *Journal of Craniofacial Surgery*, 28(2), 413–417.

Fairbanks, G. (1960). *Voice and Articulation Drillbook* (2nd ed.). New York, NY: Harper.

Ferreira, G.Z., Bressmann, T., Dutka, J.C.R., Whitaker, M.E., de Boer, G., Marino, V.C.C., & Pegoraro-Krook, M.I. (2020). Analysis of oral-nasal balance after intensive speech therapy combined with speech bulb in speakers with cleft palate and hypernasality. *Journal of Communication Disorders*, 85, Article Number 105945.

Fletcher, S.G. (1970). Theory and instrumentation for quantitative measurement of nasality. *Cleft Palate Journal*, 7, 601–609.

Fletcher, S.G. (1972). Contingencies for bioelectronic modification of nasality. *Journal of Speech and Hearing Disorders*, 37(3), 329–346.

Fletcher, S.G. (1976). 'Nasalance' vs. listner judgements of nasality. *Cleft Palate Journal*, 13(1), 31–44.

Fletcher, S.G. (1978). *Diagnosing Speech Disorder from Cleft Palate*. New York, NY: Grune & Stratton.

Fletcher, S.G. (1979). Response to article on TONAR calibration (Weinberg, Noll and Donohue). *Cleft Palate Journal*, 16(2), 162–163.

Fletcher, S.G., & Bishop, M.E. (1970). Measurement of nasality with TONAR. *Cleft Palate Journal*, 7, 610–621.

Fletcher, S.G., & Daly, D.A. (1976). Nasalance in utterances of hearing-impaired speakers. *Journal of Communication Disorders*, 9(1), 63–73.

Fletcher, S.G., Sooudi, I., & Frost, S.D. (1974). Quantitative and graphic analysis of prosthetic treatment for "nasalance" in speech. *Journal of Prosthetic Dentistry*, 32(3), 284–291.

Galek, K.E., & Watterson, T. (2017). Perceptual anchors and the dispersion of nasality ratings. *Cleft Palate-Craniofacial Journal*, 54, 423–430.

Gauster, A., Yunusova, Y., & Zajac, D. (2010). The effect of speaking rate on velopharyngeal function in healthy speakers. *Clinical Linguistics and Phonetics*, 24(7), 576–588.

Gildersleeve-Neumann, C.E., & Dalston, R.M. (2001). Nasalance scores in noncleft individuals: Why not zero? *Cleft Palate-Craniofacial Journal*, 38(2), 106–111.

Ha, S., Jung, S., & Koh, K.S. (2018). Effect of vowel context on test-retest nasalance score variability in children with and without cleft palate. *International Journal of Pediatric Otorhinolaryngology*, 109, 72–77.

Ha, S., Sim, H., Zhi, M., & Kuehn, D.P. (2004). An acoustic study of the temporal characteristics of nasalization in children with and without cleft palate. *Cleft Palate-Craniofacial Journal*, 41(5), 535–543.

Hardin, M.A., Van Demark, D.R., Morris, H.L., & Payne, M.M. (1992). Correspondence between nasalance scores and listener judgments of hypernasality and hyponasality *Cleft Palate-Craniofacial Journal*, 29(4), 346–351.

Heller-Murray, E.S., Mendoza, J.O., Gill, S.V., Perkell, J.S., & Stepp, C.E. (2016). Effects of biofeedback on control and generalization of nasalization in typical speakers. *Journal of Speech, Language, and Hearing Research*, 59(5), 1025–1034.

Horii, Y. (1980). An accelerometric approach to nasality measurement: A preliminary report. *Cleft Palate Journal*, 17(3), 254–261.

Horii, Y., & Lang, J.E. (1981). Distributional analyses of an index of nasal coupling (HONC) in stimulated hypernasal speech. *Cleft Palate Journal*, 18(4), 279–285.

Hutchinson, J.M., Robinson, K.L., & Nerbonne, M.A. (1978). Patterns of nasalance in a sample of gerontologic subjects. *Journal of Communication Disorders*, 11, 469–481.

Jiang, R.-S., & Huang, H.-T. (2006). Changes in nasal resonance after functional endoscopic sinus surgery. *American Journal of Rhinology*, 20(4), 432–437.

Karakoc, O., Akcam, T., Birkent, H., Arslan, H.H., & Gerek, M. (2013) Nasalance scores for normal-speaking Turkish population. *Journal of Craniofacial Surgery*, 24(2), 520–522.

Karakoc, O., Timur Akcam, M., Genc, H., Birkent, H., Binar, M., & Gerek, M. (2015). Do pharyngeal surgeries for snoring and obstructive sleep apnea have an impact on nasalance scores? *Journal of Craniofacial Surgery*, 26(7), 2213–2216.

Karling, J., Larson, O., Leanderson, R., Galyas, K., & De Serpa-Leitao, A. (1993). NORAM – An instrument used in the assessment of hypernasality: A clinical investigation. *Cleft Palate-Craniofacial Journal*, 30(2), 135–140.

Keuning, K.H.D.M., Wieneke, G.H., & Dejonckere, P.H. (2004). Correlation between the perceptual rating of speech in Dutch patients with velopharyngeal insufficiency and composite measures derived from mean nasalance scores. *Folia Phoniatrica et Logopaedica*, 56, 157–164.

Keuning, K.H.D.M., Wieneke, G.H., Van Wijngaarden, H.A., & Dejonckere, P.H. (2002). The correlation between nasalance and a differentiated perceptual rating of speech in Dutch patients with velopharyngeal insufficiency. *Cleft Palate-Craniofacial Journal*, 39(3), 277–284.

Kim, D.H., Hong, Y.-K., Jeun, S.-S., Park, J.-S., Kim, S.W., Cho, J.H., Park, Y.J., Lee, H.J., Yeon-Shin H., & Kim, S.W. (2017). Effects of changes in nasal volume on voice in patients after endoscopic endonasal transsphenoidal surgery. *American Journal of Rhinology and Allergy*, 31(3), 177–180.

Kim, E.Y., Yoon, M.S., Kim, H.H., Nam, C.M., Park, E.S., & Hong, S.H. (2012). Characteristics of nasal resonance and perceptual rating in prelingual hearing impaired adults. *Clinical and Experimental Otorhinolaryngology*, 5(1), 1–9.

Kim, Y.H., Lee, S.H., Park, C.W., & Cho, J.H. (2013). Nasalance change after sinonasal surgery: Analysis of voice after septoturbinoplasty and endoscopic sinus surgery. *American Journal of Rhinology and Allergy*, 27(1), 67–70.

Kudo, K., Takagi, R., Kodama, Y., Terao, E., Asahito, T., & Saito, I. (2014). Evaluation of speech and morphological changes after maxillary advancement for patients with velopharyngeal insufficiency due to repaired cleft palate using a nasometer and lateral cephalogram. *Journal of Oral and Maxillofacial Surgery, Medicine, and Pathology*, 26(1), 22–27.

Kuehn, D.P., & Moller, K.T. (2000). The state of the art: Speech and language issues in the cleft palate population. *Cleft Palate-Craniofacial Journal*, 37(4), 348.

Kummer, A.W. (2008) *Cleft Palate and Craniofacial Anomalies: Effects on Speech and Resonance* (2nd ed.). Clifton Park, NY: Delmar.

Kummer, A.W. (2011). Disorders of resonance and airflow secondary to cleft palate and/or velopharyngeal dysfunction. *Seminars in Speech and Language*, 32(2), 141–149.

Küttner, C., Schönweiler, R., Seeberger, B., Dempf, R., Lisson, J., & Ptok, M. (2003). Objektive Messung der Nasalanz in der deutschen Hochlautung: Ein Vergleichskollektiv zur Beurteilung funktioneller Ergebnisse bei Lippen-Kiefer-Gaumen-Spalten. *HNO*, 51(2), 151–156.

Laczi, E., Sussman, J.E., Stathopoulos, E.T., & Huber, J. (2005). Perceptual evaluation of hypernasality compared to HONC measures: The role of experience. *Cleft Palate-Craniofacial Journal*, 42(2), 202–211.

Lee, A., & Browne, U. (2013). Nasalance scores for typical Irish English-speaking adults. *Logopedics, Phoniatrics, Vocology*, 38(4), 167–172.

Lehes, L., Horn, R., Lippus, P., Padrik, M., Kasenõmm, P., & Jagomägi, T. (2018). Normative nasalance scores for Estonian children. *Clinical Linguistics and Phonetics*, 32(11), 1054–1066.

Lewis, K.E., & Watterson, T. (2003). Comparison of nasalance scores obtained from the Nasometer and the NasalView. *Cleft Palate-Craniofacial Journal*, 40(1), 40–45.

Lewis, K.E., Watterson, T., & Quint, T. (2000). The effect of vowels on nasalance scores. *Cleft Palate-Craniofacial Journal*, 37(6), 584–589.

Li, H.-Y., Lee, L.-A., Fang, T.-J., Lin, W.-N., & Lin, W.-Y. (2010). Evaluation of velopharyngeal function after relocation pharyngoplasty for obstructive sleep apnea. *Laryngoscope*, 120(5), 1069–1073.

Litzaw, L.L., & Dalston, R.M. (1992). The effect of gender upon nasalance scores among normal adult speakers. *Journal of Communication Disorders*, 25(1), 55–64.

Mandulak, K.C., & Zajac, D.J. (2009). Effects of altered fundamental frequency on nasalance during vowel production by adult speakers at targeted sound pressure levels. *Cleft Palate-Craniofacial Journal*, 46(1), 39–46.

Marino, V.C.C., Cardoso, V.M., De Boer, G., Dutka, JCR., Fabbron, E.M.G., & Bressmann, T. (2018). Normative nasalance scores for middle-aged and elderly speakers of Brazilian Portuguese. *Folia Phoniatrica et Logopaedica*, 70(2), 82–89.

Marino, V.C.C., Dutka, J.C.R., de Boer, G., Cardoso, V.M., Ramos, R.G., & Bressmann, T. (2016). Normative nasalance scores for Brazilian Portuguese using new speech stimuli. *Folia Phoniatrica et Logopaedica*, 67, 238–244.

Mayo, C.M., & Mayo, R. (2011). Normative nasalance values across languages. *ECHO*, 6(1), 22–32.

Mayo, R., Floyd, L.A., Warren, D.W., Dalston, R.M., & Mayo, C.M. (1996). Nasalance and nasal area values: A cross-racial study. *Cleft Palate-Craniofacial Journal*, 33(2), 143–149.

Mohd Ibrahim, H., Reilly, S., & Kilpatrick, N. (2012). Normative nasalance scores for the Malay language. *Cleft Palate-Craniofacial Journal*, 49(5), e61–e63.

Moll, K.L. (1964). 'Objective' measures of nasality. *Cleft Palate Journal*, 35, 371–374.

Mra, Z., Sussman, J.E., & Fenwick, J. (1998). HONC measures in 4- to 6-year-old children. *Cleft Palate-Craniofacial Journal*, 35(5), 408–414.

Nellis, J.L., Neiman, G.S., & Lehman, J.A. (1992). Comparison of nasometer and listener judgments of nasality in the assessment of velopharyngeal function after pharyngeal flap surgery. *Cleft Palate-Craniofacial Journal*, 29(2), 157–163.

Nguyen, V.T., Lehes, L., Truong, T.T.H., Hoang, T.V.A., & Jagomägi, T. (2019). Normative nasalance scores for Vietnamese-speaking children. *Logopedics, Phoniatrics, Vocology*, 44(2), 51–57.

Okalidou, A., Karathanasi, A., & Grigoraki, E. (2011). Nasalance norms in Greek adults. *Clinical Linguistics and Phonetics*, 25(8), 671–688.

Park, M., Baek, W.S., Lee, E., Koh, K.S., Kim, B.-K., & Baek, R. (2014). Nasalance scores for normal Korean-speaking adults and children. *Journal of Plastic, Reconstructive and Aesthetic Surgery*, 67(2), 173–177.

Pegoraro-Krook, M.I., Dutka-Souza, J.C.R., Williams, W.N., Teles Magalhães, L.C., Rossetto, P.C., & Riski, J.E. (2006) Effect of nasal decongestion on nasalance measures. *Cleft Palate-Craniofacial Journal*, 43(3), 289–294.

Pinborough-Zimmerman, J., Canady, C., Yamashiro, D.K., & Morales Jr., L. (1998). Articulation and nasality changes resulting from sustained palatal fistula obturation. *Cleft Palate-Craniofacial Journal*, 35 (1), 81–87.

Reddy, R.R., Reddy, S.G., Banala, B., Bronkhorst, E., Kummer, A.W., Kuijpers-Jagtman, A.M., & Bergé, S.J. (2016). Use of a modified Furlow Z-plasty as a secondary cleft palate repair procedure to reduce velopharyngeal insufficiency. *International Journal of Oral and Maxillofacial Surgery*, 45(2), 170–176.

Rieger, J., Wolfaardt, J., Seikaly, H., & Jha, N. (2002). Speech outcomes in patients rehabilitated with maxillary obturator prostheses after maxillectomy: A prospective study. *International Journal of Prosthodontics*, 15(2), 139–144.

Rochet, A.P., Rochet, B.L., Sovis, E.A., & Mielke, D.L. (1998). Characteristics of nasalance in speakers of Western Canadian English and French. *Canadian Journal of Speech-Language Pathology and Audiology*, 22, 94–103.

Scarsellone, J.M., Rochet, A.P., & Wolfaardt, J.F. (1999). The influence of dentures on nasalance values in speech. *Cleft Palate-Craniofacial Journal*, 36(1), 51–56.

Seaver, E.J., Dalston, R.M., Leeper, H.A., & Adams, L.E. (1991). A study of nasometric values for normal nasal resonance. *Journal of Speech and Hearing Research*, 34(4), 715–721.

Seltzer, A.P. (1957). The Seltzer nasometer for measuring nasal patency. *Transactions: American Academy of Ophthalmology and Otolaryngology*, 61(3), 413–415.

Shelton Jr., R.L., Knox, A.W., Arndt Jr., W.B., & Elbert, M. (1967). The relationship between nasality score values and oral and nasal sound pressure level. *Journal of Speech and Hearing Research*, 10(3), 549–557.

Shin, Y.J., Kim, Y., & Kim, H.G. (2017). The comparative study of resonance disorders for Vietnamese and Korean cleft palate speakers using nasometer. *Maxillofacial Plastic and Reconstructive Surgery*, 39(1), 9.

Soneghet, R., Santos, R.P., Behlau, M., Habermann, W., Friedrich, G., & Stammberger, H. (2002). Nasalance changes after functional endoscopic sinus surgery. *Journal of Voice*, 16(3), 392–397.

Stellzig, A., Heppt, W., & Komposch, G. (1994). Das nasometer: Ein Instrument zur Objektivierung der Hyperrhinophonie bei LKG-Patienten. *Fortschritte der Kieferorthopädie*, 55(4), 176–180.

Stewart J., & Kohlberger M. (2017). Earbuds: A method for analyzing nasality in the field. *Language Documentation & Conservation*, 11, 49–80.

Sussman, J.E. (1995). HONC measures in men and women: Validity and variability. *Cleft Palate-Craniofacial Journal*, 32(1), 37–48.

Švec, J.G., & Granqvist, S. (2018). Tutorial and guidelines on measurement of sound pressure level in voice and speech. *Journal of Speech, Language, and Hearing Research*, 61(3), 441–461.

Sweeney, T., & Sell, D. (2008). Relationship between perceptual ratings of nasality and nasometry in children/adolescents with cleft palate and/or velopharyngeal dysfunction. *International Journal of Language and Communication Disorders*, 43(3), 265–282.

Sweeney, T., Sell, D., & O'Regan, M. (2004). Nasalance scores for normal-speaking Irish children. *Cleft Palate-Craniofacial Journal*, 41(2), 168–174.

Tachimura, T., Kotani, Y., & Wada, T. (2004). Nasalance scores in wearers of a palatal lift prosthesis in comparison with normative data for Japanese. *Cleft Palate-Craniofacial Journal*, 41(3), 315–319.

Tachimura, T., Mori, C., Hirata, S.-I., & Wada, T. (2000). Nasalance score variation in normal adult Japanese speakers of mid-west Japanese dialect. *Cleft Palate-Craniofacial Journal*, 37(5), 463–467.

Trost-Cardamone, J.E. (1989). Coming to terms with VPI: A response to Loney and Bloem. *Cleft Palate Journal*, 26(1), 68–70.

Tuzuner, A., Demirci, S., Akkoc, A., Arslan, E., Arslan, N., & Samim, E.E. (2014). Nasalance scores in pediatric patients after adenoidectomy. *International Journal of Pediatric Otorhinolaryngology*, 78(4), 610–613.

Vallino-Napoli, L.D., & Montgomery, A.A. (1997). Examination of the standard deviation of mean nasalance scores in subjects with cleft palate: Implications for clinical use. *Cleft Palate Journal*, 34, 512–519.

Van Lierde, K.M., Bonte, K., Baudonck, N., Van Cauwenberge, P., & De Leenheer, E.M.R. (2008). Speech outcome regarding overall intelligibility, articulation, resonance and voice in Flemish children a year after pharyngeal flap surgery: A pilot study. *Folia Phoniatrica et Logopaedica*, 60(5), 223–232.

Van Lierde, K.M., Claeys, S., De Bodt, M., & Van Cauwenberge, P. (2004). Outcome of laryngeal and velopharyngeal biofeedback treatment in children and young adults: A pilot study. *Journal of Voice*, 18(1), 97–106.

Van Lierde, K.M., Monstrey, S., Bonte, K., Van Cauwenberge, P., & Vinck, B. (2004). The long-term speech outcome in Flemish young adults after two different types of palatoplasty. *International Journal of Pediatric Otorhinolaryngology*, 68(7), 865–875.

Van Lierde, K.M., Van Borsel, J., Moerman, M., & Van Cauwenberge, P. (2002). Nasalance, nasality, voice, and articulation after uvulopalatopharyngoplasty. *Laryngoscope*, 112(5), 873–878.

Van Lierde, K.M., Wuyts, F.L., Bonte, K., & Van Cauwenberge, P. (2006) The nasality severity index: An objective measure of hypernasality based on a multiparameter approach – A pilot study. *Folia Phoniatrica et Logopaedica*, 59(1), 31–38.

Van Lierde, K.M., Wuyts, F.L., De Bodt, M., & Van Cauwenberge, P. (2001). Nasometric values for normal nasal resonance in the speech of young Flemish adults. *Cleft Palate-Craniofacial Journal*, 38(2), 112–118.

Van Lierde K.M., Wuyts F.L., De Bodt M., & Van Cauwenberge P. (2003). Age-related patterns of nasal resonance in normal Flemish children and young adults. *Scandinavian Journal of Plasic Reconstrive Surgery and Hand Surgery*, 37, 344–350.

Watterson, T., & Lewis, K.E. (2006). Test-retest nasalance score variability in hypernasal speakers. *Cleft Palate-Craniofacial Journal*, 43(4), 415–419.

Watterson, T. (2020). The use of the Nasometer and interpretation of nasalance scores. *Perspectives*, 5(1), 155–163.

Watterson, T., Hinton, J., & McFarlane, S. (1996). Novel stimuli for obtaining nasalance measures from young children. *Cleft Palate-Craniofacial Journal*, 33(1), 67–73.

Watterson, T., Lewis, K., & Brancamp, T. (2005). Comparison of nasalance scores obtained with the Nasometer 6200 and the Nasometer II 6400. *Cleft Palate-Craniofacial Journal*, 42(5), 574–579.

Watterson, T., Lewis, K.E., & Deutsch, C. (1998). Nasalance and nasality in low pressure and high pressure speech. *Cleft Palate-Craniofacial Journal*, 35(4), 293–298.

Watterson, T., Lewis, K.E., & Foley-Homan, N. (1999). Effect of stimulus length on nasalance scores. *Cleft Palate-Craniofacial Journal*, 36(3), 243–247.

Watterson, T., Lewis, K.E., Ludlow, J.C., & Ludlow, P.C. (2008). The effect of nasal decongestion on nasal patency and nasalance scores in subjects with normal speech. *Cleft Palate-Craniofacial Journal*, 45(6), 620–627.

Watterson, T., McFarlane, S.C., & Wright, D.S. (1993). The relationship between nasalance and nasality in children with cleft palate. *Journal of Communication Disorders*, 26(1), 13–28.

Watterson, T., York, S.L., & McFarlane, S.C. (1994). Effects of vocal loudness on nasalance measures. *Journal of Communication Disorders*, 27(3), 257–262.

Weatherley-White, R.C., Dersch, W.C., & Anderson, R.M. (1964). Objective measurement of nasality in cleft palate patients: A preliminary report. *Cleft Palate Journal*, 16, 120–124.

Weinberg, B., Noll, J.D., & Donohue, M. (1979). TONAR calibration: A brief note. *Cleft Palate Journal*, 16(2), 158–161.

Whitehill, T.L. (2001). Nasalance measures in Cantonese-speaking women. *Cleft Palate-Craniofacial Journal*, 38(2), 119–125.

Williams, R.G., Eccles, R., & Hutchings, H. (1990). The relationship between nasalance and nasal resistance to airflow. *Acta Oto-Laryngologica*, 110(3–4), 443–449.

Woo, S.T., Park, Y.B., Oh, D.H., & Ha, J.-W. (2019). Influence of the nasometric instrument structure on nasalance score. *Applied Sciences*, 9(15), Article Number 3040.

Zajac, D.J., Preisser, J. (2016). Age and phonetic influences on velar flutter as a component of nasal turbulence in children with repaired cleft palate. *Cleft Palate-Craniofacial Journal*, 53(6), 649–656.

Zajac, D.J., Lutz, R., & Mayo, R. (1996). Microphone sensitivity as a source of variation in nasalance scores. *Journal of Speech, Language, and Hearing Research*, 39(6), 1228–1231.

Zemann, W., Feichtinger, M., Santler, G., & Kärcher, H. (2006). Veränderung der Nasalanz nach Le Fort-I Osteotomie. *Mund – Kiefer – und Gesichtschirurgie*, 10(4), 221–228.

25

ELECTROPALATOGRAPHY

Alice Lee

Introduction

Speech sounds are produced by moving the articulators to change the shape of the vocal tract that modifies the periodic sound of phonation generated at the laryngeal level and the outgoing airstream from the lungs. The articulators are either brought into contact to create a temporary complete obstruction, or close to each other to create a narrow constriction somewhere along the vocal tract. While some articulatory gestures can be seen easily (e.g. bilabial closure), most are produced inside the oral cavity, hence, invisible to investigators or clinicians unless specialized tools or instruments are used. One instrumental technique that captures an aspect of articulation—lingual articulation—is electropalatography (EPG).

EPG detects, visually displays and records the pattern and timing of contact between the tongue and the hard palate during speech (Hardcastle, Gibbon, & Jones, 1991). In order to capture the tongue palate contact patterns, an artificial EPG plate that fits the palate must be custom-made for each speaker or client (see Figure 25.1a). The sensors are embedded on the lingual surface of the plate, with each connected to a thin wire. The wires are gathered together and leave the mouth either at the sides or centrally depending on the design. The wires are then connected to an external processing unit (a multiplexer) that is connected to an EPG machine which is connected to a computer or a laptop. When the speaker produces a lingual sound, for example, the voiceless alveolar plosive /t/, the tongue blade and the lateral sides of the tongue are raised to make contact with the alveolar region and lateral sides of the palate respectively, to create a complete seal for building up intraoral pressure behind the place of articulation during the stop period. A closed electric circuit is formed for sensors that are touched by the tongue and this information is displayed real time on the computer screen as tongue palate contact patterns (see Figure 25.1b). Hence, EPG only shows where on the palate that the tongue touches during speech production. It does not provide information on the shape and movement of the tongue that can be captured by other instrumental techniques, such as ultrasound (see Chapter 29). However, applying our general understanding of typical lingual articulation that the tongue tip and blade articulate against the upper teeth or the alveolar ridge, the anterior section of the tongue body articulates against the hard palate, and the posterior section against the velum (Ball & Müller, 2005), we can, to a certain extent, infer the lingual gestures based on the tongue palate contact patterns captured by EPG (see Figure 25.1c and d). A few EPG

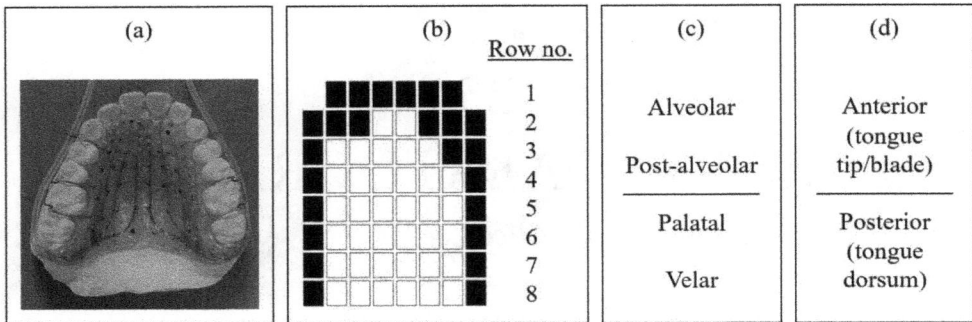

(a)	(b) Row no.	(c)	(d)
	1 2 3 4 5 6 7 8	Alveolar Post-alveolar —— Palatal Velar	Anterior (tongue tip/blade) —— Posterior (tongue dorsum)

Figure 25.1 (a) An EPG plate of the Reading system of a typical speaker; (b) a schematic representation of tongue palate contact showing a typical contact pattern (indicated by the filled boxes) for alveolar plosives /t/, /d/, /n/; (c) the phonetic regions of the palate; and (d) the part of the tongue presumed to contact the phonetic regions.

systems have been developed in the past 50+ years (outlined in the following section). They differ in detail such as the construction of the EPG plates, the number and placement location of the sensors, and other hardware and software specifications, but they share the general engineering design described above.

Brief historical background to EPG

EPG is a computerized version of an old fieldwork technique—palatography—for finding out the places of articulation for the speech sounds of a language (Hardcastle & Gibbon, 2005; Ladefoged, 2003). This method involves painting the speaker's tongue surface with some edible dark paste (e.g. mixture of cocoa powder and olive oil). When the speaker produces a lingual sound, the tongue touches the palate and the dark paste is then transferred onto the surface of the palate, showing the tongue palate contact pattern. The contact patterns of the different speech sounds are documented by inserting a mirror at an angle into the mouth and photographing the reflected contact pattern on the mirror (Ladefoged, 2003). While this traditional method is simple and does not involve complicated instruments, the procedure is quite time-consuming and it is not useful for investigating many articulatory phenomena, such as, the changes in contact patterns when the phonemes are articulated at levels other than isolation (e.g. connected speech); the gradual change in contact pattern in diphthongs; and the fine articulatory gestures involved in the different phases (approach, closure and release) of production of plosives, etc. These articulatory phenomena can be studied using EPG.

A succinct description of the history of EPG has been provided by Professor Alan Wrench (see Articulate-Instruments-Ltd, 2013) and below is a summary of the key points, supplemented with additional references. The first EPG is probably the one called "phonokinesigraph" developed by Herbert Koepp-Baker and reported in his PhD dissertation in 1938 in the United States. In the 60s, EPG was developed in Russia (Kuzmin, 1962), Japan (Shibata, 1968) and the United States (Kydd & Belt, 1964; Rome, 1964; cited by A. A. Wrench, personal communication, February 5, 2020). Then in the late 60s, Professor William Hardcastle in the United Kingdom and Professor Samuel Fletcher in the United States developed versions of the Kydd and Belt system. In the 70s, three EPG systems developed in three independent labs are available for speech research: the Reading EPG system developed in the United Kingdom, the US system and the Rion EPG developed in Japan; and around the same time, research work on developing an EPG system was being done in France and Germany as well (A. A. Wrench, personal communication, February 5, 2020).

For the Reading EPG system, the software had been rewritten a few times since the prototype in order to run it on different updated computer operating systems (see Articulate-Instruments-Ltd, 2013). The latest version, WinEPG™, with software Articulate Assistant™ that runs on Microsoft Windows, and was available from Articulate Instruments Ltd (Scobbie, Wood, & Wrench, 2004). The Reading style EPG plate contains 62 electrodes, embedded in eight horizontal rows (with 6 electrodes in the first row or row 1, and eight electrodes in row 2–8) according to identifiable anatomical landmarks (Hardcastle, Jones, Knight, Trudgeon, & Calder, 1989; see Figure 25.1a). The first row of electrodes is placed horizontally across the plate along the palatal junctures of the upper front incisors; and the last row is located on the juncture between the hard palate and the soft palate. In addition, the first four rows of electrodes are closer to each other, occupying the anterior one-third of the plate (Hardcastle et al., 1989). There is a modified version of the Reading EPG plate, the Articulate EPG plate, with the first row of electrodes placed slightly more anteriorly and the central electrodes of the last row placed slightly more posteriorly (Wrench, 2007). The Reading EPG system samples the tongue palate contact patterns at 100 Hz and the acoustic signal at 22,050 Hz simultaneously. That is, 100 EPG frames or palatograms per second, or 10 milliseconds between two consecutive EPG frames. The company also manufactured a lightweight EPG portable training unit (PTU) that gives real-time visual display of the contact patterns for treatment purposes, but recording of the contact patterns and acoustic signal is not possible (Leitch, Gibbon, & Crampin, 1998). Another UK-manufactured EPG system, Linguagraph, is currently commercially from Rose Medical Solutions Ltd. This system works with the Reading style EPG plate (Kelly, Main, Manley, & McLean, 2000).

The US EPG system was first produced by the Kay Elemetrics and the product was known as Kay Elemetrics Palatometer. The system was then produced by a different company and the equipment was called the LogoMetrix palatometer system. The current version is the SmartPalate system, manufactured by CompleteSpeech (Fabus et al., 2015). The EPG plate of this system has 124 electrodes, with two sensing bilabial closure and the rest distributed in the alveolar and postalveolar region, the lateral and the medial midline of the palatal region, and the velar region of the palate (see, e.g. Figure 1 in Appendix 1 in the paper by Fabus et al., 2015). For the Japanese system, the Rion system was used widely in Japan but the production of which discontinued in the 90s. A new EPG system, WinSTARS (EPG Research Centre, Nishinomiya, Japan), has been developed recently. It uses the Reading style EPG plate, which is plugged into a multiplexer that links to a laptop via Bluetooth (Yamamoto, 2019). A software comes with this system for real-time visual display and further analysis of the EPG data can be carried out using the Articulate Assistant™ software.

How to use EPG

EPG has been used in research to investigate different lingual articulatory phenomena in typical speakers as well as atypical articulatory gestures in children and adults with speech sound disorders due to different causes (e.g. cleft palate, speech sound disorders of unknown origin, motor speech disorders and hearing impairment; see, e.g. Lee, 2019). The technique has also been used as a tool to provide real-time visual feedback of tongue palate contact patterns to clients in speech therapy. As stated above, a custom-made EPG plate is needed for each speaker and this involves a visit to a dentist or an orthodontist to make an accurate initial alginate impression of the upper teeth (Lee, Gibbon, Crampin, Yuen, & McLennan, 2007). The dental model is then made and sent to a dental device company for making an EPG plate. However, not every dental device company makes EPG plate and circumstances might change over time, hence, EPG users, especially first-time users, are advised to contact the manufacturer of the EPG system they plan to purchase or have purchased for information on EPG plate making. When the EPG plate arrives, it is advisable to ask the clients to wear the EPG plate or a pseudo-EPG plate (i.e. an EPG plate without the sensors) to adapt to the presence of a dental device in the mouth when talking before carrying out any articulation assessment. Different adaptation processes have been used (see McLeod & Searl, 2006, for a review) and an adaptation time of 2 hours was recommended based on the results of comparisons between the speech in no-plate condition and the speech after different adaptation times (McLeod & Searl, 2006).

Because EPG is a specialist technique and that the equipment is not inexpensive, at the moment, this technique is usually only used as the last resort with clients who show persistent speech disorders that do not respond to conventional speech therapy approaches (Gibbon & Wood, 2010). Even with an EPG system already available in the clinic, there is an additional cost for tailor-making the EPG plates, hence, careful planning is suggested. There are a few factors that clinicians might want to consider before pursuing EPG therapy with a client (see, e.g. Gibbon & Wood, 2010; Lee et al., 2007). The first factor is related to dental and/or orthodontic issues. As a good fit of the EPG plate with the palate is needed, dental problems such as caries and attrition can cause poor retention of the EPG plate; and changes in dental alignment or eruption of molars can affect the fitting of the EPG plate (Lee et al., 2007). Hence, clinicians should plan EPG therapy during a stable period of dental development or at a time that the clients, especially individuals with history of craniofacial defects, will not have orthodontic treatment or maxillofacial surgery.

Another factor to consider is the motivation for EPG therapy and the compliance of the client as well as the parents if it is children clients. Furthermore, the clinicians' judgment about whether the clients will benefit from an external visual feedback and be able to link the tongue palate contact patterns that they see on the computer screen to what they do with their tongue in the mouth. There has not been any study that investigated the level of intellectual abilities or what sorts of cognitive skills are required for benefiting from external visual feedback on lingual articulation. But a few previous studies on EPG therapy for children and teenagers with Down syndrome have shown that the participants who had a minimum of age-equivalent cognitive level of 3 years were able to make use of the visual feedback of EPG to learn new articulatory gestures (Cleland, Timmins, Wood, Hardcastle, & Wishart, 2009; Wood, Timmins, Wishart, Hardcastle, & Cleland, 2019). Before using EPG in research or as a clinical tool, a good understanding of the typical tongue palate contact patterns is important. The subsection below describes the tongue palate contact patterns observed in typical speakers reported in the literature.

Tongue palate contact patterns in typical speakers

EPG registers characteristic contact patterns for lingual phonemes, such as oral and nasal alveolar plosives /t/, /d/, /n/ and velar plosives /k/, /g/, /ŋ/; alveolar fricatives /s/, /z/; postalveolar fricatives /ʃ/, /ʒ/ and affricates /tʃ/, /dʒ/; lateral approximant /l/; rhotic /ɹ/; and palatal approximant /j/ for English (e.g. Alwan, Narayanan, & Haker, 1997; Cheng, Murdoch, Goozée, & Scott, 2007; Gibbon, Yuen, Lee, & Adams, 2007; Hardcastle & Barry, 1989; Liker & Gibbon, 2008, 2018; Liker, Gibbon, Wrench, & Horga, 2007; McLeod, Roberts, & Sita, 2006;

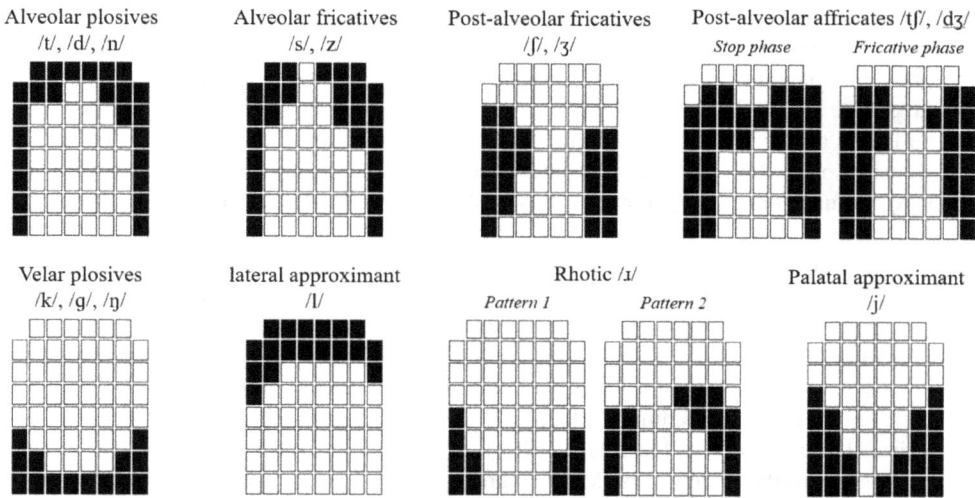

Figure 25.2 Examples of typical tongue palate contact patterns for some of the English consonants.

Narayanan, Alwan, & Haker, 1997). The distinguishing features in the contact patterns for these consonants are explained below and illustrated in Figure 25.2. For the other English consonants—oral and nasal bilabial plosives /p/, /b/, /m/; labiodental fricatives /f/, /v/; glottal fricative /h/; and approximant /w/—there is usually no tongue palate contact or minimal contact mainly in the posterior lateral margin of the palate, depending on the phonetic context.

The contact patterns for oral and nasal alveolar plosives are generally characterized by the presence of complete contact across the palate in the alveolar region and lateral sides of the palate, forming a pattern that resemble the shape of a horseshoe. For the complete contact across the palate, it can be formed by either 100% contact of (at least) a row of electrodes, or a complete contact made up of contacted electrodes in adjacent rows. A previous study compared the contact patterns of /t/, /d/ and /n/ in 15 typical speakers of English (Gibbon et al., 2007). The findings were that nearly all the plosives showed complete contact across the palate and no contact in the posterior central region of the palate. Bilateral contact occurred in more than 80% of the oral plosives produced but 55% for the nasal plosive. It was explained that the higher occurrence of bilateral contact in /t/ and /d/ was possibly because a lateral seal is needed to build up intraoral pressure for producing the oral plosives as compared to the nasal plosive (Gibbon et al., 2007). For the oral and nasal velar stops, the contact is concentrated in the velar region of the palate, with some speakers showing 100% contact in row 8 as shown in Figure 25.2.

The tongue palate contact patterns for the alveolar and postalveolar fricatives are similar to the one of the alveolar plosives, where there are bilateral contact and contact in the region relevant to the place of articulation. However, instead of a complete contact across the palate, there is a gap or no contact in the medial electrodes (see Figure 25.2). This corresponds to the findings of medial groove formation along the length of the tongue for /s/ and by the posterior section of the tongue for /ʃ/ (Stone, Faber, Raphael, & Shawker, 1992). The gap or the width of the constriction is narrower and located in the alveolar region for /s/ but wider and located in the postalveolar region for /ʃ/. The affricates consist of two components: the stop phase followed by a homorganic fricative (Ladefoged, 2006). The stop phase of the postalveolar affricates shows a contact pattern similar to that of alveolar plosives, with a bilateral contact and complete closure across the palate in the alveolar or postalveolar region depending on the phonetic context. The frication component has a pattern similar to that of postalveolar fricatives (see Figure 25.2).

The lateral approximant has been grouped into light or clear /l/ and dark /l/, with the light allophone associated with prevocalic context and the dark allophone with the postvocalic position (Narayanan et al., 1997). For light //, a contact pattern characterized by complete contact across the palate in the alveolar region and little bilateral contact is usually observed. For dark /l/, there is more variations in the contact patterns observed, with most who showed alveolar contact and some who showed no contact in the alveolar region but contact or close approximation of the tongue dorsum and the posterior part of the palate (McLeod & Singh, 2009; Narayanan et al., 1997). For the alveolar approximant or rhotic /ɹ/, a pattern of "broad lateral tongue contact along the posterior hard palate and the lack of contact centrally" has been reported in the literature (Schmidt, 2007, p. 77; see also, e.g. Alwan et al., 1997; Hitchcock, McAllister Byun, Swartz, & Lazarus, 2017; McLeod & Singh, 2009; and Figure 25.2). Some of the speakers in the reference by McLeod and Singh showed a slightly different pattern for /ɹ/, which is characterized by broader lateral contact in the palatal region and narrower lateral contact posteriorly, with no central contact (shown also in Figure 25.2). For the palatal approximant /j/, the contact pattern consists a bilateral contact extending anteriorly from the velar region to the postalveolar or even alveolar region.

Varying patterns of tongue palate contact are registered for vowels. There is usually a higher amount of contact for close vowels (e.g. /i/, /ɪ/, /ɛ/, /u/, /ʊ/ in English), with the bilateral contact extends forward from the velar region, but minimal or no tongue palate contact for open vowels (e.g. /ɑ/, /æ/, /ɒ/, /ɔ/; Gibbon, Lee, & Yuen, 2010; see also Figure 25.3). For diphthongs, depending on the "constituent" monophthongs involved, a gradual change in the contact pattern can be expected; for example, an increase in the amount of contact for /eɪ/, /aɪ/, /ɔɪ/, /aʊ/, /əʊ/ but a decrease in contact for /ɪə/ (Gibbon et al., 2010).

For the distinguishing features of typical tongue palate contact patterns of English consonants and vowels described above and the contact patterns shown in Figure 25.2 and 25.3, one can expect the observation of contact patterns with similar features in other typical speakers. However, the actual amount of contact may vary from one person to another. For example, a study that investigated the characteristics of contact pattern during closure period of velar plosive /k/ reported apparent differences in the amount of contact measured at the frame of maximum contact among seven male and female adult native speakers of English, with some speakers showing "almost twice as much contact" as the other speakers (Liker & Gibbon, 2008, p. 145). Similar finding of inter-speaker variations in the amount of contact has been reported for other consonants, such as alveolar plosives (Gibbon et al., 2007). For intra-speaker variability, children seemed to vary more than the adults in the tongue palate contact patterns between repetitions (Cheng et al., 2007). The amount of contact also varies depending on the phonetic context due to coarticulatory effect. For example, a study showed that the place of articulation and amount of contact of the voiceless velar plosive /k/ were influenced by the vowel context, with a slightly more fronted place of contact and higher amount of contact when /k/ was produced in /i/ contexts as compared to the /a/ context (Liker & Gibbon, 2008; see also Figure 25.3). However, the level of coarticulatory effect of adjacent vowel on the consonant differs between consonants; for example, one study reported that the anticipatory coarticulatory effect brought by a vowel was greater for /ɹ/, followed by /t/ and /l/, and then /k/ and /s/ (Zharkova, 2008).

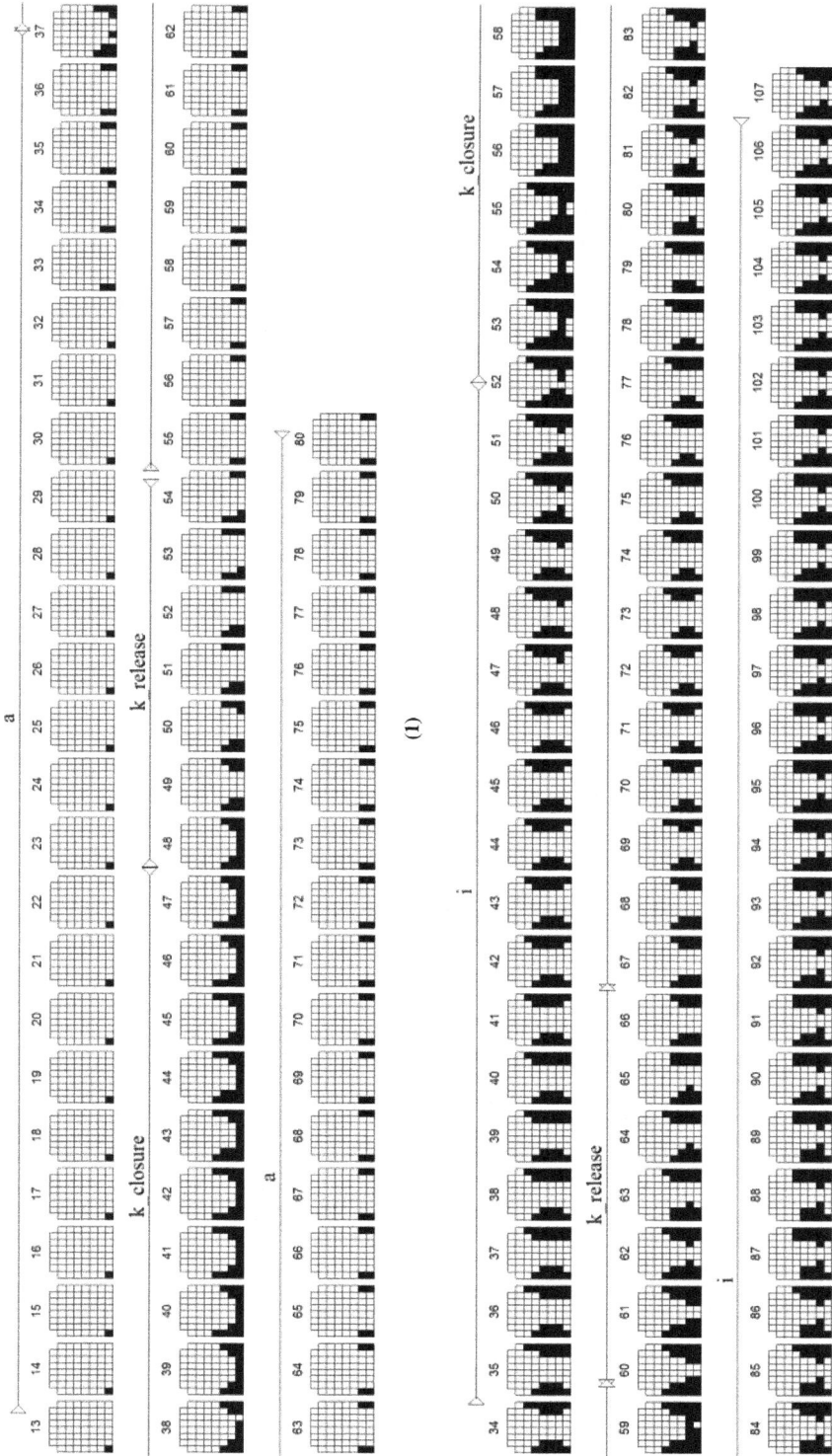

Figure 25.3 Tongue palate contact patterns of two non-sense syllable sequences (/aka/, /iki/) produced by a typical speaker, showing different amount of contact for (1) the vowels /a/ and /i/, and (2) consonant /k/ due to the coarticulatory effect of adjacent vowels.

Assessment of lingual articulation

Whether it is carrying out a research project or using EPG as a biofeedback tool in clinics, assessment of lingual articulation using EPG is only a part of an assessment protocol. A comprehensive speech evaluation should include an auditory-perceptual judgement-based assessment involving narrow or broad phonetic transcription of the speech sounds or errors produced by the clients (for further information regarding assessment see, e.g. Brosseau-Lapré & Rvachew, 2020; Velleman, 2016). The assessment materials can be a published articulation test, or a list of speech stimuli (e.g. words, phrases, etc.) devised by the researchers or clinicians. In the case of speech therapy using EPG, the assessment stimuli can include the targets to be treated to evaluate treatment progress, and un-treated phonemes to assess for generalization. The management protocol usually involves a pre-treatment articulation assessment, followed by a course of speech intervention using EPG to give visual feedback, and then post-treatment assessment to evaluate the treatment outcome. If possible, a mid-treatment assessment would be useful to evaluate the mid-way progress and a follow-up post-treatment to evaluate maintenance of correct articulatory gestures. In addition, in clinical intervention, understanding what the client is able and unable to produce regarding lingual gestures is essential for understanding the underlying articulatory difficulties and treatment planning.

Tongue palate contact data obtained using EPG can be analyzed by qualitative and/or quantitative measures. Data analysis usually begins with visual examination of the tongue palate contact patterns and judging whether the patterns are appropriate for the target sounds and phonetic context. This process can be documented by a qualitative description of the typical and atypical articulatory features observed (see, e.g. Hardcastle, Morgan Barry, & Clark, 1985, 1987; Lee et al., 2007). The terms used in the review by Gibbon (2004) on atypical tongue palate contact patterns observed in individuals with articulation errors associated with cleft palate (e.g. increased contact, retraction etc.) can be used to summarize the overall patterns demonstrated. Figure 25.4 shows an error contact pattern observed in a male adult speaker with speech disorders associated with cleft palate for the target /t/, reported in the study by Gibbon and Crampin (2001). The error produced was perceived as a middorsum palatal stop. Applying the knowledge on typical contact patterns for alveolar plosives, it can be described that this error pattern is showing increased contact because there should be zero contact for the

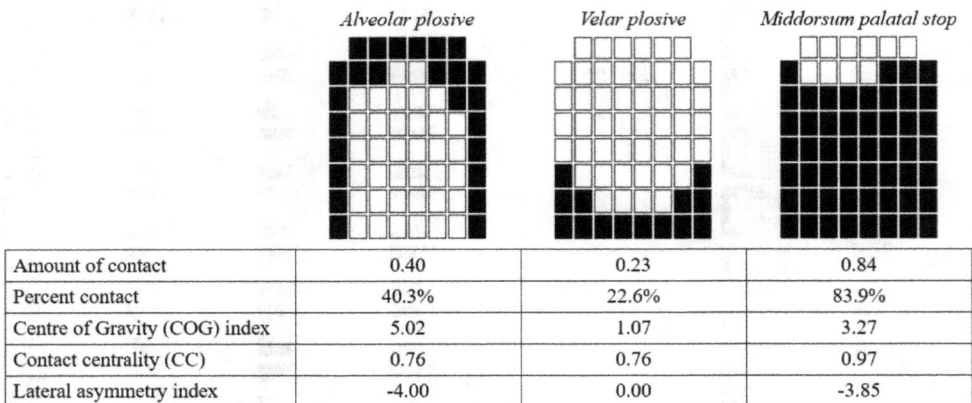

	Alveolar plosive	Velar plosive	Middorsum palatal stop
Amount of contact	0.40	0.23	0.84
Percent contact	40.3%	22.6%	83.9%
Centre of Gravity (COG) index	5.02	1.07	3.27
Contact centrality (CC)	0.76	0.76	0.97
Lateral asymmetry index	-4.00	0.00	-3.85

Figure 25.4 Results of a number of quantitative measures for two typical tongue palate contact patterns (/t/, /k/) and an error pattern (middorsum palatal stop) reported in the study by Gibbon and Crampin (2001).

medial section in the posterior half of the palate. In addition, the overall location of contact was retracted slightly because the contact mainly occurred in the postalveolar region through palatal to the velar region.

For quantitative analysis, a number of measures or indices have been used or proposed in the literature. Depending on the articulatory phenomenon investigated, these measures are usually obtained at the frame that shows maximum contact within a segment; the onset and offset of the segment and sometimes also at the temporal mid-point and a few time points equally spaced between the onset and offset. The quantitative measures can be grouped into the following categories according to the aspect of articulatory phenomena they quantify. The most commonly used measure is probably the amount of contact, or percent contact, which is a similar measure expressed in percentage. See the worked example in Figure 25.4, where the error pattern showed a percent contact that is more than twice the percent contact of the typical pattern for /t/.

The second group of indices is for quantifying the location of the main concentration of contacted electrodes across the palate or within a region of the palate. The most often used measure is the Centre of Gravity (COG) index (Jones & Hardcastle, 1995). There are a few variations of the equation for calculating the COG index (see Table 25.1), but they generally follow the idea of assigning different weightings to each row in a systematic way, so that a higher value of the index represents either more anterior or posterior place of contact. The COG values shown in Figure 25.4 were calculated using the first equation shown in Table 25.1. The alveolar plosive showed a higher value than the velar stop, differentiating anterior and posterior contact; whereas the COG index of the middorsum palatal stop is somewhere between these two phonemes because of extended contact. The other measures for indexing the location of concentration of electrodes contacted across the palate in the front/back dimension include contact anteriority (CA) and contact posteriority (CP), with versions of the equations for measuring the same within the alveolar of palatal regions (CAa, CPa and CAp, CPp respectively; Fontdevila, Pallarès, & Recasens, 1994a, 1994b); and anteriority index which was devised for the Japanese Rion system (Faber, 1989, cited in Fontdevila et al., 1994a; see Table 25.1). The concentration of contact can also be measured in the central/lateral dimension using contract centrality (CC). Figure 25.4 shows that the error pattern showed a relatively higher CC value, indicating a more central contact than the typical /t/ and /k/. Regarding the left/right symmetry of contact, it can be quantified using (lateral) asymmetry index (Scott & Goozée, 2002, cited in Cheng et al., 2007; Marchal & Espesser, 1989; see Table 25.1). As the nominator of the equation is obtained by subtracting the number of contacts on the left half of the plate from the right half, a zero value indicates equal amount of contact on both halves (e.g. the one of the velar plosive in Figure 25.4), whereas a negative value indicates a higher amount of contact on the left side (e.g. the one of the alveolar plosive and error pattern in the same figure).

The variability index (VI) measures the variability in tongue palate contact across productions of a phoneme embedded in the same utterance (Farnetani & Provaglio, 1991). The index is calculated by first obtaining a cumulative contact pattern; that is, the frequency of contact for each electrode over a number of repetitions. A frequency of contact of 0% or 100% means no variation in contact; while 50% indicates the highest variation, as the electrode was activated for half of the time. For contact frequency within the range of >50% to <100%, the value is subtracted from 100; whereas for frequency within the range of >0% to 50%, zero is subtracted from the value. Then multiply each of the converted scores above by the number of electrodes that show the score, and the sum of which is divided by the total number of electrodes on the plate to obtain the VI (absolute) index, or by the total number of contacts to calculate the

Table 25.1 A summary of EPG quantitative measures

Quantitative measure	Formula	Reference
Amount of contact	$N_{Contact} / N_{Total}$	
Percent contact	$(N_{Contact} / N_{Total}) \times 100$	
Centre of gravity (COG) index	$(0.5R_8 + 1.5R_7 + 2.5R_6 + 3.5R_5 + 4.5R_4 + 5.5R_3 + 6.5R_2 + 7.5R_1) / N_{Contact}$	Mitzutani et al. (1988, cited in Fontdevila et al., 1994a); Hardcastle, Gibbon, and Nicolaidis et al. (1991)
	$(1R_8 + 3R_7 + 5R_6 + 7R_5 + 9R_4 + 10R_3 + 11R_2 + 12R_1) / N_{Contact}$	Hardcastle, Gibbon, and Jones (1991)
	$(R_1 + 2R_2 + 3R_3 + 4R_4 + 5R_5 + 6R_6 + 7R_7 + 8R_8) / N_{Contact}$	Scott and Goozée (2002, cited in Cheng et al., 2007)
Contact anteriority (CA)	$\log [1(R_8/8) + 9(R_7/8) + 81(R_6/8) + 729(R_5/8) + 6561(R_4/8) + 59049(R_3/8) + 531441(R_2/8) + 3587227(R_1/6) + 1] / \log (4185098 + 1)$	Fontdevila et al. (1994a)
Alveolar contact anteriority (CAa)	$\log [(R_4/8) + 9(R_3/8) + 81(R_2/8) + 547(R_1/6) + 1] / \log 639$	Fontdevila et al. (1994b)
Palatal contact anteriority (CAp)	$\log [(R_8/8) + 9(R_7/8) + 81(R_6/8) + 1] / \log 92$	Fontdevila et al. (1994b)
	$\log [1(R_8/8) + 9(R_7/8) + 81(R_6/8) + 729(R_5/8) + 1] / \log (820 + 1)$	Fontdevila et al. (1994a)
Contact posteriority (CP)	$\log [1(R_1/6) + 9(R_2/8) + 81(R_3/8) + 729(R_4/8) + 6561(R_5/8) + 59049(R_6/8) + 531441(R_7/8) + 4782969(R_8/8) + 1] / \log (5380840 + 1)$	Fontdevila et al. (1994a)
Alveolar contact posteriority (CPa)	$\log [(R_1/6) + 9(R_2/8) + 81(R_3/8) + 729(R_4/8) + 1] / \log 821$	Fontdevila et al. (1994b)
Palatal contact posteriority (CPp)	$\log [(R_6/8) + 9(R_7/8) + 81(R_8/8) + 1] / \log 92$	Fontdevila et al. (1994b)
Anteriority index	$(36R_1 + 6R_2 + R_3) - [R_4 + 6R_5 + [36(R_6 + R_7) / 2]]$	Faber (1989) cited in Fontdevila et al. (1994a)
Contact centrality (CC)	$\log [1(C_1/14) + 17(C_2/16) + 289(C_3/16) + 4913(C_4/16) + 1] / \log (5220 + 1)$	Fontdevila et al. (1994a)
Alveolar contact centrality (CCa)	$\log [(C_1/6) + 9(C_2/8) + 81(C_3/8) + 729(C_4/8) + 1] / \log 821$	Fontdevila et al. (1994b)
Palatal contact centrality (CCp)	$\log [(C_1/6) + 7(C_2/6) + 49(C_3/6) + 343(C_4/6) + 1] / \log 401$	Fontdevila et al. (1994b)
Asymmetry index	$(N_R - N_L) / (N_R + N_L)$	Marchal and Espesser (1989)
Lateral asymmetry index	$[(N_R - N_L) / (N_R + N_L)] \times 100$	Scott and Goozée (2002, cited in Cheng et al., 2007)
Variability index (absolute)	$[[Count \times (100 - F_{>50-<100})] + [Count \times (F_{>0-\leq50} - 0)]] / 62$	Farnetani and Provaglio (1991)
Variability index (relative)	$[[Count \times (100 - F_{>50-<100})] + [Count \times (F_{>0-\leq50} - 0)]] / N_{Contact}$	Farnetani and Provaglio (1991)
Coarticulation index (CI)	$(|\%R_{1A} - \%R_{1B}| + |\%R_{2A} - \%R_{2B}| + |\%R_{3A} - \%R_{3B}| + |\%R_{4A} - \%R_{4B}| + |\%R_{5A} - \%R_{5B}| + |\%R_{6A} - \%R_{6B}| + |\%R_{7A} - \%R_{7B}| + |\%R_{8A} - \%R_{8B}|) / 8$	Farnetani et al. (1989, cited in 1991)
Coarticulation index (anterior zone) (CI$_{anterior}$)	$(|\%R_{1A} - \%R_{1B}| + |\%R_{2A} - \%R_{2B}| + |\%R_{3A} - \%R_{3B}| + |\%R_{4A} - \%R_{4B}|) / 4$	Fontdevila et al. (1994a)
Coarticulation index (posterior zone) (CI$_{posterior}$)	$(|\%R_{5A} - \%R_{5B}| + |\%R_{6A} - \%R_{6B}| + |\%R_{7A} - \%R_{7B}| + |\%R_{8A} - \%R_{8B}|) / 4$	Fontdevila et al. (1994a)

| Articulatory reduction index | $[(R_{1P} - R_{1C}) + (R_{2P} - R_{2C}) + (R_{3P} - R_{3C}) + (R_{4P} - R_{4C}) + (R_{5P} - R_{5C}) + (R_{6P} - R_{6C}) + (R_{7P} - R_{7C}) + (R_{8P} - R_{8C})] / 8$ | Farnetani and Provaglio (1991) |
| Trough index (TI) | $[(N_{V1i} + N_{V2i}) / 2] / N_{Ci}$ | Engstrand (1989, cited in Hardcastle, Gibbon, & Nicolaidis, 1991) |

Note: $N_{Contact}$ = total number of electrodes contacted; N_{Total} = total number of electrodes on the EPG plate; R_i = number of contacts on row i; C_i = number of contacts on column i counted from the outer columns; N_R = number of contacts on the right half of the palate; N_L = number of contacts on the left half of the palate; $F_{>50-<100}$ = frequency of contact ranged between >50% to <100%; $F_{>0-\le50}$ = frequency of contact ranged between >0% to 50%; $\%R_{1A}$ = percent contact on row i in phonetic context A; $\%R_{1B}$ = percent contact on row i in phonetic context B; R_{iP} = number of contacts on row i of the consonant prototype; R_{iC} = number of contacts on row i of the same consonant produced in connected speech; N_{V1i} = number of contacts on the row that shows the highest contact (row i) for vowel 1 in a vowel-consonant-vowel (VCV) sequence; N_{V2i} = number of contacts on the same row for vowel 2 in the VCV sequence; N_{Ci} = number of contacts on the same row for the intervocalic consonant.

VI (relative) index. Figure 25.5 shows the VI results of two hypothetical patterns, with the consistent contact patterns showing lower VI values than the varied error patterns for an alveolar fricative.

Another group of indices measures the difference in contact as a result of coarticulation, different speech styles or linguistic levels, or lingual "relaxation." The coarticulation index (CI) is the average difference in percent contact in each row between two tokens of a phoneme produced in different phonetic context; for example, /t/ produced in "a tip" versus "a tab," and /n/ in "a nip" versus "a nab" showed in the worked example in Figure 25.6 using the data reported in Gibbon et al.'s (2007) study. The CI index can also be calculated for a specific region: $CI_{anterior}$ for the alveolar and postalveolar regions (row 1–4 on the EPG plate) and $CI_{posterior}$ for the palatal and velar regions (row 5–8). As shown in Figure 25.6, the coarticulatory effect of the following vowel is greater on /n/ than on /t/ and the effect is mainly in the alveolar region. The articulatory reduction index uses an equation similar to the one of CI to quantify the difference in contact when the phoneme is produced in different context, such as at word level versus connected speech level (Farnetani & Provaglio, 1991).

The trough index (TI) is a ratio of the average amount of contacts in the row of highest contact of two identical vowels to the amount of contacts in the same row of the intervocalic

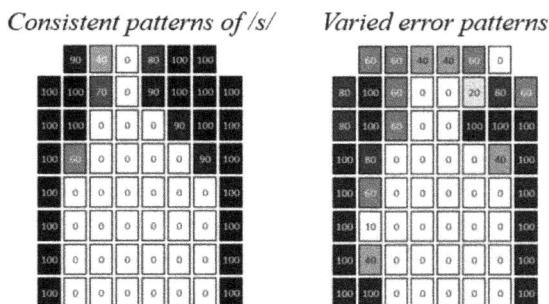

	Consistent patterns of /s/	Varied error patterns
Variability index (absolute)	2.74	8.87
Variability index (relative)	21.25	32.35

Figure 25.5 Results of variability indices for two cumulative contact patterns—one showing consistent contact and one showing varied error patterns over repetitions.

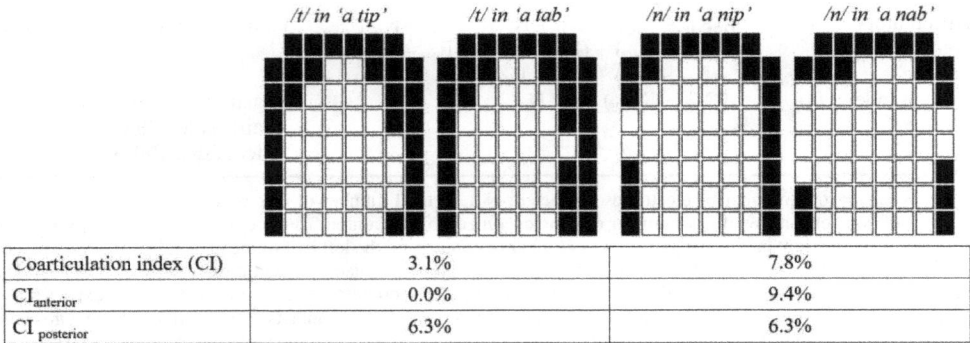

	/t/ in 'a tip' and /t/ in 'a tab'	/n/ in 'a nip' and /n/ in 'a nab'
Coarticulation index (CI)	3.1%	7.8%
CI$_{anterior}$	0.0%	9.4%
CI$_{posterior}$	6.3%	6.3%

Figure 25.6 Coarticulatory effect of following vowel (/i/ and /æ/) on the tongue palate contact for /t/ and /n/ as quantified using Coarticulation index (CI), CI$_{anterior}$ for row 1–4, and CI$_{posterior}$ for row 5–8.

consonant in a vowel-consonant-vowel sequence (Engstrand, 1989, cited in Hardcastle, Gibbon, & Nicolaidis, 1991; see Table 25.1). Figure 25.7 shows the TI calculated based on the number of contacts in row 7 for utterance "ipi" produced by a typical speaker. The value is higher than 1, indicating the tongue "relaxed" and showed a relatively lower contact during the bilabial plosive in the intervocalic position.

EPG as a biofeedback tool in speech therapy

After analyzing the results from speech assessment and examination of tongue palate contact patterns, the general error patterns that the client is showing can be worked out. For example, the case presented in the paper by Lee et al. (2007) is a child with speech sound disorders associated with cleft palate, who showed retracted place of contact for the alveolar plosives and fricatives, the affricates and the lateral approximant; but correct contact patterns for the bilabial and velar plosives, and the postalveolar fricative but limited to word level. Hence, the general direction for speech intervention for this child is to establish an anterior contact for the phonemes in error. One way to help the child achieving an anterior tongue palate contact is to make use of the correct lingual gestures that the child already had, and in this case, using /ʃ/ as a facilitative context by placing the treatment target close to the correct sound would be useful. For example, using phrases such as "fish chips" for facilitating correct pattern for /tʃ/ and "fish supper" for /s/ (Lee et al., 2007). Other principles of treatment target selection

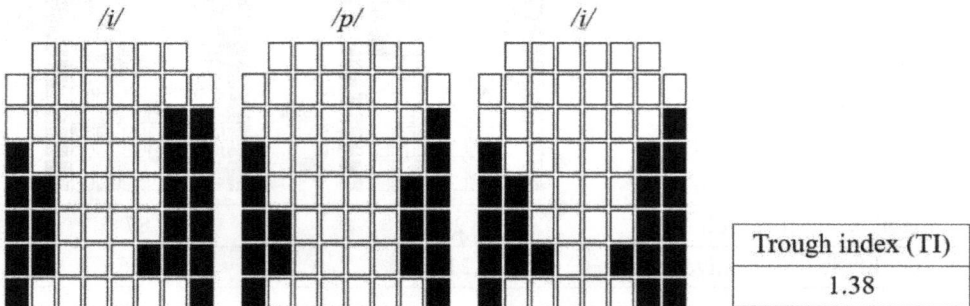

Trough index (TI)
1.38

Figure 25.7 Trough index (TI) for utterance "ipi".

used in conventional speech therapy can be used as long as they are also applicable to the case at hand.

Regarding treatment dosage and service delivery model, there has not been any study that compared different treatment dosages for EPG therapy. The treatment schedule used in previous studies is usually 2 sessions per week. For example, the study on EPG therapy with children with Down syndrome applied a schedule of two 1-hour sessions every week over 12 weeks (Wood et al., 2019); and a study on children with speech sound disorders used a schedule of two 30-minute session per week over 8 weeks (Hitchcock et al., 2017). Another study on children with history of cleft palate provided 12 one clinician-led EPG therapy session at an SLT clinic every month, supplemented with home practice using a PTU for 30 minutes per day (Fujiwara, 2007). One of the clients also had a 30-minute online EPG therapy session every week from the clinician between the monthly face-to-face SLT appointments. A recent systematic review examined the relationship between treatment intensity and treatment outcomes for speech intervention that used an external visual feedback for children with SSD of unknown origin or due to a motor speech problem (Hitchcock, Swartz, & Lopez, 2019). A total of 29 treatment studies in the form of case studies, case series, or single-case experimental design were included in the review, with five of them used EPG, six used visual acoustic, and 18 used ultrasound. The study showed that both treatment intensity (measured using the cumulative intervention index—a product of dose-by-dose frequency by total intervention duration; Warren, Fey, & Yoder, 2007) and dose alone showed a weak but statistically significant positive correlation with the treatment outcomes. Moreover, duration alone showed a weak but statistically significant negative correlation with the treatment outcomes. The results seemed to indicate that a high dose is useful as it allows plenty of opportunities for the clients to practice the new articulatory gestures during the therapy sessions, and a more intensive therapy schedule over a shorter span is preferred to the same number of sessions spread over an extended period (Hitchcock et al., 2019). Repetitive and intensive practice has been recommended for speech intervention using EPG (Gibbon & Wood, 2010). Although a small number of EPG studies were included in this review and that participants were limited to a certain group of children, their recommendations can be used as a general guide before more specific research findings for EPG therapy for different clinical groups are available.

Speech therapy using EPG usually starts with an introduction session to familiarize the clients with the equipment—the way it works and to establish the link between the tongue palate contact patterns shown on a computer screen with they do with their tongue when they say different sounds or make different lingual gestures (Gibbon & Wood, 2010; Hitchcock et al., 2017). For developing the speech stimuli, aside from making use of the strategy of facilitative context if applicable, it is useful to start with speech tasks with a motor complexity level which is just above the current level of the clients and then increase the complexity level as they progress (Gibbon & Wood, 2010). In terms of feedback, the application of the principles of motor learning (Maas et al., 2008) has been recommended for EPG and other instrumental techniques for giving external biofeedback. There are two types of feedback: knowledge of performance (KP) and knowledge of results (KR). KP is about informing the clients of how they have performed; for example, pointing out that they are able to make a horseshoe shape on the palatogram on the computer screen for the treatment on establishing an anterior and bilateral contact for an alveolar plosive. KR is for letting the clients know if their production is correct or not; for example, simply telling the clients that they have made a correct pattern for /t/ or /d/. KP is useful at the start of intervention for establishing new articulatory behaviors, while KR is useful for consolidating the correct gestures once the clients have understood what is required for the target sound.

Evidence regarding efficacy of EPG therapy

Previous EPG treatment studies were mostly single-case studies, case series and controlled studies, and in general, they have shown positive improvement of different levels in most of the clients after the course of therapy. A survey was carried out to find out the clinical opinions from 10 SLTs working in Scotland about clients they had treated with EPG between 1993 and 2003 (Gibbon & Paterson, 2006). Results of 60 clients were reported and the breakdown of the cause of SSD is 45% for cleft palate, 32% for SSD of unknown origin, and 23% with mixed etiologies. The SLTs reported that most of the clients had improved their articulation to some extent and almost all had increased awareness of their own articulation difficulties following EPG therapy. However, one aspect of intervention—generalization—has been shown to be difficult to achieve (Gibbon & Paterson, 2006; Lohmander, Henriksson, & Havstam, 2010). The latest bigger-scale EPG treatment study is probably the single-blinded, parallel randomized controlled trial (RCT) that included 27 children with Down syndrome, who were randomly assigned to one of three treatment groups: speech therapy using EPG for visual feed-back, speech therapy based on conventional approach, and no therapy (Wood et al., 2019; see also Cleland et al., 2009; Wood, Wishart, Hardcastle, Cleland, & Timmins, 2009). The finding of this study was that although three groups showed "gains in accuracy of production imme-diately post-therapy, as measured by PCC [percentage consonants correct] … Reassessment at 3 and 6 months post-therapy revealed that those who had received therapy based directly on EPG visual feedback were more likely to maintain and improve on these gains compared with the other groups" (Wood et al., 2019, p. 234).

A Cochrane Systematic Review was carried out to examine the evidence regarding efficacy of EPG therapy for individuals with history of cleft palate specifically (Lee, Law, & Gibbon, 2009). The review was published in 2009 and updated in 2017. The review identified one RCT carried out by Michi and colleagues who reported the findings of fewer therapy sessions needed to achieve the treatment goals for the EPG therapy and frication display method (a real-time trace of level of frication energy produced), followed by EPG therapy, and conventional speech treatment (Michi, Yamashita, Imai, Suzuki, & Yoshida, 1993). However, the strength of evidence provided by this RCT is limited by a number of methodological shortcomings, including a very small sample size (two participants in each treatment arm), lack of blinding of outcome assessor(s), few quantitative outcome measures used, and treatment results not reported as planned.

Previous EPG studies of speech disorders

Some of the previous EPG studies of speech disorders have been cited above, so here is a review of important studies or useful papers for those who are interested to read more about EPG. The first one is an EPG bibliography where it lists EPG studies written in English, and it presents the publications in terms of those related to the description of different EPG systems; general bibliography of EPG studies in English; and the bibliography of clinical applications of EPG (Gibbon, 2013). The second resource is reviews on the atypical tongue palate con-tact patterns that have been reported in the literature for two clinical groups: speech sound disorders of unknown origin (Gibbon, 1999) and cleft palate (Gibbon, 2004; Gibbon & Lee, 2010). Regarding using EPG as a treatment tool, the following papers or book chapters are recommended: Lee et al. (2007); Gibbon and Wood (2010); Gibbon and Lee (2011); and Lee, Harding-Bell and Gibbon (2019). Finally, there is a resource book that provide tongue palate contact pattern for all English consonants and monophthongs obtained from one typical speaker of English (McLeod & Singh, 2009).

Conclusion

EPG has provided us important information on lingual articulation along the transverse plane that we often have forgotten about (McLeod, 2011). EPG has also been shown to be a useful tool to provide insight on the underlying articulatory difficulties that led to speech errors. This raises our awareness of the possibility of the presence of atypical lingual gestures that we cannot perceive. Even without access to an EPG system, we can still apply what we learned about typical and atypical lingual articulation to hypothesize about the underlying cause of articulation problems.

References

Alwan, A.A., Narayanan, S.S., & Haker, K. (1997). Toward articulatory-acoustic models for liquid approximants based on MRI and EPG data. Part II. The rhotics. *Journal of the Acoustical Society of America*, *101*(2), 1078–1089.

Articulate-Instruments-Ltd. (2013). A history of EPG. Retrieved from http://www.articulateinstruments.com/a-history-of-epg/?LMCL=vU4WtS&LMCL=viFdWn&LMCL=vU4WtS

Ball, M. J., & Müller, N. (2005). *Phonetics for communication disorders*. New York, NY: Routledge.

Brosseau-Lapré, F., & Rvachew, S. (2020). *Introduction to speech sound disorders*. San Diego: Plural Publishing Inc.

Cheng, H. Y., Murdoch, B. E., Goozée, J. V., & Scott, D. (2007). Electropalatographic assessment of tongue-to-palate contact patterns and variability in children, adolescents, and adults. *Journal of Speech, Language, & Hearing Research*, *50*, 375–392.

Cleland, J., Timmins, C., Wood, S. E., Hardcastle, W. J., & Wishart, J. G. (2009). Electropalatographic therapy for children and young people with Down's syndrome. *Clinical Linguistics & Phonetics*, *23*(12), 926–939.

Fabus, R., Raphael, L., Gatzonis, S., Dondorf, K., Giardina, K., Cron, S., & Badke, B. (2015). Preliminary case studies investigating the use of electropalatography (EPG) manufactured by CompleteSpeech® as a biofeedback toolin intervention. *International Journal of Linguistics and Communication*, *3*(1), 11–23.

Farnetani, E., & Provaglio, A. (1991). Assessing variability of lingual consonants in Italian. *Quaderni del Cantro di Studio per le Ricerche di Fonetica del C.N.R.*, *10*, 117–145.

Fontdevila, J., Pallarès, M. D., & Recasens, D. (1994a). The contact index method of electropalatographic data reduction. *Journal of Phonetics*, *22*(2), 141–154.

Fontdevila, J., Pallarès, M. D., & Recasens, D. (1994b). Electropalatographic data collected with and without a face mask. *Journal of Speech & Hearing Research*, *37*(4), 806–812.

Fujiwara, Y. (2007). Electropalatography home training using a portable training unit for Japanese children with cleft palate. *Advances in Speech-Language Pathology*, *9*, 65–72.

Gibbon, F. E. (1999). Undifferentiated lingual gestures in children with articulation/phonological disorders. *Journal of Speech, Language, and Hearing Research*, *42*(2), 382–397.

Gibbon, F. E. (2004). Abnormal patterns of tongue-palate contact in the speech of individuals with cleft palate. *Clinical Linguistics & Phonetics*, *18*(4–5), 285–311.

Gibbon, F. E. (2013). Bibliography of electropalatographic (EPG) studies in English (1957–2013). Retrieved from http://www.articulateinstruments.com/EPGrefs.pdf

Gibbon, F. E., & Crampin, L. (2001). An electropalatographic investigation of middorsum palatal stops in an adult with repaired cleft palate. *Cleft Palate-Craniofacial Journal*, *38*(2), 96–105.

Gibbon, F. E., & Lee, A. (2010). Producing turbulent speech sounds in the context of cleft palate. In S. Fuchs, M. Toda, & M. Żygis (Eds.), *Turbulent sounds: An interdisciplinary guide* (pp. 303–341). Berlin: de Gruyter.

Gibbon, F. E., & Lee, A. (2011). Articulation – Instruments for research and clinical practice. In S. Howard & A. Lohmander (Eds.), *Cleft palate speech: Assessment and intervention* (pp. 221–238). Chicester, West Sussex, UK: Wiley-Blackwell.

Gibbon, F. E., Lee, A., & Yuen, I. (2010). Tongue-palate contact during selected vowels in normal speech. *Cleft Palate-Craniofacial Journal*, *47*(4), 405–412.

Gibbon, F. E., & Paterson, L. (2006). A survey of speech and language therapists' views on electropalatography therapy outcomes in Scotland. *Child Language Teaching and Therapy*, *22*(3), 275–292.

Gibbon, F. E., & Wood, S. E. (2010). Visual feedback therapy with electropalatography. In A. L. Williams, S. McLeod, & R. J. McCauley (Eds.), *Interventions for speech sound disorders in children* (pp. 509–536). Baltimore, MD: Paul H. Brookes Publishing Co.

Gibbon, F. E., Yuen, I., Lee, A., & Adams, L. (2007). Normal adult speakers' tongue palate contact patterns for alveolar oral and nasal stops. *Advances in Speech-Language Pathology*, *9*(1), 82–89.

Hardcastle, W. J., & Barry, W. (1989). Articulatory and perceptual factors in/l/vocalisations in English. *Journal of the International Phonetic Association*, *15*(2), 3–17.

Hardcastle, W. J., Gibbon, F., & Nicolaidis, K. (1991). EPG data reduction methods and their implications for studies of lingual coarticualtion. *Journal of Phonetics*, *19*, 251–266.

Hardcastle, W. J., & Gibbon, F. E. (2005). Electropalatography as a research and clinical tool: 30 years on. In W.J. Hardcastle & J. Mackenzie Beck (Eds.), *A Figure of speech: A festschrift for John Laver* (pp. 39–60). Mahwah, NJ: Lawrence Erlbaum Associates.

Hardcastle, W. J., Gibbon, F. E., & Jones, W. (1991). Visual display of tongue-palate contact: Electropalatography in the assessment and remediation of speech disorders. *British Journal of Disorders of Communication*, *26*(1), 41–74.

Hardcastle, W. J., Jones, W., Knight, C., Trudgeon, A., & Calder, G. (1989). New developments in electropalatography: A state-of-the-art report. *Clinical Linguistics & Phonetics*, *3*(1), 1–38.

Hardcastle, W. J., Morgan Barry, R. A., & Clark, C. J. (1985). Articulatory and voicing characteristics of adult dysarthric and verbal dyspraxic speakers: An instrumental study. *British Journal of Disorders of Communication*, *20*(3), 249–270.

Hardcastle, W. J., Morgan Barry, R. A., & Clark, C. J. (1987). An instrumental phonetic study of lingual activity in articulation-disordered children. *Journal of Speech & Hearing Research*, *30*, 171–184.

Hitchcock, E. R., McAllister Byun, T., Swartz, M., & Lazarus, R. (2017). Efficacy of electropalatography for treating misarticulation of/r/. *American Journal of Speech-Language Pathology*, *26*(4), 1141–1158.

Hitchcock, E. R., Swartz, M. T., & Lopez, M. (2019). Speech sound disorder and visual biofeedback intervention: A preliminary investigation of treatment intensity. *Seminars in Speech and Language*, *40*(2), 124–137.

Jones, W. J., & Hardcastle, W. J. (1995). New developments in EPG3 software. *European Journal of Disorders of Communication*, *30*, 183–192.

Kelly, S., Main, A., Manley, G., & McLean, C. (2000). Electropalatography and the Linguagraph system. *Medical Engineering & Physics*, *22*(1), 47–58.

Ladefoged, P. (2003). *Phonetic data analysis: An introduction to fieldwork ad instrumental techniques.* Oxford, UK: Blackwell Publishing.

Ladefoged, P. (2006). *A course in phonetics* (5th ed.). Boston, MA: Thomson Higher Education.

Lee, A. (2019). Electropalatography. In J.S. Damico & M.J. Ball (Eds.), *The SAGE encyclopedia of human communication sciences and disorders* (pp. 679–680). Thousand Oaks, CA: SAGE Publications, Inc.

Lee, A., Gibbon, F. E., Crampin, L., Yuen, I., & McLennan, G. (2007). The national CLEFTNET project for individuals with speech disorders associated with cleft palate. *Advances in Speech-Language Pathology*, *9*, 57–64.

Lee, A., Harding-Bell, A., & Gibbon, F.E. (2019). Diagnosis and intervention for cleft palate speech using electropalatography (EPG). In A. Harding-Bell (Ed.), *Case studies in cleft palate speech: Data analysis and principled intervention.* Guildford, Surrey, UK: J&R Press Ltd.

Lee, A., Law, J., & Gibbon, F. E. (2009). Electropalatography for articulation disorders associated with cleft palate. *Cochrane Database of Systematic Reviews 2009*(Issue 3), Art. No.: CD006854. doi:10.1002/14651858.CD006854.pub2

Leitch, E., Gibbon, F. E., & Crampin, L. (1998). Portable training for speech disorders. *Speech and Language Therapy in Practice, Winter edition*, 9–12.

Liker, M., & Gibbon, F. E. (2008). Tongue palate contact patterns of velar stops in normal adult English speakers. *Clinical Linguistics & Phonetics*, *22*(2), 137–148.

Liker, M., & Gibbon, F. E. (2018). Tongue-palate contact timing during/s/and/z/in English. *Phonetica*, *75*(2), 110–131.

Liker, M., Gibbon, F. E., Wrench, A. A., & Horga, D. (2007). Articulatory characteristics of the occlusion phase of/tʃ/compared to/t/in adult speech. *Advances in Speech-Language Pathology*, *9*(1), 101–108.

Lohmander, A., Henriksson, C., & Havstam, C. (2010). Electropalatography in home training of retracted articulation in a Swedish child with cleft palate: Effect on articulation pattern and speech. *International Journal of Speech-Language Pathology*, *12*(6), 483–496.

Maas, E., Robin, D. A., Austermann Hula, S. N., Freedman, S. E., Wulf, G., Ballard, K.J., & Schmidt, R.A. (2008). Principles of motor learning in treatment of motor speech disorders. *American Journal of Speech-Language Pathology, 17,* 277–298.

Marchal, A., & Espesser, R. (1989). L'asymétrie des appuis linguo-palatins. *Journal d'Acoustique, Societe française d'acoustique, 2,* 53–57.

McLeod, S. (2011). Speech-language pathologists' knowledge of tongue/palate contact for consonants. *Clinical Linguistics & Phonetics, 25*(11–12), 1004–1013.

McLeod, S., Roberts, A., & Sita, J. (2006). Tongue/palate contact for the production of/s/and/z/. *Clinical Linguistics & Phonetics, 20*(1), 51–66.

McLeod, S., & Searl, J. (2006). Adaptation to an electropalatograph palate: Acoustic, impressionistic, and perceptual data. *American Journal of Speech-Language Pathology, 15*(2), 192–206.

McLeod, S., & Singh, S. (2009). *Speech sounds: A pictorial guide to typical and atypical speech.* San Diego: Plural Publishing.

Michi, K., Yamashita, Y., Imai, S., Suzuki, N., & Yoshida, H. (1993). Role of visual feedback treatment for defective/s/sounds in patients with cleft palate. *Journal of Speech and Hearing Research, 36*(2), 277–285.

Narayanan, S. S., Alwan, A. A., & Haker, K. (1997). Toward articulatory-acoustic models for liquid approximants based on MRI and EPG data. Part I. The laterals. *Journal of the Acoustical Society of America, 101*(2), 1064–1077.

Schmidt, A. M. (2007). Evaluating a new clinical palatometry system. *Advances in Speech-Language Pathology, 9*(1), 73–81.

Scobbie, J. M., Wood, S. E., & Wrench, A. A. (2004). Advances in EPG for treatment and research: An illustrative case study. *Clinical Linguistics and Phonetics, 18*(6–8), 373–389.

Stone, M., Faber, A., Raphael, L. J., & Shawker, T. H. (1992). Cross-sectional tongue shape and linguopalatal contact patterns in [s], [ʃ], and [l]. *Journal of Phonetics, 20*(2), 253–270.

Velleman, S. L. (2016). *Speech sound disorders.* Philadelphia: Wolters Kluwer.

Warren, S. F., Fey, M. E., & Yoder, P. J. (2007). Differential treatment intensity research: A missing link to creating optimally effective communication interventions. *Mental Retardation and Developmental Disabilities Research Reviews, 13*(1), 70–77.

Wood, S. E., Timmins, C., Wishart, J., Hardcastle, W. J., & Cleland, J. (2019). Use of electropalatography in the treatment of speech disorders in children with Down syndrome: A randomized controlled trial. *International Journal of Language & Communication Disorders, 54*(2), 234–248.

Wood, S. E., Wishart, J., Hardcastle, W., Cleland, J., & Timmins, C. (2009). The use of electropalatography (EPG) in the assessment and treatment of motor speech disorders in children with Down's syndrome: Evidence from two case studies. *Developmental Neurorehabilitation, 12*(2), 66–75.

Wrench, A. A. (2007). Advances in EPG palate design. *Advances in Speech-Language Pathology, 9*(1), 3–12.

Yamamoto, I. (2019). Tongue-palate contact patterns for Japanese speakers with and without cleft lip and palate. *International Journal of Speech-Language Pathology, 22*(1), *70–77.* doi:10.1080/17549507. 2019.1593505

Zharkova, N. (2008). An EPG and ultrasound study of lingual coarticulation in vowel-consonant sequences. *Proceedings of the 8th International Seminar on Speech Production, Strasbourg, France,* 241–244.

26

ELECTROMAGNETIC ARTICULOGRAPHY

Pascal van Lieshout

General introduction

Humans are capable of communicating in a very unique way. They alter the resonance properties of the vocal tract to create sounds by moving oral structures that from a phylogenetic point of view primarily are tasked with chewing and swallowing (van Lieshout, 2017). According to Lieberman (Lieberman, 2003; see also van Lieshout, 2015), the exact time course of these changes is not known, but "the speech producing morphology capable of producing the full range of human speech is a species-specific human attribute that appeared in the last 150,000 years" (p. 270). Clearly, moving these structures such as lips, mandible and tongue for the purpose of producing speech puts very different demands on their motor control (van Lieshout, 2015).[1] Instead of generating a certain amount of pressure or force as needed for handling food particles, they need to move with sufficient speed and accuracy to enable a relatively fast sequence of movements that form specific constrictions inside targeted locations in the vocal tract. How fast we move these structures varies from individual to individual, but in general, we seem to move them at such a speed that the number of linguistic units we can produce (syllables or words) are close to maximum rates at which information can be conveyed in daily conversations (Coupé et al., 2019). This is quite amazing, given the fact that these oral structures are very different in terms of size, mass, muscular composition and neural innervation (Coupé et al., 2019; van Lieshout, 2015). So, it should not come as a surprise that people have always been fascinated by this motor skill and the fact that as a species we seem to learn it quite naturally without explicit instruction over a timespan roughly between birth and toward the end of puberty, depending on the kind of aspects of speech motor control one is looking at (Smith et al., 1995). Although many theories exist and try to describe the processes involved in producing speech, there are still many questions unanswered, in particular with respect to how speech motor skills develop in relation to language, cognition and other functions involved in communication, what defines the skill as such (e.g. principles of effort vs. information transfer; Coupé et al., 2019; Xu, & Prom-on, 2019), and how the brain manages to control this complex function given the high demands and differences among the various structures.

One of the main obstacles in studying speech production and its control has always been the lack of suitable tools to actually monitor and record what is going on inside the vocal tract. The acoustic signal can only provide a very indirect reflection of the underlying motor actions and in many cases, it is hard to do the inverse process of relating acoustic features to movements of articulators, although much progress has been made in this direction (e.g. Chartier et al., 2018). Thus, scientists have explored more direct methods to study the vocal tract events. Prior to 1970, one option was to use X-ray machines. X-rays are shortwave electromagnetic signals that can penetrate the skin and other organic tissues, and thus allow visualization of internal structures. However, this type of radiation comes with obvious health risks. To somewhat decrease the health risks, an innovative modification called the X-ray Microbeam was developed in the 1980s by a Japanese group (Fujimura & Haskin, 1981; Kiritani et al., 1975). In the X-ray Microbeam system, narrow X-ray beams are guided by a computer to predict the location of small gold pellets attached to surface structures of the vocal tract. Unfortunately, this was an expensive setup in terms of infrastructure and human resources needed. Currently, there is only one remaining X-ray Microbeam facility in the world located at the University of Wisconsin in Madison, USA. This seriously limits accessibility although their database has been made available to researchers (Westbury et al., 1990). Furthermore, there is still a health risk as the system uses a certain dosage of X-ray exposure.

Other developments have included systems that use ultra-frequency sound as a transmission signal to visualize structures with different sound reflective properties (Ultrasound; e.g. Bressmann, 2007) and more recently, speech researchers have been exploring the use of Magnetic Resonance Imaging techniques (Lingala et al., 2016) that also allow for visualizing intra-oral structures with minimal health risks. Another methodology that was developed in the late 1970s and early 1980s was electromagnetic articulography. This method uses a different part of the spectrum of electromagnetic signals than X-rays, also capable of penetrating soft organic tissues but without presenting a known biohazard[2].

In the next sections, I will first briefly go over the history of Electromagnetic Articulograph (EMA) systems. This is followed by a section with more details on basic measurement principles, their measurement accuracy as a tool to track movements of vocal tract structures and some examples of ways to process EMA data. Then I will provide an overview of the literature published on the use of these systems, focusing on the number, areas and types of publication and the countries from where these publications originated. This information is relevant to gauge the impact of the EMA technology in the past 15 years on research and clinical work. Finally, I will discuss some possible future developments, including a new system that combines the use of articulography with the recording of cortical brain signals as part of a single Magnetoencephalography (MEG) setup.

History of Electromagnetic Articulography (EMA)

Electromagnetic Articulography is based on the well-known principle that an electromagnetic field can induce an electrical current in a metal wire or coil. Early applications in speech research can be found in studies on breathing and jaw movements (Hixon, 1971; van der Giet, 1977). Two labs in the 1980s were instrumental in developing this technology to track movements of speech articulators. One lab was located in the USA (Perkell et al., 1992) and the other one in Germany (Schönle et al., 1987). Only the German system (AG100) became a commercially available system, which was developed by the German company Carstens MedizinElektronik GmbH. Later, other EMA systems such as the Wave system, developed by the Canadian NDI company, became available. The Wave system was the successor of the AURORA system from the same company (Kröger et al., 2008).

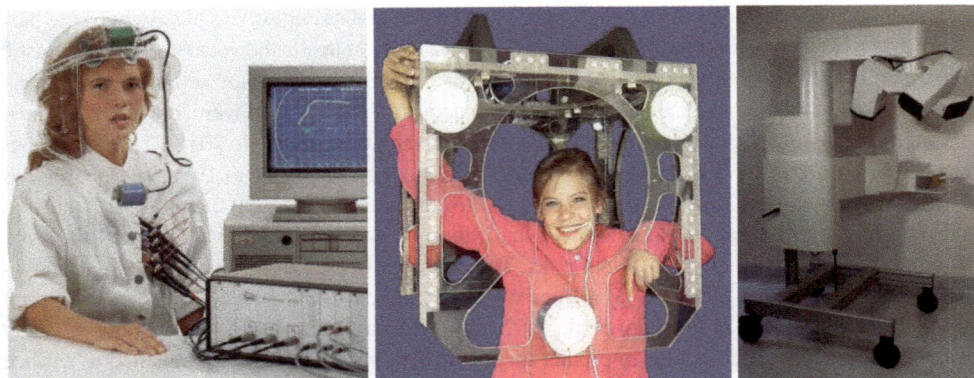

Figure 26.1 Images of the AG100 (left), AG500 (middle) and AG501 (right) systems (images used with permission from Carstens Medizinelektronik GmbH).

The original Articulograph systems were only capable of recording movements in a 2D midsagittal plane. More details on these older systems can be found elsewhere (Perkell et al., 1992; Schönle et al., 1987; for a more general overview see Van Lieshout, 2006). The 2D systems had limitations in terms of sensitivity to measurement artifacts related to movements outside the midsagittal plane or rotations of the coil as well as those related to the need to constrain head motion. For the same reasons, these systems could not provide information about meaningful lateral motion or tongue rotations or to study the specific contributions of head motion as part of communicative intent (Hoole & Nguyen, 1999; Tiede et al., 2019). Thus, the search for a system that would be able to deal with these issues was well motivated and culminated in the development of systems that are capable of recording 3 movement directions and two angular rotations (referred to in general as 5D Electro-Magnetic Articulography).The Carsten's company referred to their 5D systems as the AG500 series, with the most recent version, the AG501. Figure 26.1 shows a picture of the 3 generations of AG systems (AG100, AG500, AG501), excluding the AG200 which was basically a modified AG100.

The first paper to my knowledge that discussed the potential for a 5D system was published by Andreas Zierdt (Zierdt, 1993) who has (co)published further papers on the measurement principles, technical specifications and data processing issues (e.g. Hoole & Zierdt, 2010). Since then, several other papers have been published around the use of 5D EMA and this will be highlighted in the section below on articulography publications. As mentioned, the most recent version of the 5D EMA is the AG501 which has been shown to be very reliable in terms of accuracy of measurement, not only compared to the AG500 but also when compared to the WAVE system (Savariaux et al., 2017). This will be discussed in the next section.

Measurement principles, technical evaluations and date processing

Measurement principles

All Articulograph systems (at least from the AG line) use a set of dipole transmitters in combination with mono-axial receiver coils[3]. Each receiver coil has five degrees of freedom (3 movement directions: front/back, up/down, left/right and 2 angles, viz. azimuth and elevation).

Rotations around the main axis of the receiver coil cannot be registered which is why a receiver coil cannot be in a perpendicular position to more than 3 transmitters at any given time. The strength of the induced complex signal in a receiver coil is roughly inversely proportional to its distance (3rd power of radius) from each corresponding transmitter. The AG500's original sensors (HS220s) were replaced with sensors that have higher output with improved signal-to-noise ratio (HQ220s) in 2009. The AG501 uses sensors that have been further improved (HQ220-L120-B).

Transmitters in the AG500 are placed in a spherical configuration on a plexiglass cube with an edge length of 50 cm. The AG501 has nine transmitter coils embedded in three rectangular structures mounted above the registration volume. Frequencies of transmitters range from 7.5 to 13.75 kHz, with amplitudes ranging from 8.85 to 16.66 µT (Stella et al., 2012). Whereas the sampling rates for the AG500 and AG501 can be set to different values (up to 1250 Hz for the AG501), typical values reported in the literature mention 200 and 400 Hz. Voltages are quantized at a 16-bit resolution. The AG501 can also process signals from more receiver coils (up to 24) than the AG500.

Coil location is derived from a mathematical representation of the spatial pattern of the magnetic field in the measurement volume as determined by a standardized calibration procedure. The typical spherical shaped registration volume for the EMA systems has a radius of 150 mm. The coil position is based on a voltage to distance function derived using a narrow bandpass filter based on the frequencies associated with each transmitter. The amplitude of the induced signal in the receiver coil is compared to the estimated amplitudes based on the calculated field representation. Differences are expressed in RMS values, where for calibration purposes it is recommended to keep the RMS error at 14 digits or lower, which is roughly equivalent to a 1.12 mV difference based on the 16 digit representation of a 5V range (Stella et al., 2012; Yunusova et al., 2009). RMS errors are evaluated based on a threshold that can be changed by the user. If RMS errors exceed that threshold, the system will recalculate the differences until the RMS threshold is reached. Following the calibration procedure, the calculated RMS values are made available for inspection and validation.

The WAVE system has an unknown number of transmitter coils embedded in a field generator whose dimension is $20 \times 20 \times 7$ cm and which generates an electromagnetic registration volume of either $50 \times 50 \times 50$ cm or $30 \times 30 \times 30$ cm. It can register up to 16 receiver coils (including 5-Degrees Of Freedom reference sensors) at frequencies between 100 and 400 Hz. The size and shape of the WAVE receiver coils differ from the EMA coils. The Wave coils are not shielded in the same way as the AG coils which makes them more susceptible to external magnetic field disruptions.

The coil localization algorithm employed by the AG systems involves finding an optimal solution via a nonlinear root-finding algorithm using 6 equations (one for each transmitter) and 5 unknown variables related to the two movement and two rotational dimensions. The approximation algorithm used by AG systems is called the Newton–Raphson method which estimates the values of coil position and orientation by iteratively surveying the solution landscape of the nonlinear system while attempting to converge on a minimum solution (Hoole & Zierdt, 2010; Kaburagi et al., 2005).

Technical evaluations

Various studies have been conducted to test the measurement accuracy of the Carsten's AG and NDI-Wave systems over the past 10 years. For example, the paper by Savariaux and colleagues (Savariaux et al., 2017) provides an overview of those published between 2008 and 2013 and they themselves tested several AG and Wave systems. The most recent paper by Sigona et al. (Sigona et al., 2018) made a direct comparison between the AG500 and AG501 systems. In our own lab, we also made a direct comparison between the AG500 and the AG501 using a custom made calibration device (Lau, 2013).

From the findings of these very diverse studies some general inferences can be made regarding the stability and accuracy of the different Articulograph systems (AG500, AG501, Wave). With respect to the registration space where measurements are likely to be the most accurate, it is recommended that for the AG systems it should be within a spherically shaped volume with a radius of 100 mm (Sigona et al., 2018; Stella et al., 2012; Yunusova et al., 2009). This would roughly correspond to the size of an average human head and it should be centered around the origin of the measurement field. For the Wave system, it was found that the average tracking errors are smallest within approximately 200 mm from the field generator with a slight improvement noticed for the 300-mm^3 field volume setting (Berry, 2011; see also Savariaux et al., 2017).

To avoid crosstalk between the signals of nearby receiver coils, the manufacturer of the AG systems recommends keeping a minimum distance of 8 mm between them, although this can be difficult to achieve in experiments when coils are moving toward each other at shorter distances. The study by Stella and colleagues (Stella et al., 2012) did not find any significant influence on coil signals when they tested 15 and 30 mm inter-coil distances. It is important to note that studies that have tested the performance of AG500 and AG501 systems, typically used a fixed distance between receiver coils (Lau, 2013; Savariaux et al., 2017; 2015 et al., 2018; Stella et al., 2012; Yunusova et al., 2009).

The overall measurement accuracy of the systems varies, as one would expect. In fact, they vary even for the same system in different labs (Savariaux et al., 2017). Ideally, one would like to see measurement errors to be less than 0.5 mm and for the three systems described here, that is attainable provided one restricts measurements to within the ideal working space (see above). Moving further away from the transmitters and outside the ideal space does introduce larger errors (Lau, 2013; Savariaux et al., 2017; Sigona et al., 2018; Stella et al., 2012). This variation is illustrated in Figure 26.2, showing spatial error maps for the AG500 and AG501 (Lau, 2013). Errors in general do not seem to be related to movements of the receiver coils as such (Kroos, 2012; Lau, 2013; Savariaux et al., 2017). For the AG500, some (relatively large magnitude) errors have been related to the algorithm used to derive positions based on the measured amplitudes in relation to the magnetic field estimates (Stella et al., 2012; see also Hoole & Zierdt, 2010; Kaburagi et al., 2005).

For those studies that used speech tasks (e.g. paragraph reading, as opposed to a rotating disk or other physical object with receiver coils attached to it), the findings for the AG500 showed that 95% of the errors were within an acceptable range of values between 0.25 and 1.72 mm (Stella et al., 2012; Yunusova et al., 2009). For the Wave system a similar type of approach yielded a 95% error range between 0.08 and 0.55 mm across individuals (Berry, 2011). In the Sigona et al. (Sigona et al., 2018) paper they used repeated trials on 3 pseudo-words and found that the AG501 showed reliable data with accurate tracking of the coils, but the AG500 performed more poorly with errors appearing in a random and unpredictable manner. Kroos (2012) also compared the AG500 to a line-of-sight system (Vicon, Vicon Motion Systems) that has a higher claimed accuracy and found the averaged RMS error for the AG500 across the different conditions (based on Euclidean distance between the position estimates of the two systems) to be 1.38 mm. The angular RMS error was 50 degrees, all based on using the AG500 proprietary software. Based on the test results from all the studies mentioned here, it seems clear that the AG501 is currently the most accurate device (Kroos, 2012; Lau 2013; Savariaux et al., 2017;

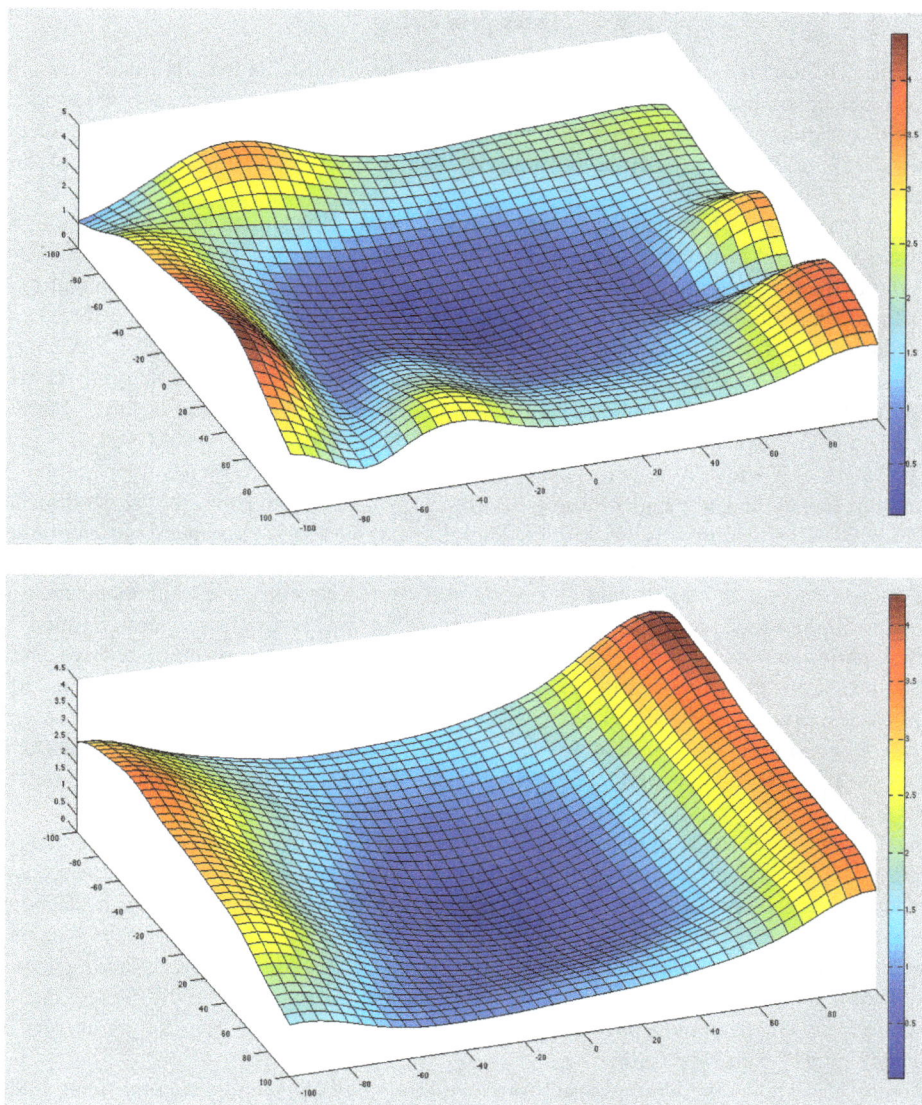

Figure 26.2   Mapping of the positional error magnitude along the x-y plane through the origin in a AG500 (top) and AG501 (bottom) system as used in the Oral Dynamics Lab at the University of Toronto. Scales are in millimeters. The vertical dimension in this surface plot represents the positional error magnitude of the point in that x-y location. Elevations (red) represent areas of high error; Troughs (blue) represent areas of low error (Lau, 2013; figures used with permission from author).

Sigona et al., 2018). However, as mentioned earlier, for the AG systems a careful calibration procedure is required in order to obtain reliable data and several authors have made recommendations on how to check for errors (e.g. Kroos, 2012; Lau, 2013; Savariaux et al., 2017; Sigona et al., 2018; Yunusova et al., 2009). For the Wave system, a user based calibration procedure is not required, which makes this system easier to use in settings where technical support is more limited (Berry, 2011).

Data processing

Regardless of the type of EMA system used, they all provide access to coordinates and angles of the receiver coil positions over time. These movement data can be further analyzed to address specific research questions. Needless to say that such questions will vary and in the sections below, I will provide more information on the broader areas of research in which articulography systems have been utilized.

Given that different labs have different needs and research questions, the way Articulograph data are processed also varies quite a bit. The manufacturers of the AG and Wave systems do provide their own software to do initial data processing. This may include calculating the coordinates and angular positions from the raw amplitudes, head movement correction, jaw movement correction and filtering. However, given the lack of a standardized EMA analysis toolbox, most labs use a custom-made software suite to extract those data that they consider to be the most relevant. Examples of those software packages can be found in the literature (e.g. MAYDAY software, Sigona, Stella, Grimaldi, & Gili Fivela, 2015; EMATOOLS, Nguyen, 2000; MVIEW; Tiede, 2005). In this chapter, I will focus on the software developed in the Oral Dynamics Lab at the University of Toronto, called EGUANA (Neto Henriques & van Lieshout, 2013). EGUANA is currently based on a Matlab (Mathworks) environment and can be used for different types of AG systems (from the original 2D AG100 to the current 5D AG501) and allows the user to extract data on a wide variety of frequently used kinematic measures (movement amplitude, velocity, duration etc.), as well as measures that are less common (e.g. cyclic spatio-temporal index or cSTI, discrete and continuous estimates of relative phase). It also provides options to do more sophisticated head and jaw movement corrections. More detailed descriptions of these measures and options as provided in EGUANA can be found in earlier publications (Neto Henriques & van Lieshout, 2013; van Lieshout & Moussa, 2000; van Lieshout et al., 2007). Eventually, we aim to make the software available to a wider range of users using an online platform.

To illustrate some of the options in EGUANA and the kind of data that can be extracted from AG recordings, I will present some graphical user interface display windows from the software. Further details can be found elsewhere (Neto Henriques & van Lieshout, 2013; van Lieshout & Moussa, 2000; van Lieshout et al., 2007). Figure 26.3 shows the main window displaying the trajectories and angular information of all receiver coils, as well as the corresponding acoustic signal for a given trial. The signals can be shown in raw format (unfiltered), filtered and with or without jaw and head movement correction. From this window, the user can select particular pairs of signals[4] to analyze further.

Figure 26.4 shows the window used for calculating a cyclic spatio-temporal index (cSTI), based on the original STI measure proposed by Anne Smith and colleagues (Smith & Goffman, 1998). For this analysis, all movement trajectories are divided into individual movement cycles based on specific amplitude and time criteria (Neto Henriques & van Lieshout, 2013; van Lieshout & Moussa, 2000; van Lieshout et al., 2007). Those cyclic segments are then overlaid on top of each other and amplitude and time normalized. Standard deviations of the overlapping signals are then calculated at 2% intervals and summed to derive the final cSTI value. cSTI is a measure of variability in producing a series of movement cycles associated with the same task.

Figure 26.5 shows an overview of all the kinematic measures that are calculated for each movement cycle (based on the previous cSTI procedure) for the selected signals. As mentioned above, some of these are fairly standard (movement range or amplitude, peak velocity, duration), while others are more specific to different models of movement control (stiffness, velocity profile index etc.; see e.g. Munhall et al., 1985; van Lieshout et al., 2007). EGUANA stores data

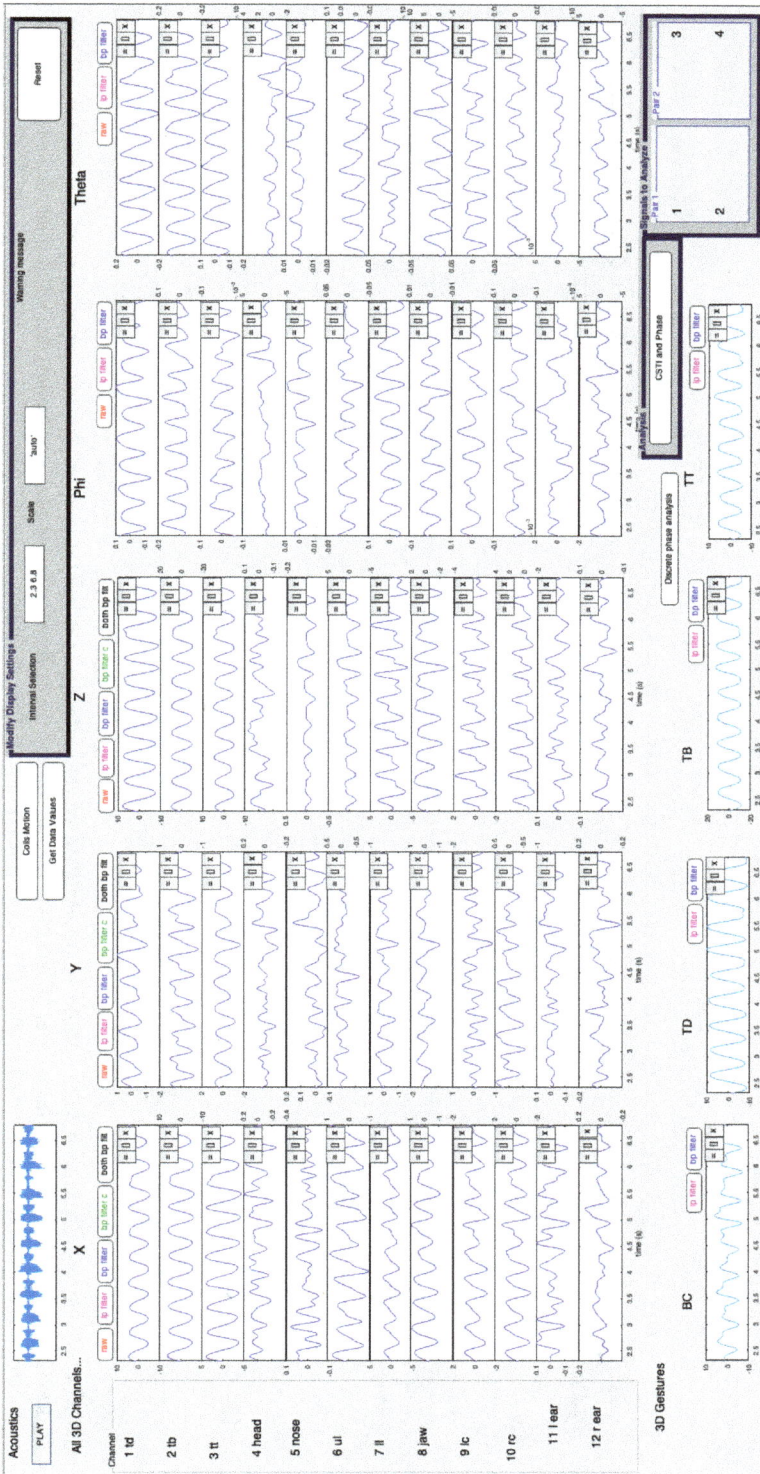

Figure 26.3 Main overview window of EGUANA (Neto Henriques & Van Lieshout, 2013; Van Lieshout & Moussa, 2000; Van Lieshout, 2006), showing the front-back (X), left-right (Y) and up-down (Z) channels plus the corresponding angular data (Phi & Theta). Also shown are the gestural data for bilabial closure (BC), Tongue Dorsum (TD), Tongue Body (TB) and Tongue Tip (TT).

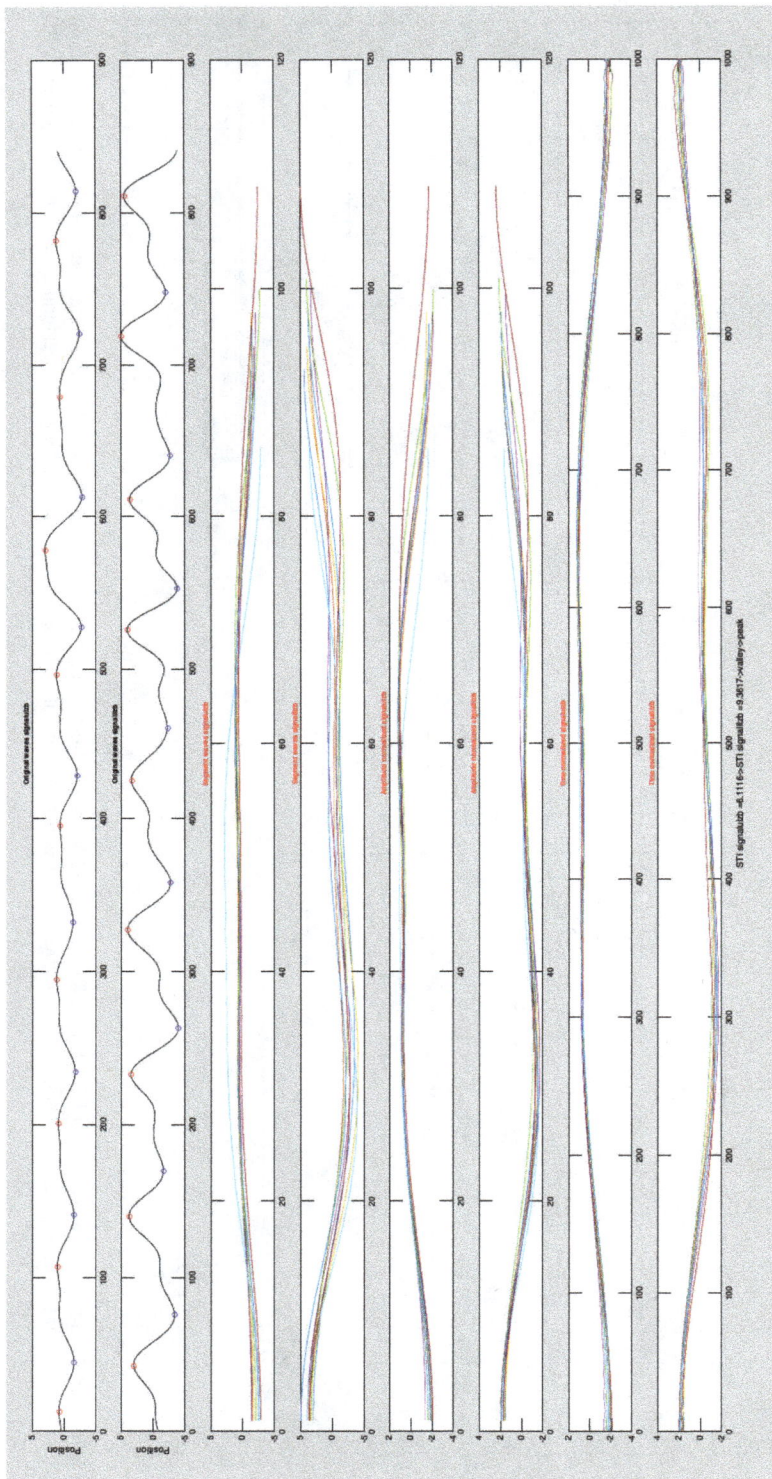

Figure 26.4 Cyclic Spatio-Temporal Index (cSTI) window of EGUANA (Neto Henriques & Van Lieshout, 2013; Van Lieshout, 2006), showing two selected channels (here: upper lip and lower lip trajectories), the markers indicating peak (red circles) and valley (blue circles) positions and the segmented raw movement cycles for each channel (3rd and 4th panel from top), their amplitude (5th and 6th panel from top) and time (7th and 8th panel from top) normalized versions. At the bottom the calculated cSTI values are shown as well.

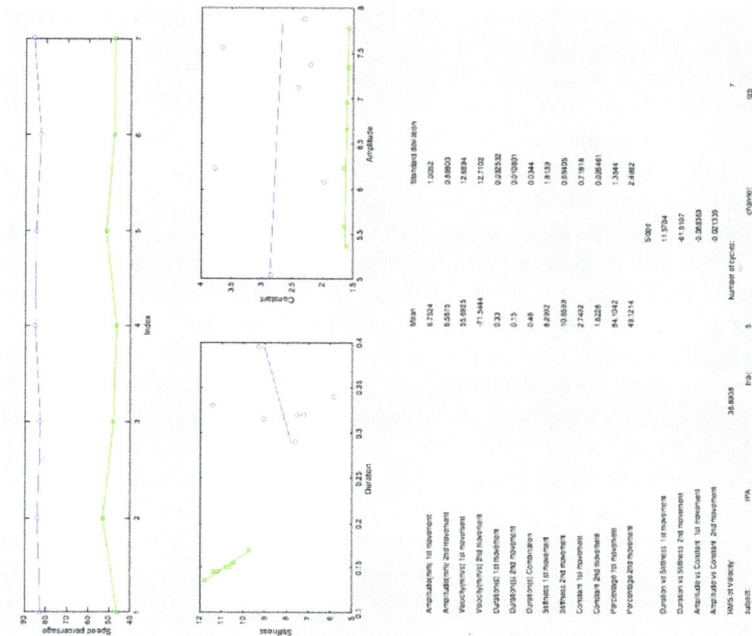

Figure 26.5 Kinematic measures window of EGUANA (Neto Henriques & Van Lieshout, 2013; Van Lieshout, P., & Moussa, W. 2000; Van Lieshout, 2006), showing various kinematic measures for the upper lip and lower lip data (as used in Figure 26.4). The panels show calculated data for each movement cycle and the panel in the right bottom of the window shows the average values across all selected cycles within a trial.

related to individual values for each cycle as well as the averaged values across an entire trial, in a user specified location.

Finally, Figure 26.6 shows data on the calculation of continuous estimates of relative phase for two signals engaged in a joint task, indicating the nature and stability of their coupling over the time course of a single trial. The signals are bandpass filtered prior to the phase calculations based on a spectral analysis to determine the frequencies in each signal with the highest power (referred to as the dominant motion primitive; van Lieshout et al., 2004). Relative phase measures are preferred over other measures of relative timing because they are not directly influenced by movement durations (Scott Kelso, 1997; van Lieshout et al., 2007), which would distort the true nature of the coupling relationship at the level of individual movement cycles. The measures shown indicate the average relative phase value and its (circular) standard deviation (see van Lieshout et al., 2007 for more details). EGUANA also calculates relative phase values (and their variability) for 1 sec epochs across the trial so researchers can focus on specific parts of a trial (e.g. before and after a switch in stimuli during a trial; van Lieshout, 2017).

In sum, using software suites like EGUANA users have access to a wide array of measures to quantify movement kinematics and coordination patterns in speech and other oral tasks (see Steele & Van Lieshout, 2004 for a description of using articulography in swallowing research). In the next section, I will provide more information on the nature and number of publications related to articulography since 2006 (for an overview of studies prior to 2006, see van Lieshout, 2006).

Published literature on Electromagnetic Articulography

In this section, I will focus on the areas of research in which articulography systems have been used and the type of publications in which these studies have been published. I also report on the number of publications and the countries where these publications originated from. The aim is to give an idea of the impact of this technology on speech research and how well these publications actually represent relevant areas of speech research across the world. Publications were searched in the Scopus database (© Elsevier), the largest database of its kind that also includes conference proceedings and is not restricted to a particular field of research. The following string of keywords was used: [articulograph*] AND [electro-magnet*] OR [EMMA] OR [EMA]. The search was restricted to papers published between 2005 and 2019, as a previous review chapter on articulography was published in 2006[5] (van Lieshout, 2006), covering the older AG100 system and publications on articulography up to and including 2005. Further restrictions on the search were made regarding document type, limiting it to journal articles, conference proceedings, book chapters and review articles. Finally, only publications published in English were included. The total number of publications found was 357, with 4 duplicates removed, leading to a final total of 353 (average of 23.5 publications/year).

Number, areas and types of publication

Based on the content of the publications, the papers are classified into four major areas of research. Four is of course an arbitrary number in itself but further refinement was not deemed useful and would make it harder to compile interpretable overviews. It also follows the classification used in the 2006 publication (van Lieshout, 2006) to maintain a certain degree of consistency.

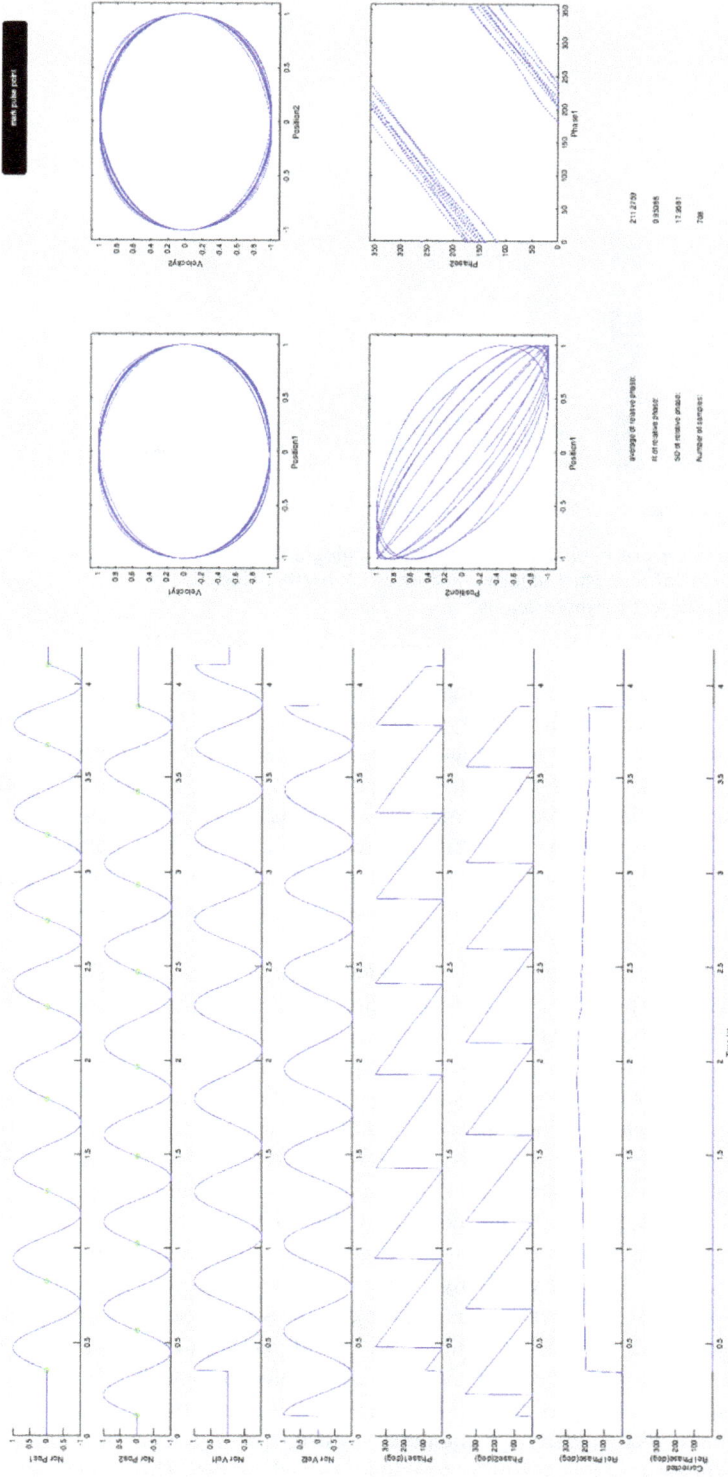

Figure 26.6 Continuous relative phase measures window of EGUANA (Neto Henriques & Van Lieshout, 2013; Van Lieshout, 2006), showing relative phase data for the upper lip and lower lip data (as used in Figure 26.4). The panels show the position data (1st and 2nd panel on left), velocity data (3rd and 4th panel on left), phase data (5th and 6th panel on left) and relative phase data (bottom panel on left). On the right-hand side, it shows position versus velocity plots for both channels (top) as well as position versus position and phase versus phase plots (bottom panel) for both channels. Finally, in the right bottom of the window the average value, circular standard deviation, converted standard deviation and number of samples used for the calculation are provided for the selected trial.

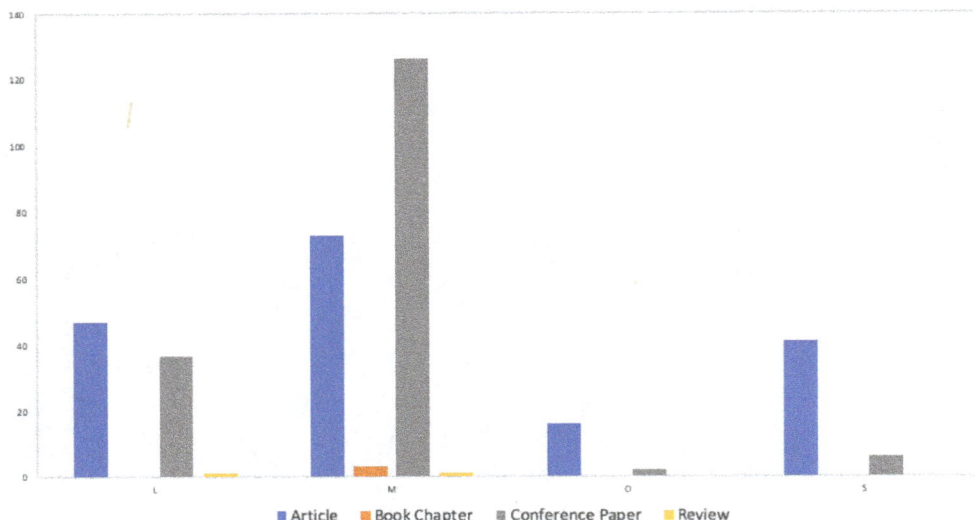

Figure 26.7   Number and type of publications related to articulography (N = 353) from 2005 to 2019, separated for the four areas of interest: Linguistic/phonetic (L); Methodology (M); Other (O); Speech-Language Pathology (S). See text for more details.

The first area concerns studies related to linguistic/phonetic questions, with a specific theoretical or experimental aim related to sound systems across a variety of languages but mostly English. The second area was related to methodological issues around the use and reliability of articulography systems. The third area was about the use of articulography with patient populations, addressing questions related to symptoms of speech/language disorders or the use of articulography as feedback tool for treatment or screening purposes. The fourth area was more a mix of studies that could not be uniquely classified into one of the other three areas, and mostly involved studies in the area of swallowing or studies that addressed the creation or use of datasets for different purposes.

Figure 26.7 shows the number of publications for each of the four main areas of research, divided into the four types of publications (journal articles, proceedings, book chapters, review articles). Percentage values (based on total of 353 publications) are presented in text.

Clearly, the largest number of publications between 2005 and 2019 were related to methodological issues (57.5%). Papers related to linguistic/phonetic questions made up for 24.1% of all papers, leaving smaller percentages for papers on clinical speech-language pathology topics (13.3%) and other areas (5.1%). The majority of papers related to methodology were published in proceedings (35.7%), with journal articles being second most used publication type (20.7%). For linguistic/phonetic papers, the divide was more evenly, with 13.5% published as journal articles and 10.5% as proceedings. For the speech-language pathology papers, the majority were published as journal articles (11.6%), with only a very small percentage (1.7%) appearing in proceedings. For the other types of publications, the majority was published as journal articles (4.5%). When collapsed across type of publication, 50.1% of all publications were published as journal articles and the rest were for the most part published in proceedings (48.4%).

The fact that methodological papers have a strong representation in proceedings is not surprising as for many fields like engineering, computer science, speech science and linguistics peer reviewed proceedings carry a near similar weight as journal articles. This is also reflected in the relatively equal percentages of proceedings and journal articles for studies related to linguistic/phonetic questions. For speech-language pathology, similar to medicine, journal articles are the more typical outlet for publication. More importantly, these numbers show that despite the fact that articulography has been around for more than 25 years, the dominant area of research still revolves around methodological issues, which in part is triggered by the fact that new(er) systems have been released in the past 10 years. Scientists are critical of new technologies and feel a strong need to verify how robust they are and how well they can address the questions relevant for speech and language research. Just the fact alone that the AG500 and AG501 systems have triggered multiple papers on the robustness and reliability of tracking receiver coil positions (see section on *Technical Evaluations*) testifies to the scrutiny imposed on these technologies. This is of course a good thing because one should never rely on manufacturer's data to go ahead and use these technologies assuming all findings can be trusted. In fact, the critique that was published on some of the issues associated with the AG500 system has motivated the development of the AG501 system that has now to be shown to be very robust and reliable and perhaps as some argued, the best articulography system currently in use (Sigona et al., 2018).

What is less comforting, however, is the fact that relatively few studies have been conducted in areas like speech-language pathology using articulography. This is partly due to the costs associated with purchasing such systems but also, no doubt, related to the demands on technical expertise for data collection and data analysis when using them. In addition, running articulography studies is labor intensive and all these factors make it often very difficult for clinical settings to adopt these sophisticated technologies. This is truly a limitation, because data about movements of speech articulators can be a crucial piece of information to assess the true nature of speech and language disorders in a variety of populations (e.g. Murdoch, 2011; van Lieshout & Moussa, 2000). The use of this technology for clinical purposes was in fact one of the original aims for the AG100 system when it was first developed in the late 1980s. The Wave system was also developed with such purpose in mind, and with no need for a time-consuming and complex calibration procedure, it had the better odds of being used in clinics. However, based on the publications surveyed this is still not happening on a scale that will support our knowledge in areas critical to clinical diagnosis and treatment. Hopefully, the next 10 years will see a change towards this much needed direction.

Countries of publications

Research using the articulography technology is not something that can happen without a strong resource infrastructure. Apart from financial support, these technologies require technical expertise for system maintenance, data collection and data analysis, as already mentioned. This means that there will be a bias toward laboratories that are situated in countries that have a well-supported research infrastructure with access to research grants at all levels (national, regional, local). Thus, it should come as no surprise that two-thirds of all publications (N = 353) originate from researchers located in North America (33.7%) and Europe (31.0%). Asia (mainly Japan and China) account for 18%, whereas other continents contribute relatively small numbers (South America: 1.5%; Australia: 9.3%) or none (Africa). Figure 26.8 provides more details for individual countries showing the number of publications in the four main areas of research.

Based on the information presented here, the top 5 countries involved in articulography research are the USA (by far), with distant second France, followed by Australia, Canada and Germany/Japan (tied). It is interesting to notice the difference in distribution of areas of research

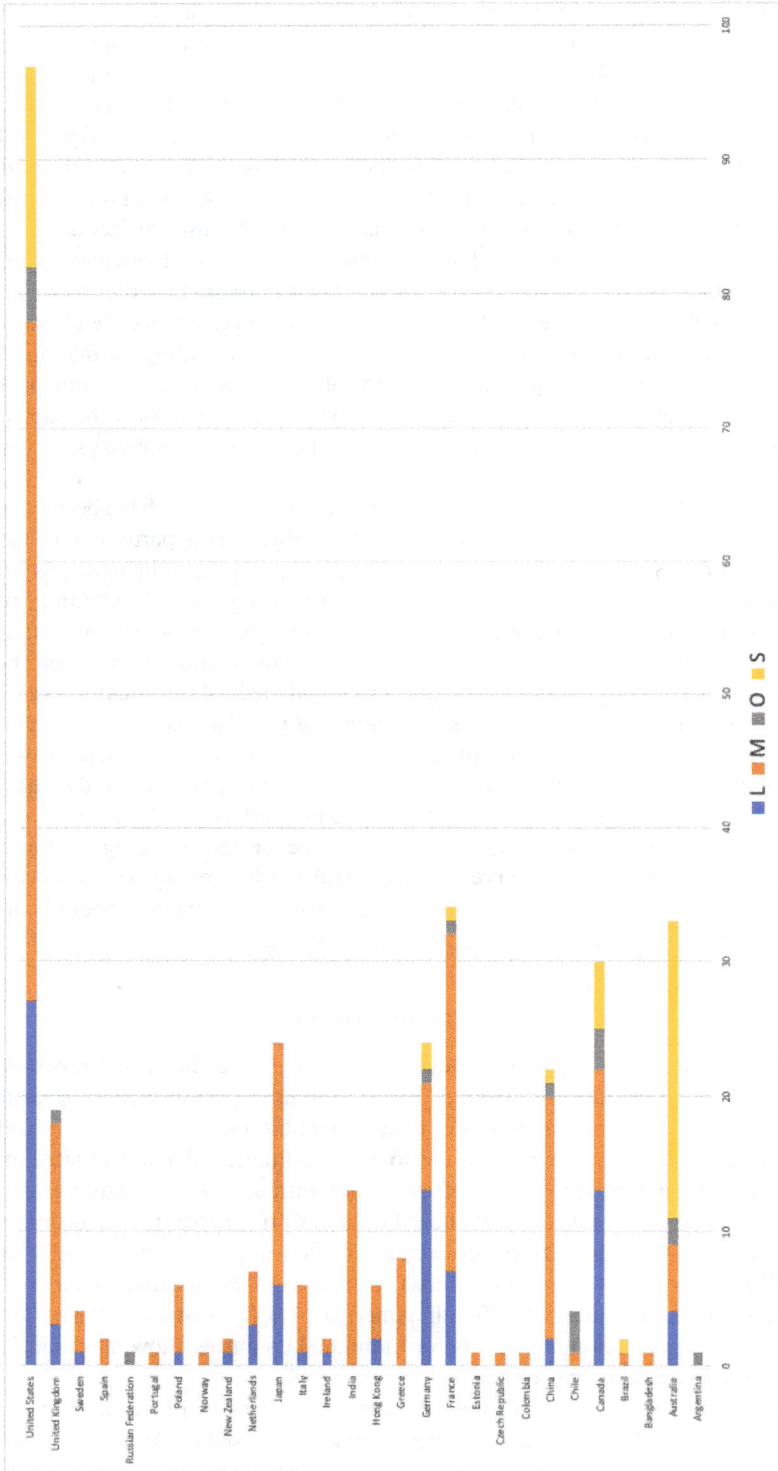

Figure 26.8 Number of publications related to articulography (N = 353) from 2005 to 2019 for individual countries of origin, separated for the four areas of interest: Linguistic/phonetic (L); Methodology (M); Other (O); Speech-Language Pathology (S). See text for more details.

across these countries. For example, Australia has a strong research funding infrastructure, but the number of speech laboratories that are doing research using articulography is relatively small. In fact, one research group at the University of Queensland in Brisbane is largely responsible for the majority of studies using articulography in the area of speech-language pathology. Also interesting is that most studies originating from Asia have a strong methodological focus, as shown for both Japan and China.

Future developments

With respect to future developments of articulography, there are a couple of noticeable trends. One is the use of more than one Articulograph for studying dyads (e.g. Lee et al., 2018). The Carstens company has created special soft- and hardware to sync an AG500 with an AG501 or two AG501 systems to allow for time-aligned recordings that can be compared directly (https://www.articulograph.de/articulograph-head-menue/dual-arrangements/). The dual setup also specifies certain requirements for keeping the two systems at a minimal distance (around 1.5–2 m) to avoid interference. Other developments from the Carstens company are to buy parts of the AG501 system (AG501-ip) that can be used in the base model without a calibration device, providing an accuracy of 0.6 mm (compared to 0.3 mm with calibration device), according to the company (https://www.articulograph.de/news-events/recent-news-and-dates/). The NDI company has also decided to replace the WAVE system with a new device, called the VOX-EMA (https://www.ndigital.com/msci/products/vox-ema/). According to the company, it provides a static positional accuracy up to 0.9 mm RMS and like the WAVE, does not need user calibration. There is no published study on this device yet, but no doubt those will appear in the near future if current trends (see previous section) are any indication.

Other developments in recent past is the development of a system that uses a Magneto-encephalographic (MEG) device to track not only electrical brain waves but simultaneously movements of the articulators during speech production (Alves et al., 2016). The system is called Magneto-articulography for the Assessment of Speech Kinematics (MASK). Based on an evaluation of an early prototype of the MASK system (Lau, 2013), the accuracy of the initial prototype of this device was not as good as that of an AG501 or WAVE system, with an average dynamic RMS error of 1.3 mm across its measurement space (which is somewhat smaller than that for AG500/AG501) and a less predictable error pattern compared to the AG systems. Again, this was based on a very early version of the MASK system and further improvements have been made. The unique part of this system is of course the fact that one can sample movements of articulators in direct temporal relationship to activity in various areas of the brain. No other technology to date can offer this type of information, allowing for a more detailed understanding of how the brain controls speech movement kinematics and coordination (Alves et al., 2016; Lau, 2013).

No doubt other developments will take place in the not so distant future. Real-time MRI systems are being developed that will allow for tracking movements of speech articulators at a sampling rate that will capture important kinematic characteristics while providing a general overview of all relevant vocal tract structures (e.g. Lingala et al., 2016). Other technologies like Ultrasound will also continue to develop to provide faster sequences of 3D images of the tongue, which can also be combined with other technologies like Articulography (e.g. Chen et al., 2019). The main issue that will remain is that as shown in the literature data above, the application of Articulography technology in clinical studies is still very limited. For one part, this again is a reflection of the resources needed to acquire, maintain and operate these devices and the analyses of their output (van Lieshout, 2006). For the other part, it is the lack of convincing evidence on a variety of populations that having access to this type of data will make a difference in how speech and language disorders can be diagnosed and treated. This is the challenge that faces researchers who so far have been for a large part preoccupied with determining the more technical aspects of these devices (as shown in the overview above). More data are needed and in order to provide larger numbers in support of claims that show the relevance of these objective measurements, labs across the world need to come together to standardize data collection and analysis practices. There are some initiatives underway like the AG Wiki user platform (https://www.articulograph.de/customer-data/wiki-community-area/). More needs to be done because the number of active users of Articulography will always be relatively small and the populations that can be included will also be in relatively small numbers when confined to a single location. There are lots of opportunities. Let's hope there will also be leadership to move these goals forward.

Notes

1 Obviously, there have been changes in other parts of the speech production system as well, in particular with respect to the vocal folds and their anatomical location, as well as control of the breathing apparatus to serve the relatively new speech function in humans. However, in this chapter I will primarily focus on structures involved in articulation, that is, the ability to form constrictions to modify vocal tract resonance properties.
2 The Electromagnetic Articulograph (EMA) uses electromagnetic fields (EMF) to track the movements of "sensors" or transducer coils attached to speech articulators (e.g. lips, tongue, etc.). For the original AG100 which uses slightly smaller extreme low frequency (ELF) electromagnetic fields (EMF) values compared to the newer systems, an independent study by Hasegawa-Johnson (Hasegawa-Johnson, 1998) has shown that the strengths of the magnetic fields are well below the maximum permissible exposure that is specified by the American National Standards Institute and is comparable to EMF's generated by household electrical appliances like hairdryers. According to the WHO Fact Sheet N205: "Magnetic Field Studies: There is little confirmed experimental evidence that ELF magnetic fields can affect human physiology and behavior at field strengths found in the home or environment. Exposure of volunteers for several hours to ELF fields up to 5 mT had little effect on several clinical and physiological tests, including blood changes, ECG, heart rate, blood pressure and body temperature" (http://www.who.int/mediacentre/factsheets/fs205/en/). According to the information summarized on the website of the WHO, a modern computer screen at operating distance has a value lower than 0.7 µT. Values for common household appliances range from 0.01 to 20 µT at a distance of 30 centimeters (http://www.who.int/peh-emf/about/WhatisEMF/en/index3.html). EMA systems produce ELF magnetic fields in the order of 1.25µT (= 0.00125 mT).
3 I will focus on AG systems here, as the design specifications of the hardware in the WAVE system are proprietary and not described in any publicly available documents (Berry, 2011; Savariaux et al., 2017).
4 In EGUANA one always has to pick pairs of signals involved in the same type of vocal constriction task (e.g. upper lip and lower lip in bilabial closure) to measure coordination variables such as relative phase.
5 An English version of this paper is available through Researchgate (https://www.researchgate.net/publication/323561185_The_use_of_Electro-Magnetic_Midsagittal_Articulography_in_oral_motor_research)

References

Alves, N., Jobst, C., Hotze, F., Ferrari, P., Lalancette, M., Chau, T., van Lieshout, P., & Cheyne, D. (2016). An MEG-compatible electromagnetic-tracking system for monitoring orofacial kinematics. *IEEE Trans Bio-Med Eng*, *63(8)*, 1709–1717.
Berry, J.J. (2011). Accuracy of the NDI Wave Speech Research System. *J Speech Lang Hear Res*, *54(5)*, 1295–1301.

Bressmann, T. (2007). Ultrasound imaging and its application in speech-language pathology and speech science. *Perspectives on Speech Science and Orofacial Disorders*, *17*(2), 7–15.

Chartier, J., Anumanchipalli, G.K., Johnson, K., & Chang, E.F. (2018). Encoding of articulatory kinematic trajectories in human speech sensorimotor cortex. *Neuron*, *98*(5), 1042–1054.e4.

Chen, W.-R., Tiede, M., Kang, J., Kim, B., & Whalen, D.H. (2019). An electromagnetic articulography-facilitated deep neural network model of tongue contour detection from ultrasound images. *J Acoust Soc Am*, *146*(4), 3081.

Coupé, C., Oh, Y., Dediu, D., & Pellegrino, F. (2019). Different languages, similar encoding efficiency: Comparable information rates across the human communicative niche. *Sci Adv,5*(9), eaaw2594.

Fujimura, O., & Haskin, M.E. (1981). X-ray microbeam system with a discrete-spot target. In *Proc. SPIE 0273, Application of Optical Instrumentation in Medicine IX*, 244–253.

Hasegawa-Johnson, M. (1998). Electromagnetic exposure safety of the Carstens articulograph AG100. *J Acoust Soc Am*, *104*(4), 2529–2532.

Hixon, T.J. (1971). Magnetometer recording of jaw movements during speech. *J Acoust Soc Am*, *49*(1A), 104.

Hoole, P., & Nguyen, N. (1999). Electromagnetic articulography. In W. Hardcastle & N. Hewlett (Eds.), *Coarticulation: Theory, Data and Techniques* (Cambridge Studies in Speech Science and Communication, pp. 260–269). Cambridge: Cambridge University Press.

Hoole, P., & Zierdt, A. (2010). Five-dimensional articulography. In B. Maassen & P. van Lieshout (Eds.), *Speech Motor Control: New Developments in Basic and Applied Research* (pp. 331–350). Oxford, UK: Oxford University Press.

Kaburagi, T., Wakamiya, K., & Honda, M. (2005). Three-dimensional electromagnetic articulography: A measurement principle. *J Acoust Soc Am*, *118*(1), 428–443.

Kiritani, S., Ito, K., & Fujimura, O. (1975). Tongue-pellet tracking by a computer-controlled x-ray microbeam system. *J Acoust Soc Am*, *57*(6 Pt 2), 1516–1520.

Kröger, B.J., Pouplier, M., & Tiede, M.K. (2008). An evaluation of the Aurora system as a flesh-point tracking tool for speech production research. *J Speech Lang Hear Res*, *51*(4), 914–921.

Kroos, C. (2012). Evaluation of the measurement precision in three-dimensional Electromagnetic Articulography (Carstens AG500). *J Phonetics*, *40*(3), 453–465.

Lau, C. (2013). *Validation of the magneto-articulography for the assessment of speech kinematics (MASK) system and testing for use in a clinical research setting*. Unpublished Master of Health Sciences Thesis, University of Toronto.

Lee, Y., Gordon Danner, S., Parrell, B., Lee, S., Goldstein, L., & Byrd, D. (2018). Articulatory, acoustic, and prosodic accommodation in a cooperative maze navigation task. *PloS One*, *13*(8), e0201444.

Lieberman, P. (2003). Motor control, speech, and the evolution of human language. In M.H. Christiansen & S. Kirby (Eds.), *Language Evolution* (pp. 255–271). Oxford, UK: Oxford University Press.

Lingala, S.G., Sutton, B.P., Miquel, M.E., & Nayak, K.S. (2016). Recommendations for real-time speech MRI. *Journal of Magnetic Resonance Imaging*, *43*(1), 28–44.

Munhall, K.G., Ostry, D.J., & Parush, A. (1985). Characteristics of velocity profiles of speech movements. *J Experimental Psychology. Human Perception and Performance*, *11*(4), 457–474.

Murdoch, B.E. (2011). Physiological investigation of dysarthria: Recent advances. *Int J Speech Lang Pathol*, *13*(1), 28–35.

Neto Henriques, R., & van Lieshout, P. (2013). A comparison of methods for decoupling tongue and lower lip from jaw movements in 3D articulography. *J Speech Lang Hear Res*, *56*(5), 1503–1516.

Nguyen, N. (2000). A MATLAB toolbox for the analysis of articulatory data in the production of speech. *Behavior Research Methods, Instruments, & Computers: A Journal of the Psychonomic Society, Inc*, *32*(3), 464–467.

Perkell, J.S., Cohen, M.H., Svirsky, M.A., Matthies, M.L., Garabieta, I., & Jackson, M. T.T. (1992). Electromagnetic midsagittal articulometer systems for transducing speech articulatory movements. *J Acoust Soc Am,92*(6), 3078–3096.

Savariaux, C., Badin, P., Samson, A., & Gerber, S. (2017). A comparative study of the precision of carstens and northern digital instruments electromagnetic articulographs. *J Speech Lang Hear Res*, *60*(2), 322–340.

Schönle, P.W., Gräbe, K., Wenig, P., Höhne, J., Schrader, J., & Conrad, B. (1987). Electromagnetic articulography: Use of alternating magnetic fields for tracking movements of multiple points inside and outside the vocal tract. *Brain Lang*, *31*(1), 26–35.

Scott Kelso, J.A. (1997). *Dynamic patterns: The Self-organization of Brain and Behavior*. Cambridge: MA. MIT Press.

Sigona, F., Stella, A., Grimaldi, M., & Gili Fivela, B. (2015). MAYDAY: A software for multimodal articulatory data analysis. In A. Romano, M. Rivoira, & I. Meandri (Eds.), *Aspetti prosodici e testuali del raccontare: Dalla letteratura orale al parlato dei media* (pp. 173–184). Proc. X Convegno Nazionale dell'Associazione Italiana di Scienze della Voce (AISV), Torino, Italia.

Sigona, F., Stella, M., Stella, A., Bernardini, P., Fivela, B.G., & Grimaldi, M. (2018). Assessing the position tracking reliability of Carstens' AG500 and AG501 electromagnetic articulographs during constrained movements and speech tasks. *Speech Commun*, *104*, 73–88.

Smith, A., & Goffman, L. (1998). Stability and patterning of speech movement sequences in children and adults. *J Speech Lang Hear Res*, *41*(1), 18–30.

Smith, A., Goffman, L., & Stark, R. (1995). Speech motor development. *Seminars in Speech and Language*, *16*(2), 87–99.

Steele, C.M., & Van Lieshout, P.H.H.M. (2004). Use of electromagnetic midsagittal articulography in the study of swallowing. *J Speech LangHear Res*, *47*(2), 342–352.

Stella, M., Bernardini, P., Sigona, F., Stella, A., Grimaldi, M., & Fivela, B.G. (2012). Numerical instabilities and three-dimensional electromagnetic articulography. *J Acoust Soc Am*, *132*(6), 3941–3949.

Tiede, M. (2005). *MVIEW: Software for Visualization and Analysis of Concurrently Recorded Movement Data*. New Haven, CT: Haskins Laboratories.

Tiede, M., Mooshammer, C., & Goldstein, L. (2019). Noggin Nodding: Head movement correlates with increased effort in accelerating speech production tasks. *Frontiers in Psychology*, *10*, 2459.

van der Giet, G. (1977). Computer-controlled method for measuring articulatory activities. *J Acoust Soc Am*, *61*(4), 1072–1076.

Van Lieshout, P.H.H.M. (2006). La utilización de la articulografia mediosagital electromagnética en la investigación sobre movilidad oral. In E. Padrós-Serrat (Ed.), *Bases diagnósticas terapéuticas y posturales del funcionalismo craneofacial* (pp. 1140–1156). Madrid: Ripano Editorial Médica.

van Lieshout, P.H.H.M. (2015). Jaw and lips. In M.A. Redford (Ed.), *The Handbook of Speech Production* (pp. 79–108). Chichester, UK: John Wiley & Sons, Inc.

van Lieshout, P.H.H.M. (2017). Coupling dynamics in speech gestures: Amplitude and rate influences. *Experimental Brain Research. Experimentelle Hirnforschung. Experimentation Cerebrale*, *235*(8), 2495–2510.

van Lieshout, P.H.H.M., Bose, A., Square, P.A., & Steele, C.M. (2007). Speech motor control in fluent and dysfluent speech production of an individual with apraxia of speech and Broca's aphasia. *Clinical Linguistics & Phonetics*, *21*(3), 159–188.

Van Lieshout, P., Hulstijn, W., & Peters, H.F.M. (2004). Searching for the weak link in the speech production chain of people who stutter: A motor skill approach. In B. Maassen, R. Kent, H.F.M. Peters, P. Van Lieshout, & W. Hulstijn (Eds.), *Speech Motor Control In Normal And Disordered Speech* (pp. 313–356). Oxford, UK: Oxford University Press.

Van Lieshout, P., & Moussa, W. (2000). The assessment of speech motor behaviors using electromagnetic articulography. *The Phonetician*, *81*(1), 9–22.

Westbury, J., Milenkovic, P., Weismer, G., & Kent, R. (1990). X-ray microbeam speech production database. *J Acoust Soc Am 88*(S1), S56–S56.

Xu, Y., & Prom-on, S. (2019). Economy of effort or maximum rate of information? Exploring basic principles of articulatory dynamics. *Frontiers in Psychology*, *10*, 2469.

Yunusova, Y., Green, J.R., & Mefferd, A. (2009). Accuracy assessment for AG500, electromagnetic articulograph. *J Speech Lang Hear Res*, *52*(2), 547–555.

Zierdt, A. (1993). Problems of electromagnetic position transduction for a three-dimensional articulographic measurement system. *Proc. Institut für Phonetik und sprachliche Kommunikation der Universitat München*, 31.

27
MAGNETIC RESONANCE IMAGING

Vikram Ramanarayanan and Christina Hagedorn[1]

Magnetic resonance imaging (MRI) has enabled examination of shaping along the entirety of the vocal tract during speech production, providing a means for observing and quantifying the "choreography" of the articulators, in space and time (in the case of real-time MRI), including structural/morphological characteristics of speakers in conjunction with their articulation dynamics and acoustics (Narayanan, Nayak, Lee, Sethy, & Byrd, 2004). Importantly, MRI offers a clear advantage over other instrumentation methods with respect to patient safety, relative non-invasiveness of imaging and the ability to image in 3D or simultaneously in multiple arbitrary 2D planes. On the other hand, MRI is typically more expensive and less accessible—with particular consequences for field studies—as compared to other sensing modalities.

Introduction

The utility of magnetic resonance imaging for speech research

Magnetic resonance imaging (MRI) is an especially useful tool with which to study speech production given that it (i) allows for visualization of the entire vocal tract, (ii) is minimally invasive in nature, and (iii) does not subject experimental participants to ionizing radiation. MRI requires only that the participant read phrases from a projected screen, or speak spontaneously in response to a spoken or textual cue, oftentimes lying supine in the scanner bore. See Figure 27.1.

Examination of the entirety of the vocal tract during speech production provides a means for observing and quantifying movement of the vocal tract articulators (e.g. lips, tongue tip, tongue dorsum, velum, epiglottis, vocal folds), both during sustained speech sound production, in the case of static MRI, and dynamically, in space and time, in the case of real-time MRI. In allowing the experimenter to observe movement of all parts of the vocal tract over time, in 3D or in multiple 2D planes (e.g. sagittal, coronal, etc.), real-time MRI offers a considerable advantage over flesh-point tracking methods (e.g. X-ray microbeam, electromagnetic articulography), which allow for movement analysis of only specific flesh-points within the vocal tract. That all active speech articulators can be viewed simultaneously makes MRI an ideal tool with which to investigate coordination patterns among the articulators, helping researchers address long-standing

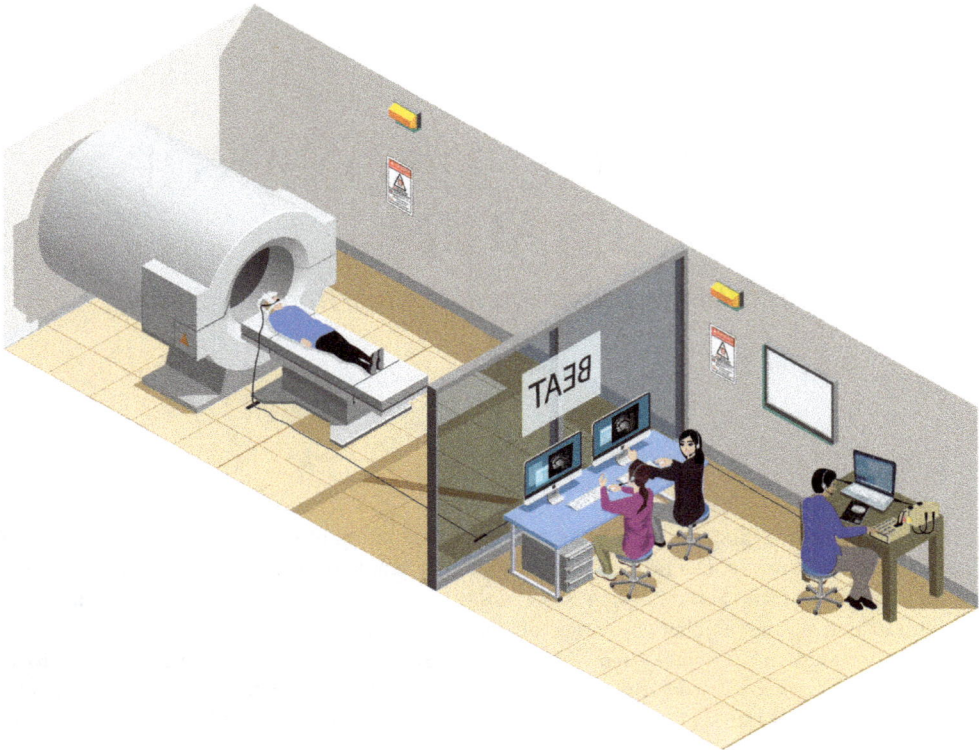

Figure 27.1 Schematic of the MRI data collection setup. The image depicts three experimenters in the control room (a principal investigator, an MRI operator, and an audio operator, respectively, from left to right in the bottom half of the image) inspecting images from a patient who has just successfully completed a scanning session (top half of the image). The images are recorded along with synchronous audio of the patient's speech via a fiberoptic microphone attached to a head coil while the patient responds to stimuli back-projected onto a screen (in this example, the word "beat"), viewed through a mirror setup positioned over the eyes.

questions in the area of motor speech disorders, especially. Moreover, the global view of the vocal tract provided by MRI encompasses both the static, hard structures (e.g. hard palate, pharyngeal wall), against which active articulators move, and the active articulators, themselves. This allows not only for the relationship between variations in the structural morphology of an individual's vocal tract and the articulatory-kinematic patterns produced to be examined, but also for investigation of articulatory—acoustic relations based on vocal tract area and volume functions, over time.

Magnetic resonance imaging is minimally invasive in that it does not require sensors or appliances to be adhered to, or make contact with, the participant's vocal tract, as is the case for other articulatory data collection modalities, including electropalatography (EPG), electromagnetic articulography (EMA), X-ray microbeam, Vicon, Optitrack and ultrasound (Ramanarayanan et al., 2018). The minimally invasive nature of MRI is particularly beneficial when investigating the speech of patients, in that it helps mitigate the risk of exacerbating damage to vulnerable tissue (e.g. post-surgically, in the case of individuals who have undergone glossectomy or cleft-palate repair). Additionally, the likelihood that any part of the experimental apparatus will significantly perturb speech movements so as to cause the participant to use atypical or more variable speech movement patterns is virtually nonexistent (in contrast to EPG, EMA, etc.), contributing further to the utility of MRI for studying patient populations, which typically exhibit inherently high degrees of articulatory variability. That MRI exposes participants to no ionizing radiation is also especially beneficial, particularly in investigating the speech of patients who may frequently undergo medical procedures involving radiation (e.g. X-ray, computed tomography (CT) scan, radiation therapy) and children, who are most susceptible to the health risks of radiation, due to the intrinsically high radiosensitivity of developing organs and tissues.

Challenges in the utilization of magnetic resonance imaging for speech research

While MRI offers the aforementioned advantages for speech imaging, its drawbacks must also be considered, particularly when working with patient populations. While certain limitations of MRI restrict the body of individuals that can be safely imaged, other constraints have serious implications for data collection and analysis from the researcher's perspective.

Although MRI is particularly well-suited to image individuals in the patient population, certain factors have the potential to render individuals ineligible for participation in MRI studies. Individuals with implanted pacemakers or defibrillators are typically excluded from MRI studies, due to the risk of the alternating magnetic fields, the basic mechanism upon which MRI relies, causing interference with these devices. Relatedly, while it is not unsafe for individuals with small pieces of metal in the mouth (e.g. amalgam fillings, bonded retainers, etc.) to undergo MRI scanning, the presence of metal may compromise image quality. Degradation of image quality due to the presence of metal is largely participant-dependent and oftentimes presents inconsistently, even within single data collection sessions (Lingala, Sutton, Miquel, & Nayak, 2016; Toutios & Narayanan, 2016).

Additional factors that may deter individuals from participating in MRI studies include the presence of claustrophobia, general anxiety, or fear of being confined in the scanner bore for the duration of the study. Relatedly, young children and adolescents may be even less agreeable to participating in these studies, in which they will be separated from caregivers and encounter an unfamiliar environment (i.e. the scanner bore, housed within a hospital room) and all that it entails (e.g. loud and irregular scanner noise, restriction of body movement, relying on a two-way intercom system to speak with experimenters and caregivers, etc.).

That the teeth are not directly identifiable using MRI, due to their composition, is a limitation of this modality that does not directly impact the participant population, but rather, data analysis. This makes investigation of articulatory patterns involved in the production of alveolar and postalveolar fricatives—some of the most articulatorily complex segments—particularly challenging, using MRI. However, various methods of superimposing images of the teeth onto MRI images during the post-processing stage have been implemented (Ng et al., 2011; Takemoto, Kitamura, Nishimoto, & Honda, 2004).

A further consideration is that MRI data is acquired from individuals lying supine in the scanner bore, rather than in the upright posture assumed when producing most natural speech. While research suggests that differences between speech patterns produced in supine and upright positions exist (Engwall, 2003; Subtelny, Oya, & Subtelny, 1972), the effect of posture on speech is subtle, and is likely not cause for concern when interpreting MRI data (Tiede, Masaki, & Vatikiotis-Bateson, 2000). Nonetheless, some recent studies (Honda & Hata, 2007; Perry, 2011) have demonstrated the utility of upright scanners in investigating speech production, hence eliminating this concern.

Finally, a major obstacle to acquiring MRI data involves limited accessibility to the equipment and trained technicians needed to carry out the data collection protocol. Access to MRI scanners is oftentimes prohibitively costly, and the availability of such scanners for research applications (even when the cost is not prohibitively high) depends largely on geographical location. Further, availability of and costs associated with MRI technicians responsible for carrying out the data collection protocol (involving the identification of the desired scan plane(s), selection of the appropriate pulse sequence, etc.) must be considered when assessing the feasibility of MRI for studying speech production. Moreover, the post-processing and temporal reconstruction of raw MRI data and the development of novel techniques used in the quantitative analysis of MRI data requires the expertise of engineers and other professionals and is often computationally intensive.

The rest of this chapter is organized as follows: we first take the reader through how MRI technology has evolved over the past few years, viewed through the lens of applicability to clinical phonetics. Next, we describe the practical considerations a researcher or clinician must take into account while collecting such data. We then present a sampling of the insights such MRI technology can provide to various kinds of clinical phonetics applications. Finally, we conclude with an outlook on the future of such technologies.

Evolution of the technology

Magnetic resonance imaging (MRI) is a medical imaging technique in which the signal intensity depends on the density of hydrogen nuclei in a tissue element and the atomic properties of the protons within each such molecule. MR techniques involve the use of strong magnetic fields to align the magnetic moments of the hydrogen nuclei and the use of high radio-frequency impulses to set them into resonance. Consequently, it is suited to produce images of soft tissue in the body that contain water and therefore hydrogen nuclei, such as the tongue and lips, as opposed to bony tissue (as in the case of X-ray tomography techniques).

Several early studies leveraged MRI to image the vocal tract. Baer, Gore, Gracco, and Nye (1991) recorded speech corresponding to four vowels from two male participants while obtaining simultaneous axial, coronal, or midsagittal MR slice images of their vocal tracts. Other studies consequently expanded this to examine the vocal tract shaping of various sounds using MRI, for instance, vowels (Baer et al., 1991; Greenwood, Goodyear, & Martin, 1992; Moore, 1992), nasals (Dang, Honda, & Suzuki, 1993) and fricatives (Narayanan, Alwan, & Haker, 1995). Static MRI provides rich spatial information about the articulators at only one point in time and so is conducive to studying only sustained articulations, such as vowels, liquids, nasals, and fricatives (Narayanan et al., 1995; Story, Titze, & Hoffman, 1996). Based on the same technology, cine MRI attempts to reconstruct the dynamics of articulation by collecting static configurations of the vocal tract over several productions of a single item, and sequencing them to render an approximation of real-time production (see, for example, Stone, Davis, Douglas, Aiver, et al., 2001a,b; Takemoto, Honda, Masaki, Shimada, & Fujimoto, 2006).

Over the past two decades, real time MRI, elaborating traditional medical MRI, has played a critical role in studying a variety of biological movement patterns, including cardiac motion (Nayak & Hu, 2005) and joint kinematics (Zhang, Gersdor, & Frahm, 2011). Engineers and speech scientists have collaboratively applied rtMRI technology to the study of speech production (Bresch, Kim, Nayak, Byrd, & Narayanan, 2008; Kim, Narayanan, & Nayak, 2009; Narayanan et al., 2004).

In contrast to static MRI and cine MRI, rtMRI does not require participants to produce several repetitions of each token but rather allows for fast acquisition rates (e.g. 83 frames per second or higher, Lingala et al., 2017) on single tokens. rtMRI for speech has been shown to effectively shed light on a wide variety of phenomena in both typical and disordered speech production that would not be possible to investigate using tools providing more limited spatio-temporal information about vocal tract shaping (Carignan, Shosted, Fu, Liang, & Sutton, 2015; Perry, Kuehn, Sutton, & Fang, 2017).

Over the past decade, rtMRI data collection and post-processing methodologies have undergone tremendous advances. As noted above, temporal acquisition rates have reached 83 frames per second (f.p.s) (Toutios & Narayanan, 2016), which is sufficiently high to capture exceptionally fast articulatory movements, such as those produced during trill consonants. These high temporal acquisition rates also allow for fine-grained analysis of articulatory coordination (i.e. reflecting spatio-temporal coupling of distinct articulatory gestures) that may differ between typical and clinical populations.

In addition to increased temporal resolution, recent advances have allowed for spatial resolution to be improved, as well, such that imaging may take place in virtually any plane desired. While much of the pioneering work in studying speech using rtMRI relied on midsagittal vocal tract slices, recent developments have allowed for the simultaneous acquisition of multiple slices (e.g. parasagittal, axial, coronal, transverse, oblique) (Kim, Proctor, Narayanan, & Nayak, 2012; Lingala et al., 2015, Fu et al., 2015, 2017; Iltis et al., 2015; Lingala et al., 2016).

While rtMRI typically has an intrinsically lower frame rate than the other modalities, recent advances in parallel imaging and sparse reconstruction have helped to significantly improve the temporal resolution of acquired data including multiplane imaging (Fu et al., 2017, 2015; Iltis et al., 2015; Lingala et al., 2016). Very recent developments in acquisition techniques have allowed for three-dimensional imaging, which provides volumetric data that can be applied to the study of vocal tract shaping during complex segment production (Lim et al., 2019). For example, using 3D acquisition, researchers can study subtle changes in tongue volume and deformation patterns involved in the production of the liquid [l], which requires a stretching action of the tongue, as both tongue tip and tongue dorsum gestures are made while one or both sides of the tongue are lowered, allowing lateral airflow.

Technology use and considerations

This section first describes a typical MRI data collection setup in a clinical phonetics or speech research setting. We follow this up with a discussion on considerations that need to be taken into account for post-processing and denoising the speech data collected from the highly noisy MRI scan environment.

Data collection considerations

The MRI data collection process typically involves taking the following considerations into account:

- *Participant Briefing and Consent*. This process involves explaining to the participant the objective of the study and what it involves, and obtaining their informed consent to collect and use data. During this process, participants are also required to fill out an MRI safety form to confirm that there is no metal inside their bodies that could adversely affect either their health (e.g. presence of pacemakers) or the study (e.g. artifacts produced by certain fillings/metal in the mouth) during the MRI scan.

- *Participant Positioning*. Once participants have understood and signed their informed consent forms, they are again instructed to ensure that there is no metal on their persons before they are requested to lie down on the MRI scan bed. Once this is done, we recommend padding the participant's head to ensure comfort, as well as to minimize head movement and rotation.
- *Microphone Setup*. Once the participant is lying supine in the scanner, we position a fiber-optic microphone firmly next to the speaker's mouth to record the participant's speech during the scan.
- *Stimulus Presentation*. To present experimental stimuli visually to the participant, one can use a mirror setup in the scanner (positioned appropriately above the participant's eyes) in conjunction with a screen opposite the bore and a projector from the scan room back-projecting stimuli onto it. See Figure 27.1.
- *Image and Audio Recording Preparation*. Before the actual scan process begins, the MRI operator typically uses the console in the control room to select an appropriate scan plane (or set of planes, in the case of multiplane or 3D imaging) and image scanning software protocol (technically called a "pulse sequence") that encodes the spatial and temporal resolution of the MRI data to be collected, based on the design specifications of the experiment.[2]
- *Time Considerations*. The subject onboarding, setup of microphone, settling in of the participant in the scanner, and setup of the stimulus projection screen apparata takes approximately 30–45 minutes, in addition to the regular data collection.

Audio denoising

MRI scanners produce high-intensity noise in the audible frequency range that corrupts speech recordings. This degrades the audio signal recorded such that acoustic analysis of the speech content is difficult, if not impossible, necessitating additional steps to improve the audio quality. Another motivation for denoising speech corrupted with scanner noise arises from the need to enable communication between participants and clinicians and researchers during the data acquisition session.

Bresch and Narayanan (2009) proposed a solution to this problem that uses two fiber optical microphones—one inside the magnet near the participant's mouth to record his/her speech, and a separate microphone located away from the participant and outside the magnet, but inside the scanner room, placed such that it captures almost exclusively the ambient noise and not the participant's speech. This system allows the simultaneous capture of audio and the MR images and ensures absolute synchronicity for spontaneous speech and other vocal productions, including singing. Later innovations in audio denoising eliminated this need for a second microphone outside the scanner. Such innovations, including the development of multiple signal processing and machine learning algorithms to process and enhance such noisy speech is important, particularly given the wide range of noises produced by multiple imaging protocols of interest, such as those that image multiple plans simultaneously, 3D imaging, etc. In such cases, some sequences are easier to denoise than others. For a more detailed discussion on MRI audio denoising as well as the current state of the art, please see Vaz, Ramanarayanan, and Narayanan (2018).

Applications of magnetic resonance imaging to clinical research

Before being used to investigate atypical speech production, MRI was, and continues to be used to shed light on phenomena exhibited by typical speakers of a variety of languages. Example videos of such phenomena can be found at a publicly accessible website[3] containing links to real-time MRI clips corresponding to all speech sounds of American English, made available by the Speech Production and Articulation kNowledge (SPAN) group at the University of Southern California (Toutios et al., 2016). This rich repository facilitates the use of rtMRI data by speech scientists and clinicians alike for instructional and clinical purposes.

Over and above its applicability in imaging typical speech production, rtMRI has been particularly useful for investigating several speech disorders originating at distinct levels of the motor speech system (see Table 27.1). For example, while congenital aglossia, glossectomy procedures and craniofacial anomalies, such as cleft palate, act as structural perturbations to the speech production system, Apraxia of Speech (AoS) arises due to breakdown at the planning and programming level of speech motor control, and vocal fold paralysis, in some cases, may manifest due to nerve damage.

rtMRI has revealed that both individuals with aglossia, a congenital disorder in which a person is born without a tongue, and individuals with oral cancer who have undergone partial removal of the tongue by means of a glossectomy procedure utilize compensatory strategies to produce target speech sounds for which they can no longer form the typical articulatory movements. Specifically, speakers lacking a tongue tip due to congenital aglossia have been observed to produce target coronal constrictions with a bilabial constriction (McMicken et al., 2017). Interestingly, the authors noted that the target coronal stops [t] and [d], produced bilabially by the speaker, were perceptually distinct from target bilabial stops [p] and [b], produced using the same articulators. Further investigation by Toutios, Byrd, Goldstein, and Narayanan (2017) revealed that though both target coronals and target bilabials were produced bilabially by the patient, the articulations corresponding to each differed in subtle but important ways. The target coronal constrictions were produced with an elongated bilabial constriction and a wide pharyngeal region, as compared to the target bilabial constrictions. A follow-up acoustic simulation experiment, modeling the acoustics produced under these distinct articulation conditions, demonstrated that the specific combination of compensatory strategies utilized by the patient (i.e. elongation of the bilabial region and widening of the pharynx) created a marked acoustic difference between the respective outputs of the model, consistent with the perceptual differences observed between the target bilabials and target coronals, produced bilabially, by the patient.

The use of compensatory articulation is not limited to individuals with aglossia, but rather has also been evidenced in patients who have received surgical treatment of lingual cancer. Hagedorn et al. (2014, 2017) demonstrated that one individual with oral cancer who underwent resection of oral (anterior) lingual tissue produced target coronals stops using compensatory labiodental constrictions (Figure 27.2), and produced target coronal fricatives using compensatory tongue dorsum constrictions. This work also revealed that an individual who underwent removal of both oral (anterior) and base of tongue (posterior) tissue produced target coronal stops compensatorily, using simultaneous coronal and labial constrictions (see Figure 27.2). Using tagged cine-MRI, work by Stone et al. (2014) investigating motion patterns in /i/ to /s/ transitions in typical speakers and patients who had undergone partial glossectomy revealed differences in the strategies utilized by patients and typical speakers in the production of /s/.

In addition to being capable of identifying structural impairments of the tongue, and consequential compensatory patterns, rtMRI has also been used to assess and quantify impairment in the structure and control of the velum, responsible for modulating separation of the oral and nasal cavities. Drissi et al. (2011) demonstrated, using rtMRI, the ability to calculate the elevation angle of the velum in relation to the hard palate, the velar eminence angle, defined as the angle formed by the velum, itself, and used as an index of velic flexibility, and percentage reduction of anterior-posterior pharyngeal lumen diameter, in children with suspected velopharyngeal impairment (VPI). More recent work by Perry et al. (2020) demonstrated that

Table 27.1 Exemplar clinical applications that have particularly benefitted from MRI-based analysis

Clinical population	Description	Findings	Relevant publications
Congenital aglossia	Absence of the entire tongue at birth	Compensatory behavior in consonant production	McMicken et al. (2017), Toutios et al. (2017)
Partial glossectomy	Removal of part of the tongue (typically a component of treatment for oral cancer)	Compensatory behavior in consonant production	Hagedorn et al. (2014, 2017), Stone et al. (2014)
Apraxia of speech	Motor speech disorder affecting the planning and programming of speech sequences	Covert intrusion errors in repeated and spontaneous speech	Hagedorn et al. (2017)
Suspected velopharyngeal insufficiency	Impairment in achieving closure of the velum to the pharyngeal wall during target oral segments	MRI enabled calculation of the elevation angle of the soft palate in relation to the hard palate, the velar eminence angle and the percentage of reduction of the antero-posterior diameter of the pharyngeal lumen	Drissi et al. (2011)
Typical individuals (phonatory behavior)	Periods of vocal fold adduction and abduction	MRI capable of distinguishing adducted and abducted positions of vocal folds	Sorensen et al. (2018)
DiGeorge syndrome	Also known as 22q11.2 Deletion Syndrome; May result in underdevelopment of several body systems	Individuals with 22q11.2 Deletion Syndrome have tensor veli palatini muscles that are significantly shorter, thinner and less voluminous than typical individuals	Perry et al. (2020)
Cleft palate (repair)	Presence of an opening in the hard palate due to lack of fusion of the palatine prominences during development in the womb	Individuals with repaired cleft palate exhibit significantly shorter hard palate height and length, shorter levator muscle length, shorter intravelar segment, more acute levator angles of origin, shorter and thinner velum, and greater pharyngeal depth, though normal resonance.	Perry et al. (2018)
Submucous cleft palate	Presence of an opening in the hard structures of the hard palate due to lack of fusion of the palatine prominences underneath the fused mucous membrane (soft tissue) during development in the womb	MRI capable of identifying submucous cleft palate	Perry, Kuehn, Wachtel, Bailey, and Luginbuhl (2012)

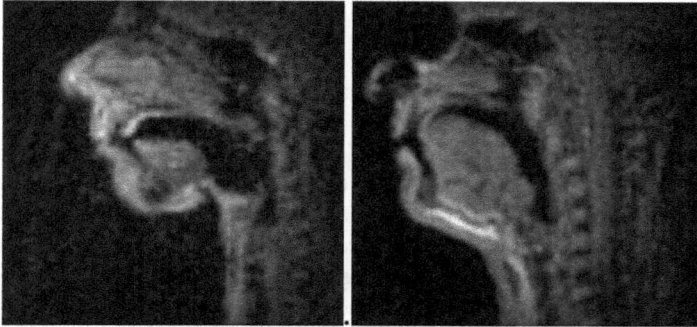

Figure 27.2 Glossectomy patient (left) produces target coronal stop /d/ compensatorily, by forming both labial and coronal constrictions; Typical speaker (right) produces /d/ by creating only a coronal constriction. (With permission of ASHA.)

individuals with the congenital 22q11.2 Deletion Syndrome exhibit tensor veli palatini muscles that are significantly shorter, thinner and less voluminous than typical individuals. Earlier work by the same group revealed that individuals with cleft palate exhibit significantly shorter hard palate height and length, shorter levator muscle length, shorter intravelar segment, more acute levator angles of origin, shorter and thinner velum and greater pharyngeal depth, though normal resonance (Perry et al., 2018). MRI has also been demonstrated to successfully detect submucous cleft palate, in which a cleft of the bony structure of the palate is covered by intact soft tissue (Perry et al., 2012). rtMRI has proven useful in imaging not only the supralaryngeal articulators, but the vocal folds, by scanning in the transverse plane, as well. Recent work by Sorensen et al. (2018) demonstrated the ability of rtMRI to identify, based on both manual segmentation of air-tissue boundaries and on an automatic pixel intensity detection method, periods of vocal fold adduction and abduction that can be used to differentiate typical and atypical phonatory behavior, and be applied to the diagnosis and management of vocal fold paralysis.

Finally, rtMRI has been used to shed light on aspects of acquired Apraxia of Speech (AoS) never before observed using other imaging modalities. Specifically, Hagedorn et al. (2017) provided evidence that while most errors made during both spontaneous speech and repeated speech (in a speak-after-me shadowing task) would traditionally be described as substitution errors based on acoustics alone, the errors involve synchronous production of a target gesture (e.g. a tongue tip constriction for /t/) and an intrusive gesture (e.g. a tongue dorsum constriction during /t/) (see Figure 27.3). Accordingly, these errors would more accurately be described as intrusion errors.

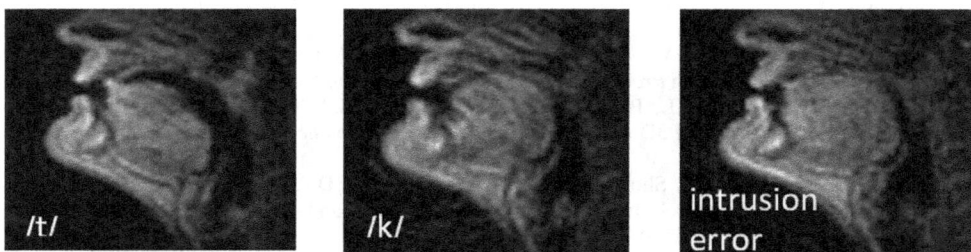

Figure 27.3 Intrusion errors in a patient with apraxia of speech. (With permission of ASHA.)

Conclusion

MRI is a particularly useful tool with which to study both typical and atypical speech production in that it provides a global view of the vocal tract, is minimally invasive to the participant, and does not subject the participant to ionizing radiation. Challenges in the implementation of MRI research do exist, however. Notably, MRI safety considerations limit the population that can be imaged, and post-processing tools are necessary to address loud and irregular acoustic scanner noise that may interfere with analysis of the speech data. Recent advances in MRI have led to high temporal frame rates and spatial resolution, facilitating analysis of the complex and quickly-unfolding dynamic events in speech production. Research has demonstrated that MRI is capable of providing both theoretical and clinical insight on speech production patterns associated with a wide range of clinical populations, including individuals with cleft palate, congenital aglossia, and apraxia of speech, among many others. While many speech disorders have been investigated using MRI, others (e.g. the dysarthrias) have not. As such, widening the range of disorders examined using this methodology and the novel analytical techniques associated with it will certainly be an important direction for future research.

Notes

1 Both authors contributed equally to the writing of this chapter.
2 For more details on various pulse sequences used to collect MRI data, please see Lingala et al. (2016). The choice of pulse sequence affects the data collection significantly in many ways. Some are noisier than others. Others involve careful choices of either higher spatial or temporal resolution that typically trade off against each other due to signal processing constraints.
3 http://sail.usc.edu/span/rtmri_ipa

References

Baer, T., Gore, J.C., Gracco, L.C. & Nye, P.W. (1991). Analysis of vocal tract shape and dimensions using magnetic resonance imaging: Vowels. *The Journal of the Acoustical Society of America, 90*(2), 799–828.

Bresch, E., Kim, Y.-C., Nayak, K., Byrd, D. & Narayanan, S. (2008). Seeing speech: Capturing vocal tract shaping using real-time magnetic resonance imaging [exploratory dsp]. *IEEE Signal Processing Magazine, 25*(3), 123–132.

Bresch, E. & Narayanan, S. (2009). Region segmentation in the frequency domain applied to upper airway real-time magnetic resonance images. *IEEE Transactions on Medical Imaging, 28*(3), 323–338.

Carignan, C., Shosted, R.K., Fu, M., Liang, Z.-P. & Sutton, B.P. (2015). A realtime MRI investigation of the role of lingual and pharyngeal articulation in the production of the nasal vowel system of French. *Journal of Phonetics, 50*, 34–51.

Dang, J., Honda, K. & Suzuki, H. (1993). MRI measurements and acoustic investigation of the nasal and paranasal cavities. *The Journal of the Acoustical Society of America, 94*(3), 1765–1765.

Drissi, C., Mitrofano_, M., Talandier, C., Falip, C., Le Couls, V. & Adamsbaum, C. (2011). Feasibility of dynamic MRI for evaluating velopharyngeal insufficiency in children. *European Radiology, 21*(7), 1462–1469.

Engwall, O. (December, 2003). A revisit to the application of MRI to the analysis of speech production-testing our assumptions. In *Proc of 6th International Seminar on Speech Production* (Vol. 43, p. 48).

Fu, M., Barlaz, M.S., Holtrop, J.L., Perry, J.L., Kuehn, D.P., Shosted, R.K., ... Sutton, B.P. (2017). High-frame-rate full-vocal-tract 3D dynamic speech imaging. *Magnetic Resonance in Medicine, 77*(4), 1619–1629.

Fu, M., Zhao, B., Carignan, C., Shosted, R.K., Perry, J.L., Kuehn, D.P., ... Sutton, B.P. (2015). High-resolution dynamic speech imaging with joint low-rank and sparsity constraints. *Magnetic Resonance in Medicine, 73*(5), 1820–1832.

Greenwood, A.R., Goodyear, C.C. & Martin, P.A. (1992, Dec). Measurements of vocal tract shapes using magnetic resonance imaging. *IEE Proc. I - Communications, Speech and Vision, 139*(6), 553–560.

Hagedorn, C., Lammert, A., Bassily, M., Zu, Y., Sinha, U., Goldstein, L. & Narayanan, S.S. (2014). Characterizing post-glossectomy speech using real-time MRI. In *International Seminar on Speech Production, Cologne, Germany* (pp. 170–173).

Hagedorn, C., Proctor, M., Goldstein, L., Wilson, S.M., Miller, B., Gorno-Tempini, M.L. & Narayanan, S.S. (2017). Characterizing articulation in apraxic speech using real-time magnetic resonance imaging. *Journal of Speech, Language, and Hearing Research, 60*(4), 877–891.

Honda, Y. & Hata, N. (2007). Dynamic imaging of swallowing in a seated position using open-configuration MRI. *Journal of Magnetic Resonance Imaging, 26* (1), 172–176.

Iltis, P.W., Frahm, J., Voit, D., Joseph, A.A., Schoonderwaldt, E. & Altenmüller, E. (2015). High-speed real-time magnetic resonance imaging of fast tongue movements in elite horn players. *Quantitative Imaging in Medicine and Surgery, 5*(3), 374.

Kim, Y.-C., Narayanan, S.S. & Nayak, K.S. (2009). Accelerated three-dimensional upper airway MRI using compressed sensing. *Magnetic Resonance in Medicine, 61*(6), 1434–1440.

Kim, Y.-C., Proctor, M.I., Narayanan, S.S. & Nayak, K.S. (2012). Improved imaging of lingual articulation using real-time multislice MRI. *Journal of Magnetic Resonance Imaging, 35*(4), 943–948.

Lim, Y., Zhu, Y., Lingala, S.G., Byrd, D., Narayanan, S. & Nayak, K.S. (2019). 3D dynamic MRI of the vocal tract during natural speech. *Magnetic Resonance in Medicine, 81*(3), 1511–1520.

Lingala, S.G., Sutton, B.P., Miquel, M.E. & Nayak, K.S. (2016). Recommendations for real-time speech MRI. *Journal of Magnetic Resonance Imaging, 43*(1), 28–44.

Lingala, S.G., Zhu, Y., Kim, Y.-C., Toutios, A., Narayanan, S. & Nayak, K.S. (2015). High spatio-temporal resolution multi-slice real time MRI of speech using golden angle spiral imaging with constrained reconstruction, parallel imaging, and a novel upper airway coil. *Proc ISMRM 23rd Scientific Sessions, 689.*

Lingala, S.G., Zhu, Y., Kim, Y.-C., Toutios, A., Narayanan, S. & Nayak, K.S. (2017). A fast and flexible MRI system for the study of dynamic vocal tract shaping. *Magnetic Resonance in Medicine, 77*(1), 112–125.

McMicken, B., Salles, F., Von Berg, S., Vento-Wilson, M., Rogers, K., Toutios, A. & Narayanan, S.S. (2017). Bilabial substitution patterns during consonant production in a case of congenital aglossia. *Journal of Communication Disorders, Deaf Studies & Hearing Aids, 5*, 175.

Moore, C.A. (1992). The correspondence of vocal tract resonance with volumes obtained from magnetic resonance images. *Journal of Speech, Language, and Hearing Research, 35*(5), 1009–1023.

Narayanan, S., Nayak, K., Lee, S., Sethy, A. & Byrd, D. (2004). An approach to real-time magnetic resonance imaging for speech production. *Journal of the Acoustical Society of America, 115*, 1771.

Narayanan, S.S., Alwan, A.A. & Haker, K. (1995). An articulatory study of fricative consonants using magnetic resonance imaging. *Journal of the Acoustical Society of America, 98*(3), 1325–1347.

Nayak, K.S. & Hu, B.S. (2005). The future of real-time cardiac magnetic resonance imaging. *Current Cardiology Reports, 7*(1), 45–51.

Ng, I., Ono, T., Inoue-Arai, M., Honda, E., Kurabayashi, T. & Moriyama, K. (2011). Application of MRI movie for observation of articulatory movement during a fricative /s/ and a plosive /t/ tooth visualization in MRI. *The Angle Orthodontist, 81* (2), 237–244.

Perry, J.L. (2011). Variations in velopharyngeal structures between upright and supine positions using upright magnetic resonance imaging. *The Cleft Palate-Craniofacial Journal, 48*(2), 123–133.

Perry, J.L., Kotlarek, K.J., Spoloric, K., Baylis, A., Kollara, L., Grischkan, J.M., … others (2020). Differences in the tensor veli palatini muscle and hearing status in children with and without 22q11. 2 deletion syndrome. *The Cleft Palate-Craniofacial Journal, 57*(3), 302–309.

Perry, J.L., Kotlarek, K.J., Sutton, B.P., Kuehn, D.P., Jaskolka, M.S., Fang, X., … Rauccio, F. (2018). Variations in velopharyngeal structure in adults with repaired cleft palate. *The Cleft Palate-Craniofacial Journal, 55*(10), 1409–1418.

Perry, J.L., Kuehn, D.P., Sutton, B.P. & Fang, X. (2017). Velopharyngeal structural and functional assessment of speech in young children using dynamic magnetic resonance imaging. *The Cleft Palate-Craniofacial Journal, 54*(4), 408–422.

Perry, J.L., Kuehn, D.P., Wachtel, J.M., Bailey, J.S. & Luginbuhl, L.L. (2012). Using magnetic resonance imaging for early assessment of submucous cleft palate: A case report. *The Cleft Palate-Craniofacial Journal, 49*(4), 35–41.

Ramanarayanan, V., Tilsen, S., Proctor, M., Töger, J., Goldstein, L., Nayak, K.S. & Narayanan, S. (2018). Analysis of speech production real-time MRI. *Computer Speech and Language, 52*, 1–22.

Stone, M., Davis, E.P., Douglas, A.S., Ness Aiver, M.N., Gullapalli, R., Levine, W.S. & Lundberg, A.J. (2001a). Modeling tongue surface contours from cine-MRI images. *Journal of Speech, Language, and Hearing Research, 44*(5), 1026–1040.

Stone, M., Davis, E.P., Douglas, A.S., Ness Aiver, M., Gullapalli, R., Levine, W.S. & Lundberg, A. (2001b). Modeling the motion of the internal tongue from tagged cine-MRI images. *The Journal of the Acoustical Society of America*, *109*(6), 2974–2982.

Stone, M., Langguth, J., Woo, J., Chen, H., Prince, J. (2014). Tongue motion patterns in post-glossectomy and typical speakers: A principal components analysis. *Journal of Speech, Language and Hearing Research 57*(3): 707–717.

Story, B.H., Titze, I.R. & Hoffman, E.A. (1996). Vocal tract area functions from magnetic resonance imaging. *The Journal of the Acoustical Society of America*, *100*(1), 537–554.

Subtelny, J.D., Oya, N. & Subtelny, J. (1972). Cineradiographic study of sibilants. *Folia Phoniatrica et Logopaedica*, *24*(1), 30–50.

Takemoto, H., Honda, K., Masaki, S., Shimada, Y. & Fujimoto, I. (2006). Measurement of temporal changes in vocal tract area function from 3D cine-MRI data. *The Journal of the Acoustical Society of America*, *119*(2), 1037–1049.

Takemoto, H., Kitamura, T., Nishimoto, H. & Honda, K. (2004). A method of tooth superimposition on MRI data for accurate measurement of vocal tract shape and dimensions. *Acoustical Science and Technology*, *25*(6), 468–474.

Tiede, M.K., Masaki, S. & Vatikiotis-Bateson, E. (2000). Contrasts in speech articulation observed in sitting and supine conditions. *In Proceedings of the 5th Seminar on Speech Production, Kloster Seeon, Bavaria* (pp. 25–28).

Toutios, A., Byrd, D., Goldstein, L. & Narayanan, S.S. (2017). Articulatory compensation strategies employed by an aglossic speaker. *The Journal of the Acoustical Society of America*, *142*(4), 2639–2639.

Toutios, A., Lingala, S.G., Vaz, C., Kim, J., Esling, J.H., Keating, P.A., ... others (2016). Illustrating the production of the international phonetic alphabet sounds using fast real-time magnetic resonance imaging. In *Interspeech* (pp. 2428–2432).

Toutios, A. & Narayanan, S.S. (2016). Advances in real-time magnetic resonance imaging of the vocal tract for speech science and technology research. *APSIPA Transactions on Signal and Information Processing*, *5*, e6.

Vaz, C., Ramanarayanan, V. & Narayanan, S. (2018). Acoustic denoising using dictionary learning with spectral and temporal regularization. *IEEE/ACM Transactions on Audio, Speech, and Language Processing*, *26*(5), 967–980.

Zhang, S., Gersdor_, N. & Frahm, J. (2011). Real-time magnetic resonance imaging of temporomandibular joint dynamics. *The Open Medical Imaging Journal*, *5*, 1–9.

28

VIDEO TRACKING IN SPEECH

Christian Kroos

Introduction

Human speech has a visual component. Although we do not need to see the face of a speaker to understand what has been said, being able to do so increases the amount of speech information available to us, in particular, in acoustically noisy conditions. Everyday evidence comes from what has traditionally been called "lip reading," that is, from the ability of, e.g. severely hearing-impaired people to pick up substantial parts of a conversation, and also from intentionally silent speech signaling ("read my lips"). The term "lip reading," however, is slightly misleading as the information conveyed visually is not confined to the movement of the lips but comprises at least the lower half of the face if not even the entire facial surface (Vatikiotis-Bateson, Munhall, Hirayama, Lee, & Terzopoulos, 1996). There has been ongoing effort in auditory-visual speech research to replace the term with "speech reading" and the latter will be used in this chapter.

Auditory-visual speech research is an active research field with its own dedicated conference (AVSP – International Conference on Auditory-Visual Speech Processing), but the majority of the work is conducted outside the clinical area. During the last five or so decades the emphasis has been on two focal points of the observable impact of visual speech:

1. The gain in intelligibility through the visual modality, be it in acoustically clean or noisy conditions or with the acoustic modality completely missing ("silent speech reading");
2. Auditory-visual interference, in particular in the form of auditory illusions.

In the latter category, the best known and arguably most spectacular phenomenon of auditory-visual speech is an illusion called the McGurk Effect (McGurk & MacDonald, 1976). A video of a speaker uttering the syllable /ga/ dubbed with the acoustic syllable /ba/, aligned at the stop consonant release, creates convincingly the perception of auditory /da/ in the viewer. The illusion is particularly powerful, because the observer can make the auditory perception flip back and forth by opening and closing the eyes when watching the video or—even simpler—by locking at and away from the video. The astonishing realization is: What you hear changes with what you see.

Since its discovery in the late 1970s hundreds of scientific papers have been published—a Google Scholar search at the time of writing of this chapter with the exact phrase "McGurk effect" resulted in 7,260 hits. Every aspect of the illusion appeared to have been examined only to find new surprising intricacies, not yet researched and understood. For instance, the McGurk effect pertains also to certain other syllable combinations (MacDonald & McGurk, 1978), is to some degree robust against a temporal misalignment of the visual and the auditory stimuli with an asymmetrical sensitivity (Munhall, Gribble, Sacco, & Ward, 1996), creates a strong after-effect (Bertelson, Vroomen, & De Gelder, 2003), tolerates the removal of the central part of the visual signal (Kroos & Dreves, 2008), can also be caused by interference from a haptic stimulus (Fowler & Dekle, 1991), and might not (Saldaña & Rosenblum, 1993) or might (Kroos & Hogan, 2009) be specific to speech—to list only a few facets.

The gain in intelligibility mentioned above is very well researched, too, starting in the 1950s (Sumby & Pollack,1954). From testing the improvement with different interfering noise categories to estimating the contribution of parts of the face to gauging the maximum amount of information humans can extract (see Grant & Bernstein, 2019, for a recent review).

Neither the gain in intelligibility nor the illusions resulting from auditory-visual interference are fully understood. They touch on fundamental issues of how human speech production and perception is structured and controlled and rival theories in those domains put forward diverging explanations. For instance, if phonetic targets are assumed to be the articulatory speech gestures, visual speech is simply the speech gesture made visible instead of being made audible. If the phonetic targets are assumed to be acoustic in nature, then some learned association is postulated and usually an auditory-visual integration mechanism, although even the existence of the latter is sometimes contested. Attempts to quantify the amount of information came likewise to substantially varying results (e.g. Auer Jr, 2009).

From the above it should be clear that currently strong limits exist on how much of the articulatory process can be recovered through video tracking in speech. Although we have not yet seen the newest machine learning methods, which do exceed human performance in some areas, applied in full to this problem, it is unlikely that they will able to remove the limitations in the near future if at all. This does not diminish the usefulness of (auditory-)visual speech and measuring face motion in a variety of settings. After all, it offers the rare opportunity to investigate (to some degree) speech and its disorders separate from auditory processing.

Note that the term "video tracking" used in the title of the chapter is meant in a broad sense covering all methods that use a camera, not just standard video capture. Not included are tracking systems that use different signal acquisition procedures even if they result in sequences of images. X-ray movies, real-time Magnetic Resonance Imaging (MRI) or ultrasound techniques are not covered, neither are tracking methods which might also be applied for visual speech measurement but again employ different data acquisition methods such as Electromagnetic Articulography (EMA). Some of the considerations with regard to video tracking might be applicable to these other methods nevertheless. We will use the terms "tracking" and "capture" interchangeably, but refer to "measurements" only if the tracking results in numerical data points that are independent of the tracking system, the speaker, the recording situation and the setup. In today's computer-based systems this is the case more often than not, although for visualization and to a lesser degree animation purposes it might not be required.

Face motion capture

Background

Historically, attempts of measuring face motion have been focused on emotional face expressions. As early as the middle of the nineteenth century, Guillaume-Benjamin Duchenne attempted to record face motion with the recently invented photographic camera. The strongest impetus came, however, much later in the 1970s from the work of Ekman and Friesen (Ekman & Friesen, 1971) and their comparative studies of emotional facial expressions across the diverse cultures of the world. They adopted the facial motion coding system developed by the Swedish anatomist Carl-Herman Hjortsjö and developed it further into the Facial Action Coding System (FACS): A unified framework for face motion analysis based on anatomical structures. FACS constitutes a quasi-quantitative method, the action units are limited and discrete and to characterize their activation a strength level (one out of five) can be assigned to them. Active action units and their strength, however, had to be manually asserted by trained coders who looked at video sequences or still images, but FACS delivered a decisive motivation and a coding basis for subsequent engineering attempts to automate the tracking process.

Although being a known phenomenon, (auditory-)visual speech received far less attention. This is partly due to technical reasons. Speech consisting of relatively fast movements with critical timing requirements necessitates methods with sufficiently high temporal resolution unless only static configurations are examined with the inflicted loss in ecological validity in research and reduced usefulness in clinical settings. Emotional face expressions on the other hand can be studied on a much slower scale. FACS mentioned above, for instance, assumes that each of the configurations can be sustained for some time.

Given the more difficult capture situation, it appears to be recommended to formulate the tracking problem explicitly before describing the instrumentation that is available to solve it. All the difficulties encountered in face motion capture in everyday practical work can be traced back to the underlying fundamental problem of tracking the facial surface and with a proper understanding of it, difficulties can be addressed and often completely avoided.

Problem formulation

On the visually observable surface the human face consists of the facial skin. Very broadly speaking, the skin layer is followed toward the inside by mixed layers consisting of adipose tissue, fibrous connective tissue such as tendons and ligaments and facial muscles and underneath them the bone structure of the scull. The muscles of the face have a complex layout and interact with each other as well as with muscles of the oral, pharyngeal and laryngeal regions with the interactions extending as far as the sternum. Some of them have multiple, spatially separate insertion points and some of them are part of the intricate motor equivalence system formed via the hyoid bone, the only free-floating bone in the human body.

The action of the mandible strongly impacts the observable lower half of the facial surface. The mandible itself is a rigid structure attached to the scull at the temporomandibular joint and therefore can be fully described as rigid body motion with six motion parameters (three translational and three rotational). However, the motion parameters would need to be inferred from the visually observable movement of the chin and the (within limitations) independently movable layers of skin, fat tissue and muscles render this difficult.

The goal of the tracking is to determine the change in location of a set of measurement points or regions of interest on the facial surface from time $t-1$ to time t. We assume the time variable to be discrete and it usually amounts to video frames and we will refer to frames in the reminder of the chapter. Using light-based cameras only the intensity values of pixels are available, though they might have several color channels and they might be acquired outside the visible light range, e.g. in the infrared spectrum. The location of a pixel in the camera image is linked to a real-world spatial location through the projective geometry of the camera including nonlinear distortions by the lens system. Formulas have been derived to compute the spatial location—reversing perspective transformation—but the depth dimension is in general lost. As a consequence, almost all tracking systems use several cameras to recover the missing dimension. This is beneficial in the case of occlusions, too, and occlusions are almost unavoidable, e.g. with any nonfrontal posture of the head relative to the camera the nose will occlude a part of the face. For the tracking results to be meaningful, it is required that the measurements points or areas of interest are the same from one frame to the next, i.e. that they are not reset every frame but determined at the beginning of the continuous tracking process and, ideally, that they are constant across recordings and maybe even speakers.

To further complicate matters, most camera-based capture systems available for speech motion capture outside the video and movie animation industry are not head-mounted. Thus, from the camera's or cameras' point of view the entire face changes with any head motion. The observable changes of the facial surface are a mixture of the impact of global head motion and intrinsic local face motion and, thus, in order to obtain useful results, the impact of head motion almost always has to be compensated for.

Based on the previous paragraphs, the problem can now be stated as follows:

Estimate the spatial location of a set of predetermined, fixed points or patches of the facial surface in head-centered coordinates for all frames of a recording.

Methods and systems

As might have been already become clear, face motion tracking is not an easy problem. In standard video some parts of the face appear visually highly structured such as the lip boundaries, while others such as the cheeks often expose little detail. To exacerbate the problem, lighting changes can have a dramatic impact on the latter areas. Accordingly, face motion tracking applications explored two different approaches: One tried to solve the problem as it is despite the inherent difficulties, the other attempted to circumvent it by using markers attached to the face. The latter has achieved by far more reliable results and has been mostly in use in speech face motion tracking with the former catching up only in recent years owing to breakthroughs in machine learning. Due to their unconstrained applicability, marker-free methods might, however, soon become the leading approach, despite that they are often limited to the image plane while marker-based methods usually return results in all three spatial dimensions.

A notable third approach consists in projecting a grid of light onto the speaker's face during the recording. *Structured light* approaches then track the deformation of the grid caused by protruding or receding elements of the face, e.g. lip rounding or spreading, over time. However, they do not correct for head movements and do not return measurement points fixed to the facial surface, rendering them substantially less useful.

Marker-based methods

Principles

Markers are easier to track since they can be designed to be visually distinct from the facial surface, either in color, shape or reflectance and most of the time in a combination of those properties. In the case of active markers, they even emit signals themselves. In practice, they are required to be sparsely distributed over the face, i.e. a minimum distance between adjacent marker needs to be observed. Having the markers reasonably scattered solves the problem of identifying them individually across frames. Tracking methods rely hereby on the assumptions that a marker does not move much from one frame to the next, i.e. in the incoming frame, the marker is assumed to be still in the vicinity of its previous location and—rather importantly—closer to its previous location than any other marker. Obviously, this assumption only holds if the video frame rate is high enough and since high frame rates increase the processing demands—often to the limits of the available hardware, violations are common. The mandible can move fast and a lip movement in the same direction, e.g. for a bilabial closure, would add to the speed, making the combined frame-to-frame displacements rather large given standard video rates. More sophisticated tracking algorithms involve therefore predicting the future location based on the current movement direction and velocity. In particular, the Kalman filter, named after its inventor, provides a mathematically optimal way to integrate a model-based prediction and actual measurement data. However, in the case of face motion, predictions can fail, too. They require marker acceleration to change smoothly, which occasionally is not the case, because of a collision of the lips bringing their movement to an abrupt halt, or because of a sudden head movement in the opposite direction as an ongoing jaw movement. By and large, however, marker-based tracking methods return reliable results. Tracking resolution and signal-to-noise ratio is dependent of course on the system type and setup.

Availability

There is a considerable number of commercial devices available for face motion tracking, e.g. Optotrak, Vicon, Elite, Qualisys. None of them were developed solely for this particular purpose, but usually for tracking biological motion in general, e.g. arm and hand movements for grasping analysis, full body motion for gait analysis, etc. They are, however, either suitable from the onset or employ special adaptations, e.g. smaller markers to enable face motion tracking. Figure 28.1 shows 50 face-tracking Vicon markers (3 mm diameter) attached to the author's face and three head tracking markers (9 mm diameter) mounted on a head band. The flashlight of the cameras demonstrates the high reflectance of the markers.

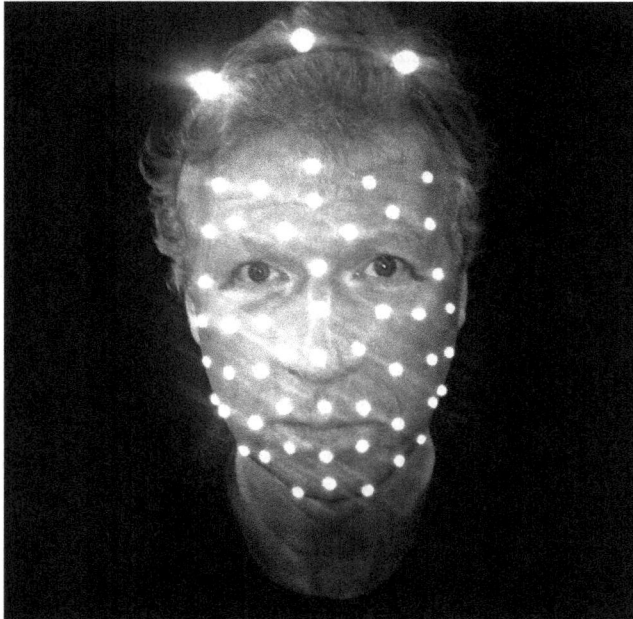

Figure 28.1   Face motion tracking with markers.

Marker-free methods

Principles

The advantages of avoiding the use of markers are evident: No tethering, no need to attach markers, which might interfere with natural face motion, and no physical loss of markers. As mentioned before these advantages come with considerable costs in the form of tracking difficulties. Early attempts focused therefore on facial *features*, visually clearly distinguishable parts of the face such as the lips, eyebrows, eyelids, nose and lower outline of the chin. *Feature tracking* alleviates tracking problems, but restricts the results to those predefined features and often employs strong assumptions about the facial structures to be tracked.

Early attempts used a pixel-based computational method called *optical flow*. The approach assumed that the intensity value (three of them in a digital color image: red, green and blue) of a tracked object do not change from one frame to the next. Since there is only one scalar constraint to determine the two velocity components of the pixel movement, this is an *ill-posed* problem. There might be many pixels with identical intensity values, both in local neighborhoods and across the image. Furthermore, the invariance assumption does not hold if lighting changes occur. These difficulties were addressed by introducing additional constraints to the method and some limited success was achieved (e.g. Wu, Kanade, Cohn, & Li, 1998).

Later approaches tried to avoid optical flow because of the inherent problems. In general, solution attempts involved the use of more information than just single pixels, either (a) larger patches of the facial surface as rendered in its image plane projection or (b) full appearance models. As an example for (a), Kroos, Kuratate, & Vatikiotis-Bateson (2002) used patches of the facial surface surrounding the nodes of a mesh grid superimposed on the image and fitted to the face. With a coarse-to-fine strategy applied both to the mesh and the image (via multi-resolution analysis using the discrete wavelet transform), the locations changes of the nodes were tracked. As an example for (b), Xiao, Baker, Matthews, & Kanade (2004) employed a combination of two-dimensional and three-dimensional active appearance models and used a real-time fitting algorithm to register head orientation and face motion changes.

Appearance model already made use of stochastic properties of objects in images and of faces in particular and learned some of the parameters of the model from the data. This trend dominated the majority of the approaches ever since, most of them involving *Hidden Markov Models*, in which the transition probabilities of the states of the tracked entities from one frame to the next were learned beforehand from large data sets and the most likely path through the potential transitions in the image sequence under investigation determined via a dynamic programming algorithm.

In recent years, an exceptional jump in performance has been observed with the advent of *deep learning* (Goodfellow, Bengio, & Courville, 2016), a machine learning method using Artificial Neural Networks (ANN) with multiple layers. ANNs learn a given task from large data sets without much human interference and without requiring an understanding of the peculiarities of a solution found. They are inspired by biological neurons, but constitute a strong mathematical abstraction and simplification of their biological models.

ANNs gained popularity throughout the 1970s and 80s, but fell out of favor later because their deep variants, meaning networks with many layers, could not be successfully trained owing to a lack in understanding of the underlying principles. In addition, theoretical results pointed out that more than one layer (besides input and output) might not be necessary. This changed in the first decade of the current century: Better training methods were developed and the theoretical result turned out to be too abstract to be applicable to real-world tasks. The renaissance of deep ANNs was helped by the fact that huge data sets became commonplace and computational processing power increased not at least through the heavy parallel processing capabilities of GPUs (Graphical Processor Units).

For image-based object and scene recognition Convolutional Neural Networks (CNNs), which apply a cascade of parallel learnable two-dimensional filters, turned out to be most successful. For time series data, for which temporal long-term dependencies need to be learned, Recurrent Neural Networks (RNNs) were found to be most suitable, in particular specific variants that can handle a common problem, the vanishing gradient problem, such as Long Short-Term Memory networks (LSTMs). Marker-free video-based tracking of face motion can be considered a combination of an image problem—the face in a single frame—and a time series problem—frames over time.

At the time of writing, the application of deep learning methods explicitly for face motion tracking is still at its infancy. One of the reasons is that for popular tasks such as emotional face expression recognition, no intermediate tracking step is required but the image or image sequence is submitted in its raw form to the network and classification is directly accomplished. All that is needed is a large dataset labeled appropriately with the emotion displayed in the video. A similar situation can be found in (audio-)visual automatic speech recognition. The trained networks certainly track face movements, but if not forced otherwise, the tracking information is inaccessibly buried in the intermediate representations of the input data in the hidden layers of the networks. The capture also pertains only to motion that is relevant to performance improvement on the specific task, i.e. emotional expression recognition or speech recognition. The tracking results are unlikely to constitute a veridical representation of all movements of the entire face.

It is foreseeable that in the near future deep learning will be applied to a much larger degree to the tracking problem itself and that commercial software will be developed. Very large networks as they have become common recently with up to hundreds of millions of artificial synapses are likely to learn autonomously the fundamental properties of human face motion and underlying anatomical and functional relations from video sequences alone, although they will then bury the relationship information opaquely in their connection weights and only provide the capture results and, ideally, estimations of the underlying articulation.

Availability

There are many stereo cameras commercially available and they sometimes come with face tracking software. Due to their often considerable price tag, line of motion tracking devices developed for computer games, in particular, the Kinect (developed by PrimeSense) have become popular in research and as sensing systems in, for instance, robotics. Extensive open-source libraries exist and are well maintained such as the OpenCV library but require in general a higher degree of technical knowledge for their application.

Data processing

Raw motion capture data are rarely useful for clinical applications. As a minimum they have to be compensated for head motion unless the speakers head was sufficiently restrained during the recording, e.g. with a head rest. Due to the bone structure of the skull, the human head can be treated mathematically as rigid structure and thus can be fully described with six motion parameters. If the tracking includes at least three measurement points that are not affected by skin movements, the parameters can be estimated using the General Procrustes Method (Gower, 1975). Due to unavoidable measurement errors, it is recommended to use more than the mathematical minimum number of three markers to obtain an overdetermined system of equations, which tends to average out the errors. Since head motion compensation affects all face markers and impacts them in an unequal manner due to the rotation components, errors in the head motion estimation propagate and might bias the face motion capture results.

Note that head movements in themselves might be of interest and were linked to speech articulation. However, to recover veridical head motion parameters, the center of rotation needs to be known. In humans there is no single point for the center of rotation as there is no single joint connecting the head to the torso: Head motions are accomplished by the combined action of eight joints of complex geometry of the upper and lower cervical spine (Zatsiorsky, 1998). An approximation with an appropriately located single point will still give good results, though. Furthermore, for computationally compensating the impact of head motion the true rotation center is not needed. All that is required is an (affine) transformation that transforms the face coordinates from a world-centered coordinate system—usually determined by the focal point and focal axis of the (single) camera or set arbitrarily in a system calibration step—to a head-centered coordinate system. This implies that movements of the entire torso also do not matter in this context while of course they affect the estimations of true head motion.

Marker-based tracking methods provide flesh point results. Figure 28.2 shows a sample of the movement of a midsagittal lip marker in the longitudinal dimension aligned with the acoustic time signal and spectrogram of the uttered sentence.

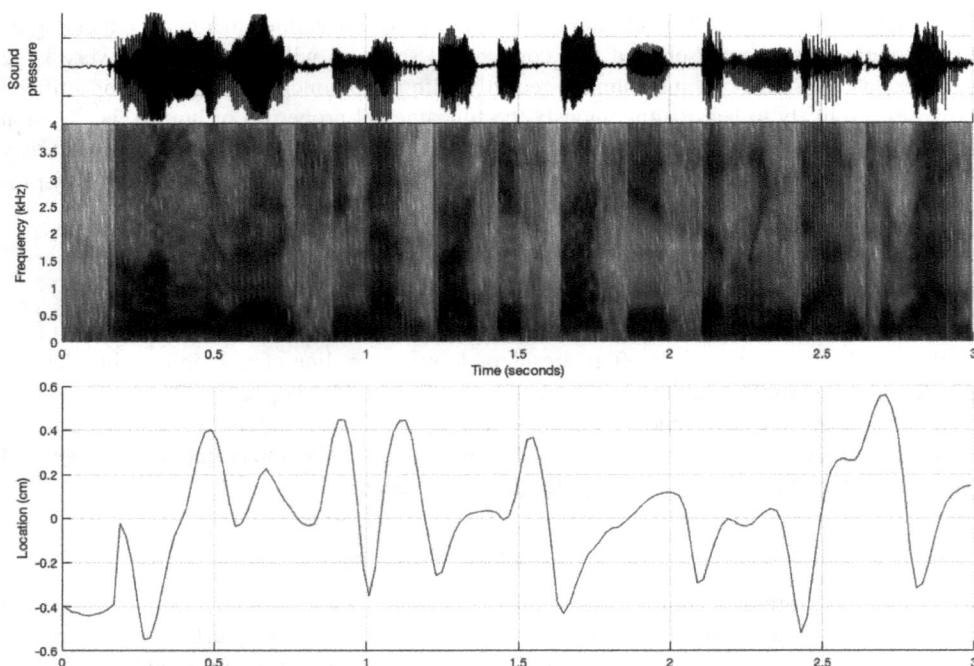

Figure 28.2   Lower lip tracking sample.

The motion signals can be directly used to determine velocities and accelerations. The same holds for marker-free method if they track fixed points of the facial surface. However, one needs to keep in mind that the resulting point trajectories are always affected by tracking noise and that velocities and accelerations are not mathematical derivatives but based on discrete differences in marker location across two or more frames. Thus, they tend to be noisy, the effect accumulating when moving toward higher derivatives. Accelerations are often already badly affected and, one level higher, the change in acceleration, called *jerk*, an important target variable in biological motion, is even more so. Accordingly, often trajectory smoothing is required.

There are many approaches to this problem, all of them have at least one free parameter for the user to set, although for biological motion reasonable defaults or recommendations are usually available. To name only two methods:

- The Savitzky-Golay filter (Press & Teukolsky, 1990) provides very reasonable results and is easy to apply;
- Functional Data Analysis (Ramsay & Silverman, 2006), which models a signal by combining a set of weighted base functions, is more flexible and can be fine-tuned to the smoothing needs, but requires more background knowledge.

The results from feature tracking methods are advantageous for visual inspection, although it is of course doubtful whether they can add anything that an experienced practitioner cannot extract from the raw video. Since they usually return shapes, they require in general another processing step, e.g. computing the center of gravity of a shape. These processed results might be particularly helpful if the procedure is tailored to a specific measurement of interest, e.g. the ratio of longitudinal to transversal lip opening as a dimensionless indicator for lip spreading and rounding.

Practical considerations

Ideally one would be able to recover the entire articulation process simply by filming the speaker using standard video and subsequently running some capture and detection software on the stored video sequence. This is currently out of reach and it might never become possible unless all articulatory information is indeed fully reflected in the observable facial surface and neck area. Given the fine adjustments of articulatory structures deep in the pharyngeal and laryngeal regions (e.g. changes in the settings of the vocal cords and the arytenoids, the epiglottis, the tongue root, the velum), this appears unlikely, although future processing methods might be able to detect minute changes in the observable structures and map them correctly to the underlying articulation.

Accordingly, entire domains, such as determining the degree of nasalization, are excluded from visual analysis. Even looking at more accessible domains, some problems surface regularly in video tracking in speech, but can often mitigated by choosing the most suitable tracking system and software and taking proper precautions in the setup and during recording.

Choice of system

The general differences between the systems have been already discussed. These inherent system properties will often determine the choice, e.g. whether or not markers can be used for the intended purpose. However, a couple of other criteria need to guide the selection as well.

For the intended application,

- The tracking resolution of individual measurement points, both in spatial and temporal respect, must be sufficiently high;
- The minimum distance between measurement points (markers or virtual tracking points) must be sufficiently small;
- The spatial arrangement in the examination room must allow for the proper positioning of the camera or multiple cameras and for some systems the lighting needs to be controlled;
- Items or devices that might occlude parts of the speakers face, either temporarily or for the entire duration of the recording, must be considered—the ability to handle occlusions varies substantially across systems;
- Items or surfaces in the visual field of the camera(s) that strongly reflect light, either temporarily or for the entire duration of the recording, must be taken into consideration – the most common source of mis-tracking in marker-based systems are reflections from shiny surfaces that resemble a marker from the system's point of view.

Head motion tracking

The importance of minimizing the error in the head motion tracking was pointed out before, including the recommendation to use more than three markers in marker-based systems. Determining locations that are not affected by skin movements (face, neck or scalp), however, is not easy. The nasion provides a point for most but not all speakers. In general, headbands made from elastic fabric with the marker sewn onto them provide the best solution albeit one which is far from being perfect. Obviously, the markers on the headband can be affected by motions of the forehead skin and the entire headband might slip during a recording.

Usually, one would prefer to obtain the face motion tracking results as measurements in a fixed coordinate reference system aligned with the primary anatomical axis of the head. In marker-based systems, it can be accomplished with simple calibration devices. This can be any rigid structure that allows the attachment of at least three markers and a temporary fixation to the head, e.g. in the form of a bite-block. In marker-free methods there are approaches to obtain the reference system algorithmically via an implicit analysis of face motion invariants in the locations of facial landmarks.

Marker placements in marker-based systems

The selection of marker locations depends, of course, crucially on the intended application. Constraints are imposed by the required minimum distance of neighboring markers, attachment suitability of the area, numbers of markers available and peculiarities of the regions of interest. This becomes particularly evident at the lips. Due to their importance in speech and their movement range and shape flexibility, it would be preferable to track them with a high number of markers. Some areas of the lips, however, are likely to be affected by occlusions: Markers placed too far toward the inside might disappear in the mouth during certain movements while for locations toward the vermillion border, markers might be only partially visible during strong lip rounding. Even more problematic, paired markers on longitudinally similar locations on the lower and upper lip might come very close to each other or even in direct contact with each other during lip closure. The tracking system might not be able to distinguish them and swap marker identity: The marker that had been tracked so far as the upper lip marker becomes the lower lip marker and vice versa. This is known as trajectory crossover and requires laborious manual correction in the post-processing. As a consequence, it is difficult if not impossible to determine lip closure directly with marker-based systems. As a workaround, markers can be placed close to the vermillion border and the closure distance between paired upper and lower lip markers determined in a calibration recording of the speaker with a relaxed closed mouth without any lip compression. To reliably detect incomplete lip closures, however, this might still not be sufficient.

Some areas of the face are more correlated with each other than others. Highly correlated areas—as for instance the cheeks—can be tracked with fewer markers or virtual measurement points. High correlations, however, do not exclude the possibility that the non-correlated amount of the variance is more than simply variability induced by tissue constraints and, thus, might—albeit small in amplitude—indeed contain viable speech information that is not observable elsewhere.

Tracking the mandible

Direct measurements of all six movement parameters of the mandible are not achievable with video tracking. At best they can be inferred from tracking of the chin. If only the degree of jaw opening is required (usually a combination of a rotational movement around the transversal axis and a translational movement in the anterior direction), a single marker attached directly underneath the front of the chin yields useable results in particular when combined with other makers at the chin line, which are considerably more lateral positioned. The same holds for the averaged results of a multitude of virtual measurement points on the chin line in marker-free methods. The results will not be precise, though, since some lip movements such as strong protruding motions have an impact on the skin across the entire chin.

Tracking noise

All systems suffer from tracking noise. Most of the time this is not an issue, either because the noise magnitude is too small to be relevant or because the noise can be removed through trajectory smoothing. However, if the recording situation is less than ideal this can change quickly, independently of how good the nominal signal-to-noise ratio of the system might be. Of particular concern is the situation where phenomena or symptoms under investigation are characterized by small movement amplitude changes or discontinuities. Under certain circumstances (problematic lighting, reflecting surfaces or items in the visual field) the capture results might oscillate between two or more most likely locations. Usually these are neighboring locations and thus the tracking ambiguity creates the impression of a tremor. Similarity goes both ways and thus, clearly, a physiological tremor can closely resemble tracking noise and be filtered out through trajectory smoothing if the smoothing strength is set inappropriately.

References

Auer Jr, E.T. (2009). Spoken word recognition by eye. *Scandinavian Journal of Psychology*, *50*(5), 419–425.

Bertelson, P., Vroomen, J. & De Gelder, B. (2003). Visual recalibration of auditory speech identification: a McGurk aftereffect. *Psychological Science*, *14*(6), 592–597.

Ekman, P. & Friesen, W.V. (1971). Constants across cultures in the face and emotion. *Journal of Personality and Social Psychology, 17*(2), 124–129.

Fowler, C.A. & Dekle, D.J. (1991). Listening with eye and hand: Cross-modal contributions to speech perception. *Journal of Experimental Psychology: Human Perception and Performance, 17*(3), 816–828.

Goodfellow, I., Bengio, Y. & Courville, A. (2016). *Deep Learning*. Cambridge, MA; London, UK: MIT press.

Gower, J.C. (1975). Generalized procrustes analysis. *Psychometrika, 40*(1), 33–51.

Grant, K.W. & Bernstein, J.G. (2019). Toward a model of auditory-visual speech intelligibility. In A.K. Lee, M.T. Wallace, A.B. Coffin, A.N. Popper & R.R. Fay, *Multisensory Processes: The Auditory Perspective* (pp. 33–57). Cham: Springer.

Kroos, C. & Dreves, A. (2008). McGurk effect persists with a partially removed visual signal. In R. Göcke, P. Lucey & S. Lucey, Paper presented at *International Conference on Auditory-Visual Speech Processing, AVSP 2008*, (pp. 55–58). Moreton Island, QLD, Australia: ISCA.

Kroos, C. & Hogan, K. (2009). Visual influence on auditory perception: Is speech special? In B.-J. Theobald & R. Harvey, Paper presented at *International Conference on Auditory-Visual Speech Processing, AVSP 2009*, (pp. 70–75). Norwich, UK: ISCA.

Kroos, C., Kuratate, T. & Vatikiotis-Bateson, E. (2002). Video-based face motion measurement. *Journal of Phonetics, 30*(3), 569–590.

MacDonald, J. & McGurk, H. (1978). Visual influences on speech perception processes. *Perception & Psychophysics, 24*(3), 253–257.

McGurk, H. & MacDonald, J. (1976). Hearing lips and seeing voices. *Nature, 264*(5588), 746–748.

Munhall, K.G., Gribble, P., Sacco, L. & Ward, M. (1996). Temporal constraints on the McGurk effect. *Perception & Psychophysics, 58*(3), 351–362.

Press, W.H. & Teukolsky, S.A. (1990). Savitzky-Golay smoothing filters. *Computers in Physics, 4*(6), 669–672.

Ramsay, J.O. & Silverman, B.W. (2006). *Functional Data Analysis*. New York, NY: Springer.

Saldaña, H.M. & Rosenblum, L.D. (1993). Visual influences on auditory pluck and bow judgments. *Perception & Psychophysics, 54*(3), 406–416.

Sumby, W.H. & Pollack, I. (1954). Visual contribution to speech intelligibility in noise. *The Journal of the Acoustical Society of America, 26*(2), 212–215.

Vatikiotis-Bateson, E., Munhall, K.G., Hirayama, M., Lee, Y.V. & Terzopoulos, D. (1996). The dynamics of audiovisual behavior in speech. In D.G. Stork, M.E. Hennecke & D.G. Stork (Ed.), *Speechreading by Humans and Machines: Models, Systems, and Applications*. Berlin, Heidelberg: Springer.

Wu, Y.T., Kanade, T., Cohn, J. & Li, C.C. (1998). Optical flow estimation using wavelet motion model. *Sixth International Conference on Computer Vision* (pp. 992–998). IEEE.

Xiao, J., Baker, S., Matthews, I. & Kanade, T. (2004). Real-time combined 2D + 3D active appearance models. In Proceedings of the 2004 IEEE Computer Society Conference on Computer Vision and Pattern Recognition, 2, (pp. 535–542). Washington, DC: IEEE Computer Society.

Zatsiorsky, V.M. (1998). *Kinematics of Human Motion*. Champaign, IL: Human Kinetics.

29

ULTRASOUND TONGUE IMAGING

Joanne Cleland

Introduction

Ultrasound has been used as a diagnostic medical tool since 1956. In 1969 Kelsey, Minifie and Hixon proposed using ultrasound to image the tongue (Ultrasound Tongue Imaging: UTI) as a safer alternative to X-ray imaging for viewing the articulators in both typical and disordered speech production. UTI is an instrumental articulatory technique that can be used to view and record movements of the surface of the tongue from the root to near the tongue tip. This chapter will describe ultrasound equipment and analysis followed by an overview of the type of speech errors which can be viewed with UTI.

Ultrasound refers to soundwaves beyond the range of human hearing. In diagnostic medical ultrasound, a probe (also known as transducer) consisting of a piezoelectric crystal emits pulses of ultrasonic soundwaves between 2 and 5 MHz through the tissues of the body. Soundwaves have reflective properties, therefore after each pulse is emitted there is a short delay before an echo is received from reflecting surfaces. This echo is converted to a strength and distance and plotted to give an image, allowing us to view the boarders of tissues of different density.

There are two main applications of UTI in clinical phonetics. The first is to use the real-time dynamic images as a biofeedback tool (see Cleland and Preston, 2021, for an overview) for treating children and adults with speech sound disorders. In this application, the speaker sees their own tongue moving in real time and, guided by a Speech-Language Pathologist, uses that information to modify incorrect articulations. To use ultrasound in this way the clinician need only have a basic B-mode medical ultrasound system and a suitable probe. This is in contrast with the second application of UTI, which is for phonetic research or detailed assessment of speech disorders. In order to study the complex dynamics of speech, methods of synchronizing ultrasound with the acoustic signal at a fast enough frame rate to capture speech events are required. There are now many studies using ultrasound as a tool for studying typical speech, with common applications including sociophonetic research into tongue-shapes for /r/ and vowel changes (see for example, Lawson, Scobbie & Stuart-Smith, 2011). Advances in ultrasound hardware coupled with advances in software for analyzing ultrasound have led to ultrasound becoming standard equipment in the phonetics lab. However, clinical phonetic applications are only now emerging, perhaps because researchers have focused mainly on the biofeedback applications in clinical populations.

Ultrasound equipment

Ultrasound equipment consists of a probe (transducer) and central processing unit connected to either a stand-alone unit of the type seen in hospitals, or, more commonly in the phonetics laboratory, a PC or laptop. A variety of probes are available from ultrasound manufacturers. However, to be useful for measuring tongue movement the probe must both fit under the speaker's chin and image at adequate depth (the distance the ultrasonic waves can penetrate through the body, normally around 70–90mm is required) with an adequate field of view to image as much of the tongue as possible (Lee, Wrench, & Sancibrian, 2015). The most commonly used probes are microconvex and 20-mm convex probes. The microconvex is smaller and fits well under small children's chins, allowing more of the tongue tip to be viewed, however imaging at depth can be poor. A convex probe gives a brighter image at depth, making it more suitable for larger children and adults. Figure 29.1 shows the field of view as imaged by both types of probes.

Frame rate is also important. It is possible to achieve frame rates >300 Hz, however, imaging at this frame rate comes at the cost of spatial resolution and field of view. Wrench and Scobbie (2011) discuss the frame rates required for imaging high velocity articulations such as clicks and conclude that the optimum frame rate required is 60 to 200 Hz. In clinical phonetic applications the lower frame rate is adequate unless users specifically want to study clicks or trills. It should be noted that some ultrasound systems used in biofeedback research have frame rates much lower than 60 Hz and are therefore unlikely to be useful for studying speech dynamics from recorded data, although they are very useful for viewing tongue movements live. More recent systems used in biofeedback studies, for example the Micrus/Sonospeech system (see www. articulateinstruments.com), supply frame rates of around 100 Hz and are therefore suitable for both biofeedback and clinical phonetic applications.

There are two key technical considerations when using UTI for clinical phonetic applications. The first is synchronizing the ultrasound to the acoustic signal and recording both for playback and analysis. The second is determining, or deciding not to determine, a coordinate space for the resultant tongue shapes. A coordinate space can only be determined by either fixing the probe relative to the head using a headset or correcting for probe movement using motion tracking. In contrast, hand-holding the probe is convenient for the phonetician and likely to be more comfortable for speakers. However, the data will consist of a series of tongue curves which are not located in the same coordinate space because it is impossible to hold the probe completely still by hand. Even consecutive frames may have small differences in translation and rotation of the tongue shape. It is also quite likely that the probe will drift to an off-center position, leading to a view which is not mid-sagittal and prone to artifacts. Some researchers use a small camera or mirror as a method of

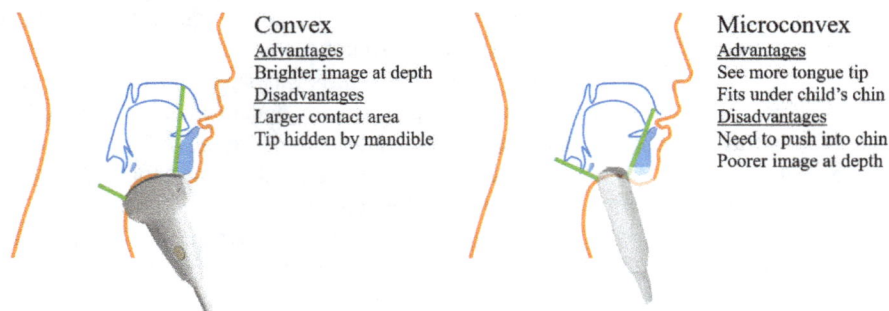

Figure 29.1   Comparison of convex (left) and microconvex probes (right). (With thanks to Alan Wrench for supplying the image.)

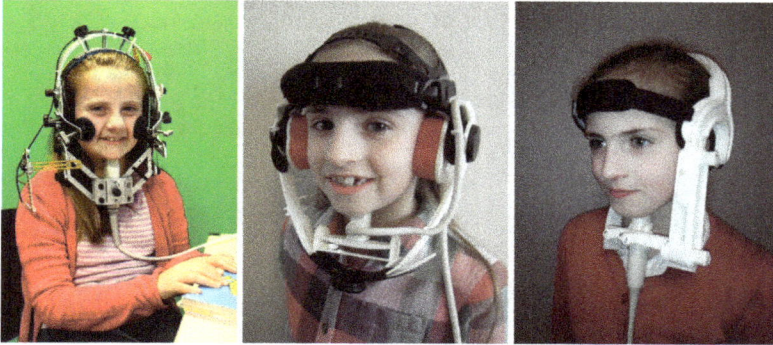

Figure 29.2 Headsets from Articulate Instruments Ltd. used in clinical studies arranged from left to right chronologically.

checking that the probe is roughly in the midline and it is possible to use data acquired in this way either for qualitative observations or by applying scaler metrics which are not sensitive to translation and rotation. These types of metrics give numeric values based on single tongue curves and are sensitive to tongue-shape features such as the amount of tongue bunching and/or the number of tongue inflections (see below). However, such metrics still presume that the probe is held in the midline and may not be sensitive to twisting (yaw and pitch) or lateral displacement. An alternative approach is to stabilize the probe relative to the head or correct for head movement. Several research labs have systems for doing so, though not all have been used for clinical research. The Haskins Optically Corrected Ultrasound System (HOCUS, Whalen et al., 2005) uses a spring loaded holder for the ultrasound probe and optical tracking to correct for speaker head movement. A similar system, Sonographic and Optical Linguo-labial Articulation Recording system (SOLLAR, Noiray et al., 2018) adapts this technology into a child-friendly spaceship-themed set up. Both systems require attaching tracking dots to the speaker's head and probe and require two experimenters for data collection. Neither of these systems have yet been used for clinical phonetic research, though it would be possible to do so. Other labs stabilize the probe using a headrest or headset and have developed in-house software for analyzing data which is often made freely available (see for example www.ultraspeech.com or UltraCATS, Gu et al., 2004). A complete ultrasound system for phonetic research and biofeedback is available from Articulate Instruments Ltd. (www.articulateinstruments.com). This small portable system is a USB device which connects to a PC or laptop. Software, Articulate Assistant Advanced™, can record synchronized ultrasound, audio, and lip camera data (and other channels such as electropalatography if desired). This system has been used in several clinical phonetic studies and intervention studies. In contrast to the optically corrected systems, the Articulate Instruments system makes use of a probe stabilizing headset. This allows the user to ensure that measurements of tongue shape are not affected by probe movement but has the disadvantage that it can become heavy over time and may restrict jaw movement. Figure 29.2 shows headsets used in clinical studies in Scotland.

Understanding the ultrasound image in typical speakers

The surface of the tongue can be imaged in either a mid-sagittal or coronal view. Ultrasound is absorbed by bone and does not travel though air, therefore in both these types of images the mandible and/or hyoid bone casts a dark shadow and the air boundary at the surface of the tongue is a bright white line. Because ultrasound is reflected soundwaves, users should be aware that the

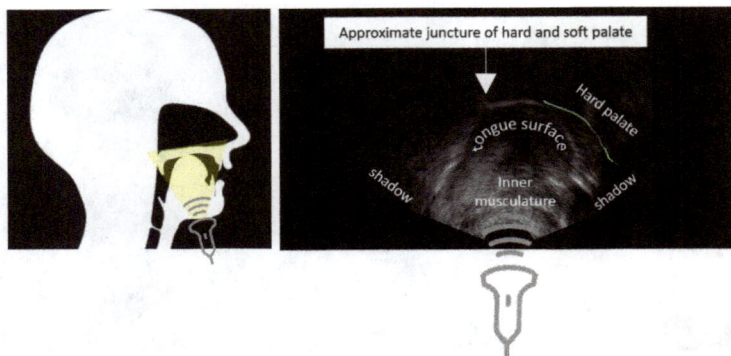

Figure 29.3 Mid-sagittal ultrasound image taken from the maximum point of contact of [k]. Tongue tip is to the right.

ultrasound image is not a photograph, rather it is vulnerable to artifacts which can be difficult to interpret, especially if the probe is off-center or indeed if the speaker has very unusual anatomy. The hard palate and the pharyngeal wall are not visible in the ultrasound image. It is possible to obtain a tracing of the hard palate by asking the speaker to swallow some water. This tracing can then be super-imposed on the image if the speaker is wearing a probe-stabilizing headset or if a system for correcting for head movement is used. If the probe is held by hand then it is not possible to add a hard palate reference trace due to probe movement. Figure 29.3 shows an ultrasound image taken from the maximum point of articulation of [k]. Most UTI studies use the mid-sagittal view with the tongue tip to the right. Unlike electromagnetic articulography and electropalatography (EPG), the image shown is an anatomically correct representation of the tongue from near the tongue tip to near the root. It can be used to image all lingual articulations, although the shadow from the mandible can obscure the tongue tip, making dentals, interdentals and linguolabials difficult to see in their entirety. Ultrasound holds advantages over EPG for imaging vowels and post-velar articulations since EPG shows only tongue-palate contact from the alveolar ridge to the boundary of the hard and soft palate. However, ultrasound typically only images a single mid-sagittal (or coronal) slice, therefore features such as tongue bracing is better imaged with EPG. 3D ultrasound systems are available, but they are as yet unable to image with the temporal resolution 2D systems are capable of.

An understanding of ultrasound tongue shapes in typical speakers is required in order to inter-pret ultrasound images from clinical populations. This is especially true when making quali-tative judgements about potentially disordered tongue shapes in speakers with motor speech disorders or unusual anatomy (for example, speakers who have had partial glossectomy). The ultrasound image is not normalized, therefore the display for each speaker shows a slightly different size and shape of tongue. Because of this, there are a large number of speaker-dependent factors involved in interpreting ultrasound. Moreover, the lack of normalization highlights the wide-range of tongue shapes that are possible. For example, American English /r/ may have at least six different possible tongue shapes (Boyce et al., 2015). Tongue-shapes for vowels will also differ greatly, even within one language, due to both dialect features and speaker-specific anatomy. This makes comparing ultrasound images between speakers a challenge, with most phonetic studies choosing to look at intra-speaker measures. Nevertheless, there are some com-monalities in tongue-shapes for specific speech sounds. The www.seeingspeech.com website provides a very useful clickable IPA chart of ultrasound movies collected from two different speakers. Table 29.1 shows example ultrasound images from a range of consonants compared to MRI images from the same speaker.

Table 29.1 Ultrasound (left) and MRI (right) images for a range of consonants from the IPA

Articulation	Ultrasound	MRI
Alveolar Stop [t]		
Alveolar fricative [s]		
Postalveolar fricative [ʃ]		
Retroflex approximant [ɹ]		
Dark l [ɫ]		

(*Continued*)

Table 29.1 (Continued)

Articulation	Ultrasound	MRI
Palatal fricative [ç]		
Velar Stop [k]		
Uvular stop [q]		
Pharyngeal fricative [ħ]		

Analyzing ultrasound data

The type of analyses that are possible depend on the type of ultrasound system used to acquire the data. Most types of analysis involve first tracking the surface of the tongue and fitting a spline with a number of discreet data points to the surface. Until fairly recently phoneticians fitted splines to ultrasound images by hand using specialist software (for example, Articulate Assistant Advanced (AAA), or UltraCats). This was a time consuming process and as such necessitated choosing only a limited number of frames for analysis, for example choosing only

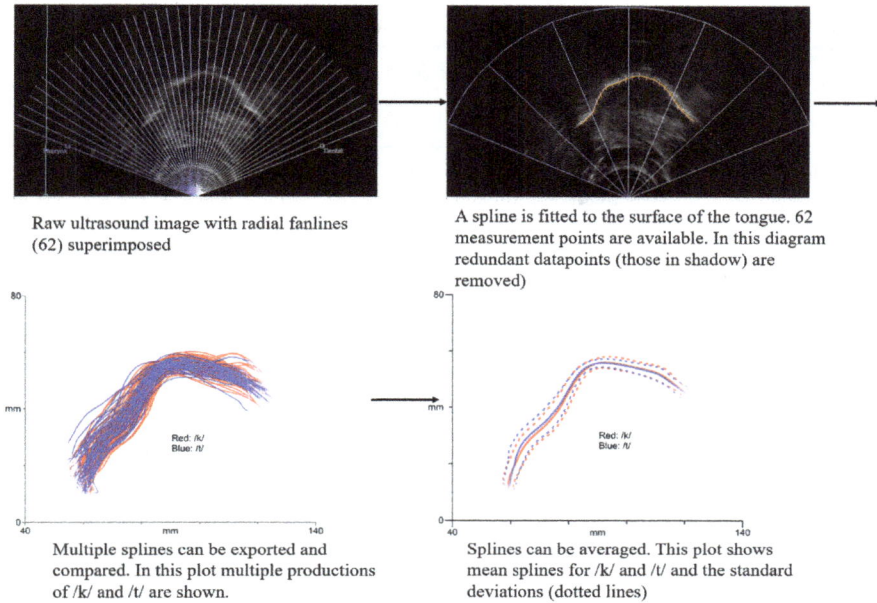

Raw ultrasound image with radial fanlines (62) superimposed

A spline is fitted to the surface of the tongue. 62 measurement points are available. In this diagram redundant datapoints (those in shadow) are removed)

Multiple splines can be exported and compared. In this plot multiple productions of /k/ and /t/ are shown.

Splines can be averaged. This plot shows mean splines for /k/ and /t/ and the standard deviations (dotted lines)

Figure 29.4 Example of ultrasound analysis. Panel 1 (top left) shows the raw ultrasound image with fanlines emanating from the probe. Panel 2 (top right) shows a spline fitted to the surface of the tongue with measurement (data) points represented by orange spokes along each fanline. Panel 3 (bottom left) shows multiple splines from individual productions of /t/ and /k/ superimposed and panel 4 shows these same splines averaged.

the burst of stops or midpoint of fricatives. There are now a number of algorithms available for fitting splines to the tongue surface automatically (including in AAA software), or semi-automatically, allowing all ultrasound frames to be used if dynamic analysis is required. Once splines are fitted, either polar or Cartesian coordinates can be exported and used to compare tongue shapes quantitatively. Polar coordinates are often used since the probe can be used as the origin and splines can be fitted along radial fanlines. Figure 29.4 gives an example of data acquired using the Articulate Instruments Ltd ultrasound system with headset stabilization. The top left panel shows 62 fanlines emanating from the probe. First, the phonetician annotates the speech data using either acoustic or articulatory landmarks. In this example, the phonetician has annotated stop closures at the burst. Next, a spline is automatically fitted to the surface of the tongue (panel 2). From here either the coordinates can be exported and compared statistically or multiple splines can be compared visually (panel 3). If headset stabilization is used, it is possible to average multiple splines for comparison (panel 4), see Articulate Assistant Advanced "t-test function". If headset stabilization is not used (either because it is not available or because it is not desirable for young children or speakers with clinical diagnoses) then coordinates are exported and scaler metrics are used to compare tongue-shapes. For example, the Dorsum Excursion Index (DEI, Zharkova, 2013) can be used to compare the degree of tongue dorsum movement between two different target phonemes, irrespective of translation and rotation.

Table 29.2 summarizes the key indices which have been used in the literature to quantify or compare tongue shapes with reference to papers using them on clinical populations. It is important to note that even if probe stabilization is not used it is often still important that the UTIs are acquired with both the mandible and hyoid shadow in view. This is because

Table 29.2 Ultrasound metrics used to quantify disordered speech

Measure	Description	Independent of head movement	Example use
T-test function (Articulate Instruments Ltd)	Determines whether there is a statistically significant difference between two sets of tongue curves along a fanline.	No	Identification of covert contrast in children with persistent velar fronting (Cleland et al., 2017)
Mean nearest neighbour difference (Zharkova & Hewlett, 2009)	Quantifies the difference between two tongue curves	No	Coarticulation and stability in people who stutter (Belmont, 2015)
Dorsum excursion index (DEI) (Zharkova, 2013)	Quantifies the extent of excursion of the tongue dorsum, conceptually represented by the point on the tongue curve located opposite the middle of the straight line between two curve ends	Yes	Identification of covert contrast in velar fronting (McAllister Byun et al., 2016)
LOC$_{a-i}$ (Zharkova, 2015)	Quantifies excursion of the tongue in relation to the back of the tongue.	Yes	Covert contrast of s and ʃ (both stopped to dental) (Zharkova et al., 2017)
Curvature degree Curvature position (Aubin & Menard, 2006)	Quantifies the extent of maximal excursion within a single tongue shape Determines where on the tongue curve the excursion is	Yes	Covert contrast of s and ʃ (Zharkova et al., 2017)
Procrustes analysis (Dawson et al., 2016)	Gives the sum of the squared differences between two tongue shapes, following translation, rotation and scaling	Yes	Tongue complexity in vowel production in speakers with Down Syndrome compared to resting state (Carl, 2018)
Modified curvature index (Dawson et al., 2016)	Quantifies curvature degree and number of inflections in a tongue shape	Yes	Tongue complexity in vowel production in speakers with Down Syndrome (Carl, 2018)
Discrete Fourier transformation (Dawson et al., 2016)	Differentiation of tongue shapes between targets	Yes	Differentiation of tongue shapes for target vowels in speakers with Down syndrome (Carl, 2018)
Number of inflections (NINFL) (Preston et al., 2019)	Count of the number of tongue curvature changes in a single tongue contour	Yes	Tongue complexity in rhotic distortions (Preston et al., 2019)
Peak velocity (Heyde et al., 2015)	Calculates displacement and velocity of tongue movement along a single measurement vector	No	Kinematic analysis in people who stutter (Heyde et al., 2015)

KT crescent (Scobbie & Cleland, 2017)	Quantifies dorsal velar constriction spatially in relation to a same-speaker alveolar baseline	Yes	Degree of separation between /k/ and /t/ in a child with persistent velar fronting (Cleland & Scobbie, 2018)
Width measure and tongue length (Roxburgh, 2018)	Quantifies the mean and maximum distances between two curves measured radially from the probe origin. Zones of significance are compared to the proportion of visible tongue length.	Yes	Degree of separation between velar and alveolar consonants in children with submucous cleft palate (Roxburgh, 2018)
Anteriority index 3D Ultrasound (Bressmann et al., 2005)	Volumetric index indicating relative position of the main mass of intrinsic tongue tissue in the oral cavity	No	Tongue protrusion following partial glossectomy (Bressmann et al., 2005)
Concavity index 3D Ultrasound (Bressmann et al., 2005)	Measures how convex or concave the shape of the tongue is along the whole length of the tongue volume	No	Tongue grooving following partial glossectomy (Bressmann et al., 2005)
Asymmetry index. 3D Ultrasound (Bressmann et al., 2005)	Volumetric measure of the difference in lateral tongue height between each side of the tongue	No	Tongue symmetry following partial glossectomy (Bressmann et al., 2005)
Tongue displacement (Bressmann et al., 20116)	Cumulative displacement of maximum tongue height measured radially	No	Tongue displacement during production of /r/ before and after intervention (Bressmann et al., 2016)

most measures require the phonetician to determine end points of the tongue spline and this is not possible if the probe is rotated such that a large portion of the tongue front or root is not in view.

Clinical populations

As a biofeedback tool UTI has been used most often with children with residual speech sound errors; persistent speech sound disorders; Childhood Apraxia of Speech; hearing impairment; cleft lip and palate; and Down syndrome (Sugden et al., 2019). It is less used as a biofeed-back tool for adults with acquired disorders, though it has been used with adults with acquired apraxia of speech (Preston & Leaman, 2014) and glossectomy (Blyth et al., 2016; Girod-Roux et al., 2020). As a clinical phonetic tool UTI has potential utility in any studies where the phonetician believes that studying tongue movement directly is likely to add important information that phonetic transcription cannot provide. Therefore, it is mostly likely to be of use for investigating motor speech disorders; articulation disorders including cleft lip and palate; and dysfluency. For children with surface-level phonological impairments it can be important in uncovering subtle underlying motor speech constraints. Ultrasound is also used to identify subtle speech differences in speakers with visual impairments (Ménard et al., 2013), how-ever, since visually impaired speakers do not present with a speech disorder this population is beyond the scope of this chapter.

Speech errors revealed by ultrasound

Clinical phonetic applications of UTI broadly fall into four different types: (1) Comparisons with typical speakers, (2) identification of covert errors/supplementing phonetic transcription, (3) identification of covert contrasts, and (4) quantifying change post-intervention.

Comparisons with typical speakers

Studies comparing the speech of clinical populations to typical speakers using UTI are relatively sparse to date. Ultrasound offers the potential to answer theoretical questions about the nature of tongue movements in disordered speakers, yet normative data with which pathological data could be compared is relatively rare, especially in studies of children. UTI studies of typical speakers tend to answer specific questions, for example studies of coarticulation, rather than provide information about a wide variety of tongue movements. Nevertheless a few studies have attempted to compare ultrasound metrics between typical speakers and speakers from clinical groups. Heyde et al. (2016) compared peak velocity and duration of onset and offset of consonantal closure between persons who stutter and typical speakers. They demonstrated that persons who stutter display different behavior in the consonantal offset. In a number of studies comparing typical speakers with partial glossectomy patients, Bressmann and colleagues have used 3D ultrasound to measure the functional topography of the tongue prior to surgery with the hope of predicting post-surgical outcomes (see for example Bressmann, Uy, & Irish, 2004). Using scaler metrics (see Table 29.2) Carl (2018) demonstrated that speakers with Down syndrome show reduced tongue shape curvature and complexity of some vowels compared to typical speakers.

An alternative approach to comparing clinical populations to typical speakers is to compare speakers with reduced intelligibility to speakers from the same clinical group with normalized speech. Cleland et al. (2019) report on error types identified using UTI in 39 children with cleft lip and palate. Many of the children presented with few or no errors in their speech. Given the anatomical differences in cleft lip and palate, children with normalized speech serve as a better control group than typical speakers. The error types identified in this study are explored in detail in the next section.

Covert errors/supplementing phonetic transcription

There is a long history of using instrumental phonetic techniques to supplement phonetic transcription and describe covert errors. Cleland et al. (2019) demonstrated that using ultrasound to aid phonetic transcription leads to improved inter-rater reliability and reveals errors such as double articulations that were missed during traditional phonetic transcription. These covert errors are subtle unexpected articulations which suggest underlying motor constraints but do not lead to loss of contrast or pattern phonologically. For example, Cleland et al. (2017) describe a case study of a child called Rachel with persistent velar fronting who produced oral stops using a variety of different tongue shapes (retroflexes, undifferentiated gestures and typical alveolar gestures) which appeared random, rather than phonologically patterned. These error types are important because they can provide useful diagnostic information, in Rachel's case a potential motor speech disorder. Similarly, Bressmann et al. (2011) describe Sandra, a nine year old with cleft lip and palate, who alternated inaudible alveolar and velar gestures during attempts at /k/ which were transcribed as [?], again this information is important because it shows that Sandra is attempting appropriate lingual movements.

Ultrasound can also be used to confirm perception based transcription in a more objective way, for example, backing errors show as clear raising of the tongue dorsum. Table 29.3

Table 29.3 Ultrasound errors, example and expected (Ext)IPA transcriptions; darker line denotes palate

Error type	Description	Ultrasound example	Expected IPA transcription
1 Increased contact	Raising of tongue body and tip/blade toward or in contact with the hard palate		Simultaneous alveolar + postalveolar + palatal
2 Retraction to velar or palatal	Anterior target retracted to velar or palatal		Velar or palatal
3 Retraction to uvular*	Any velar or pre-velar target retracted to uvular		Uvular
4 Retraction to pharyngeal*	Any uvular or pre-uvular target retracted to pharyngeal		Pharyngeal
5 Fronted	Posterior target is fronted to palatal, post-alveolar, or alveolar		Alveolar, post-alveolar, or palatal
6 Complete Closure	No visible groove in the coronal view.		Any lateral sibilant
7 Undershoot*	No contact with palate		"lowered" diacritic, or approximant
8 Double Articulation	Simultaneous production of two consonants: normally alveolar-velar		Any double articulation, e.g. [k͡t] or [p͡t]
9 Increased Variability	Different tongue-shapes per repetition	*(dynamic analysis required)*	Different transcriptions across repetitions
10 Abnormal Timing	Mis-directed articulatory gestures or release of articulations with abnormal timing	*(dynamic analysis required)*	Any diacritic denoting timing such as lengthening marks
11 Retroflexion	Tongue tip retroflexion during any non-retroflex target		Any retroflex consonant

*An earlier version of these error types appeared in Cleland et al. (2019) without retraction to uvular and pharyngeal and where undershoot is called "open pattern."

summarizes both types of ultrasound errors as reported so far in studies of children in the Ultrasuite corpus (Eshky et al., 2019). Errors are classified broadly in line with Gibbon's 2004 taxonomy of error types identified using electropalatography in the speech of children with cleft lip and palate. Since ultrasound shows tongue shape rather than tongue palate contact, "open pattern," an EPG pattern where there is no tongue-palate contact, can be sub-divided into retraction to uvular or pharyngeal, or articulatory undershoot. Retroflex productions can also be identified using ultrasound. It is important to note that not all the error types are mutually exclusive, for example, it is possible for one segment to be retracted, variable and have unusual timing. The error types are described in more detail below.

Increased contact

Undifferentiated lingual gestures are an error type found in children with persistent SSD of unknown origin (Gibbon, 1999) where the child fails to adequately differentiate the tongue tip/blade and tongue dorsum, instead moving the whole tongue in a single undifferentiated gesture. This type of error is indicative of a problem with speech motor control and thus is important from a diagnostic and therapeutic point of view. In UTI undifferentiated gestures show as a raising of the whole tongue body, usually during an alveolar or velar target. If a hard palate has been superimposed on the image then increased or complete contact can be seen from the alveolar to velar region.

Retraction errors

Retraction errors involve production of an alveolar (or sometimes labial or labiodental) target at a more posterior place of articulation. These errors are often found in the speech of children with cleft lip and palate where compensatory backing articulations are very common (see for example Bressmann et al., 2011). These errors are typically not covert in nature, i.e. the phonetician is able to accurately transcribe an error as palatal, velar, uvular or pharyngeal. However, ultrasound analysis can lead to more accurate transcription and confirmation of place of articulation by viewing the image.

Fronted placement

Speakers who produce a target velar at an alveolar place of articulation can be seen to have fronted placement on the UTI. These errors are often phonological in nature, for example velar fronting, a common developmental phonological error, where /k/ is produced as [t] (see Cleland et al., 2017). Fronting of /k/ to a midpalatal plosive can also be observed in speakers with cleft lip and palate (Bressmann et al., 2011). Again, these errors are likely to be overt and therefore the ultrasound offers confirmatory, rather than additional information.

Complete closure

This error type is viewed in the coronal plane. In this view raising and lowering of the sides of the tongue are visible. During production of a grooved fricative such as /s/ the sides of the tongue are raised and the center grooved, producing a wing-shaped UTI. In a complete closure error both the sides and center of the tongue are raised in a dome-shaped UTI. For /s/ and /ʃ/ productions these errors will typically sound like lateral or palatal fricatives. These errors are a common residual (articulatory) speech sound error and UTI confirms phonetic transcription, rather that adds to it. A similar error, loss of concavity, is described by Bressmann et al. (2015) in speakers with lingual hemiparesis. It is not straightforward to determine from coronal ultrasound which place of articulation the complete closure occurs at because, unlike mid-sagittal views, there is no standard method of obtaining a particular coronal slice. The probe can be angled (usually by hand) to point more toward the tip or root to give some indication of the coronal slice being viewed. Alternatively, 3D ultrasound could be used to determine both place of articulation and degree of grooving.

Undershoot

In an undershoot error the tongue approaches the hard palate but fails to make contact. These types of errors are commonly described in the literature on dysarthria using other articulatory techniques, however, despite UTI being applied to patients with dysarthria in one of the first studies of disordered speech (Shawker & Sonies, 1984) it has been under-used with this population. Errors may be transcribed as weak or lowered articulations, with the ultrasound providing important information about the magnitude of undershoot. This type of error is also seen in children with Childhood Apraxia of Speech or during the therapeutic process where a child moves their tongue in the direction of an articulatory target but fails to make contact.

Double articulation

Double articulations are normally covert errors or covert contrasts. They involve two simultaneous primary places of articulation such as velar + alveolar or bilabial + velar. In the latter example, the phonetician usually transcribes a bilabial because it is visually salient, UTI provides extra information which is diagnostically important. Gibbon (2004) suggests these labio-lingual double articulations may occur as an intermediate step between an incorrect backing pattern and a correct bilabial production in children with cleft lip and palate, suggesting that presence of this error may indicate positive change in a child's speech system. Bressmann et al. (2011) also report one speaker with cleft lip and palate who used a glottal+pharyngeal double articulation for /k/. Alveo-velar double articulations are harder to identify using ultrasound because they can look very similar to increased contact. Identifying a small pocket of air between the alveolar and velar region is challenging because it relies on very good probe stabilization and spatial resolution.

Increased variability

Increased sub-phonemic variability may be indicative of a subtle motor speech disorder. In this error type the speaker produces multiple repetitions of the same speech sound with greater variability than a typical speaker. This is essentially a covert error, because typically the phonetician will transcribe each repetition using the same phonetic symbol but dynamic ultrasound analysis reveals subtle articulatory variability. Figure 29.5 shows variable productions of /k/ from one child produced during a diadochokinesis task. Single spline tracings from the burst of each production show variation in the place of the tongue shape, despite all productions being transcribed as [k].

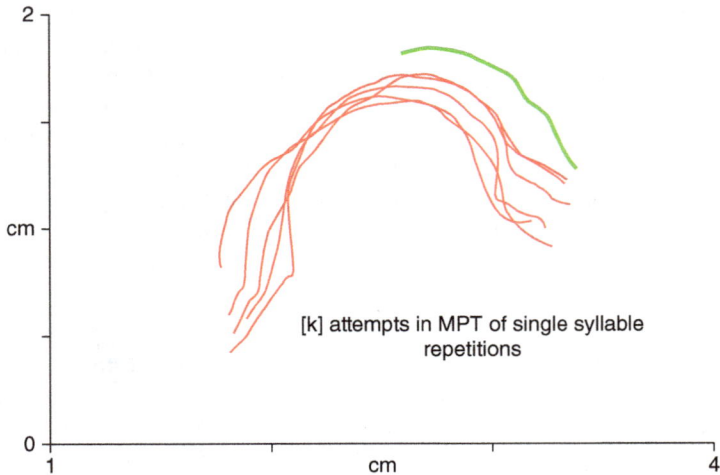

Figure 29.5 Example variability in tongue shape for six consecutive productions of [k].

Abnormal timing

Ultrasound can reveal timing errors such as abnormally long closures or misdirected gestures which may indicate difficulties with motor planning or programming. Dynamic analysis is required to identify these errors. They may be transcribed as lengthened stop closures (for example), however, even visual inspection of the ultrasound can reveal steady tongue-state during silences or long stop closures. These may also be observed in speakers with disfluencies.

Retroflex productions

Retroflexion is visually salient on ultrasound. In Cleland et al.'s (2017) case study of Rachel, retroflex stops for both alveolar and velar targets were identified from the UTI but these productions had not been transcribed as retroflex, suggesting a covert error. It is unclear why children might produce retroflexes in error in a language such as English where retroflexes only occur in the late acquired articulatory complex /r/ target. Another study, Cleland et al. (2015) suggested that one child with persistent velar fronting produced a retroflex stop for /k/ only in a stimulability task where he was instructed to try to produce [k], in this case the explanation for the error could be a conscious effort from the child to produce a more posterior articulation.

Covert contrast

The term covert contrast is used to describe differences in perceptually neutralized contrasts which can be identified instrumentally. For example, a Speech-Language Pathologist may identify that a child is unable to make a contrast between /t/ and /k/, producing both as [t], however acoustic or articulatory analysis may show small differences between these target phonemes. This is important diagnostically because a child with a covert contrast may have a motor speech problem rather than a phonological one. Two studies have attempted to identify covert contrasts using UTI (Cleland et al., 2017 and McAllister Byun et al., 2016) and a further paper (Zharkova, Gibbon & Lee, 2017) gives suggestions of metrics for identifying covert contrast and a case study of a typically developing child with covert contrast between /s/ and /ʃ/. Identifying covert

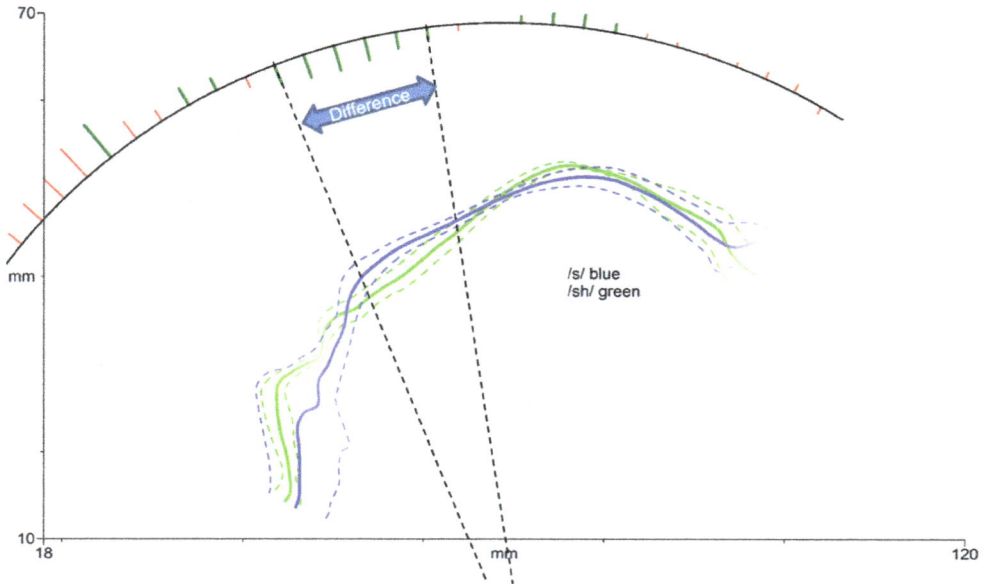

Figure 29.6 Averaged /s/ (blue) and /ʃ/ (green) productions showing difference in the tongue root despite both being transcribed as [ʃ].

contrasts in children with speech sound disorders first requires recording the child saying minimal pair words containing the target phonemes (or at least words where the vowel environment is controlled) preferably multiple times. Figure 29.6 shows average tongue shapes for /s/ and /ʃ/ in a child with cleft lip and palate, both were transcribed as [ʃ]. By comparing the tongue shapes visually we can see that although the tongue shapes overlap in the anterior region, there is an area in the root where the shapes are differentiated. The t-test function in AAA confirms a statistical difference, this child therefore has a covert contrast between these phonemes.

The Cleland et al. (2017) and McAllister Byun et al. (2016) papers both attempted to find covert contrast in children with velar fronting. This particular phonological process is common in the speech of typically developing children, but can persist. In both studies children with velar fronting were recorded saying multiple words with velar and alveolar targets and these were then compared to determine if there were any differences in tongue shape between the two target phonemes. The McAllister Byun study also employed acoustic analysis. By comparing tongue shapes for /t/ and /k/ using the in-built t-test function in AAA software, Cleland et al. (2017) showed that the children in their study showed no evidence of covert contrast. McAllister Byun et al. (2016) employed the ratio metric, DEI, in their study of two children with perceptually neutralized velars and found evidence of convert contrast in one child. These studies exemplify the two different approaches to analyzing ultrasound data: Cleland et al. (2017) using headset stabilization to compare sets of tongue curves directly and McAllister Byun et al. (2016) using a scaler metric which can be calculated independent of translation and rotation.

Quantifying change post-intervention

The majority of studies using ultrasound as a biofeedback tool use perceptual measures to quantify change post-intervention (Sugden et al., 2019). As well as being easier to undertake, perceptual measures have ecological validity. A small number of studies have used ultrasound metrics to measure change post-intervention. This has the advantage of being free from listener-bias and has the potential to be automated. Cleland et al. (2015) use the t-test function within AAA to show quantifiable differences in tongue shape after intervention for seven children with a variety of speech sound errors. This approach is suitable for measuring changes in any intervention target which involves changing the shape or position of the tongue, which is likely to be the case for all ultrasound visual biofeedback therapy. However, it requires collecting assessment data with a probe stabilizing headset and aligning sessions using a hard palate trace and therefore may not be suitable for all intervention studies, particularly with younger children.

An alternative approach is to use scaler metrics to measure changes. A number of those shown in Table 29.2 would be appropriate to use with specific targets. For example, DEI would be a good choice for measuring changes post-intervention for children with fronting or backing patterns. The NINFL metric has been used to measure changes in tongue complexity post intervention for children with rhotic distortions (Preston et al., 2019), showing that after intervention children adopt more complex tongue shapes and that this correlates well with perceptual accuracy.

Conclusion

Ultrasound Tongue Imaging is a safe and useful technique for viewing and quantifying tongue shape and movement. When tongue movements are viewed in real time it is a useful biofeedback tool in the speech pathology clinic, showing promise of being effective in remediating persistent or residual speech sound disorders (Sugden et al., 2019). In the clinical phonetics lab ultrasound is a relatively new tool, having been hampered in the past by low frame rates; difficulties synchronized ultrasound to audio; and difficulties analyzing the resultant data. Technological advances have led to several different ultrasound systems and software now being available at affordable prices. This coupled with the ease of acquisition of ultrasound data, even in small children, suggests that this technique is set to become standard equipment for clinical phoneticians.

Ultrasound can be used to identify all of the errors described in the electropalatography literature (Cleland et al., 2019) and advances in metrics for describing ultrasound data illustrate the potential to use this technique to measure tongue movement in a wide variety of clinical populations, either for answering theoretical questions or measuring progress during biofeedback intervention.

References

Articulate Instruments Ltd, (2012). *Articulate Assistant Advanced User Guide: Version 2.14.* Edinburgh, UK: Articulate Instruments Ltd.

Aubin, J., & Ménard, L. (2006). Compensation for a labial perturbation: An acoustic and articulatory study of child and adult French speakers. In H.C. Yehia, D. Demolin, & R. Laboissière (Eds.), *Proceedings of the 7th International Seminar on Speech Production* (pp. 209–216), Ubatuba, Brazil.

Belmont, A. (2015). *Anticipatory coarticulation and stability of speech in typically fluent speakers and people who stutter across the lifespan: An ultrasound study Master of Science thesis.* University of South Florida.

Blyth, K.M., Mccabe, P., Madill, C., & Ballard, K.J. (2016). Ultrasound visual feedback in articulation therapy following partial glossectomy. *J Commun Disord, 61,* 1–15.

Boyce, S., Tiede, M., Espy-Wilson, C. Y., & Groves-Wright, K. (2015). Diversity of tongue shapes for the American English rhotic liquid. In The Scottish Consortium for ICPhS 2015 (Ed.), *Proceedings of the 18th International Congress of Phonetic Sciences.* Glasgow, UK: the University of Glasgow. ISBN 978-0-85261-941-4. Paper number 847.1-4 retrieved from http://www.internationalphoneticassociation.org/icphs-proceedings/ICPhS2015/Papers/ICPHS0847.pdf

Bressmann, T., Koch, S., Ratner, A., Seigel, J., & Binkofski, F. (2015). An ultrasound investigation of tongue shape in stroke patients with lingual hemiparalysis. *J Stroke Cerebrovasc Dis*, *24*(4), 834–839.

Bressmann, T., Harper, S., Zhylich, I., & Kulkarni, G.V. (2016). Perceptual, durational and tongue displacement measures following articulation therapy for rhotic sound errors. *Clin Linguist Phon*, *30*(3-5), 345–362.

Bressmann, T., Radovanovic, B., Kulkarni, G.V., Klaiman, P., & Fisher, D. (2011). An ultrasonographic investigation of cleft-type compensatory articulations of voiceless velar stops. *Clin Linguist Phon*, *25*(11-12), 1028–1033.

Bressmann, T., Thind, P., Uy, C., Bollig, C., Gilbert, R.W., & Irish, J.C. (2005). Quantitative three-dimensional ultrasound analysis of tongue protrusion, grooving and symmetry: Data from 12 normal speakers and a partial glossectomee. *Clin Linguist Phon*, *19*(6–7), 573–588.

Bressmann, T., Uy, C., & Irish, J.C. (2005). Analysing normal and partial glossectomee tongues using ultrasound. *Clin Linguist Phon*, *19*(1), 35–52.

Carl, M. (2018). *Vowel Production in Down Syndrome: An Ultrasound Study*. Unpublished PhD dissertation. City University New York, New York.

Cleland, J., Lloyd, S., Campbell, L., Crampin, L., Palo, J.P., Sugden, E., Wrench, A., & Zharkova, N. (2019). The impact of real-time articulatory information on phonetic transcription: ultrasound-aided transcription in cleft lip and palate speech. *Folia Phoniatr Logop*, *72*(2), 120–130.

Cleland, J., & Preston, J. (2021). Biofeedback interventions. In A.L. Williams, S. McLeod, R.J. McCauley (Eds.) *Interventions for Speech Sound Disorders in Children* (2nd Ed.; pp. 1–50). Baltimore: Paul H Brookes Pub Co.

Cleland, J., & Scobbie, J.M. (2018). Acquisition of new speech motor plans via articulatory visual biofeedback. In S. Fuchs, J. Cleland, and A. Rochet-Cappelan (Eds.). *Speech Perception and Production: Learning and Memory.* Berlin: Peter Lang

Cleland, J., Scobbie, J.M., Heyde, C., Roxburgh, Z., & Wrench, A.A. (2017). Covert contrast and covert errors in persistent velar fronting. *Clin Linguist Phon*, *31*(1), 35–55.

Cleland, J., Scobbie, J.M., & Wrench, A.A. (2015). Using ultrasound visual biofeedback to treat persistent primary speech sound disorders. *Clin Linguist Phon*, *29*(8–10), 575–597.

Dawson, K.M., Tiede, M.K., & Whalen, D.H. (2016). Methods for quantifying tongue shape and complexity using ultrasound imaging. *Clin Linguist Phon*, *30*(3–5), 328–344.

Eshky, A., Ribeiro, M.S., Cleland, J., Richmond, K., Roxburgh, Z., Scobbie, J., & Wrench, A. (2019). UltraSuite: A repository of ultrasound and acoustic data from child speech therapy sessions. *arXiv preprint arXiv:1907.00835.*

Girod-Roux, M., Hueber, T., Fabre, D., Gerber, S., Canault, M., Bedoin, N., … & Badin, P. (2020). Rehabilitation of speech disorders following glossectomy, based on ultrasound visual illustration and feedback. *Clin Linguist Phon, 34*, 1–18.

Gibbon, F.E. (1999). Undifferentiated lingual gestures in children with articulation/phonological disorders. *J Speech Lang Hear Res*, *42*(2), 382–397.

Gibbon, F.E. (2004). Abnormal patterns of tongue-palate contact in the speech of individuals with cleft palate. *Clin Linguist Phon*, *18*(4–5), 285–311.

Gu, J., Bressmann, T., Cannons, K., and Wong, W. (2004). *The Ultrasonographic Contour Analyzer for Tongue Surfaces (Ultra-CATS)*, University of Toronto, Toronto, ON, Canada.

Heyde, C.J., Scobbie, J.M., Lickley, R., & Drake, E.K. (2016). How fluent is the fluent speech of people who stutter? A new approach to measuring kinematics with ultrasound. *Clin Linguist Phon*, *30*(3–5), 292–312.

Kelsey, C.A., Minifie, F.D., & Hixon, T.J. (1969). Applications of ultrasound in speech research. *Journal of Speech and Hearing Research*, *12*(3), 564–575.

Lawson, E., Scobbie, J.M., & Stuart-Smith, J. (2011). The social stratification of tongue shape for postvocalic/r/in Scottish English1. *J Sociolinguist*, *15*(2), 256–268.

Lee, S.A.S., Wrench, A., & Sancibrian, S. (2015). How to get started with ultrasound technology for treatment of speech sound disorders. *Persp Speech Sci Orofac Disord*, *25*(2), 66–80.

Ménard, L., Toupin, C., Baum, S.R., Drouin, S., Aubin, J., & Tiede, M. (2013). Acoustic and articulatory analysis of French vowels produced by congenitally blind adults and sighted adults. *J Acoust Soc Am*, *134*(4), 2975–2987.

McAllister Byun, T., Buchwald, A., & Mizoguchi, A. (2016). Covert contrast in velar fronting: An acoustic and ultrasound study. *Clin Linguist Phon*, *30*(3–5), 249–276.

Noiray, A., Abakarova, D., Rubertus, E., Krüger, S., & Tiede, M. (2018). How do children organize their speech in the first years of life? Insight from ultrasound imaging. *J Speech Lang Hear Res, 61*(6), 1355–1368.

Preston, J.L., McCabe, P., Tiede, M., & Whalen, D.H. (2019). Tongue shapes for rhotics in school-age children with and without residual speech errors. *Clin Linguist Phon, 33*(4), 334–348.

Preston, J.L., & Leaman, M. (2014). Ultrasound visual feedback for acquired apraxia of speech: A case report. *Aphasiology, 28*(3), 278–295.

Roxburgh, Z. (2018). *Visualising articulation: real-time ultrasound visual biofeedback and visual articulatory models and their use in treating speech sound disorders associated with submucous cleft palate.* Unpublished PhD dissertation. Queen Margaret University, Edinburgh.

Scobbie, J.M., & Cleland, J. (2017). Area and radius based mid-sagittal measurements of comparative velarity. *Ultrafest VIII, Potsdam, Germany.*

Shawker, T.H., & Sonies Phd, B.C. (1984). Tongue movement during speech: A real-time ultrasound evaluation. *J Clin Ultrasound, 12*(3), 125–133.

Sugden, E., Lloyd, S., Lam, J., & Cleland, J. (2019). Systematic review of ultrasound visual biofeedback in intervention for speech sound disorders. *Int J Lang Commun Disord, 54*(5), 705–728.

Whalen, D.H., Iskarous, K., Tiede, M.K., Ostry, D.J., Lehnert-LeHouillier, H., Vatikiotis-Bateson, E., & Hailey, D.S. (2005). The Haskins optically corrected ultrasound system (HOCUS). *J Speech Lang Hear Res, 48*, 543–553.

Wrench, A.A., & Scobbie, J.M. (2011). Very high frame rate ultrasound tongue imaging. In Proceedings of the 9th International Seminar on Speech Production (ISSP) (pp. 155–162), Montreal, Canada

Zharkova, N. (2013). A normative-speaker validation study of two indices developed to quantify tongue dorsum activity from midsagittal tongue shapes. *Clin Linguist Phon, 27*(6–7), 484–496.

Zharkova, N. (2013). Using ultrasound to quantify tongue shape and movement characteristics. *Cleft Palate Craniofac J, 50*(1), 76–81.

Zharkova, N., Gibbon, F.E., & Lee, A. (2017). Using ultrasound tongue imaging to identify covert contrasts in children's speech. *Clinical Linguist Phon, 31*(1), 21–34

Zharkova, N., & Hewlett, N. (2009). Measuring lingual coarticulation from midsagittal tongue contours: Description and example calculations using English/t/and/ɑ/. *J Phonet, 37*(2), 248–256.

Instrumental analysis of acoustic, auditory, and perceptual phonetics

30

SOUND SPECTROGRAPHY

Chiara Meluzzi

Introduction

This chapter aims at providing the reader with a short and comprehensive introduction to the spectrographic analysis of speech and its applications in clinical linguistics. Since the development of the first sound spectrograph, also called sonograph, in the 1940s (Koenig et al., 1946), the rapid change in both instruments for data collection and sound analysis have greatly improved the potential for acoustic analysis of speech signals, enhancing our understanding of speech production and perception also in relation to sound change (Ohala, 1993). A radical innovation in spectrography has been introduced with digital signal processing (Farmer, 1997, p. 22) and the development of different software for digital audio analysis. Fujimura and Erickson (1997) recall that Potter et al. (1966) developed the first visual representation of speech: Visible Speech displayed sound as a two-dimensional time-frequency function called a spectrogram. Nowadays, there are many software available to perform spectrographic or digital audio analysis (e.g. Matlab, Python, C Speech, Speech Analyzer, Voice Vista, just to mention a few). In this chapter we will refer in particular to PRAAT (Boersma & Weenink, 2020) which is an open resource available for Windows, Macintosh, Chromebook, Raspberry Pi and Linux, with a large community of users online composed by both linguists and engineers. All the examples presented in the following sections were recorded by the author with a TASCAM DR-20 recorder, at a frequency of 44.1 kHz with a sampling rate of 16 bit (see Vogel & Reece, Chapter 18, this volume); visualization and annotation have be performed in PRAAT 6.0.37.

The chapter is organized as follows: the first section provides some basic concepts of acoustics and spectrography, thus also introducing the PRAAT software; the second section introduces the acoustic analysis of speech, by discussing how vowels, obstruents, nasals, liquids and rhotics appear on a spectrogram and which values are usually analyzed, while the third section will present some spectrographic studies in clinical phonetics.

Basic notions in the acoustics of speech signal

In general, acoustic phonetics deals with the description of different acoustic signals produced when vocal organs move during speech, thus generating the vibration of air molecules (Harrington, 2013, p. 81). The most widespread theory behind acoustic phonetics is the so-called source-filter model (Fant, 1960), which assumes an idealized vocal tract with the source being the origin of the airflow and the filter consisting of every modification of the vocal tract occurring because of the movements of the different articulatory organs. The source-filter model assumes a certain degree of linearity between speech production and acoustics; however, the quantal theory of speech production (Stevens, 1972) looks at this relationship as nonlinear and focuses on discontinuities (see also Stevens & Hanson, 2013).

When a speech sound is produced, the human acoustic apparatus perceives a series of frequencies within a certain range (16–20.000 Hz, for more details on speech perception see Pisoni, 2017, and Neger et. al., 2015, Janse and Rietveld, Chapter 4, and McGuire, Chapter 34, this volume), transformed into electrical impulses by the basilar membrane and the Organ of Corti. The frequency is an inherent characteristic of the sound: it represents the number of oscillations made in 1 second, and it is measured in Hertz (Hz). Speech is usually between 100 and 16.000 Hz. Another common measure is the amplitude of a sound wave (or waveform): it is conventionally expressed in decibel (dB) and represents the increase or decrease of air pressure at a given point during phonation (Ladefoged, 1962).

Sounds can be cataloged as pure or complex sound waves; complex waves can be again divided between harmonic and non-harmonic sounds, the last possibly being with or without harmonic components. In the acoustic analysis of speech, it is important to remember that we are dealing with complex waves. Pure sounds repeat the same oscillatory movement periodically in time, and this movement is represented by a single sinusoid curve expressible with a single frequency; unfortunately, these sounds do not appear in nature, but they can be produced artificially (e.g. by a programmed script). Complex wave sounds, such as human speech, can in turn have harmonics or be without harmonics. The first typology of complex sounds can have a periodicity but without a sinusoidal trend: they consist in a sum of various simple wave sounds. A third category is represented by aperiodic wave sounds, which are usually referred to as noise events. Moreover, in analyzing speech we deal with either complex or aperiodic waves, but also silence, which is the absence of vibration of the vocal folds, identifiable as lack of information on the spectrogram. In the next section we will see all these notions applied in detail, but to give an example for each category, vowels represent complex wave sounds with a harmonic component, fricatives represent noise, while voiceless plosives are characterized by a silence corresponding to the holding phase before the release of the articulators.

In comparison to noise or silence, complex wave sounds are the most studied in speech acoustics, because they are continuous sounds and present certain physical features that are directly connected with both the articulatory characteristics of the vocal tract and the physiology of the speaker. Complex waves consist of a sum of simple waves, each of them being a multiple of the fundamental frequency (F0), also called first harmonic. In articulatory terms, the F0 defines the number of vocal fold vibrations in a specific unit of time, and, as a consequence, F0 can be found only for voiced sounds. The fundamental frequency is one of the principal features of a speech sound, and it is also used in studying voice quality (see Garellek, 2019). It is also primarily linked to the perception of voice pitch, alongside with other factors (e.g. intensity, see Fujimura & Erickson, 1997). Complex wave forms can contain specific harmonic components, which are integer multiples of the fundamental frequency. An example of a complex sound with harmonic components is the central note of the piano, with an energy peak at 440 Hz and the other harmonics as multiples of the first one (i.e. 880 Hz, 1720 Hz and so on).

Moreover, the first harmonic (F0), like every other harmonic, is inversely related to the length of the tube, and this means that the lower the articulatory tube the higher the harmonics. The principle is the same as a comparison of a violin with a cello, and, thus, women have higher frequency values than men. It is generally assumed that the idealized epilaryngeal tube of a male speaker has an average length of about 17.5 cm.

As said, in the source-filter model every modification of the vocal tract has effects on the pressure and the frequency of the airflow. Channel restrictions, also called "nodes," increase the frequency by amplifying the sound wave in peaks called resonances or formants, whereas channel openings or "anti-nodes" create a frequency drop and a weakening of the harmonics, thus generating anti-resonance in the vocal tract filter known as anti-formants (Fujimura & Erickson, 1997). The position of nodes and antinodes in the articulation of a sound generates formants and anti-formants, whose values help distinguishing the different sounds, as we will see more fully for vowels.

Before moving to the characteristics specific of each sound class, a few words must be devoted to the visual representation called spectrographic analysis. In particular, a distinction must be applied between "spectrum" and "spectrogram," two terms sometimes confusing and confused.

In acoustic phonetics, a spectrum of frequencies is a visual representation of a single point in time of a speech sound, in the frequency domain. As reconstructed by Fulop (2011, p. 2), the term spectrum was first used by seventeenth century scientists studying light, and applied to sound analysis only two centuries later. This occurred first when J. Fourier demonstrated that sound signals are complex wave sounds composed of a sum of simple waves, and then in 1936 when Lewis proposed a new spectrum for studying vocal resonance. Conversely, a spectrogram is a representation of the spectrum which also accounts for time. In Figure 30.1 the word "spectrography" is shown, as visualized in PRAAT: in the upper box, the spectrum presents the frequency on the x-axis and the amplitude on the y-axis; in the lower box, the spectrogram has the time on the x-axis, the frequency on the y-axis, whereas the degree of darkness of the image represents the differences in amplitude.

Although this may seem simple, it is important to keep in mind that spectra (as well as spectrograms) are mathematically derived from sound signals. As we said, spectrum analysis has its core in Fourier's demonstration of how a periodic function could be expressed as the sum of exponential component functions, called harmonics of the function (Fulop, 2011, p. 18).

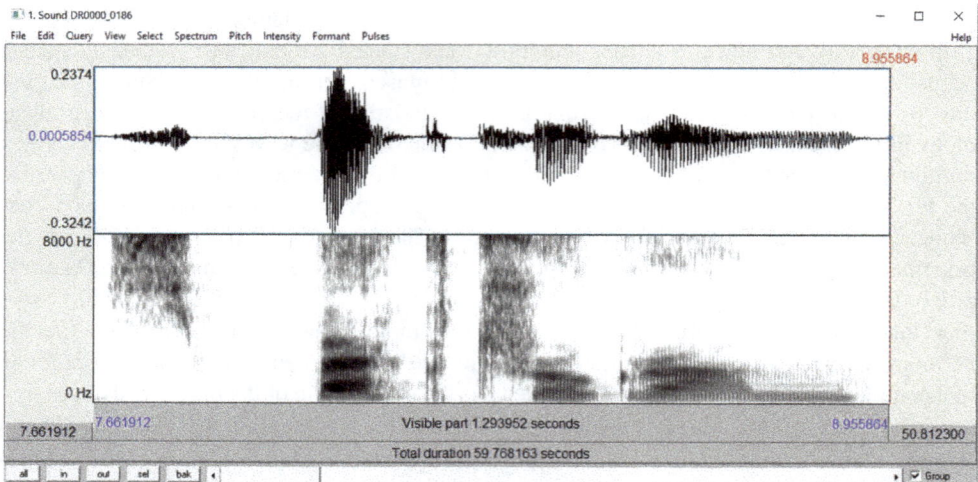

Figure 30.1 Spectrum and spectrogram representation of the word "spectrography" as visualized in PRAAT.

Therefore, we can have different spectra and spectrograms according to the techniques adopted. The most common spectrum is a power spectrum obtained through a Fast Fourier Transform (FFT spectra), taken at a specific location on the waveform and with frequency values on the x-axis and intensity on the y-axis (see also Fulop, 2011, p. 26–34). Conversely, there are spectra which are not based on waveforms, that is on an amplitude-time function, but on what is called an envelope, that is the display of total distribution of frequencies in a sound signal (Farmer, 1997, p. 23). Spectral envelopes are used in the Linear Predictive Coding (LPC) formula, which generates LPC spectra. Other techniques could be applied to model vowel spectra, such as the principal components analysis (PCA, Klein et al., 1970) or the discrete cosine transformation (DCT, Zahorian & Jagharghi, 1993): PCA accounts better for data with a high variance, in which formant tracking could be difficult, like in child speech (see Palethorpe et al., 1996), whereas DCT coefficients have proven to be very accurate in distinguishing different vowels in particular in automatic speech recognition (Milner & Shao, 2006). As for spectrograms, an important distinction has to be made between wideband and narrowband spectrograms: the main difference is the transmission rate, since wideband spectrograms support a higher transmission rate than narrowband ones. Conversely, narrowband spectrograms provide better frequency resolution than wideband ones (see also Farmer, 1997; Harrington, 2013; Fulop, 2011).

The reader will find more useful information and explanations in introductory manuals to acoustics starting from the classic Joss (1948), and then the works by Peter Ladefoged (e.g. Ladefoged, 1964). More recent manuals in acoustic phonetics include (but are not limited to) Fulop (2011), in particular on the difference between power spectra, Stevens (2000), and the chapter by Harrington (2013). On PRAAT, the vast majority of resources are available on the software's website (http://www.fon.hum.uva.nl/praat/); other manuals are also listed and available from the same website, including tutorials on how to perform automatic analysis through PRAAT scripts.

Spectrographic analysis of speech

Spectrographic analysis of speech is still a growing field of research. Although articulatory analysis has seen a rapid development in both techniques and methods, there is still a demand for integrating the acoustic and articulatory analysis, in particular in clinical phonetics. Acoustic analysis remains widely used since it has some major advantages over articulatory fieldwork studies, the main ones being the affordability of instruments for performing both data elicitation and the following visualization and analysis. Since it is a noninvasive technique, speech samples can be easily recorded at different points in time and with many different subjects. Obviously, sample dimension together with research and annotation protocols depend on the accuracy of the research questions: this topic has been widely addressed in experimental phonetics, and also recently in clinical linguistics and phonetics (see Müller & Ball, 2017, in particular the chapter by Vesna Milder, Mildner, 2017).

In this section, different sound classes will be discussed with their spectrographic characteristics, and with the main methodologies applied in phonetic literature for their analysis. As noted at the beginning of the chapter, all examples provided belong to the voice of the author, thus a 33-year-old female Italian-L1 speaker, and data are visualized and annotated in PRAAT 6.1.09 (Boersma & Weenink, 2020). At the end of each session, a brief overview is provided on the most recent works in clinical phonetics involving the sounds concerned, leaving to the following section a more comprehensive analysis of advances in spectrography for speech pathology. Since there are already different and comprehensive reviews of acoustic studies in speech pathology, in this section only the most recent publications will be included.

The reader will find an accurate presentation of works on spectrography prior to the new millennium in Farmer (1997), with important updates made by Ball and Lowry (2001), Windsor et al. (2012) and, finally, Katz (2019). Further suggested readings are also the manuals by Ladefoged (2005), Stevens (2000), Fulop (2011) and also Fry (2009) for a series of introductory readings on this topic; Di Paolo and Yaeger Dror (2011) and Thomas (2010) also present insights from a sociophonetic perspective into acoustic analysis for different sound classes together with the most common acoustic measures adopted.

Vowels

Together with Voice Onset Time (VOT) for obstruents (see below), vowels are one of the most studied variables in phonetic research and all the related subfields like sociophonetics and clinical phonetics. The reader will find a useful guide on vowel analysis from both an acoustic and a kinematic perspective as well as applications in speech pathology in the handbook edited by Ball and Gibbon (2013). At the end of this section, more references will also be provided.

From an articulatory perspective, in the production of vowels there is no constriction of the epilaryngeal tube, thus the airflow is modified according to the degree of proximity between the tongue and the palate, both in the vertical axe (high vs. low tongue movement) and in the horizontal axe (front vs. back movement). These two movements of the tongue shrink and broaden the channel at different points, thus creating different effects of resonance and anti-resonance: for instance, if the shrinking happens near a velocity node, that is where the pressure is at its maximum, the frequency of resonance increases. Conversely, if the shrinking happens in the proximity of an antinode, that is where the oral pressure is at its minimum, the frequency of resonance decreases. Figure 30.2, inspired by Giannini and Pettorino' work (1992, p. 127), offers a visual representation of the phonatory mechanism in the production of the three cardinal vowels [i]/[a]/[u] with the position of nodes and antinodes with respect to first and second formant.

In practical terms, this means that the shape of the tongue during the production of a vowel characterizes the acoustic frequencies of the soundwave according to the distribution of nodes and antinodes and the relative constrictions or openings of the channel. This correlates to the different frequencies of the formants. In particular, the first formant (F1) relates to the degree of opening of the vowels, with [a] having the highest F1 and the high vowels [i] and [u] the lowest, and the second formant (F2) is proportionally related to the degree of anteriority, thus [i] showing the highest values and [u] the lowest.

Moreover, it is worth remembering that a third factor affects the production of vowels, namely the degree of protrusion of the lips, with the well-known division between rounded versus unrounded vowels (Ladefoged & Maddieson, 1990). This distinction could be phonologically implemented in different languages but could also be determined by an idiosyncrasy of the speaker or by a pathological condition.

Figure 30.3 shows how vowels appear on the waveform and the spectrogram as visualized in PRAAT: the example considers again the three cardinal vowels [a], [i] and [u] pronounced in isolation. By using the function "Formants > Show formants," red dots will appear on the spectrogram (Figure 30.3b) showing, as the name suggests, the position and movement of all the visible formants, with analysis based on LPC. This visualization could be helpful for beginners to start visualizing formants and formant trajectories, but also it will help in understanding if the software (and, as a consequence, the possible automatic scripts) is working correctly or if there is some overlap or issues in the automatic process of formant recognition. For instance, in a thesis about vowels produced by hearing impaired adult speakers that I supervised (D'Aco, 2019), the automatic F2 values of [u] were drastically higher than the expected 850 Hz for an Italian male adult

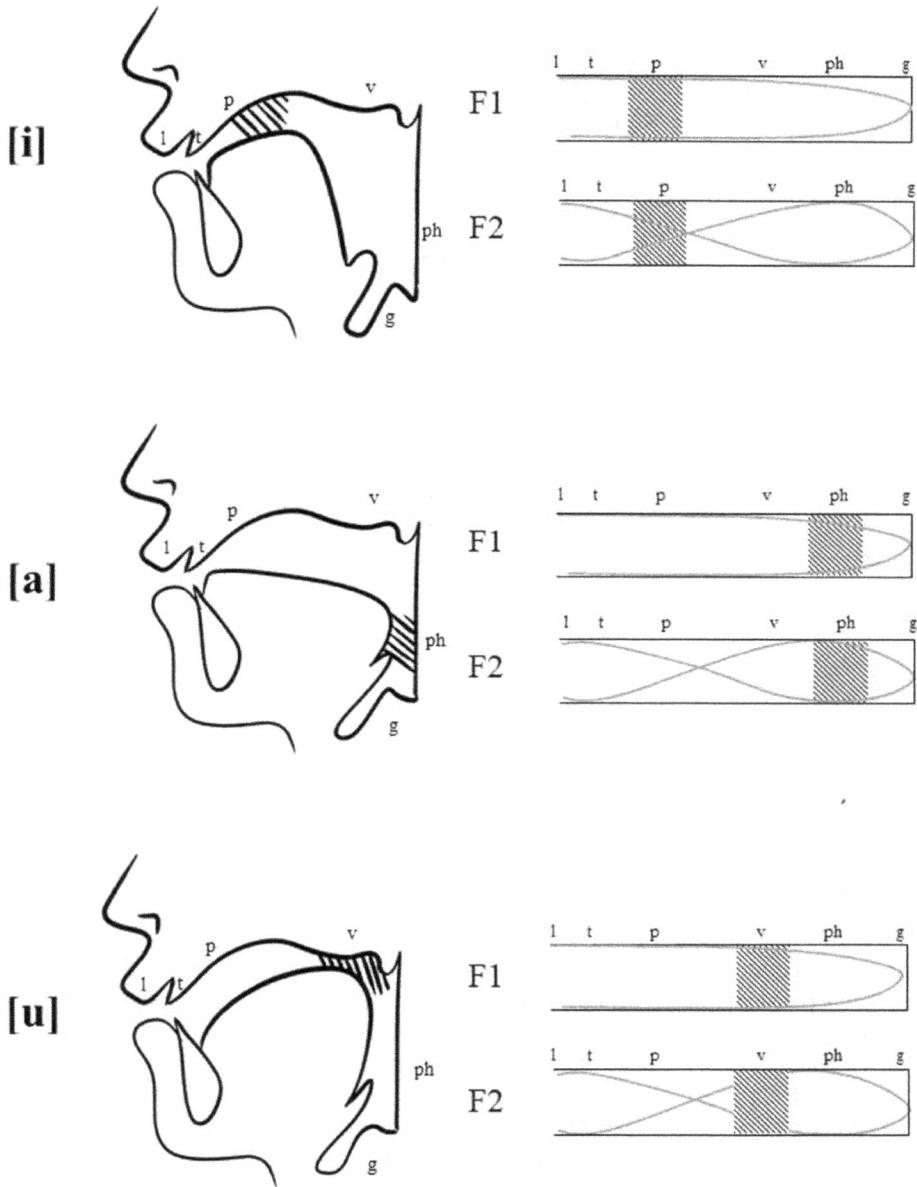

Figure 30.2 The epilaryngeal channel and F1/F2 variation during the production of [i], [a] and [u] Lips (l); Teeth (t); Palate (p); Velum (v); Pharynx (ph); Glottis (g).

speaker (Giannini & Pettorino, 1992). A visual inspection of the formants automatically identified on PRAAT revealed that F1 and F2 were too near to each other to be perceived as coincident by the software. Therefore, the reported automatic values for F2 were the frequencies of the third formant (F3). The moral of the story is that a manual check is always necessary before moving to the analysis, especially when working on pathological speech.

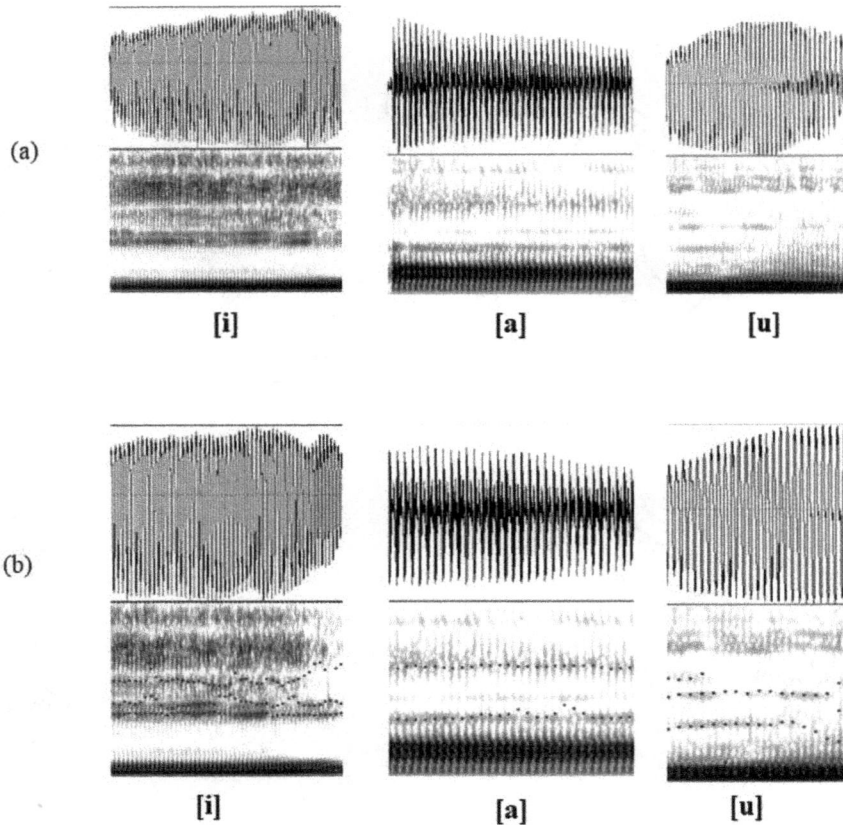

Figure 30.3 (a) Spectrum and spectrogram of the vowels [i], [a] and [u] in PRAAT; (b) The automatic display of vowel formants in PRAAT (red dots).

Many works have provided reference formant values for different languages, often considering the realization of male speakers in their 30s without cognitive, hearing or speaking impairments (e.g. Ladefoged, 1996; Hillenbrand et al., 1995 for American for English, Giannini & Pettorino, 1992 for Italian). It is important to keep in mind that female voices, as well as children's speech, will show generally higher formants values, since they depend on the length of the epilaryngeal channel, and that this length has an inverse proportion with formant values (see above). In clinical phonetics, it is, thus, particularly important to consider if the epilaryngeal tube has possibly suffered modifications that could affect formants (as well as F0, Harrington, 2013) in comparison to control groups. This makes questionable whether and to what extent it is possible to compare values across speakers. Over the years, different normalization procedures have been implemented, in both acoustic and linguistic fields: the most widespread formula remains Lobanov (1971), albeit others prefer to normalize Hertz values to the Bark scale (Traunmüller, 1990). However, some scholars have warned against the acritical use of normalization procedures, since they all tend to reduce the variability within the sample, leading to over-generalizations especially if the sample dimension is not wide enough (as it is often the case in clinical phonetics). Adank (2003) and Van der Harst (2011) both offer a critical discussion on normalization procedures and their pros and cons.

Three main kinds of acoustic analysis could be conducted on vowels: target-analysis, dynamic analysis and vowel space analysis. Target analysis (also referred to as static analysis) is usually the most common: formants values are extracted at the midpoint of the vowels under investigation (usually stressed ones), in order to avoid coarticulatory problems with the adjacent consonants. Obviously, if your investigation focuses on C-to-V or V-to-C coarticulation (e.g. Recasens, 1999, 2014; Rubertus & Noiray, 2018 on children's speech), then you might prefer a target point closer to the boundary between the two acoustic intervals. Conversely, dynamic analysis usually involves the extraction of formant values at different time points (5 or 7, depending on vowel length) at equal distance between each other. This kind of data allows the analysis of vowel trajectory over phonation till the reach (and maintenance) of the target phone, i.e. the arrival at a steady-state. Examples of dynamic analysis in clinical phonetics have focused on speech pathologies involving articulatory motor problems (e.g. Ziegler & von Cramon, 1986; Maassen et al., 2001). A third common measurement is the so-called vowel space: this can be calculated using the Euclidean distance between F1 and F2 (Nycz & Hall-Lew, 2013, p. 3), with values proportionally associated with distance between target phones in the vowel space. Moreover, vowel space can be used to test vowel reduction (Wright, 2004).

A useful method to visually inspect formant variation, in particular for dynamic analysis and for investigating the vowel space, is to plot formant values in a Cartesian space, with F2 on the x-axis and F1 on the y-axis. Although many different software packages are available for providing such graphic representations, a useful and free tool is the online application Visible Vowels (Heeringa & Van de Velde, 2018), which also automatically provides different formant normalizations. Figure 30.4 shows a possible output of a small vowel sample plotted on Visible Vowels (from Cenceschi et al., 2021).

Neumeyer et al. (2010) applied vowel space in their analysis of the productions of two groups of young and adult speakers with cochlear implants and their respective control groups. Speakers produced five German long vowels /a:, e:, i:, o:, u:/ in real disyllabic words in a sentence-reading task. Vowels were represented dynamically (see Harrington et al., 2008 for the methodology) and then the Euclidean distance from each vowel token to the center of the vowel space was calculated. Vowel space has also been used to compare the productions of speakers with and without Parkinson's disease (Rusz et al., 2011; Whitfield & Mehta, 2019; Exner, 2019), dysarthric speech (Le et al., 2017), speech of people with hearing impairment (Nicolaidis & Sfakiannaki, 2007 on Greek data), and apraxia of speech (den Ouden et al., 2018; Galkina et al., 2018).

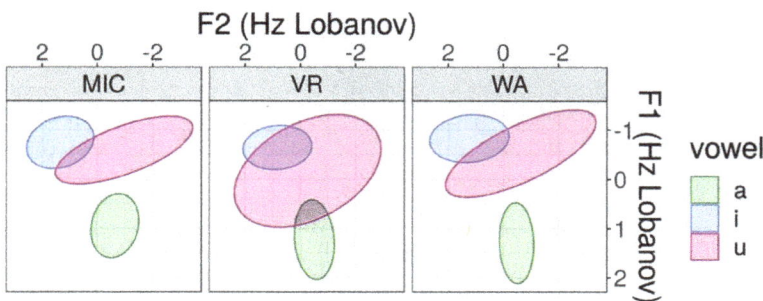

Figure 30.4 The visualization of three vowel spaces created in Visible Vowels, according to recording modality and with automatic Lobanov's normalization (data from Cenceschi et al., 2021).

Obstruents

Obstruent sounds include both stops (or plosives) and fricatives, and they are both also called "true" consonants (Fujimura & Erickson, 1997). They are characterized by a constriction along the acoustic channel, which could be either complete (for stops) or partial (for fricatives). Obstruents can also be realized with or without vibration of the vocal folds, thus resulting in voiced or voiceless sounds. It is worth remembering, especially for those who work in speech pathology, that a certain degree of devoicing, both in stops and fricatives, could be language-specific, thus not necessarily linked to articulatory problems (Thomas, 2010, p. 125–127). The reader will find useful references on devoicing, both in phonetics and speech pathology, in Ball and Müller (2016).

Stops are characterized by a complete closure of the vocal tract involving a strong contact between articulators, either lips or tongue-palate, and an abrupt release of the airflow. This articulatory configuration is reflected in the spectrum (and the spectrogram), where stops are clearly identifiable by a moment of silence followed by a spike or burst (Figure 30.5). Fujimura and Erickson (1997) also note that in the case of dorsal stops more than one burst could be

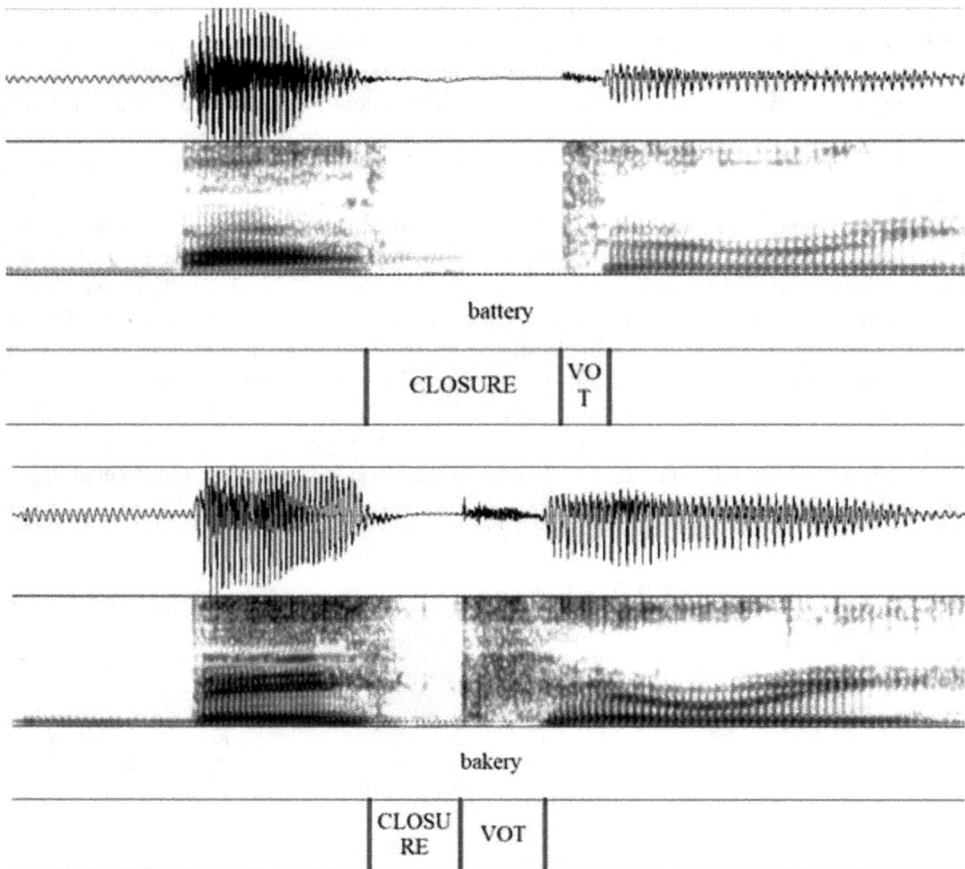

Figure 30.5 (Above) The spectrum and spectrogram of [t:] in the word *battery*. (Below) The spectrum and spectrogram of [k] in the word *bakery*. The second tier shows the annotations of closures and VOTs.

visible. Moreover, since each stop may be at a different place of constriction (lips for labials, tongue tip for apicals, and tongue body for dorsals), it is possible to detect the place of articulation thanks to formant transitions in the adjacent vowels (see Stevens, 2000, and Delattre et al., 1955 for the so-called "formant loci"). Geminated stop consonants are realized through a lengthening of the closure phase (as in Figure 30.5 above); a shortening of the preceding vowel is also attested in comparison to singleton contexts (Esposito & Di Benedetto, 1999).

The analysis of stops usually considers the F2 transition of the following vowel, and the so-called Voice Onset Time (VOT). VOT is defined as the temporal interval between the articulatory release of the stop, including the spike, and the onset, measured at the appearance of the F2, of the following vowel (Lisker & Abramson, 1964). VOT and F2 movement indicate the place of articulation of the different plosives: in particular, the longer the VOT the more posterior the occlusive. In Figure 30.5, it is possible to notice that [k] has a longer VOT as compared to the [t] produced by the same speaker. VOT also reflects the temporal difference between aspirated and nonaspirated dental voiceless stops (see Foulkes & Docherty, 1999 for a systematic review in British English dialects).

In speech pathology, plosives have been acoustically investigated with respect to the voicing contrast in people with Parkinson's disease (Whitfield et al., 2018), or in people with cleft lip and cleft palate (Sudro & Prasanna, 2019). Stop-gap duration, closure length, burst and VOT have been studied in children with speech disorders: for instance Eshghi et al. (2017) present an analysis of stops produced by Persian children with cleft palate, Goswami et al. (2020) take into account burst onset and VOT in dysarthric speech.

Fricatives are also articulated with a constriction between the two main articulators, again either lips or tongue-palate, but in this case the air continues to flow in the channel by creating a characteristic turbulence due to the place and shape of the constriction. This turbulent noise results in an aperiodic wave on the spectrum, which constitutes the principal characteristics of fricatives (Fulop, 2011 p. 97). Different fricatives can be identified by the concentration of energy at different frequencies, with dental [s] having higher values than [ʃ], as shown in Figure 30.6. If present, voicing results in the vibration of the vocal folds, visible in the voicing bar at the lowest frequency, as for voiced stops. A general reduction of the intensity on the spectrogram is natural for voiced fricatives compared to voiceless one, because the periodically interrupted airflow modulates the overall amplitude of the spectrogram (Fujimura & Erickson, 1997; see also Harrington, 2013).

Apart for duration measures, the analysis of fricatives generally results in either the analysis of power spectra (Hughes & Halle, 1956) or in the measurements of spectral moments (Forrest et al., 1988). The first uses different overlapping FFT analysis windows in order to achieve an average spectrum of the fricative, and then extracts the frequency at which the spectrum shows the highest amplitude. This procedure is called spectral peak location (Jongman et al., 2000), and it is directly related, in absence of lip rounding, to the frontness of the consonant. Thus, alveodental [s] shows higher values than postalveolar [ʃ]. To some extent similar, although based on a different method and formula, is the analysis of spectral moments introduced by Forrest et al., 1988; spectral moment analysis can be performed either in Hertz or in Bark. Among the four spectral moments (Harrington, 2013, p. 107), the first two are the most important in the analysis of fricatives (Farmer, 1997). The first spectral moment (m_1) is also called the center of gravity, and this refers to the frequency at which the spectral energy is predominantly concentrated (see Figure 30.6). The second spectral moment (m_2) refers to the spectral standard deviation, that is the distribution of the energy along the frequency axis. Taken together, these two values, and in particular m_1, are used to estimate the place of articulation of different fricatives, even when there are very subtle differences (Jongman et al., 2000). Whatever the

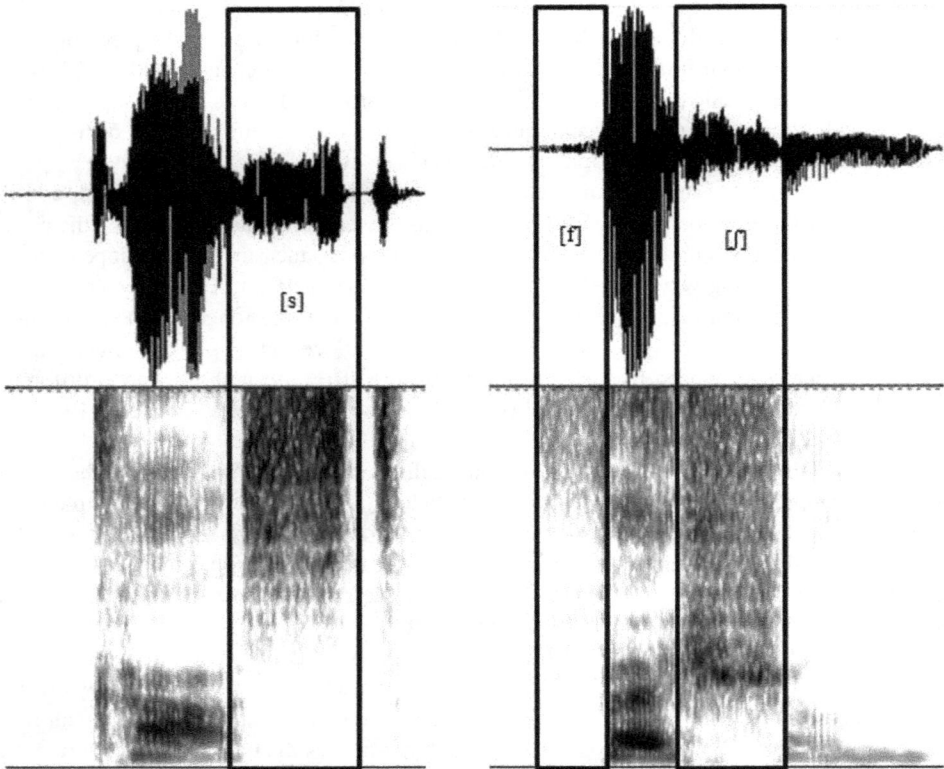

Figure 30.6   (Left) Fricative [s] in the word *cast*. (Right) Fricative [f] and [ʃ] in the word *fashion*. Boxes isolate the target consonants.

chosen method, it is worth remembering that, if measured in Hertz, acoustic values are affected by speakers' biological characteristics (e.g. male vs. female speakers). Indeed, fricatives have also shown sex-related acoustic differences (Nittrouer, 1995; Fox & Nissen, 2005), although they have not been so widely investigated as have vowels (but see Fuchs et al., 2010).

In speech pathology, fricatives have been studied in both adults and children with speech sound disorders (SSD). For instance, Maas and Mailend (2017) focus on children with SSD in the production of /s/ and /ʃ/: they consider the center of gravity and the degree of C-to-V co-articulation to analyze whether and to what extent the difference between the two places of articulation is maintained. Hernandez and Chung (2019) also analyze fricatives as a possible index for classifying speech disorders, in particular dysarthria.

Nasals and liquids

Although their articulation is very different, nasals and liquids tend to show similar characteristics on the spectrogram, since both these sonorants are characterized by formants and anti-formants (Fujimura & Erickson, 1997). Figure 30.7 shows the PRAAT spectra and spectrogram of an alveolar nasal [n] and a palatal lateral [l].

In the articulation of nasal consonants, the acoustic tube consists of a main system (the oral cavity) and a subsystem (the nasal cavity). Obviously, the tongue-palate contact in the first

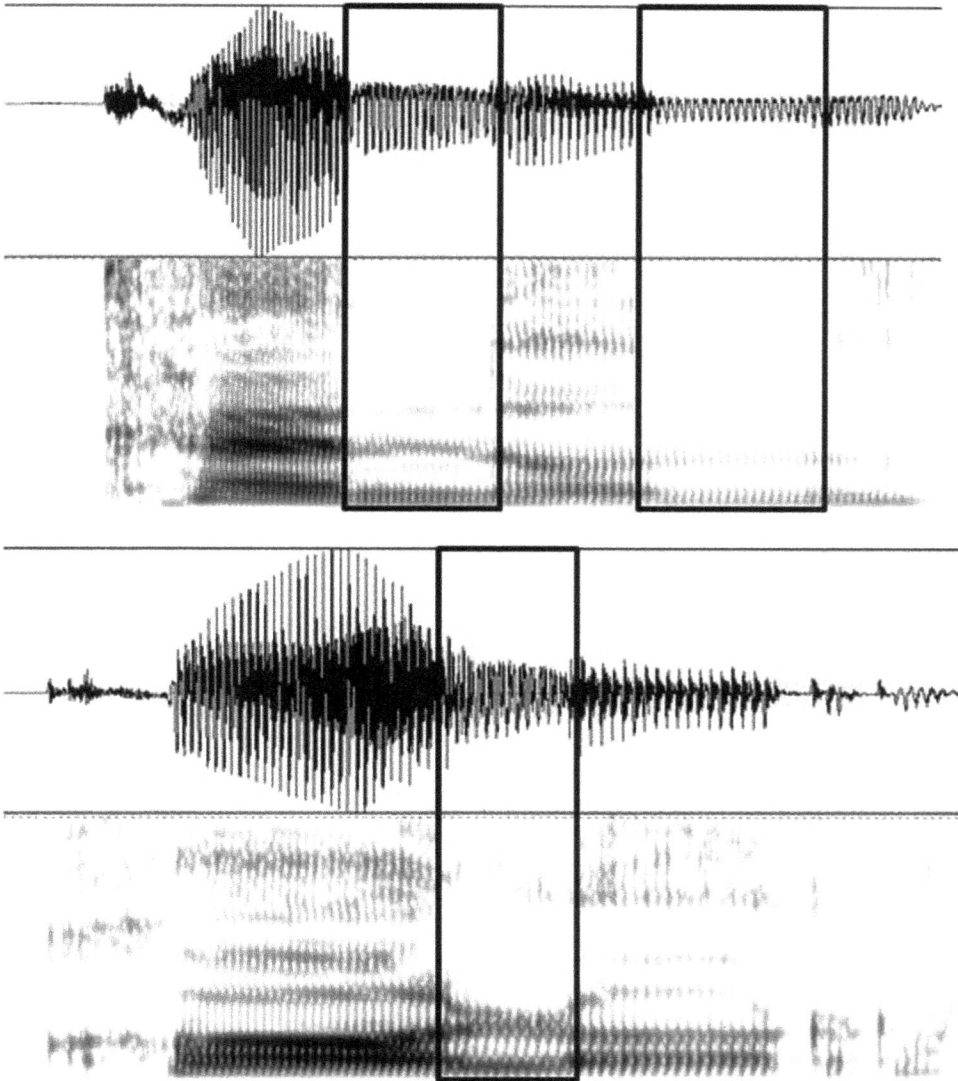

Figure 30.7 (Above) Alveolar nasals [n] in the word *cannon*. (Below) Alveolar lateral [l] in the word *color*. The black boxes isolate the two nasals and the lateral.

cavity creates modification in the airflow thus contributing to differentiating the various nasals. On the spectrogram (Figure 30.7) intervocalic nasal consonants can be recognized by abrupt spectral discontinuities, which are also considered to help determining the place of articulation of the different nasals (Stevens, 2000). Harrington (2013, pp. 112–113) presents a detailed discussion of nasal formant and anti-formant values in vocal tract models, together with a review of some of the main studies on perceptual cues for differentiating among nasals (e.g. Ohde et al., 2006). The main point to remember is that it is more difficult to determine the place of articulation for a nasal than for an obstruent if one refers only to formant transitions of the adjacent vowels. Indeed, vowels following nasals tend to be completely or partially nasalized

(Hattory et al., 1958; Chen, 1997; and also Cheng & Jongman, 2019 for an up-to-date review on both nasals and laterals).

Laterals are acoustically characterized by high values of F3 resulting from the "side pocket" created by the sideways tilting of the tongue (Thomas, 2010, p. 126). In the analysis of laterals, however, F2 is the key factor for distinguishing different places of articulation, in particular between "clear" [l] and "dark" [ɫ] in various languages (e.g. Recasens & Espinosa, 2005, on Spanish and Catalan; Carter & Local, 2007, on Newcastle-upon-Tyne English; Wang, 2016, on Sudanese). The palatal lateral [ʎ] is widespread in Romance language and its study usually involves an analysis of F1 and F3 (see Colantoni, 2004 for a review).

In speech pathology, analysis of nasal consonants has been primarily conducted in relation to articulatory problems involving velopharyngeal dysfunctions, as in the case of cleft palate (Ferreira et al., 2020), aphasia (Kurowski et al., 2007) and apraxia of speech (Marczyk et al., 2017). Laterals have been investigated in relation to loss or reduction of motor control. A good example and an up-to-date review is offered by Kuruvilla-Dugdale et al. (2018): the authors consider talkers with amyotrophic lateral sclerosis producing both vowels and consonants at different degrees of motor complexity, with laterals ranked 5 in a 6-points scale.

Rhotics

One of the most complex sound groups, both for speakers and for phoneticians, are the so-called R sounds (rhotics, or simply Rs). Since Lindau's (1985) study it has been evident that Rs include many different articulatory realizations, including approximants and fricatives. This is reflected in the way rhotics appear on the spectrogram. Taps and trills are the most common realizations of a rhotic (Ladefoged & Maddieson, 1996), and they are produced either with a contact between the tongue tip and the alveolar ridge (for alveolars) or by a vibration of the uvula against the tongue dorsum (for uvulars; see Laver, 1994; Thomas, 2010, p. 129; and Wiese, 2001 for uvular trill variants). In the case of trills more than one constriction is present (Delattre & Freeman, 1968), with a high degree of interspeaker variation (Espy-Wilson et al., 2000).

Taps and trills are also relatively easy to recognize on the spectrogram. Figure 30.8 shows the realization of a rhotic as a tap [ɾ] or as a trill [r:] in two intervocalic contexts. Contrary to previous examples, in this case Italian words have been selected, since in Italian there is a phonological distinction between intervocalic taps and trills, the first occurring as singletons and the latter as geminates. Spectrographically, during the realization of the trills there are multiple tongue-palate contacts (at least two), with a short vocoid in-between, also called a *svarabhakti* vowel.

Rhotics can also be realized as approximants or as fricatives. For instance, Belgian French shows the presence of uvular fricatives both as voiced [ʁ] and voiceless [χ] (Demolin, 2001), and standard German has a uvular approximant (Wiese, 2001). As for all other fricatives, voicing is spectrographically signaled by the periodic vocal fold vibration at the low frequencies.

In analyzing rhotics, one could first consider how to annotate these phones, since we have seen that they can appear as either taps, trills, approximants or fricatives, all with different places of articulation. Obviously, it is possible to annotate rhotics as a whole, and label them as belonging to one of the previously discussed variants. However, it may be interesting to consider a possible more detailed annotation, as proposed by Celata et al. (2016, 2018). Within this annotation protocol, rhotics are considered sequences of gestures of closure (tongue contact)

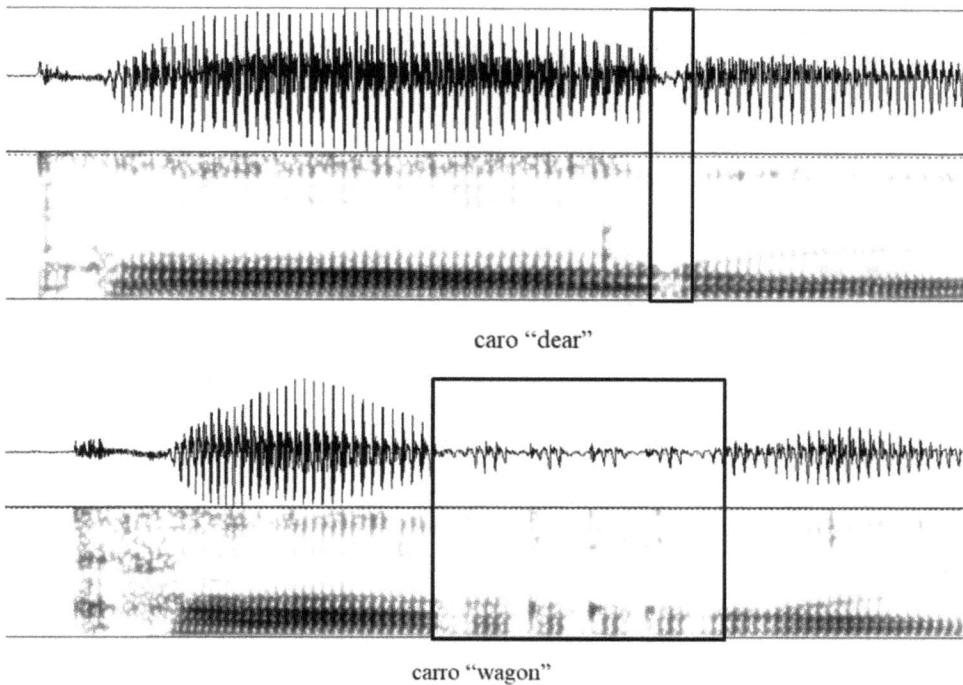

caro "dear"

carro "wagon"

Figure 30.8 (Above) Rhotic realized as a tap in the Italian word *caro* "dear." (Below) Rhotic realized as trill in the Italian word *carro* "wagon." The black boxes isolate the rhotics.

and aperture (tongue lowering, thus resulting in a vocoid). Figure 30.9 magnifies the rhotics of Figure 30.8 and their annotation, following this protocol.

The tap in the word *caro* "dear" is realized with a single gesture of closure, thus consisting of a single phase, without any annotation on the left or on the right. The label "t_c_1_e" specifies this information: "t" states the rhotic type (a tap), "c" the gesture (a closure), "1" the number of the gestural phase (in this example, the first and only one) and "e" denotes "empty," meaning that this is a monophasic rhotic. Conversely, the word *carro* "cart" presents a three-phases rhotic, two closures and one aperture. In this case, the first label is changed to "r" indicating that the whole rhotic is a trill, and the two closures are annotated as "c_1" and "c_2," respectively. The final letter indicates whether there are other labels on the right ("r," r_c_1_r), on both sides ("f" for "full," r_a_1_f), or on the left ("l," r_c_2_l). Therefore, by looking at the last annotated segment, it is immediately clear how many phases of closure or aperture have been performed during phonation. Although this annotation protocol is a bit longer to manage and to perform during manual annotations of data, it provides more information at the annotation level and opens the possibility of further different analyses on rhotic length and formant variation.

The acoustic analysis of rhotics includes segment duration and formant frequency. In particular, F3 is considered to be the best predictor of the rhotic type of articulation: F3 mean values fall between 1300 and 1950 Hertz for American English (Espy-Wilson et al., 2000, but different data are reported by Hagiwara, 1995; see Thomas, 2010, p. 134–135 for a discussion). During production of rhotics, lip rounding could play a role and it is reflected in lower values of both F2 and F3 at the onset of the rhotic segment (King & Ferragne, 2019 and Howson, 2018 for a dynamic analysis).

431

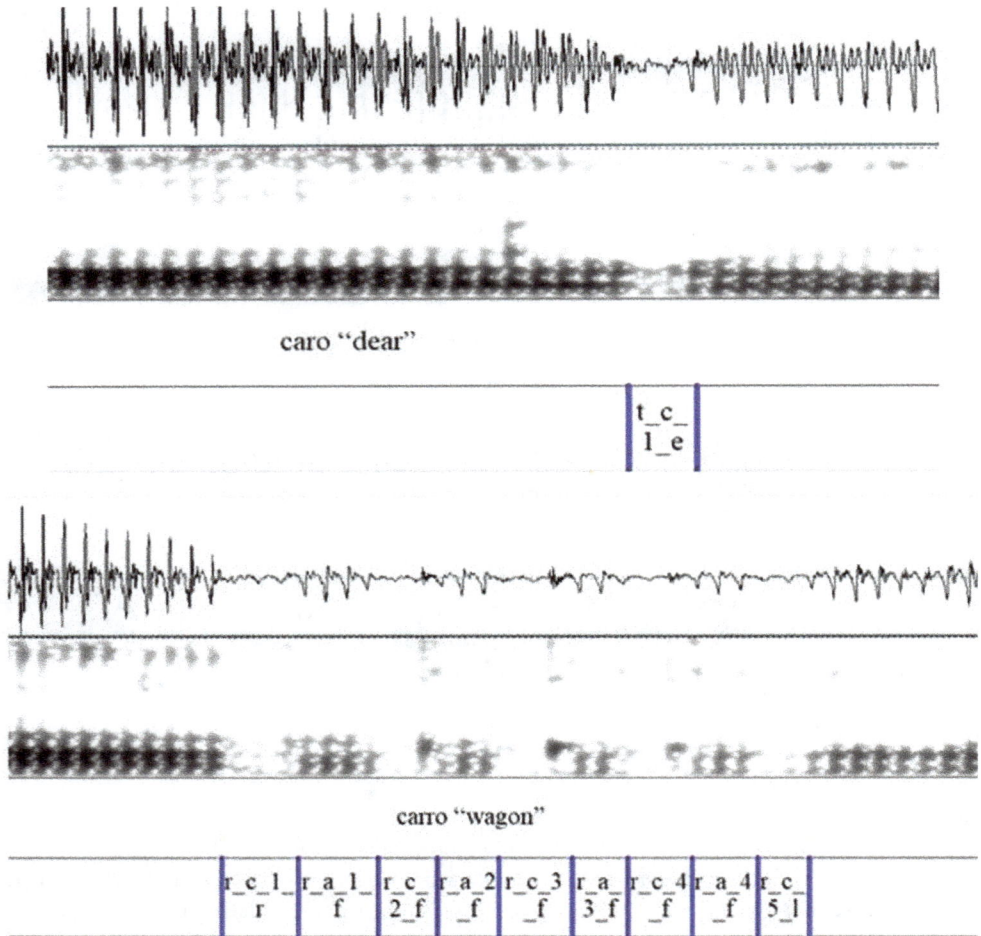

caro "dear"

carro "wagon"

Figure 30.9 (Above) Rhotic realized as a tap in the Italian word *caro* "dear." (Below) Rhotic realized as trill in the Italian word *carro* "wagon." Annotations follow the protocol of Celata et al. (2016, 2018).

Over the years, phonetic research has highlighted how rhotics are prone to sociolinguistic variation (Scobbie, 2006). In speech pathology, rhotics have been studied with respect to language acquisition in L1, thus in children with and without speech disorders (Ball et al., 2001; Chung & Pollock, 2019; Romani et al., 2017). Preston and Edwards (2009) analyzed adolescents between 10 and 14 years-old with residual speech errors. Preston and Leece (2017) provided an up-to-date literature review on rhotics in apraxia of speech, including both spectrographic and articulatory analysis.

Some generalizations

Spectrographic analysis is a powerful instrument for the quantitative investigation of speech. Although it is nowadays quite economical to perform, in terms of both hardware and software, being able to differentiate between different sounds on the spectrogram requires practice and a

Table 30.1 Main measures usually analyzed in the phonetic literature for different sound classes

Sound class	Main measures	Other measures
Vowels	F1–F2	Vowel space
Stops	VOT	Burst, closure length
Fricatives	center of gravity	other spectral moments; relation between spectral moments
Nasals	F1-F2-F3	nasalization of adjacent vowels
Laterals	F3	
Rhotics	F3	F2, rhotic type

clear annotation protocol in order to avoid hypo- or hyper-categorization. Moreover, one needs to decide on which acoustic variable(s) to focus, thus also partially adapting the annotation protocol for this purpose (e.g. in the case of rhotics).

As for different acoustic measurements, Table 30.1 summarizes the principal acoustic cues investigated in speech science and, in particular, in clinical phonetics and speech pathology.

The discussion presented here has not considered the possibilities of spectrographic analysis of voice quality, for example, and other acoustic cues need to be considered in this case. For instance, Jotz et al. (2002) investigated voice disorders in Brazilian vowels as produced by boys with dysphonia or lesion of the vocal fold. Apart from formant values, the authors also extracted noise-to-harmonics ratio (NHR). This last value is considered an index of vocal aging, together with F0 (Ferrand, 2002). Sound spectrography is not, obviously, limited to the introductory remarks presented here, which hopefully constitute a good basis for the reader to start the exploration of the possibilities of acoustic analysis in speech pathology.

Spectrography in clinical phonetics: An overview of recent developments

This section aims at offering a brief overview of more recent developments in spectrographic analysis as applied to clinical phonetic research. A sample of studies of various different speech pathologies will be presented and a special effort is made to include more recent studies, published from 2014 onward. Obviously, the studies presented here are not comprehensive of all the work done so far in the spectrographic analysis of pathological speech, but they are highly representative of some current developments within this field.

Stuttering

Stuttering has been widely investigated in both adults' and children's speech. Although nowadays articulatory techniques are applied to the investigation of stuttered speech (e.g. Didirková et al., 2019; Lenoci & Ricci, 2018, among others) acoustic features were and still are widely used for discriminating the speech characteristics of people who stutter (PWS) from those of fluent speakers. Many studies in the 1980s and 1990s considered formant frequencies, in particular F2, to be a good index for discriminating stuttered versus fluent speech (e.g. Prosek et al., 1987; Howell & Vause, 1986; Robb & Blomgren, 1997). Second formant transitions have been recently investigated in various languages. Dehqan et al. (2016) compare F2 transitions in 10 Farsi male adult PWS as opposed to non-stuttering peers. Even when perceptually similar to fluent speech, the F2 of PWS took longer to reach vowel steady state, but had an overall similar F2 slope. The authors claimed that these results were linked to the different speech motor timing associated with stuttering (see Van Lieshout, 1995), and that this is language-independent. Indeed, similar results have been attested for Bulgarian by Padareva-Ilieva & Georgieva (2018) and are aligned with previous findings in the speech of both adult and children who stutter (e.g. Subramanian et al., 2003).

Other studies on PWS focus on the role of the fundamental frequency in determining the degree of speech naturalness (Schmitt, 2016; Klopfenstein et al., 2020 for a systematic review of the literature). VOT is considered another key feature: for instance, Bakhtiar et al (2019) considered VOT, lexical tones and vowel quality in a perception task in Cantonese, given to 15 children who stuttered and 15 who did not stutter. Their results showed that stuttering slows down the response time during categorical phonemic perception.

Dysarthria

Dysarthric speech could have several causes, including Parkinson's disease (see Smith et al., 2019, and also below), and it is possible to classify different types and degrees of dysarthria (Darley et al., 1975). Acoustic correlates of dysarthric speech included F0 movements in accented versus unaccented syllables, as well as in the overall phrasal contour (Astruc & Prieto, 2006; Lowit et al., 2014; Ramos et al., 2020), but also formant variation in V-to-C coordination and VOT. For instance, Rowe and Green (2019) consider dysarthric speech resulting from amyotrophic lateral sclerosis (ALS); they tested 7 speakers with ALS producing [pataka] as many times as possible in one breath, and measured the proportion of VOT to syllable duration as well as F2 slope. Their results were compared with 18 control speakers and this confirmed that VOT is a good indicator for dyscoordination between supra and subglottal gestures, which is also attested by a reduction of F2 slope in people with ALS. These results are in line with previous literature on dysarthric speech, in particular concerning the second formant (e.g. Kent et al., 1989; Kim et al., 2009; Yunusova et al., 2008, 2012).

Recently, Hernandez and Chung (2019) have also proposed that fricatives and their acoustic correlates could be good indicators for the automatic classification of dysarthric speech. They measured the word-initial fricatives /s, z, ʃ/ in 10 English speakers with dysarthria caused by cerebral palsy, together with 9 control speakers. Their results show that the spectral properties and segmental duration of fricatives correlate with the severity of dysarthric speech (see also Yılmaz et al., 2019 for automatic speaker recognition applied to speech pathology). Other acoustic predictors were included in Allison and Hustad's (2019) research on pediatric dysarthria associated with cerebral palsy; the authors present a comprehensive review of the acoustic literature, and presented the results of their own experiment with 20 five year-old children with cerebral palsy repeating words and sentences. They then extract acoustic measurements correlating with articulatory imprecision, such as F2 range of diphthongs, proportions of observable bursts in plosives, duration of closure interval voicing and articulation rate. Their results show that F2 range in diphthongs is a promising indicator for identifying the emergence of dysarthria in children with cerebral palsy.

Apraxia and aphasia

In both apraxia of speech (AOS) and aphasia, VOT and vowels have been two of the most studied acoustic variables in different languages. Indeed, VOT is linked to timing and coordination of supralaryngeal articulators, thus being particularly prone to being disrupted in cases of AOS and also aphasia. Compensatory strategies are usually developed by speakers in order to achieve the target consonant, especially in the case of word-initial voiced ones. One of the first works by Blumstein et al. (1980) showed how VOT is a good indicator of AOS. This result has been confirmed by further studies on the topic (e.g. Mauszycki et al., 2007; Whiteside et al., 2012). Recently, Marczyk et al. (2017) investigated Spanish speakers with apraxia when articulating the initial voiced stops /b, d, g/, by measuring voicing lead, voicing lag and nasal murmur. Their hypothesis was that nasalization helps in articulating voicing as a compensatory strategy. Their results confirm that negative VOT is a cue in detecting these compensatory mechanisms, which involved the use and permanence of nasality.

So far, studies on vowels in AOS have not given straightforward results, at least in terms of absolute duration of the vocalic segments (den Ouden et al., 2018, p. 903). Conflicting results have emerged also from the analysis of vowel formants: whereas Maas et al. (2015) found significant differences between formants in AOS and unimpaired speech, no difference emerged in the adults studied by Jacks et al. (2010).

A recent work by Verhaegen et al. (2020) focused on VOT in six French speakers with aphasia. They found no great differences between Broca's and Wernicke's aphasic speech, since in both types of client there was a blurring of the voiced-voiceless opposition in stop production; huge within-speaker variation was also detected. These results were in line with previous work on English and Catalan speakers with aphasia (e.g. Baqué et al., 2015; Nespoulous et al., 2013). Haley et al. (2000) focused on fricatives in the speech of both clients with AOS and aphasia. By measuring spectral moments on voiceless fricatives, they observed lower accuracy in place of articulation leading to a reduced distinction between alveolar and palatal fricatives. Other recent developments in the acoustic analysis of aphasic speech include the automatic detection of phonemic and neologistic paraphasias (Le et al., 2017), as well as automatic segmentation of aphasic speech (Le et al., 2018).

Cognitive impairment: Alzheimer and dementia

As for dysarthric speech, recent developments in the research of people with Alzheimer and dementia concentrate on finding acoustic predictors of the disease through automatic speech recognition. Nagumo et al. (2020) present a comprehensive analysis of 8779 participants with different cognitive profiles, from healthy to global cognitive impairment; they measured both temporal features (e.g. pauses, sentence duration length) and formant features in vowels. Through a machine learning model they show that acoustic features could be used to discriminate between healthy control and impaired speech, but also between mild and global cognitive impaired speakers.

Concerning temporal markers, similar results were also obtained on Hungarian by Gosztolya et al. (2019). This work is interesting because it considered spontaneous speech rather than controlled utterances derived from sentence-reading or repetition tasks. Their corpus of 150 speakers with different degrees of cognitive impairment constitutes the Hungarian MCI-mAD database. Liu et al. (2019) also presented results from the analysis of spontaneous speech of Mandarin speakers in order to detect the development of dementia-related pathologies. They considered a set of temporal and acoustic features, and, although they do not focus on one specific acoustic feature, they confirmed that acoustic cues could predict when the deterioration of the disease took place.

Parkinson's disease

The neurodegenerative Parkinson's disease (PD) is commonly associated with a progressive impairment of motor functions, like hypokinesia and also dysarthria. Acoustic correlates have usually been detected in vowel contrast or vowel space, because of deficits in movements of both the tongue and the jaw. Conflicting results emerge from studies comparing the two-dimensional F1 × F2 vowel space of speakers with PD with respect to controls. For instance, Tjaden et al. (2013) highlighted a reduction of the vowel space in speakers with PD, whereas no statistical significance was found by Sapir et al. (2010). Whitfield and Goberman (2014) critically reviewed work in this area, and pointed out that maybe this difference was linked to methodological issues. Formant values have usually been extracted at the steady-state (mid-point) of the vowels, whereas a more dynamic approach should be adopted in dealing with PD speech. In this regard, Mefferd and Dietrich (2019) presented a kinematic and acoustic experiment conducted on 17 speakers with PD and 17 controls balanced for sex and age. The speakers were recorded while reading various times a sentence containing the diphthong /aɪ/ in the word *kite*. The acoustic measures considered were F2 minimum and maximum and their corresponding F1 values, as well as Euclidean distance in the F1-F2 planar space, which was considered an index of acoustic vowel contrast (Mefferd & Green, 2010). The results showed a greater reduction of acoustic vowel contrast in speakers with PD than in controls, but with great variation among the PD subjects. This was possibly due to different stages of speech decline or, as the authors also argue, to the nature of the task (sentence repetition).

Segment duration has also been shown to be significantly reduced in speakers with PD in comparison to controls (e.g. Lam & Tjaden, 2016). The voicing contrast is also difficult to manage for speakers with PD, thus VOT is a good marker of severity of the disease (see Whitfield et al., 2018). In a recent study by Whitfield and Gravelin (2019), the authors observed a difference in between and within word silences, thus moving the acoustic analysis (of both segment duration and F0) to the interface between segmental and suprasegmental level.

Hearing disorders

In studying pre- and post-lingual onset of deafness a major role is played by age of occurrence of the hearing loss and age of implantation of any cochlear device (Dunn et al., 2014). Many studies have focused on the analysis of the speech of speakers with and without implants, from both a spectrographic and a perceptual point of view. Acoustic analysis of children's production is usually associated with perceptual discrimination tests, quite often through Deep Neural Networks (DNN) for automatic recognition of the speaker. For instance, Arias-Vergara et al. (2019) present the results of an experiment on 60 German adult speakers (20 prelinguals, 20 postlinguals, 20 controls): they analyzed the manner of articulation of nasals, sibilants, fricatives, voiceless and voiced stops, with phone-attribution achieved through DNN. Their results show that fricatives were particularly sensitive to distinguishing cochlear implanted users from controls.

Binos et al. (2020) present the result of a longitudinal study on the vocalizations of children with cochlear implants. Their results show a longer average duration of vowels of cochlear implanted children than controls. Similar results emerged from 8–9 year old children with cochlear implants (Uchanski & Geers, 2003; Neumeyer et al., 2010). A similar pattern emerged also in the speech of adults with cochlear implants (see Nicolaidis & Sfakiannaki, 2007 on Greek). Horga and Liker (2006) demonstrated a lowering of F1 and F2 and a reduction of the vowel space of subjects with profound hearing loss compared with cochlear implant users; they also show that 12 months after implantation formant values of the subjects with hearing loss had shifted toward normative values. In the same work, no variation was detected for VOT and closure duration in plosives and fricatives.

Voicing duration is another well-documented feature in the literature on subjects with hearing deficits (e.g. McGarr & Löfqvist, 1982; Lenden & Flipsen, 2007). VOT is generally shorter in the case of hearing problems than with normal-hearing individuals (Liker et al., 2007), but Gautam et al. (2019) suggested that VOT was subject to rapid changes after implantation. In a study on Greek children, Koupka et al. (2019) presented new data to support this evidence: voiceless stops were produced with a significantly shorter VOT in cochlear implanted children than in controls, but the opposite happened for prevoicing in voiced plosives.

Conclusion

This chapter aims at presenting the basis of spectrographic analysis and its possible applications in speech pathology. Although the review of the studies offered in the previous section was not exhaustive, it was intended to be a comprehensive state of the art for understanding the possibilities of spectrographic analysis as applied to various speech and hearing disorders.

The spectrographic analysis of speech has provided a great improvement in our understanding of both speech production and perception, and recent developments like Deep Neural Network are pushing our possibilities even further. Acoustic analysis is still one of the most economical way to collect data from a large sample of speakers. It is true that nowadays the development of a great number of different techniques and instrumentation (ultrasound, electropalatography, electromagnetic articulography, and so forth) is increasing the interest in articulatory analysis. Furthermore, it is obviously true that not all articulatory information (e.g. jaw movements) could be traced in the acoustic signal to the same fine-grained degree. It has been suggested in some recent studies in clinical phonetics, though, that we should aim for integrated research protocols, in order to combine articulatory and acoustic data coming from the same subject during speech.

Apart from the proposed integration of spectrography with articulatory analysis, current and further perspectives in spectrographic research in clinical phonetics include focusing on languages other than English, in particular from minorities, together with the inclusion of bilingual speakers with different speech pathologies. Moreover, a new and enthralling perspective is represented by the application of automatic detection software packages (see Buttigieg et al., Chapter 35, this volume) associated with deep learning techniques for the automatic detection of possible pathological features in speech, and the classification of the severity of the disorders.

References

Adank, P. M. (2003). *Vowel normalization. A perceptual acoustic study of Dutch vowels*. Wageningen, The Netherlands: Ponsen & Looijen.

Allison, K. M., & Hustad, K. C. (2018). Acoustic predictors of pediatric dysarthria in cerebral palsy. *Journal of Speech, Language, and Hearing Research, 61*(3), 462–478.

Arias-Vergara, T., Orozco-Arroyave, J. R., Cernak, M., Gollwitzer, S. Schuster, M., & Nöth, E. (2019). Phone-attribute posteriors to evaluate the speech of cochlear implant users. *AGE, 50*, 3108–3112.

Astruc, L., & Prieto, P. (2006). Acoustic cues of stress and accent in Catalan. *ExLing*, 73–76.

Ball, M.J., & Gibbon, F.E. (Eds.). (2013). *Handbook of vowels and vowel disorders*. London, England: Psychology Press.

Ball, M.J., & Lowry, O.M. (2001). *Methods in clinical phonetics*. London, England: Whurr.

Baqué, L., Marczyk, A., Rosas, A., & Estrada, M. (2015). Disability, repair strategies and communicative effectiveness at the phonic level: Evidence from a multiple-case study. *Neuropsycholinguistic Perspectives on Language Cognition, 14*, 144–165.

Binos, P., Thodi, C., Vogazianos, P., Psillas, G., & Constantinidis, J. (2020). An acoustic and auditory analysis of vocants in infants with cochlear implants. *Logopedics Phoniatrics Vocology, 1*, 1–7.

Blumstein, S. E., Cooper, W. E., Goodglass, H., Statlender, S., & Gottlieb, J. (1980). Production deficits in aphasia: A voice-onset time analysis. *Brain and Language, 9*(2), 153–170.

Boersma, P., & Weenink, D. (2020). Praat: doing phonetics by computer [Computer program]. Version 6.1.09, retrieved 26 January 2020 from http://www.praat.org/.

Carter, P., & Local, J. (2007). F2 variation in Newcastle and Leeds English liquid systems. *Journal of the International Phonetic Association, 37*(2), 183–199.

Celata, C., Meluzzi, C., & Ricci, I. (2016). The sociophonetics of rhotic variation in Sicilian dialects and Sicilian Italian: corpus, methodology and first results. *Loquens, 3*(1), 025.

Celata, C., Vietti, A., & Spreafico, L. (2018). An articulatory account of rhotic variation in Tuscan Italian. Synchronized UTI and EPG data. In M. Gibson, & J. Gil (Eds.), *Romance Phonetics and Phonology* (pp. 91–117). Oxford, England: Oxford University Press.

Cenceschi, S., Meluzzi, C., & Nese, N. (accepted). A preliminary phonological investigation on the potential forensic exploitation of WhatsApp audio messages. In G. Romito (Ed.), *Studi AISV 7*. Milano, Italy: OfficinaVentuno.

Chen, M.Y. (1997). Acoustic correlates of English and French nasalized vowels. *Journal of the Acoustical Society of America*, 102, 2360–2370.

Cheng, R., & Jongman, A. (2019). Acoustic analysis of nasal and lateral consonants: The merger in Eastern Min. *The Journal of the Acoustical Society of America, 145*(3), 1828–1828.

Chung, H., & Pollock, K. E. (2019). Acoustic Characteristics of Rhotic Vowel Productions of Young Children. *Folia Phoniatrica et Logopaedica, 1*, 1–12.

Colantoni, L. (2004). Reinterpreting the CV transition. Emergence of the glide as an allophone of the palatal lateral. In J. Auger, J.C. Clements, & B. Vance (Eds.), *Contemporary Approaches to Romance Linguistics* (pp. 83–102). Amsterdam, The Netherlands: John Benjamins.

D'Aco, M. (2019). Analisi fonetica di parlanti ipoacusici a confronto con normoudenti, University of Pavia, Italy: BA thesis.

Darley, F.L., Aronson, A.E., & Brown, J.R. (1975). *Motor Speech Disorders*, Philadelphia, PA: Saunders.

Delattre, P., & Freeman, D.C. (1968). A dialect study of American r's by x-ray motion picture. *Linguistics*, 6(44), 29–68.

den Ouden, D. B., Galkina, E., Basilakos, A., & Fridriksson, J. (2018). Vowel formant dispersion reflects severity of apraxia of speech. *Aphasiology, 32*(8), 902–921.

Di Paolo, M. & Yaeger-Dror, M. (Eds.). (2011). *Sociophonetics: a student's guide*, London: Routledge.

Didirkova, I., Le Maguer, S., Hirsch, F., & Gbedahou, D. (2019) Articulatory behaviour during disfluencies in stuttered speech. *ICPhS, 19*, 1–5.

Dunn, C.C., Walker, E. A., Ole-son, J., Kenworthy, M., Van Voorst, T., Tomblin, J.B., Ji, H., Kirk, K.I., McMurray, B., & Hanson, M. (2014). Longitudinal speech perception and language performance in pediatric cochlear implant users: The effect of age at implantation. *Ear and hearing, 35*(2),148–160.

Eshghi, M., Preisser, J. S., Bijankhan, M., & Zajac, D. J. (2017). Acoustic-temporal aspects of stop-plosives in the speech of Persian-speaking children with cleft lip and palate. *International journal of speech-language pathology, 19*(6), 578–586.

Esposito, A., & Di Benedetto, M.G. (1999). Acoustical and perceptual study of gemination in Italian stops. *The Journal of the Acoustical Society of America, 106*(4), 2051–2062.

Espy-Wilson, C.Y., Boyce, S.E., Jackson, M., Narayanan, S., & Alwan, A. (2000). Acoustic modeling of American English/r/. *Journal of the Acoustical Society of America, 108*, 343–56.

Exner, A.H. (2019). *The effects of speech tasks on the prosody of people with Parkinson disease*, Purdue University, IN: PhD thesis.

Fant, G. (1960). *The acoustic theory of speech production*. The Hague, the Netherlands: Mouton the Gruyter.

Farmer, A. (1997). Spectrography. In M. Ball & C. Code (Eds.), *Instrumental Clinical Phonetics* (pp. 22–63). London, England: Whuarr.

Ferrand, C.T. (2002). Harmonics-to-noise ratio: an index of vocal aging. *Journal of voice, 16*(4), 480–487.

Ferreira, G.Z., Bressmann, T., Dutka, J.D.C.R., Whitaker, M.E., de Boer, G., de Castro Marino, V.C., & Pegoraro-Krook, M.I. (2020). Analysis of oral-nasal balance after intensive speech therapy combined with speech bulb in speakers with cleft palate and hypernasality. *Journal of communication disorders*, 85,105945.

Fox, R.A., & Nissen, S.L. (2005). Sex-related acoustic changes in voiceless English fricatives. *Journal of Speech, Language, and Hearing Research, 48*, 735–765.

Fry, D.B. (Ed.). (2009). *Acoustic phonetics: a course of basic readings.* Cambridge, England: Cambridge University Press.

Fuchs, S., Toda, M., & Żygis, M. (Eds.). (2010). *Turbulent sounds: An interdisciplinary guide.* Berlin, Germany: Walter de Gruyter.

Fujimura, O., & Erickson, D. (1997). *Acoustic phonetics.* In W.J. Hardcastle & J. Laver (Eds.), *The handbook of phonetic sciences* (pp. 65–115). London, England: Blackwell.

Fulop, S. A. (2011). *Speech spectrum analysis.* Berlin, Germany: Springer Science & Business Media.

Galkina, E., Basilakos, A., & Fridriksson, J. (2018). Vowel Formant Dispersion Reflects Severity of Apraxia of Speech. *Aphasiology, 32*(8), 902–921.

Garellek, M. (2019). The phonetics of voice. In W.F. Katz, & P.F. Assmann (Eds.), *The Routledge handbook of Phonetics* (pp. 75–196). New York, NY: Routledge.

Gautam, A., Naples, J.G., & Eliades, S.J. (2019). Control of speech and voice in cochlear implant patients. *The Laryngoscope, 129*(9), 2158–2163.

Giannini, A., & Pettorino, M. (1992). *La fonetica sperimentale.* Napoli, Italy: Liguori.

Goswami, U., Nirmala, S. R., Vikram, C. M., Kalita, S., & Prasanna, S.R.M. (2020). Analysis of Articulation Errors in Dysarthric Speech. *Journal of psycholinguistic research, 49*(1), 163–174.

Hagiwara, R. (1995). *Acoustic realizations of American/r/as produced by women and men.* Los Angeles, CA: UCLA, PhD thesis.

Haley, K. L., Ohde, R. N., & Wertz, R. T. (2000). Precision of fricative production in aphasia and apraxia of speech: A perceptual and acoustic study. *Aphasiology, 14*(5–6), 619–634.

Harrington, J., Kleber, F., & Reubold, U. (2008). Compensation for coarticulation,/u/-fronting, and sound change in standard southern British: An acoustic and perceptual study. *The Journal of the Acoustical Society of America, 123*(5), 2825–2835.

Harrington, J. (2013). Acoustic Phonetics. In W.J. Hardcastle, J. Laver, & F.E. Gibbon (Eds.), *The Handbook of Phonetic Sciences* (2nd ed. pp. 81–129). London, England: Wiley-Blackwell.

Hattory, S., Yamamoto, K., & Fujimura, O. (1958). Nasalization of vowels in relation to nasals. *Journal of the Acoustical Society of America, 30*, 267–274.

Heeringa, W., & Van de Velde, H. (2018). Visible Vowels: a Tool for the Visualization of Vowel Variation, *Proceedings CLARIN Annual Conference 2018, 8–10 October, Pisa, Italy.* CLARIN ERIC.

Hernandez, A., & Chung, M. (2019). Dysarthria Classification Using Acoustic Properties of Fricatives. *Proceedings of SICSS,* 16.

Hillenbrand, J., Getty, L.A., Clark, M.J., & Wheeler, K. (1995). Acoustic characteristics of American English vowels. *The Journal of the Acoustical society of America, 97*(5), 3099–3111.

Howson P. (2018). Rhotics and palatalization: an acoustic examination of Upper and Lower Sorbian. *Phonetica, 75*(2), 132–150.

Horga, D., & Liker, M. (2006). Voice and pronunciation of cochlear implant speakers. *Clinical linguistics & phonetics, 20*(2–3), 211–217.

Howell, P., & Vause, L. (1986). Acoustic analysis and perception of vowels in stuttered speech. *Journal of Acoustic Society of America, 79*, 1571–1579.

Jongman, A.R., Wayland, S., & Wong, S. (2000). Acoustic characteristics of English fricatives. *Journal of the Acoustical Society of America, 108*, 1252–63.

Joss, M. (1948). Acoustic Phonetics, *Supplement to Language*, 24.2.

Jotz, G. P., Cervantes, O., Abrahão, M., Settanni, F.A.P., & de Angelis, E.C. (2002). Noise-to-harmonics ratio as an acoustic measure of voice disorders in boys. *Journal of voice, 16*(1): 28–31.

Katz, W.F. (2019). New horizons in clinical phonetics. In W.F. Katz, & P.F. Assmann (Eds.), *The Routledge Handbook of Phonetics* (pp. 526–569). New York, NY: Routledge.

Kent, R.D., Kent, J.F., Weismer, G., Martin, R.E., Sufit, R.L., Brooks, B.R., & Rosenbek, J.C. (1989). Relationships between speech intelligibility and the slope of second-formant transitions in dysarthric subjects. *Clinical Linguistics & Phonetics, 3*(4), 347–358.

Kim, Y., Weismer, G., Kent, R.D., Duffy, J.R., & Green, J.R. (2009). Statistical models of F2 slope in relation to severity of dysarthria. *Folia Phoniatrica Et Logopaedica: Official Organ of the International Association of Logopedics and Phoniatrics (IALP), 61*, 329–335.

King, H., & Ferragne, E. (2019). The contribution of lip protrusion to Anglo-English/r: Evidence from hyper-and non-hyperarticulated speech, *Interspeech,* ISCA, 3322–3326.

Klein, W., Plomp, R., & Pols, L.C.W. (1970). Vowel spectra, vowel space and vowel identification. *Journal of the Acoustical Society of America, 48*, 999–1009.

Klopfenstein, M., Bernard, K., & Heyman, C. (2020). The study of speech naturalness in communication disorders: A systematic review of the literature. *Clinical linguistics & phonetics*, *34*(4), 327–338.

Koenig, W., Dunn, H.K., & Lacy, L.Y. (1946). The sound spectrograph. *Journal of the Acoustical Society of America*, *18*, 19–49.

Koupka, G. A., Okalidou, A., Greece, T., Nicolaidis, K., Konstantinidis, I., & Kyriafinis, G. (2019). Production of the Voicing Contrast by Greek Children with Cochlear Implants. *ICNLSP*, 114.

Kurowski, K.M., Blumstein, S.E., Palumbo, C.L., Waldstein, R.S., & Burton, M.W. (2007). Nasal consonant production in Broca's and Wernicke's aphasics: Speech deficits and neuroanatomical correlates. *Brain and language*, *100*(3), 262–275.

Kuruvilla-Dugdale, M., Custer C., Heidrick, L., Barohn, R., & Govindarajan, R. (2018). A phonetic complexity-based approach for intelligibility and articulatory precision testing: A preliminary study on talkers with amyotrophic lateral sclerosis. *Journal of Speech, Language, and Hearing Research*, *61*(9), 2205–2214.

Ladefoged, P. (1962). *Elements of acoustic phonetics*. Chicago, IL: Phoenix.

Ladefoged, P. (1996). *Elements of acoustic phonetics*. Chicago, IL: University of Chicago Press.

Ladefoged, P. (2005). *Vowels and consonants*. Oxford, England: Blackwell.

Ladefoged, P., & Maddieson, I. (1990). Vowels of the world's languages. *Journal of Phonetics*, *18*(2), 93–122.

Lam, J., & Tjaden, K. (2016). Clear speech variants: An acoustic study in Parkinson's disease. *Journal of Speech, Language, and Hearing Research*, *59*(4), 631–646.

Laver, J. (1994). *Principles of phonetics*. Cambridge, England: Cambridge University Press.

Le, D., Licata, K., & Provost, E.M. (2017). Automatic Paraphasia Detection from Aphasic Speech: A Preliminary Study, *Interspeech*, 294–298.

Le, D., Licata, K., & Provost, E.M. (2018). Automatic quantitative analysis of spontaneous aphasic speech. *Speech Communication*, *100*, 1–12.

Lenden, J. M., & Flipsen, P. (2007). Prosody and voice characteristics of children with cochlear implants. *Journal of Communication Disorders*, *40*, 66–81.

Lenoci, G., & Ricci, I. (2018). An ultrasound investigation of the speech motor skills of stuttering Italian children. *Clinical linguistics & phonetics*, *32*(12), 1126–1144.

Liker, M., Mildner, V., & Sindija, B. (2007). Acoustic analysis of the speech of children with cochlear implants: a longitudinal study. *Clinical Linguistics & Phonetics*, 21: 1–11.

Lindau, M. (1985). The story of/r/. In V. Fromkin (Ed.), *Phonetic Linguistics: Essays in Honor of Peter Ladefoged* (pp. 157–168). Orlando, CA: Academic Press.

Liu, Z., Guo, Z., Ling, Z., Wang, S., Jin, L., & Li, Y. (2019). Dementia Detection by Analyzing Spontaneous Mandarin Speech. *Dementia*, *84*, 74–3.

Lowit, A., Kuschmann, A., & Kavanagh, K. (2014). Phonological markers of sentence stress in ataxic dysarthria and their relationship to perceptual cues. *Journal of Communication Disorders*, *50*, 8–18.

Maas, E., & Mailend, M.L. (2017). Fricative contrast and coarticulation in children with and without speech sound disorders. *American Journal of Speech-Language Pathology*, *26*(2), 649–663.

Maassen, B., Nijland, L., & Van Der Meulen, S. (2001). Coarticulation within and between syllables by children with developmental apraxia of speech. *Clinical Linguistics & Phonetics*, *15*(1–2), 145–150.

Marczyk, A.K., Meynadier, Y., Gaydina, Y., & Solé, M.J. (2017). Dynamic acoustic evidence of nasalization as a compensatory mechanism for voicing in Spanish apraxic speech. *International Seminar on Speech Production*, 225–236.

Mauszycki, S.C., Dromey, C., & Wambaugh, J.L. (2007). Variability in apraxia of speech: A perceptual, acoustic, and kinematic analysis of stop consonants. *Journal of Medical Speech-Language Pathology*, *15*, 223–242.

McGarr, N.S., & Löfqvist, A. (1982). Obstruent production by hearing-impaired speakers: Interarticulator timing and acoustics. *Journal of the Acoustical Society of America*, *72*, 34–42.

Mefferd, A.S., & Green, J.R. (2010). Articulatory-to-acoustic relations in response to speaking rate and loudness manipulations. *Journal of Speech, Language, and Hearing Research*, *53*(5), 1206–19.

Mefferd, A.S., & Dietrich, M.S. (2019). Tongue-and jaw-specific articulatory underpinnings of reduced and enhanced acoustic vowel contrast in talkers with Parkinson's Disease. *Journal of Speech, Language, and Hearing Research*, *62*(7), 2118–2132.

Mildner, V. (2017). Experimental and quasi-experimental research in clinical linguistics and phonetics. In Müller, N., & Ball, M.J. (Eds.), *Research methods in clinical linguistics and phonetics. A practical guide* (pp. 28–47). London, England: Wiley-Blackwell.

Milner, B., & Shao, X. (2006). Clean speech reconstruction from MFCC vectors and fundamental frequency using an integrated front-end. *Speech communication*, *48*, 697–715.

Müller, N., & Ball, M. (Eds.). (2017). *Research methods in clinical linguistics and phonetics. A practical guide*. London, England: Wiley-Blackwell.

Neger, T., Janse, E., & Rietveld, T. (2015). Correlates of older adults' discrimination of acoustic properties in speech. *Speech, Language and Hearing*, *18*(2), 102–115.

Nespoulous, J.L., Baqué, L., Rosas, A., Marczyk, A., & Estrada, M. (2013). Aphasia, phonological and phonetic voicing within the consonantal system: Preservation of phonological oppositions and compensatory strategies. *Language Sciences*, *39*(1), 117–125.

Neumeyer,V., Harrington, J., & Draxler, C. (2010). An acoustic analysis of the vowel space in young and old cochlear-implant speakers. *Clinical Linguistics and Phonetics*, *24*(9), 734–741.

Nicolaidis, K., & Sfakiannaki, A. (2007). An acoustic analysis of vowels produced by Greek speakers with hearing impairment. *Proceedings of 16th International Congress of Phonetic Sciences*, 1969–1972.

Nittrouer, S. (1995). Children learn separate aspects of speech production at different rates: Evidence from spectral moments. *Journal of the Acoustical Society of America*, *97*, 520–530.

Nycz, J., & Hall-Lew, L. (2013). Best practices in measuring vowel merger. *Journal of the Acoustical Society of America*, *20*(1), 2–19.

Ohala, J.J. (1993). The phonetics of sound change. In C. Jones (Ed.), *Historical linguistics: problems and perspectives* (pp. 243–251). London, England: Routledge,.

Ohde, R.N., Haley, K., & Barne, C. (2006). Perception of the [m]-[n] distinction in consonant-vowel (CV) and vowel-consonant (VC) syllables produced by child and adult talkers. *Journal of the Acoustical Society of America*, *119*, 1697–1711.

Padareva-Ilieva, G., & Georgieva, D. (2018). F2 Transition Measurement in Bulgarian Adults who Stutter and who do not Stutter. *Foreign Language Teaching*, *45*(3), 243–251.

Palethorpe, S., Wales, R., Clark, J.E., & Senserrick, T. (1996). Vowel classification in children. *Journal of the Acoustical Society of America*, *100*, 3843–51.

Pisoni, D.B. (2017). Speech 9 Perception: Research, Theory, and Clinical Application. In E.M. Fernández, & H. Smith Cairns (Eds.), *The Handbook of Psycholinguistics* (pp. 193–212). London, England: Wiley Blackwell.

Potter, R.K., Kopp, G.A., & Kopp, H.G. (1966). *Visible Speech*. New York, England: Dover.

Preston, J.L., & Edwards, M.L. (2009). Speed and accuracy of rapid speech output by adolescents with residual speech sound errors including rhotics. *Clinical Linguistics & Phonetics*, *23*(4), 301–318.

Preston, J.L., & Leece, M.C. (2017). Intensive treatment for persisting rhotic distortions: A case series. *American journal of speech-language pathology*, *26*(4), 1066–1079.

Prosek, R., Montgomery, A., Walden, B., & Hawkins, D. (1987). Formant frequencies of stuttered and fluent vowels. *Journal of Speech and Hearing Research*, *30*, 301–305.

Ramos, V. M., Hernandez-Diaz, H.A.K., Huici, M.E.H.D., Martens, H., Van Nuffelen, G., & De Bodt, M. (2020). Acoustic features to characterize sentence accent production in dysarthric speech. *Biomedical Signal Processing and Control*, *57*, 101750.

Recasens, D. (1999). Lingual coarticulation. *Coarticulation: Theory, data and techniques*, *4*, 80–104.

Recasens, D. (2014). *Coarticulation and sound change in Romance*. New York, NY: John Benjamins Publishing Company.

Recasens, D., & Espinosa, A. (2005). Articulatory, positional and coarticulatory characteristics for clear/l/ and dark/l: evidence from two Catalan dialects. *Journal of the International Phonetic Association*, *35*(1), 1–25.

Robb, M., & Blomgren, M. (1997). Analysis of F2 transitions in the speech of stutterers and nonstutterers. *Journal of Fluency Disorders*, *22*, 1–16.

Romani, C., Galuzzi, C., Guariglia, C., & Goslin, J. (2017). Comparing phoneme frequency, age of acquisition, and loss in aphasia: Implications for phonological universals. *Cognitive neuropsychology*, *34*(7–8), 449–471.

Rowe, H.P., & Green, J.R. (2019). Profiling Speech Motor Impairments in Persons with Amyotrophic Lateral Sclerosis: An Acoustic-Based Approach. *Proceedings of Interspeech*, 4509–4513.

Rubertus, E., & Noiray, A. (2018). On the development of gestural organization: A cross-sectional study of vowel-to-vowel anticipatory coarticulation. *PloS one*, *13*(9), e0203562.

Rusz, J., Cmejla, R., Ruzickova, H., & Ruzicka, E. (2011). Quantitative acoustic measurements for characterization of speech and voice disorders in early untreated Parkinson's disease. *The Journal of the Acoustical Society of America*, *129*(1), 350–367.

Sapir, S., Ramig, L.O., Spielman, J.L., & Fox, C. (2010). Formant centralization ratio: A proposal for a new acoustic measure of dysarthric speech. *Journal of Speech, Language and Hearing Research*, *53*(1), 114–125.

Scobbie, J.M. (2006). (R) as a variable. In K. Brown (Ed.), *Encyclopedia of language & linguistics, Second Edition*(pp. 337–344). Oxford, England: Elsevier.

Smith, C.H., Patel, S., Woolley, R.L., Brady, M.C., Rick, C.E., Halfpenny, R., & Au, P. (2019). Rating the intelligibility of dysarthic speech amongst people with Parkinson's Disease: a comparison of trained and untrained listeners. *Clinical linguistics & phonetics*, *33*(10–11), 1063–1070.

Stevens, K.N. (1972). The quantal nature of speech: evidence from articulatory-acoustic data. In E. Davis, & D.P. Denes (Eds.), *Human Communication: A unified view* (pp. 51–66). New York, NY: McGraw Hill.

Stevens, K.N. (2000). *Acoustic phonetics*. New York, NY: MIT press.

Stevens, K.N., & Hanson, H.M. (2013). Articulatory-Acoustic relations as the bias of Distinctive Contrasts. In W.J. Hardcastle, J. Laver, & F.E. Gibbon (Eds.), *The Handbook of Phonetic Sciences. Second Edition*(424–453). London, England: Wiley-Blackwell.

Subramanian, A., Yairi, E., & Amir, O. (2003). Second formant transitions influent speech of persistentand recovered preschool children who stutter. *Journal of Communication Disorders*, *36*, 59–75.

Sudro, P.N., & Prasanna, S.M. (2019). Modification of Devoicing Error in Cleft Lip and Palate Speech. *Proceedings of Interspeech*, 4519–4523.

Thomas, E. (2010). *Sociophonetics: an introduction*. New York, NY: Macmillan International Higher Education.

Traunmüller, H. (1990). Analytical expressions for the Tonotopic Sensory Scale. *Journal of the Acoustical Society of America*, *88*, 97–100.

Uchanski, R., & Geers, A. (2003). Acoustic characteristics of the speech of young cochlear implant users: a comparison with normal-hearing age-mates. *Ear Hearing*, *24*, 90–105.

Van der Harst, S. (2011). *The vowel space paradox. A sociophonetic study*. Leiden, The Netherlands: LOT.

Van Lieshout, P.H. (1995). *Motor planning and articulation in fluent speech of stutterers and nonstutterers*. Nijmegen: The Netherlands: University Press Nijmegen.

Verhaegen, C., Delvaux, V., Fagniart, S., Huet, K., Piccaluga, M., & Harmegnies, B. (2020). Phonological and phonetic impairment in aphasic speech: an acoustic study of the voice onset time of six French-speaking aphasic patients. *Clinical linguistics & phonetics*, *34*(3), 201–221.

Wang, M. (2016). Research on the Acoustic Realization of Lateral in Sudanese. *International Journal of Engineering Research and Development*, *12*(10), 44–48.

Windsor, F., Kelly, M.L., & Hewlett, N. (Eds.). (2012). *Investigations in clinical phonetics and linguistics*. New York, NY: Taylor & Francis.

Whiteside, S.P., Robson, H., Windsor, F., & Varley, R. (2012). Stability in voice onset time patterns in a case of acquired apraxia of speech. *Journal of Medical Speech-Language Pathology*, *20*, 17–28.

Whitfield, J.A., & Goberma, A.M. (2014). Articulatory–acoustic vowel space: Application to clear speech in individuals with Parkinson's disease. *Journal of Communication Disorders*, *51*, 19–28.

Whitfield, J.A., Reif, A., & Goberman, A.M. (2018). Voicing contrast of stop consonant production in the speech of individuals with Parkinson disease ON and OFF dopaminergic medication. *Clinical Linguistics & Phonetics*, *32*(7), 587–594.

Whitfield, J.A., & Mehta, D.D. (2019). Examination of clear speech in Parkinson disease using measures of working vowel space. *Journal of Speech, Language, and Hearing Research*, *62*(7), 2082–2098.

Whitfield, J.A., & Gravelin, A.C. (2019). Characterizing the distribution of silent intervals in the connected speech of individuals with Parkinson disease. *Journal of communication disorders*, 78, 18–32.

Windsor, F., Kelly, M.L., & Hewlett, N. (Eds.). (2013). *Investigations in Clinical Phonetics and Linguistics*. London, England: CRC Press.

Wright, R. (2004). Factors of lexical competition in vowel articulation. *Papers in laboratory phonology* 6, 75–87.

Yılmaz, E., Mitra, V., Sivaraman, G., & Franco, H. (2019). Articulatory and bottleneck features for speaker-independent ASR of dysarthric speech. *Computer Speech & Language*, *58*, 319–334.

Yunusova, Y., Weismer, G., Westbury, J.R., & Lindstrom, M.J. (2008). Articulatory movements during vowels in speakers with dysarthria and healthy controls. *Journal of Speech, Language, and Hearing Research, 5*, 596–611.

Yunusova, Y., Green, J.R., Greenwood, L., Wang, J., Pattee, G.L., & Zinman, L. (2012). Tongue movements and their acoustic consequences in amyotrophic lateral sclerosis. *Folia Phoniatrica Et Logopaedica, 64*, 94–102.

Zahorian, S., & Jagharghi, A. (1993). Spectral shape versus formants as acoustic correlates for vowels. *Journal of the Acoustical Society of America, 94*, 1966–82.

Ziegler, W., & Von Cramon, D. (1986). Disturbed coarticulation in apraxia of speech: Acoustic evidence. *Brain and Language, 29*(1), 34–47.

31

PURE TONE AUDIOMETRY AND SPEECH AUDIOMETRY

Fei Zhao and Robert Mayr

Patients seeking care from a speech and language therapist (SLT) for speech and language disorders may present with hearing problems, mostly due to aging or having hearing impairment at birth (Welling & Ukstins, 2015). Because hearing ability is important for language and communication, SLTs play an essential role in minimizing the communication difficulties caused by hearing loss in individuals with speech and language disorders. Considering the scope of practice of SLTs, as set out by the Royal College of Speech and Language Therapists (RCSLT, 2018), this chapter provides a general introduction to pure tone audiometry and speech audiometry for clinicians with practical guidance. Its ultimate purpose is to equip SLT students and clinicians with a sufficient level of understanding of hearing and hearing impairment to carry out and interpret the outcomes obtained from a range of hearing assessments using pure tone signals and speech materials.

Introduction to pure tone audiometry

Pure tone audiometry (PTA) is a hearing sensitivity assessment method that measures a person's ability to hear pure tones at various sound frequencies. It was developed in the early 1940s and is widely used in clinical, occupational and educational settings (Kramer & Brown, 2019). The results obtained from PTA tests provide diagnostic information on the type and degree of hearing impairment in individuals, which, in turn, can be suggestive of possible underlying ear pathologies.

To conduct a PTA test in a clinical setting, a soundproof booth or a sound-attenuated room and a calibrated diagnostic audiometer are essential. Figure 31.1 shows an example of a typical setting for a pure tone audiometric test. Soundproof booths are used to minimize the influence of ambient noise on measurement results, ensuring an optimally controlled testing environment. According to the pure tone audiometry testing procedure recommended by the British Society of Audiology (BSA) (2018a), the ambient noise level should be under 30–35 dBA in a clinical setting, which roughly corresponds to the noise level during whispering. The procedure of conducting the PTA test will be discussed in detail below.

Because the PTA test has high test-retest reliability and validity in terms of diagnosis for certain ear pathologies, it is the most routinely used hearing test in ENT and Audiology clinics, and widely acknowledged as a "gold standard" in comparison to other audiological measurements when assessing an individual's hearing status (Katz,2014; Kramer & Brown, 2019). PTA contributes significantly toward diagnosis and differential diagnosis for auditory disorders.

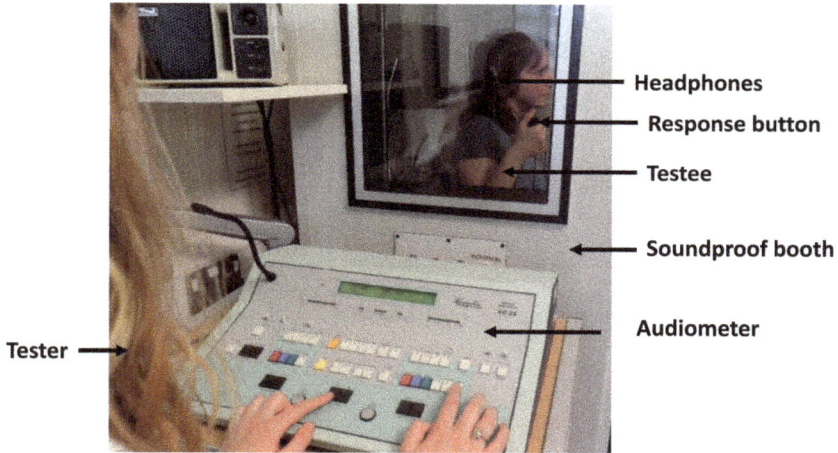

Figure 31.1 An example of a pure tone audiometric test in a sound-attenuated booth.

Audiograms

Because audibility of the human ear varies across different frequencies in terms of sound pressure level (i.e. dB SPL), for the purposes of convenience hearing level in dB (i.e. dB HL) is used to measure audibility in PTA instead of sound pressure level (dB SPL). As illustrated in Figure 31.2, an audiogram is a graphic representation of the audibility across the audiometric frequency range. Specifically, it depicts the frequency characteristics and dynamic range (i.e. between minimum sound and the loudest sound to be tolerated) in human ears. Audiograms encompass a frequency range between 125 and 8,000 Hz (x-axis),

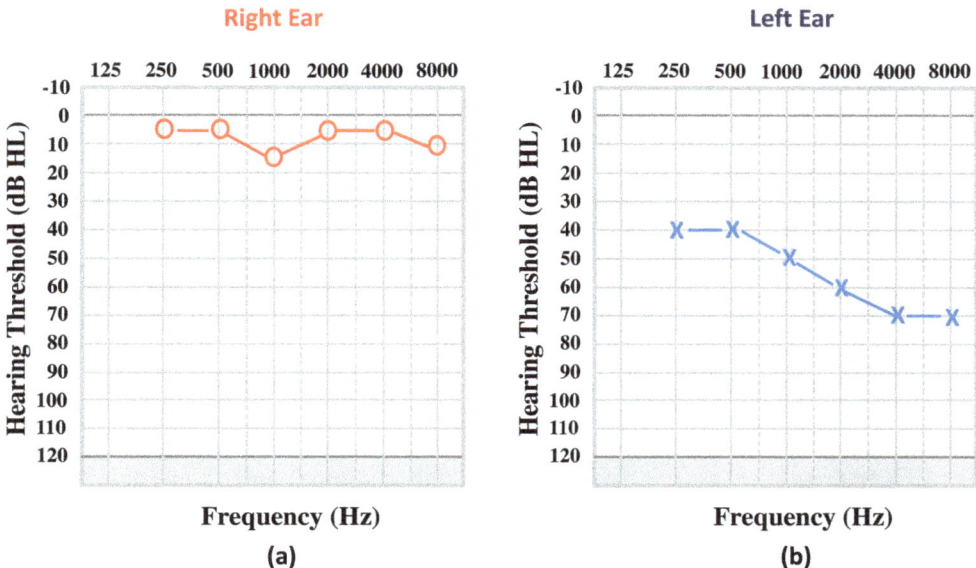

Figure 31.2 Examples of audiograms showing (a) normal hearing and (b) mild to moderate hearing loss.

Table 31.1 Pure tone audiometric measurements and symbols (Adapted from BSA recommended procedure, 2018a)

	Right ear		Left ear	
	Unmasked	*Masked*	*Unmasked*	*Masked*
Air conduction (AC)	O		X	
Bone conduction (BC)	Δ	[	Δ	]
Uncomfortable level		L	⌐	⌐

Note 1: Some of the symbols used in audiological software packages may differ from those recommended here. This is acceptable as long as the results are clear and unambiguous.

Note 2: Air-conduction symbols should be connected with continuous straight lines and bone-conduction symbols should be joined with broken lines.

and hearing level in dB (y-axis), ranging from−10 to 120 dB HL. Note that 0 dB HL refers to the level of a sound with reference to the standardized average threshold of audibility that occurs in normal listeners (Stach, 2019). The curve on the audiogram indicates the quietest sound levels the testee can hear. A curve close to the 0 dB HL line indicates normal hearing, as shown in Figure 31.2a, while a curve far below 0 dB HL indicates the need for a louder sound to be heard, thus indicating mild to moderate hearing loss, as shown in Figure 31.2b.

As shown in the audiograms above, the hearing threshold at a specific frequency obtained from the PTA is expressed as dB hearing level (i.e. dB HL), which can be plotted on an audiogram using specifically defined symbols to ease interpretation (Table 31.1).

Understanding hearing threshold measurements in PTA testing

The definition of hearing threshold is the minimum sound pressure level at which a sound of a specific frequency can be perceived by a given listener, i.e. the quietest possible sound that a subject can hear at a given frequency. *Air Conduction (AC)* refers to the incoming sound waves travelling through the ear canal to the eardrum, causing the eardrum to vibrate. These vibrations, in turn, cause movement of the ossicles (i.e. malleus, incus and stapes) that are connected to the eardrum on one side and to the inner ear on the other. The movement of the ossicles causes basilar membrane vibrations in the cochlea, which is sensed by the nerve cells. These nerve cells send electrical impulses through the auditory nerve to the brain. In contrast, *Bone Conduction (BC)* is defined as the transmission of sound waves to the inner ear through the vibrating bones of the skull for perceiving the sound, instead of sound being conveyed through air via the ear canal.

In people with normal auditory anatomic structure, AC is the main route for all sound to be transmitted; BC sound transmission occurs constantly, but only becomes noticeable when the external canals are blocked or the bone transducer is placed directly against the skull. For PTA testing, AC is usually measured using calibrated supra-aural headphones or insert phones (Figures 31.3a and 31.3b). For BC measurement, bone transducers are placed on the mastoid (Figure 31.3c). The difference between the AC and BC hearing threshold is called the A-B gap (ABG). The value of ABG is the most important diagnostic feature to distinguish

(a)

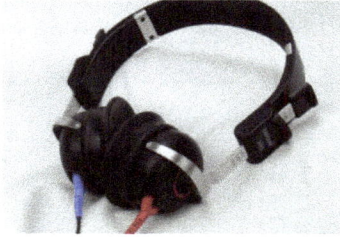

(b)

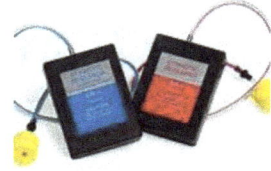

(c)

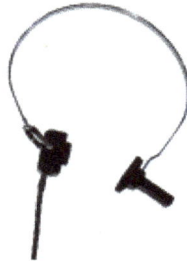

Figure 31.3 Examples of transducers used for pure tone audiometry testing; red colored side of headphones is used for right ear, blue colored side for left ear. (a) An example of TDH39-type Headphones (used with permission by MedRx http://www.medrx-usa.com); (b) An example of insert phones (used with permission of Etymotic https://www.etymotic.com); (c) An example of a bone vibrator (used with permission of Echodia http://echodia.fr/en/).

between conductive and sensorineural hearing loss. Its clinical indications will be discussed further below.

Using masking in PTA

Although SLTs may not perform a PTA themselves, in particular the complicated hearing threshold measures used when applying a masking procedure, it is useful for them to understand the rationale behind the use of masking. This theoretical knowledge will help SLTs in the interpretation of audiometric test results and their implications.

When measuring the hearing level of the affected ear, the test sound has to be fairly loud to be detectable. To avoid the non-test ear (NTE) hearing the sound, masking is needed during pure-tone audiometry because the measured hearing threshold may not be the true hearing level of the test ear (TE). As shown in Figure 31.4, there are several conditions that should be considered for masking. It is generally agreed that narrow band noise centered at the test frequency is the most efficient masker of pure tones (BSA, 2018a; Welling & Ukstins, 2015).

a) Condition 1: AC$_{TE}$ - AC$_{NTE}$ >= 40 dB

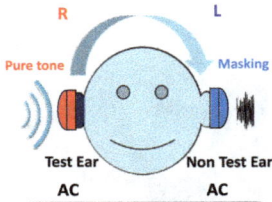

The 40-dB criterion is used because this is the smallest expected value for cross-lateralization of air-conducted tones.
AC$_{TE}$ - AC$_{NTE}$ >= **40 dB**

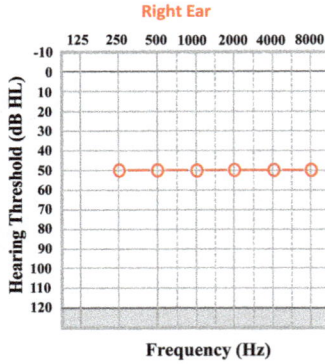

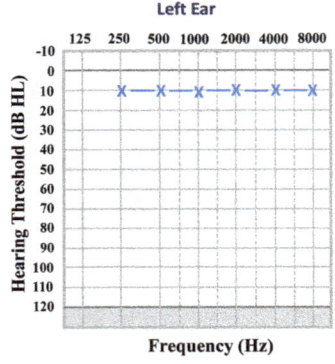

b) Condition 2: AC$_{TE}$ - BC$_{NTE}$ >= 40 dB

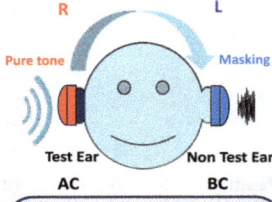

The presentation level at the test ear exceeds the unmasked bone-conduction threshold of the non-test ear by more than 40 dB.
AC$_{TE}$ - BC$_{NTE}$ >= **40 dB**

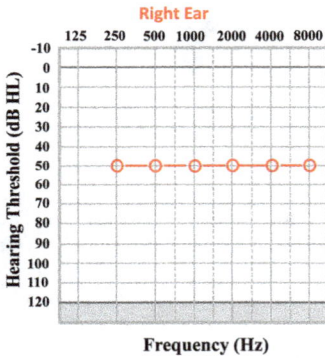

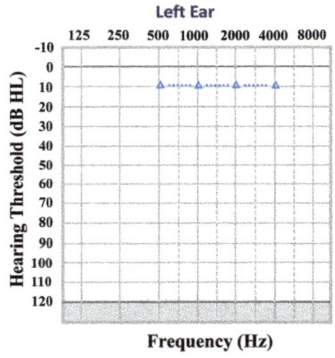

c) Condition 3: AC$_{TE}$ - BC$_{TE\ Umasked}$ >= 15 dB

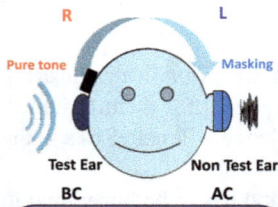

Non-test ear should be masked during bone-conduction testing anytime an unmasked air-bone gap is observed on the test ear
AC$_{TE}$ - BC$_{TE\ Umasked}$ >= **15 dB**

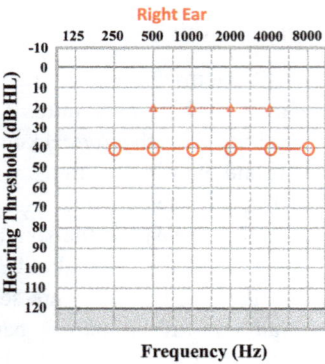

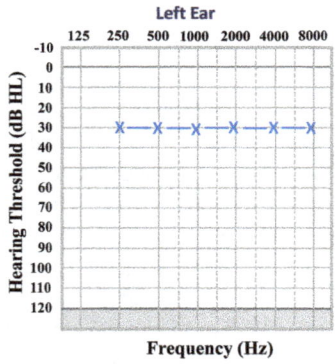

Figure 31.4　Conditions to be considered for masking in pure tone audiometry.

Performing pure tone audiometry (PTA)

PTA testing environment and setup

Because the purpose of the PTA test is to measure the minimum sound level a testee can hear, it is crucial to keep the testing environment as quiet as possible. In audiology clinics, PTA must be performed in a sound attenuated test room or soundproof booth (e.g. as shown in Figure 31.1). However, one should be aware that the hearing threshold is very likely to be elevated (i.e. worse than it should be), particularly at low frequencies when PTA is conducted in a non-sound treated room or a noisy environment.

The physical position of the testee during the PTA test is not fixed, allowing for a certain degree of flexibility. However, in order to obtain reliable hearing thresholds, the following principles ought to be adhered to: (1) The testee should be positioned so as to avoid any inadvertent visual cues by the tester, such as hand movements when operating the audiometer or facial expressions and (2) the tester should be able to clearly observe the testee's reactions without direct eye contact in case of any sign of confusion or difficulty managing the testing situation. The typical direction for arranging the testee's position is to have them facing away from the tester at an angle of 45°–90°.

Instructions for PTA testing

It is essential to give clear instructions to the testee before starting the test. According to the BSA recommended guidelines (BSA, 2018a), the instructions need to include the following information:

- The purpose of the PTA test: to test the testees' hearing by measuring the quietest sounds that they can hear. The testees should be told that they should sit quietly during the test.
- Equipment: a pair of headphones will be put around their ears and a response button will be held by the testees.
- The nature of the sound: tones with different pitches will be used, such as low-pitch "*woo*" sounds, or high-pitch "*sssss*" sounds.
- What to do when hearing the sound: As soon as a testee hears a sound, they should press a button on the response device or raise their hand. They should keep it pressed for as long as they hear the sound.
- What to do when the sound stops: They should release the button as soon as they no longer hear the sound.
- Encouragement: They should be encouraged to try hard even if the sound is very faint.
- Side to start: They need to be informed that each ear will be tested separately, starting with the better hearing side, followed by the other side.
- Possible interruption: They need to be informed that the test procedure may be interrupted or stopped if the testee feels any difficulty or discomfort during the test.
- Question: Testers ought to provide testees with an opportunity to ask any questions they may have.
- Confirmation of understanding: Testees ought to be asked to confirm that they have understood the procedure, and if not, be re-instructed.

Key steps of PTA testing

As recommended by the BSA (2018a), AC hearing thresholds are measured at octave frequencies from 250 to 8,000 Hz when using PTA in ENT/Audiology clinics, i.e. pure tone hearing thresholds are routinely measured at frequencies of 250, 500, 1,000, 2,000, 4,000 and 8,000 Hz. To establish a reliable hearing threshold, the key steps of standardized PTA testing are as follows:

- Frequencies tested: Testing starts with the better-hearing ear (according to the testee's account) at 1,000 Hz, the most sensitive frequency of the human ear; it then proceeds to 2,000 Hz, 4,000 Hz and 8,000 Hz; to ensure reliability, re-testing is conducted at 1,000 Hz and then at 500 Hz and 250 Hz before moving on to the other ear (BSA, 2018a).
- Initial intensity level to be used: The initial intensity of the sound should be presented at a higher level than the testee's estimated hearing level, such as at 40 dB HL for a normally hearing subject or approximately 30 dB above the estimated threshold for a subject with a hearing impairment, but never more than 80 dB HL. The presented tone at such a clearly audible intensity level will enable the testee to be familiarized with the sound stimulus.
- Pure tone presentations: The presentations of the tones should be 1–2 seconds in duration, with pauses of varying length (e.g. 2–4 seconds) between presentations, ensuring the patient is unable to predict the occurrence of presentations.
- Hearing threshold measurement and determination: The standard procedure for measuring hearing threshold is commonly called the "*down 10, up 5*" procedure. Figure 31.5 demonstrates the steps of establishing and determining the hearing thresholds at a particular frequency (For a more detailed testing procedure, see Kramer & Brown, 2019).

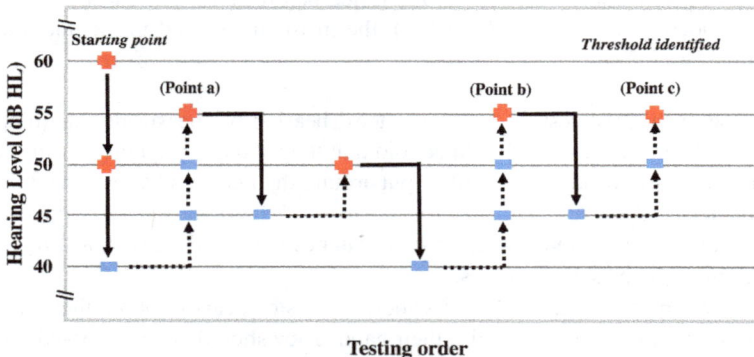

Figure 31.5   A demonstration of the steps of establishing and determining the hearing thresholds at 1,000 Hz.

Notes:

■: *Positive response*

■: *No response*

↓: *Decrease by 10 dB*

↑: *Increase by 5 dB*

Point a: 1st positive response at 55 dB HL

Point b: 2nd positive response at 55 dB HL

Point c: 3rd positive response at 55 dB HL

It should be noted that measuring hearing thresholds may be required at intermediate frequencies (e.g. 750 Hz, 15,00 Hz, 3,000 Hz and 6,000 Hz) in some cases, for example in the case of noise-induced high-frequency hearing loss.

Factors influencing the results and additional considerations

Because PTA is a subjective hearing test that requires testees to respond to stimuli when they hear a sound, like all subjective audiometric methods, a number of factors affect the accuracy and reliability of the results, for example, the test environment, background noise, familiarity of the subject with the method, concentration levels, alertness and the duration of the test. Therefore, to obtain accurate and reliable estimates of hearing thresholds, it is essential to be aware of, and avoid potential influences of such factors. In case of having unavoidable variables (e.g. background noise), test results should be noted on the audiogram in order to help interpreting the PTA results correctly.

Furthermore, for some special cases who have difficulties or are unwilling to cooperate with the PTA testing procedure, such as young children under 5 years of age, people with learning difficulties or older adults with dementia, alternative audiological measurements should be considered (BSA, 2018a; Kramer & Brown, 2019).

Interpretation of audiograms and clinical implications

To be clinically useful, the goal of PTA is to obtain accurate and reliable estimates of hearing thresholds, and consequently the audiogram provides essential diagnostic information in terms of degree of hearing loss and type of hearing loss. Moreover, the configuration of the audiogram may help to provide some indications of aetiological factors underlying the hearing loss.

Classifying degree of hearing loss and interpretation of its clinical significance

The principle underlying the classification scheme is to categorize the degrees of hearing loss based on a range from normal to profound, which indicates the extent to which the hearing loss may affect communication (ASHA, 2015; Bauch, 2014; Welling & Ukstins, 2015). According to the BSA classification system (2018a), AC hearing thresholds shown on the audiogram can be categorized in terms of either normal hearing status or different degrees of hearing loss expressed along the decibel range, i.e. normal, mild, moderate, severe and profound, as shown in Table 31.2.

It is noteworthy that there are several other classification systems to categorize the degree of hearing loss, such as those proposed by the American Speech-Language-Hearing Association (ASHA) (2018) and WHO (2012). Irrespective of the classification system used, they all provide testers with information on how to describe and interpret the degrees of hearing loss shown in the audiogram, and thus help to estimate its impact on communication and develop an appropriate intervention strategy.

It is quite common to find different degrees of hearing loss in an individual across the different frequencies shown on the audiogram (e.g. shown in Figure 31.2b). In general, it is unnecessary to assign the hearing threshold at each frequency to individual categories. The importance of the classification is to provide a general description of how the degree of hearing loss changes across frequencies. Therefore, one of the solutions is to use the average of hearing thresholds over four important frequencies to describe the overall level/degree of hearing loss. The average of one's hearing threshold is usually calculated using a set of specified frequencies, typically 500 Hz, 1,000 Hz, 2,000 Hz and 4,000 Hz, because this frequency

Table 31.2 Classification for degrees of hearing loss and their clinical implications

Classification of hearing loss	Characteristics and impact
Normal: −10 to 20 dB HL	• Able to hear quiet sounds • Occasional difficulty understanding speech in the presence of noise
Mild hearing loss: 20–40 dB HL	• Difficulty with faint or distant sounds • Increasing difficulty understanding speech in noisy situations or • Occasional non-detection of consonants
Moderate hearing loss: 41–70 dB HL*	• Ability to understand conversation if face-to-face in a quiet situation and vocabulary is controlled • Difficulty following group conversations • Inability to follow most of what is said in normal situations if hearing loss is moderately severe*
Severe hearing loss: 71–95 dB HL	• Inability to hear speech unless very loud • Severe difficulty following speech without an appropriate intervention (e.g. use of hearing aids)
Profound hearing loss: over 95 dB HL	• Inability to hear speech at all without an appropriate intervention (e.g. hearing aid or cochlear implantation) • Reliance on visual cues, such as lip-reading or sign language

*: This category can sometimes be further classified as *Moderate (41 to 55 dB HL)* and *Moderately severe hearing loss (56 to 70 dB HL)*.

range represents many speech sounds. In this case, the formula for calculating the average of hearing threshold is as follows:

The average of hearing threshold = $(HL_{500} + HL_{1000} + HL_{2000} + HL_{4000})/4$

For example, the average of hearing threshold in Figure 31.2b is 55 dB HL, which would be considered within the moderate range. Moreover, the average of hearing threshold is also helpful when comparing one ear to the other in order to determine an individual's better side for hearing.

Classifying type of hearing loss and interpretation of its clinical implications

As described in Chapter 3, the three main types of hearing loss are *conductive, sensorineural and mixed*. On the basis of audiograms, the different types of hearing loss can be diagnosed by appropriately interpreting the AC and BC hearing thresholds measured using PTA.

Conductive Hearing Loss (CHL) is a reduction in hearing sensitivity due to a disorder of the outer or middle ear. It results from mechanical attenuation of the sound waves in the outer or middle ear, preventing sound energy from reaching the cochlea. The typical audiogram of an individual with CHL shows abnormal AC hearing thresholds but normal BC hearing thresholds and the ABG is greater than 10 dB. As shown in Figure 31.6, the AC hearing thresholds across all frequencies are abnormal, ranging from 40 dB HL to 45 dB HL, while the BC hearing thresholds across frequencies are normal between 0 and 10 dB HL, with the ABG greater than 10 dB. The commonly seen ear disorders associated with CHL are earwax blockage, tympanic perforation, acute otitis media and otitis media with effusion.

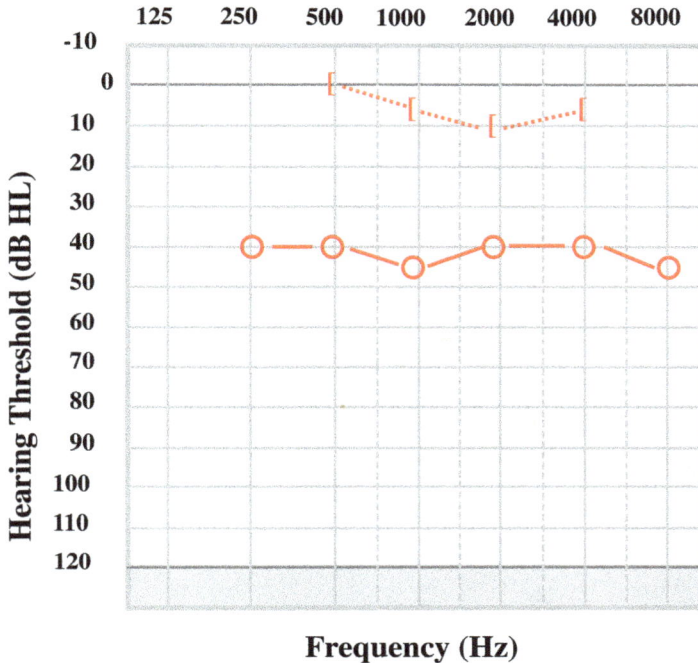

Figure 31.6 Example of an audiogram showing conductive hearing loss (CHL).

Sensorineural Hearing Loss (SNHL) is a reduction in hearing sensitivity due to a disorder of the inner ear. It results from defective function of the cochlea or the auditory nerve, and prevents neural impulses from being transmitted to the auditory cortex of the brain. The typical audiogram of an individual with SNHL shows both abnormal AC and BC hearing thresholds, and the ABG is less than 10 dB. As shown in Figure 31.7, AC and BC hearing thresholds across frequencies are abnormal, ranging from 35 dB HL to 45 dB HL and the ABG is less than 10 dB. The commonly seen cases with SNHL are age-related hearing loss and noise-induced hearing loss.

Mixed Hearing Loss is a reduction in hearing sensitivity due to a combination of a disorder of the outer or middle ear and the inner ear. In cases of mixed hearing loss, the typical audiogram shows that both AC and BC hearing thresholds are in the abnormal range, with the ABG generally greater than 10 dB (Figure 31.8).

Classification of audiogram configurations and interpretation of its clinical implications

The graph shown on audiograms indicates the configuration of hearing loss, which can be categorized as either symmetrical or asymmetrical when comparing the right ear and the left ear. A symmetrical configuration of hearing loss refers to the same or similar severity and shape of hearing loss in each ear. Individuals with age-related hearing loss usually show symmetrical configuration of hearing loss (Figure 31.9). In contrast, an asymmetrical configuration of hearing loss is defined as a difference of 15 dB between the right and left ears

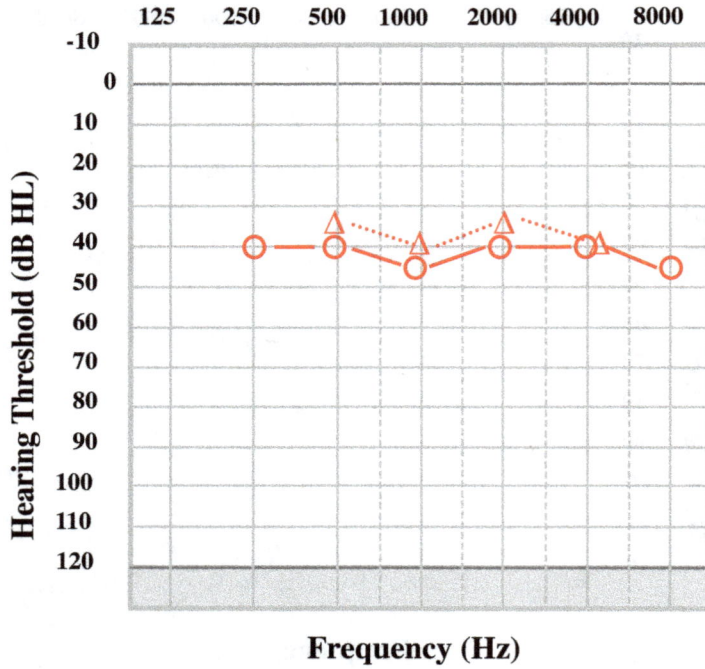

Figure 31.7   Example of an audiogram showing sensorineural hearing loss (SNHL).

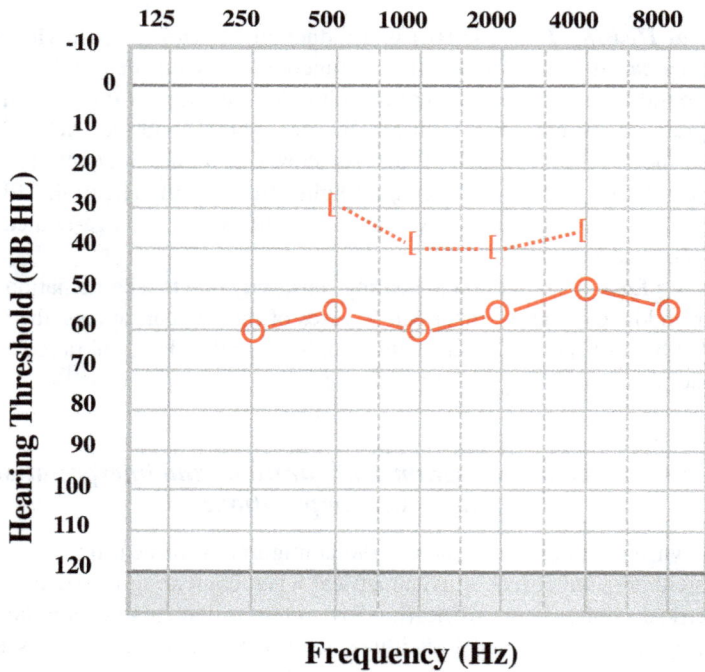

Figure 31.8   Example of an audiogram showing mixed hearing loss.

Right Ear

Left Ear

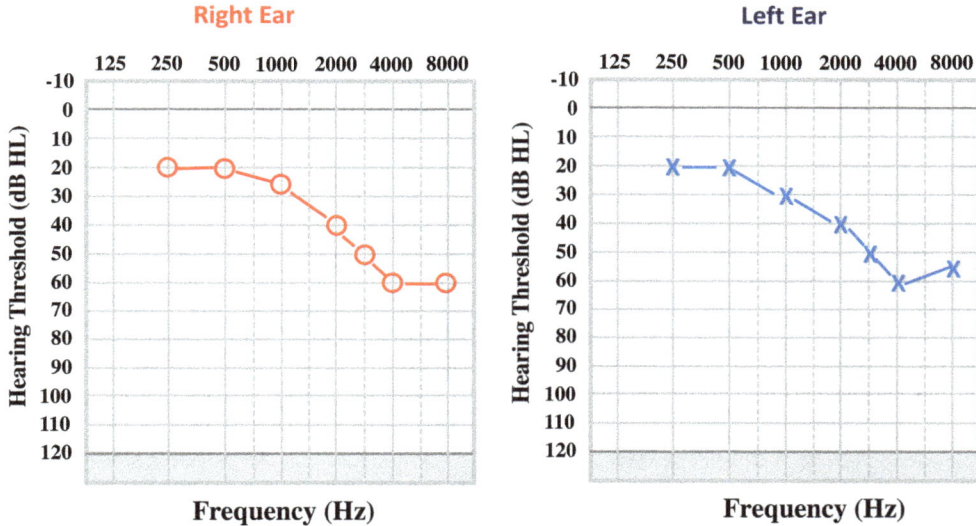

Figure 31.9 Example of an audiogram showing a symmetrical sensorineural hearing loss.

at three contiguous frequencies. Further investigation is always required, even in the absence of hearing loss, because an asymmetrical configuration of hearing loss may be indicative of a benign tumor called ***acoustic neuroma*** (or ***vestibular schwannoma***) (Figure 31.2). This diagnosis is particularly likely in the presence of additional symptoms, notably vertigo and tinnitus.

Furthermore, according to the audiometric configuration, different shapes or patterns of audiogram may be identified, such as ***flat, ski-sloping and cookie-bite (or U-shaped)*** audiometric configurations (Figure 31.10). For example, individuals with a flat audiometric configuration (Figure 31.10a) have the same or a similar degree of hearing loss across different points along the frequency range, whereas individuals with a sloping configuration exhibit normal hearing or a mild degree of hearing loss at low frequencies, moderate loss at mid-frequency range and severe hearing loss at the higher frequencies (Figure 31.10b). More importantly, several audiometric configurations can provide an indication of the possible etiological causes for hearing loss. For example, studies have shown that a cookie-bite (or U-shaped) audiometric configuration (Figure 31.10c) is associated with a certain type of autosomal dominant hereditary hearing loss (Mazzoli, Kennedy, Newton, Zhao & Stephens, 2001). Such information can support genetic counseling. In addition, a notched audiometric configuration of hearing loss between 3,000 Hz and 6,000 Hz typically indicates the cause of damage to be noise exposure (Figure 31.10d).

Speech audiometry

Speech audiometry is an important clinical tool to assess the impact of hearing loss on a person's ability to recognize and understand the speech signal they are hearing. It generally confirms pure tone audiometry results, but is recognized as a complementary measure to pure tone audiometry because PTA only shows hearing sensitivity to pure tones. It cannot represent the sounds we listen to in real-world environments. Furthermore, because speech perception involves a complex neurological and psychological process, speech audiometry

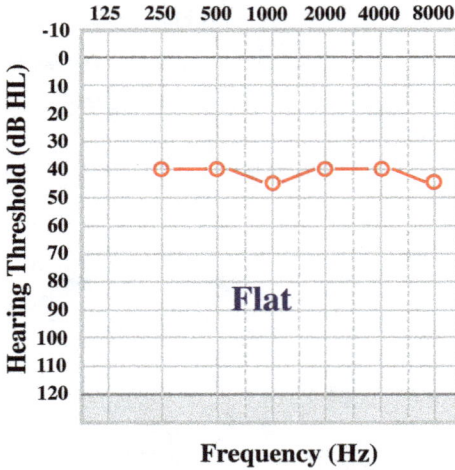

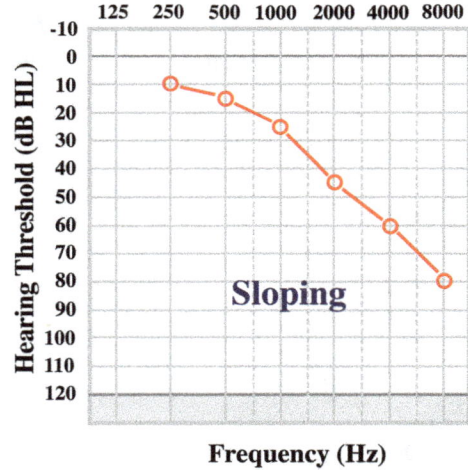

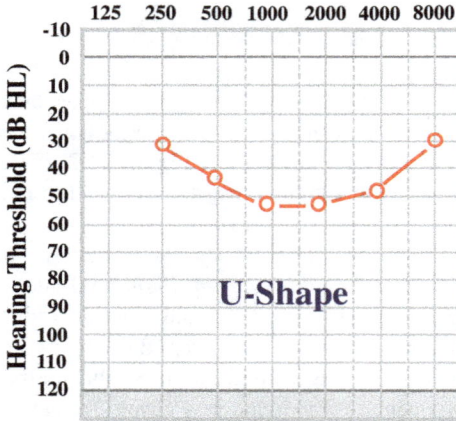

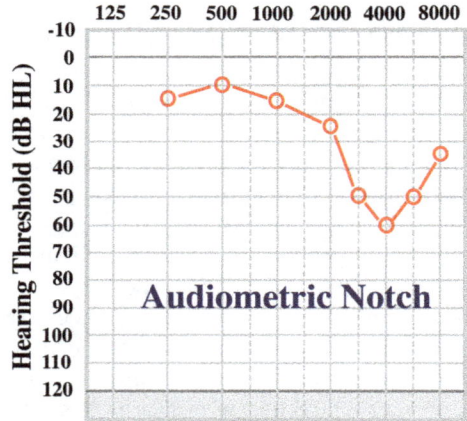

Figure 31.10 Examples of audiograms showing different configurations. (a) Example of a flat audiogram. (b) Example of a sloping audiogram. (c) Example of a U-Shape audiogram. (d) Example of an audiogram with a notch.

provides additional information in terms of a hearer's ability to recognize and discriminate speech, which may not simply be related to their degree of pure tone hearing loss (Kramer & Brown, 2019; Welling & Ukstins, 2015). Therefore, the major clinical contributions of speech audiometry are

- To assess speech intelligibility using specific types of speech stimuli in order to aid the identification of the degree and type of hearing loss and its impact on communication difficulty, particularly the difficulty of understanding speech in a quiet environment or in the presence of background noise.

- To provide valuable information on the diagnosis of certain central auditory pathologies (e.g. tumor of the auditory nerve, central auditory processing disorders).
- To evaluate the outcomes during audiological interventions, such as hearing aid fitting or cochlear implantation.

Speech materials used for speech audiometry

Speech materials used for speech audiometry can be open-set (e.g. using live voice) or closed-set (e.g. using standardized words or sentences). The digits or single words given by live voice can be used as open-set speech materials for speech audiometry. It is very easy and flexible to use, particularly in the absence of technical facilities. However, test results thus obtained may be difficult to quantify. The use of closed-set speech materials, in contrast, involves testees being given a set of standardized words or sentences to listen to either through headphones or in free field. Their task is then to repeat what they have heard.

There are many different standardized words or sentences used for speech audiometry around the world. English materials include spondaic word lists (e.g. hotdog, football), phonemically balanced word lists or sentences. One of the most widely used of these is the AB short wordlist test first developed by Arthur Boothroyd in 1968, a type of *Speech Recognition Test* (SRT). The AB test consists of 15 wordlists, with each list containing 10 phonemically balanced mono-syllabic words and each word having the same phonemic composition, i.e. three phonemes constructed as consonant–vowel–consonant. Therefore, each word list contains the same 30 phonemes in different combinations. The scoring system for the AB test is based on how many phonemes are correctly repeated by the end of each word list being tested. Three points are assigned to each word in the AB word lists, i.e. one for each phoneme. Only when a phoneme is entirely correct, does it obtain a score of 1. The wordlist and scoring procedure is illustrated in Table 31.3. For example, if the test word is SH-I-P (/ʃɪp/) and the testee's response is T-I-P ([tɪp]), they obtain a score of 2 out of 3.

Instructions for speech audiometry testing and the scoring system

As with the PTA test, it is also essential to give clear instructions to testees for speech audiometry tests. They need to be informed that instead of pressing a button to give a response, they are

Table 31.3 AB Wordlist 1 and example of scoring system

Word	Testee's response	Score	%
Ship	*Tip*	2	7
Rug	*Jug*	2	7
Fan	*Sun*	1	3
Cheek	*Eat*	1	3
Haze	*Aid*	1	3
Dice	*Eyes*	1	3
Both	*Boat*	2	7
Well	*Will*	2	7
Jot	*Jot*	3	10
Move	*Moon*	2	7
TOTAL		17/30	57

Note: **Score for Wordlist 1 = 57%**

requested to repeat a word said by the tester during the speech audiometry test. The instruction would typically be as follows:

> *"I am going to test your hearing by using a series of words. Please repeat the word you have heard. If you are not sure of the word or have only heard part of the word, please repeat as much of it as you can. Try to respond to every word you have heard."*

Understanding of SRT results and their implications

The SRT is the most commonly used speech audiometry method in ENT/Audiology clinics. It is performed by requiring the subject to repeat standard word lists delivered through headphones or speakers at varying intensities. The SRT threshold is determined by measuring the lowest level at which a testee can correctly identify words at least 50% of the time (Kramer & Brown, 2019), as demonstrated in Curve A in Figure 31.11.

The SRT is generally comparable to the results obtained from the PTA. In addition, characteristics of the SRT curve have diagnostic value in differentiating different types of hearing loss. For example, in the case of conductive hearing loss, the response curve has a normal "S" shape (Curve B in Figure 31.11), showing a shift to the right compared to the

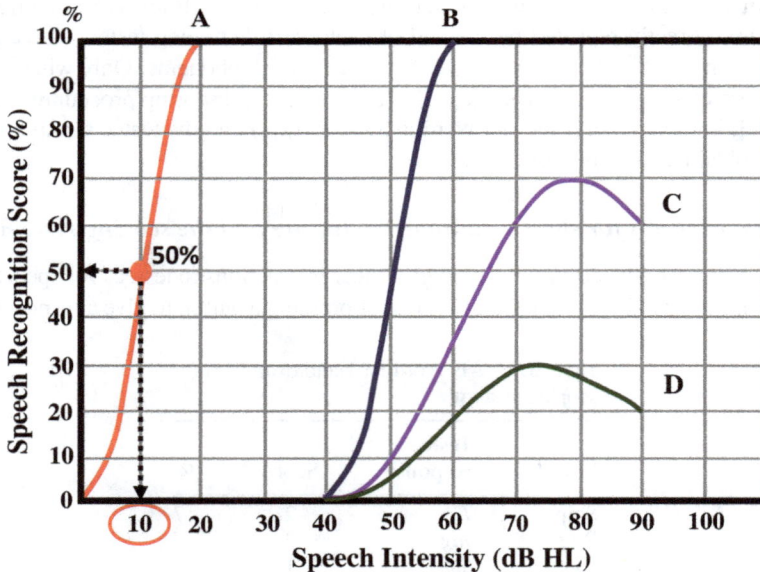

Figure 31.11   SRT characteristics in normal hearing and hearing impaired subjects.

Notes:

Curve A: Example of an SRT curve obtained from a testee with normal hearing.

Curve B: Example of an SRT curve obtained from a testee with conductive hearing loss.

Curve C: Example of an SRT curve obtained from a testee with sensorineural hearing loss.

Curve D: Example of an SRT curve obtained from a testee with retro-cochlear pathology.

normal reference curve without deformation. It means that a good speech recognition score (e.g. close to 100% correct) can be achieved when the intensity of the speech signal increases. In contrast, in the case of sensorineural hearing loss, although there is also an increase in the speech recognition score when the intensity of speech signal increases, the SRT curve typically shows deformations in higher intensity regions, indicating distortions (a roll-over effect, i.e. with increasing intensity, the percentage of correctly identified words decreases), although it may be normal elsewhere (Curve C in Figure 31.11). Curve C indicates that a moderate-severe sensorineural hearing loss can cause speech intelligibility with distortion occurring at intensities greater than 80 dB HL.

Finally, one of the major contributions of speech audiometry is to help diagnose retro-cochlear pathology on the basis of the unique SRT pattern shown in Curve D of Figure 31.11. As the figure shows, the speech recognition scores are very poor, no matter the increases in speech intensity. Therefore, SRT tests are an essential component within the test battery for identifying possible central auditory pathologies, particularly when speech intelligibility scores are significantly poorer than can be explained by pure-tone thresholds.

Applications of speech audiometry in audiological rehabilitation and other considerations

Because testing signals used in speech audiometry represent the sounds we listen to in real-world environments, speech audiometry is applied in a variety of ways in the typical hearing aid fitting protocol as part of pre-fitting selection, hearing aid fitting verification and rehabilitative counseling (Pittman, Stewart, Willman & Odgear, 2017). Numerous measures of Speech-in-Noise (SiN) tests (e.g. HINT (Hearing In Noise Test); Quick Speech In Noise (QuickSIN); The Acceptable Noise Level Test (ANLT)) are of particular value in assessing the efficacy of hearing aid fitting (BSA, 2018b; Nabelek, Tampas, & Burchfeld, 2004; Nabelek, Freyaldenhoven,Tampas, Burchfeld, & Muenchen, 2006; Saunders & Forsline, 2006).

Due to the complexity of speech audiometry in terms of testing materials and involvement of neurological processing, in comparison to PTA, more variables may affect reliability of the measurement results, such as difficulty to calibrate speech signals, the measurement technique, age, cognitive function and language ability. As a result, alternative speech test materials need to be considered in some cases to adapt the individual's age, cognitive function and language ability. Moreover, further investigation should be considered if there is a mismatch between the results obtained from speech audiometry and other diagnostic tests, such as equipment calibration or the reliability of responses.

Conclusion

Pure tone audiometry is a fundamental clinical tool to assess an individual's hearing status in terms of the degree, type and configuration of hearing loss. These results provide otologists and audiologists together with SLTs and other relevant healthcare professionals with important diagnostic information to determine the nature and cause of the hearing dysfunction, and thus allow clinical decisions to be made in terms of the selection of an appropriate management plan. Although speech audiometry is relatively complicated to perform, its results can be used as a more sensitive indicator than pure tone audiometry to evaluate the real social and communication difficulties experienced by hearing impaired individuals.

However, pure tone and speech audiometry involve voluntary behavioral responses from the testees. As with any such subjective measurements, there can be variability or error in the measurements, and this, in turn, can affect the certainty of the diagnosis. Therefore, other objective audiological measurements (e.g. tympanometry, auditory brainstem response tests) are needed to cross-check the results obtained from pure tone and speech audiometry.

References

American Speech-Language-Hearing Association (ASHA) (2015). *Type, degree, and configuration of hearing loss.* https://www.asha.org/uploadedFiles/AIS-Hearing-Loss-Types-Degree-Configuration.pdf. (Accessed on February 4, 2020).

Bauch, C.D. (2014). *Mayo Clinic on better hearing and balance(2nd ed.).* New York, NY: Rosetta Books.

Boothroyd, A. (1968). Developments in speech audiometry. *Sound,* 2, 3–10.

British Society of Audiology (BSA) (2018a*). Recommended procedure: Pure-tone air-conduction and bone-conduction threshold audiometry with and without masking.* https://www.thebsa.org.uk/resources/pure-tone-air-bone-conduction-threshold-audiometry-without-masking/ (Accessed on February 4, 2020).

British Society of Audiology (BSA) (2018b) *Practice Guidance: Assessment of speech understanding in noise in adults with hearing difficulties.* http://www.thebsa.org.uk/wp-content/uploads/2018/11/BSA-Practice-Guidance-Speech-in-Noise-Consultation-DRAFT-Nov-18.pdf. (Accessed on February 4, 2020).

Katz, J. (2014). *Handbook of clinical audiology (7th International Edition).* Philadelphia, PA: Lippincott Williams and Wilkins.

Kramer, S. & Brown, D.K. (2019). *Audiology: Science to practice(3rd ed.).* San Diego, CA: Plural Publishing Inc.

Mazzoli, M., Kennedy, V., Newton, V., Zhao, F. & Stephens, D. (2001). Phenotype/genotype correlation of autosomal dominant and autosomal recessive non-syndromal hearing impairment. In: Martini, A., Mazzoli, M., Stephens, D. & Read, A. (Eds.). *Definitions, protocols and guidelines in genetic hearing impairment* (pp. 79–141). London, UK: Whurr.

Nabelek, A.K., Tampas, J.W. & Burchfeld, S.B. (2004) Comparison of speech perception in background noise with acceptance of background noise in aided and unaided conditions. *Journal of Speech, Language, and Hearing Research,* 47, 1001–1011.

Nabelek, A.K., Freyaldenhoven, M.C., Tampas, J.W., Burchfeld, S.B. & Muenchen, R. A. (2006). Acceptable noise level as a predictor of hearing aid use. *Journal of the American Academy of Audiology,* 17, 626–639.

Pittman, A.L., Stewart, E.C., Willman, A.P. & Odgear, I.S. (2017). Word recognition and learning: Effects of hearing loss and amplification feature. *Trends in Hearing,* 21, 1–13.

Royal College of Speech and Language Therapists (RCSLT) (2018). *RCSLT Curriculum Guidance for the pre-registration education of speech and language therapists.* https://www.rcslt.org/-/media/Project/RCSLT/curriculum-guidance-2018.pdf (Accessed on February 4, 2020).

Saunders, G.H. & Forsline, A. (2006). The Performance-Perceptual Test (PPT) and its relationship to aided reported handicap and hearing aid satisfaction. *Ear Hear,* 27, 229–242.

Stach, B.A. (2019). *Comprehensive dictionary of audiology: Illustrated (3rd ed.).* San Diego, CA: Plural Publishing.

Welling, D.R. & Ukstins, C.A. (2015). *Fundamentals of audiology for the Speech-Language Pathologist (2nd ed.).* Burlington, VT: Jones & Barlett Publishers, Inc.

World Health Organisation (WHO) (2012). *Grades of hearing impairment.* https://www.who.int/pbd/deafness/hearing_impairment_grades/en/ (Accessed on February 4, 2020).

32

ALTERED SENSORY FEEDBACK IN SPEECH

Liam Barrett and Peter Howell

Introduction

During speech control, the brain generates a motor plan for an utterance and issues it to the articulators. Sensory consequences occur as the motor plan is performed that provide information about the utterance. This information can be returned over afferent pathways to allow discrepancies between the planned (efferent) and output (afferent) forms of speech to be detected. Monitoring for discrepancies would allow planning errors to be identified and feedback control occurs when errors are corrected (Howell, 2004a). The afferent information is carried in several sensory modalities (e.g. auditory, kinaesthetic and somatosensory). Audition is the modality used most often in feedback theories where the idea is that speakers listen to their speech output whilst it is being produced and speech is interrupted and corrected when planning errors are heard. A way of testing such theories is to perturb the auditory signal (change the temporal, spectral or intensity properties) that makes it appear that an error has occurred during articulation. Speakers then respond to correct the putative error and this disrupts speech control. Hence, speech disruption under auditory perturbations is considered to support auditory feedback theories.

Superficially, the disruptions to speech under auditory perturbations are similar to the dysfluencies that people who stutter (PWS) show in their unperturbed speech. This could arise because the correction-process that works for fluent speakers malfunctions in PWS. Furthermore, when the auditory feedback (AFB) of PWS was perturbed, fluency was enhanced (Howell,2004a for review). This was interpreted as showing that the problem PWS had in dealing with auditory feedback was corrected when the afferent signal was manipulated. The research on perturbations led to neural accounts of fluency control of speech, whilst the studies with PWS was exploited in interventions for speech control problems (Costello-Ingham, 1993, ; Goldiamond 1965; Howell, 2004b; Ryan, 1974; Max et al., 2004; Tourville & Guenther, 2011). This chapter reviews the effects temporal, spectral and intensity perturbations to auditory and vibratory feedback have on fluent speakers and PWS.

Altered sensory feedback

Procedures to alter the sensory consequences of own speech output include changes to AFB and VibroTactile Feedback (VTF). With AFB and VTF, temporal, spectral and intensity parameters can be altered separately or together. Furthermore, the sensory parameters have been manipulated in different ways (e.g. the spectrum of all, or just some, components of speech have been altered) and their impact on speech control may differ.

Temporal changes to AFB (Delayed Auditory Feedback)

Fluent speakers

Speech can be delayed relative to normal listening conditions, referred to as Delayed Auditory Feedback (DAF). Early work on DAF with fluent speakers, showed that speech errors[1] arise (Black,1951; Fairbanks, 1955; Lee, 1950), speakers increase voice level (Howell, 1990), speech is slowed, medial vowels in syllables are elongated (Howell, Wingfield & Johnson, 1988) and pitch is monotone. The way speakers respond to changes in the intensity of the DAF signal can be used to determine whether speakers treat DAF as speech or noise (Howell, 1990). When speakers heard their non-delayed speech amplified whilst speaking, voice level decreased (Howell, 1990) which indicated speakers compensated (Fletcher effect) intensity when vocal output was too loud (Lane & Tranel, 1971). However, when the intensity of speech delayed by 100 ms was increased, speakers *increase*d the intensity of their speech (Howell, 1990). This is a Lombard effect that occurs when speech is produced in noisy environments (speakers attempt to speak above the noise). The Lombard effect indicated that the delay transformed speech into a non-speech noise, rendering it unusable for feedback control. The Lombard effect in Howell (1990) was monotonic over the intensity range studied (all increases in DAF intensity increased vocal intensity). A Lombard effect also occurred when speaking along with white noise which further confirmed that the delayed speech sound under DAF was treated as noise rather than speech (Howell, 1990).

For fluent speakers, the length of the DAF delay-interval affects speech rate (Howell & Powell, 1987). The effects on speech rate differ for "short" delays (<100 ms) where speech rate reduces, and "long" delays (>100 ms) where speech rate increases (Kalinowski et al., 1996). Note that other authors classify delays as short/long at different durations (discussed below).

The length of the delay interval and/or intensity of DAF have been manipulated with PWS. In general, choice of what parameter value to use depends on effects Speech and Language Pathologists (SLPs) might want to induce when using them in interventions. For instance, DAF-delays could be chosen that slow speech rate or the level of DAF could be adjusted to increase vocal intensity.

People who stutter

Lee (1950) considered that there were similarities between the dysfluencies induced in fluent speakers when speaking under DAF and the dysfluencies that occur under normal-speaking conditions in PWS. The supposed similarity is misleading (Howell, 2011). For instance, superficially prolongations in stuttered speech are similar to the vowel-elongations noted in connection with DAF. However, prolongations usually occur on onset consonants whereas medial vowels are mainly affected under DAF (Howell et al., 1988). Thus, prolongations and vowel-elongations under DAF differ both on phone type and syllable position that is affected.

Nor is the speech of PWS like that observed when fluent speakers receive DAF: The natural speech of PWS is not louder or more monotonic as occurs when fluent speakers are given DAF (Howell, 2011).

Nevertheless, DAF improves the fluency of PWS to some extent. Early research on DAF with PWS tended to use long delays (100 ms and above) and concluded that DAF has the robust effect of removing stutters (Goldiamond, 1965; Lotzmann,1961; Nessel, 1958; Soderberg, 1969). That said, presenting long-delay DAF to PWS has undesirable side effects: The vowel-elongation noted to occur when fluent speakers speak under DAF also occurs with PWS (Howell et al., 1988). Howell (1990) reported that vocal intensity of PWS under long-delay (100 ms) led to a Lombard effect as noted with fluent speakers. This suggests that PWS process DAF at this delay as noise similar to fluent speakers. The increased vocal intensity under long-delay DAF that PWS experience, causes DAF speech to sound unnatural and the pattern persists post-intervention (Howell, 2004a; Novak, 1978). As well as external adjustments to intensity, speakers can influence feedback level by speaking at different loudness levels. If speech is at a low level, fluency-enhancement does not occur (Butler & Galloway, 1957). The intensity level of the delayed speech is important in accounting for differences in susceptibility to DAF across speakers, considered below (Howell & Archer, 1984).

Speech rate, vocal intensity and stuttering rate of PWS depend on the delay selected (Howell, 1990; Lotzmann, 1961; Soderberg, 1969). In the early studies on PWS, delays were employed that produced maximum disruption to fluent speakers (100–200 ms). Although long-delay DAF-speech reduces stuttering symptoms, the ancillary disfluencies that occur (drawls, loud speech, flat pitch and slow speech) are noticed by listeners (Geetha et al., 2017; Stuart & Kalinowski, 2004) and, as noted, may persist in post-intervention speech (Novak,1978). This has implications about how to employ DAF in interventions for PWS as one type of speech dysfluency may be replaced with another form.

The finding that the effects of DAF differ between long and short delays with fluent speakers is supported by studies on PWS. Kalinowski et al. (1996) proposed that DAF-delays less than 100 ms were "short" and that delays of 75 ms and 50 ms were optimal for improved speech rate and fluency. In unpublished work, Howell systematically varied delays below 100 ms and observed the impact on vocal output intensity when feedback intensity was adjusted at each delay. Delays under 30 ms led to a Fletcher effect whilst longer delays led to a Lombard effect. This suggested that the delayed sound was only treated as speech at delays up to 30 ms (somewhat shorter than Kalinowski et al., 1996 proposed).

Contemporary prostheses and research equipment delivers short-delay DAF (Howell, 2004a), typically 20–60 ms (Kalinowski et al., 1993). Short-delay DAF improves speech naturalness compared to long-delay DAF (Kalinowski et al., 1996) and maintains the fluency-enhancing effects observed under long-delay DAF (Antipova et al., 2008; Kalinowski et al.,1993; Kalinowski et al., 1996; Sparks et al., 2002; Stuart et al., 2004; Van Borsel et al., 2003). The improved naturalness probably arises because short-delay DAF (Kalinowski et al., 1996), like synchronous spectrally-changed speech (Howell et al.,1987), does not affect speech control as described for long-delay DAF. The findings that certain forms of AFB, including short-delay DAF, improve fluency when there is no global change in speech rate suggests that slowing speech is not the operative mechanism behind improvements in fluency of PWS. It has been claimed that short-delay DAF produces effects on speech fluency, rate and naturalness that are as good as other forms of altered sensory feedback (Kalinowski, et al., 1993; Macleod, et al., 1995) although this has been contested (Howell & Sackin, 2000, 2002; Kalveram, 2001; Kalveram & Jäncke,1989).

Clinical work using DAF with PWS

Short-delay DAF would be preferred if this form has equivalent effects to long-delay DAF in terms of stuttering reduction but does not slow speech rate nor increase vocal intensity. In the light of this, it is surprising that Van Borsel et al. (2003) found that PWS preferred delays of 93–147 ms when using a DAF-prosthesis over a 3-month period. Soderberg (1969) also reported PWS preferred long-delay DAF whereas Kalinowski et al. (1996) and Lotzmann (1961) reported a preference for short-delay DAF. We recommend that delay length should be optimized for PWS by allowing them to adjust delay between 0 and 250 ms.

The fluency-enhancing effects of DAF occur predominantly whilst stimulation is delivered (Lincoln et al., 2006) which confirms its prosthetic role. This allows users to choose when to use their prostheses (e.g. at interviews or when speaking in public). Long-delay DAF can also be used as a way of reducing speech rate in multi-component interventions (Atkinson-Clement et al., 2015; Ryan, 1974). One such intervention that uses DAF (Basi et al., 2016; Bothe et al., 2006) is Ryan's (1974) treatment program where the DAF component is based on Goldiamond's (1965) work.

Moreover, ways of promoting carry-over with DAF and other AFB-prostheses merit further investigation (Howell, 2004a). PWS do not need AFB altered all of the time since stuttering is intermittent. Hence, targeting altered AFB on sections of speech where there are stuttering symptoms may be sufficient to reduce dysfluency as the fluency-enhancing effects happen immediately (Howell, 2004b). Another alternative would be to reduce dosage by ramping intensity of altered AFB down after a dysfluency provided speech is fluent and switch it to its full level when the next episode of stuttering occurs (leaky integrator). Additionally, presenting altered AFB on every stuttering symptom might not be optimal for promoting long-term fluency (Howell, 2004b). The Partial Resistance to Extinction Effect or "PREE" (Hochman & Erev, 2013) indicates better retention of behaviors when reinforcement is given intermittently according to a specified schedule rather than on every occurrence. Therefore, with respect to PWS, it may be preferable to deliver fluency-inducing AFB only on a proportion of moments of stuttering that could promote retention of altered AFB's fluency-enhancing effects to unaided speech. This could be implemented if a prosthesis was controlled by an automatic recognizer that identifies stuttering symptoms (Howell et al., 1997a & Howell et al., 1997b) which is preset to deliver altered AFB on a proportion of the dysfluencies detected. Reed and Howell (2000) proposed a framework for implementing such procedures, but empirical work needs to be conducted. The present situation is that altered AFB is usually presented continuously whilst clients speak, which according to the above analysis may not be the best way of promoting retention of fluent behavior.

A potentially more serious issue than fluency improvements only occurring whilst DAF is delivered, is the claim that speakers "adapt" (lose sensitivity) to DAF and other AFB manipulations. Adaptation has similarities with the remission of stuttering noted in connection with other treatments (Weidig, 2005). The supposed adaptation under AFB would benefit from examining work on why fluent participants show differences in susceptibility to DAF (Howell & Archer, 1984). It is assumed that the reasons for fluctuations that occur across individuals (susceptibility) are related to those that happen within an individual across occasions (supposed adaptation in some PWS). Intra-individual differences in susceptibility to DAF in fluent speakers are due to adjustments of own-voice level (Howell, 2004b). Put simply, if speakers silently-mouthed utterances, there would be no auditory signal to delay and no effect of the manipulation, whereas speakers who try to shout over the DAF, enhance the altered sound. PWS using prostheses long-term may subconsciously adapt voice intensity to lower levels to make speech easier to produce that also reduces DAF-dosage. Automatic gain-control circuits (AGCs) can be included in devices to control for variations in voice levels over occasions (Howell, 2004a). AGCs ensure AFB is at a constant level irrespective of adjustments to voice level by speakers. AGCs could be included in clinical devices as they should produce a more uniform response across speakers and time according to this analysis.

Overall, temporal delays to speech feedback have a robust effect on fluent speakers and PWS. In fluent speakers, DAF induces a range of disruptions to speech (makes it sound dysfluent in different ways to stuttered speech). Two important concepts that apply to both speaker groups are: (1) short-delay DAF produces no Lombard effect, and (2) long-delay DAF (>100 ms) is responded to as noise (speakers increase vocal intensity). The delay length may, therefore, determine how delayed feedback is processed by the speaker; with longer delays being regarded as noise that affects the sensorimotor system (increased voice level) whereas, shorter delays retain processing as speech. The effects of DAF and how these depend on delay-length and participant group require further examination. DAF provides a tool to alter certain aspects of speech production for researchers and SLPs. However, differences in susceptibility need further examination as there are interesting possibilities concerning how to maximize benefit in prostheses (AGCs). A further thing to examine with prostheses is control of DAF dosage (PREE) using procedures that incorporate automatic recognition of stutters.

Frequency altered feedback

We need to review how speech is generated to understand procedures that alter frequency components of speech. Voiced speech results in a harmonic sound complex that gives speech its pitch. The pitch percept of this sound is dominated by the lowest harmonic (the fundamental, F0). The harmonic complex also excites the resonant frequencies of the vocal tract, called formants (Rosen & Howell, 2011). The formants are numbered from the lowest resonance upward. The low-order formants (first and second, F1 and F2) are most important for speech intelligibility.

Some, or all parts of the speech spectrum can be shifted in real time using a variety of software and hardware devices. Variants include shifts of the whole spectrum (frequency shifted feedback, FSF[2]; Elman, 1981; Howell et al., 1987), F0, F1 or F2 separately (Donath, Natke & Kalveram, 2002; Houde & Jordan, 1998, 2002; Jones & Munhall, 2000, 2002; Natke & Kalveram, 2001; Purcell & Munhall, 2006a & Purcell & Munhall, 2006b). F0, F1 or F2 first have to be extracted from speech before they can be selectively shifted. DSP chips perform the computations rapidly but methods that rely on the Fast Fourier Transform (FFT) require a sample before they can start the computation. Waiting for the sample before computation takes place delays AFB (AFB would then be shifted component plus DAF). Speed-changing methods that sample amplitude fluctuations in signals digitally at a rapid rate and replay them almost instantaneously at a changed rate do not entail delays (e.g. Howell et al.'s 1987 FSF procedure). The work reviewed in this section looks at shifts of: (1) whole spectrum (FSF); (2) F0; and (3) single formants.

All types of shifted sounds can be delivered in three paradigms which address distinct questions and require different response measures: (1) sustained shift during speech (often used for eliciting fluency improvements in patient groups); (2) immediate *compensation* where an attribute of speech is shifted unpredictably for a short time (typically 500 ms). Compensation occurs when the speaker responds to offset the change; (3) *adaptive* presentation where, after baseline response is measured, a component of speech (F0, F1, F2 etc.) is gradually shifted.

The shift is sustained for a period before it is gradually changed back to baseline, which is rechecked (Purcell & Munhall, 2006a). As well as any compensation that occurs in the shift phase, the changed response may persist beyond the shift period (does not return to baseline) indicating an adaptive response to the altered component (shows that a novel speech-motor command has been learned).

Finally, the speech component manipulated in the procedures and the responses measured do not always correspond. For instance, Elman (1981) shifted the whole speech spectrum but only looked at the impact this had on F0. Other possibilities (e.g. effects on pitch responses when formants are shifted) remain to be investigated in fluent speakers as well as speakers with speech disorders. Procedure section headings refer to the response measured.

Fluent speakers

Whole spectrum and F0 perturbation

Elman (1981) investigated what impact shifting the entire speech spectrum had on F0 control. The incoming speech signal was compressed in real time during speech, which shifted it upward in frequency by approximately 10%. The perturbation induced an almost immediate opposing shift (F0 was lowered).

Such compensatory responses of F0 in fluent speakers have been replicated (Burnett et al., 1998; Chen et al., 2007; Liu & Larson, 2007). However, whilst most participants compensate (change pitch in the opposite direction to the imposed shift), some follow the change in pitch and a few show no change (Burnett et al., 1998). Such inter-individual differences have been attributed to reliance either on auditory or somatosensory feedback (Lametti et al., 2012). Whilst this proposal may account for cases where compensations or null responses occur to frequency-shifted AFB, it does not explain why a significant minority of speakers follow the shift. The latter appear to rely on auditory feedback (they respond), but the response occurs in a noncompensatory way.

No Lombard or Fletcher effect occurs when the whole speech spectrum is shifted for fluent speakers (Howell, 1990). Thus, unlike long-delay DAF, intensity is not affected by FSF.

Although FSF does not affect voice-level responses, it does affect F0 (Elman, 1981) and, hence, respiratory, laryngeal and articulatory control. Thus, Heinks-Maldonado and Houde (2005) reported a relationship between voice-level perturbation and F0: a rapid 400 ms shift in voice-level (±10dB) whilst phonating a vowel resulted in speakers compensating by decreasing or increasing the F0 of their speech output. Subsequent studies provided more detail about this response: Bauer et al. (2006) highlighted that the magnitude of the F0 response diminished as the voice-level perturbation decreased (±1dB resulted in smaller F0 compensations compared to ±3dB or ±6dB). Larson et al. (2007) investigated whether the compensatory responses to F0 shifts were influenced by shifts in vocal loudness. In three experiments, F0 frequency was shifted: (1) upward or downward during phonation; (2) vocal intensity level was increased or decreased by 3dB; and (3) the two perturbations were combined. The compensatory responses for the shifts in decreasing order were 18 cents when F0 alone was altered, 14–16 cents for simultaneous shifts of F0 and vocal intensity and 10 cents when vocal intensity alone was altered. Spectral-compensation magnitude also depended on the frequency of F0 where higher F0 values led to greater spectral-compensatory shifts and reduced response times to shifted speech (Liu & Larson, 2007). Downward F0 shifts elicit larger compensatory responses than upward shifts (Chen et al., 2007). It is unclear why direction of perturbation elicits different responses. However, these findings can be exploited in speakers with fluency problems when adjustment of F0 is required in interventions. The F0 magnitude (Larson et al., 2007) and direction response effects (Chen et al., 2007) decay rapidly after FSF is switched off (F0 returns to baseline quickly). However, FSF can have long-term effects if the perturbation is sustained for long periods of time (Munhall 2006a). Hence, procedures to promote carry-over (discussed in the section on DAF) are worth exploring.

Perturbations to F0 occur with the following materials: sustained vowels (Bauer & Larson, 2003; Hain et al., 2000; Larson et al., 2007; Sivasankar et al., 2005), glissandi (Burnett & Larson, 2002), songs (Natke et al., 2003), nonsense syllables (Donath et al., 2002; Natke et al., 2003; Natke and Kalveram, 2001) and Mandarin phrases (Jones & Munhall, 2002). Perturbation of F0 also changes the supra-segmental timing of utterances (Bauer, 2004). Furthermore, shifting feedback on one syllable affects the output of the next one (a coarticulation effect). Thus, shifting F0 either upward or downward resulted in an upward shift in F0 on the subsequent syllable (Natke & Kalveram, 2001). Similar effects occur in immediate compensation paradigms where transient shifts to F0 resulted in changes in the voice fundamental on subsequent material (Donath et al., 2002).

Formant perturbation

F1 frequencies are higher for open, than for close, vowels. F2 frequencies are higher for front, than back, vowels. Similar relationships apply with consonants but the picture is more complex because articulatory shape changes dynamically during their production. Perturbation of F1 or F2 could imply that articulation of speech is incorrect. Therefore, in an adaptation paradigm, participants should adjust to compensate for the formant perturbation (Purcell & Munhall, 2006a; Villacorta et al., 2007).

Adaptation and compensation paradigms have been used to study F1 and F2 perturbations in fluent speakers. In both cases, most speakers adjust their formant frequencies in the opposite direction to the perturbation. Again (as with FSF and F0 perturbations), there are some individuals who follow and others who do not respond (Purcell & Munhall, 2006a).

When F1 or F2 are manipulated, the magnitude of the response is proportional to the magnitude of the perturbation providing the perturbation exceeds approximately 60 Hz (Purcell & Munhall, 2006a). Specifically, larger perturbations of F1 and/or F2 result in greater changes to the corresponding F1 and/or F2 values in the resultant speech (Cai et al., 2011; Purcell & Munhall, 2006b). Unlike FSF and F0 shifts however, perturbations of F1 and F2 do not result in responses larger than about 15% of the imposed shift (Purcell & Munhall, 2006b). For F1 changes, as with F0 perturbations, downward shifts elicit larger responses than upward shifts at 16.3% and 10.6% of the applied formant shift, respectively (Purcell & Munhall, 2006b). Cai et al. (2011) reported how F1 and F2 manipulation affect their corresponding responses but did not look at non-corresponding responses.

There is no evidence whether perturbation of F1 or F2 leads speakers to alter their vocal intensity (i.e. produce a Lombard, or Fletcher, effect). It is worth checking whether speakers who compensate produce a Fletcher effect whereas those who do not compensate produce a Lombard effect (treat the shifted speech as speech, or noise, respectively). Also, it is not known whether varying intensity of F1 or F2 selectively affects the intensity of the corresponding formant or the overall intensity.

In sum, fluent speakers show both compensation and adaptation to manipulations of F1 and/ or F2. This reflects both the malleability of speech-sound representations at a neuro-motor level and the ability to accurately adjust current speech output in response to concurrent auditory information in fluent speakers. It is interesting to consider why some speakers respond to the frequency perturbation by opposing the shift, whilst others follow and yet others do nothing whatsoever. All these responses are likely to arise at low levels of neural function as people are not usually aware of frequency perturbations nor their own compensation or adaptation response.

People who stutter

Whole Spectrum and F0 perturbation

Howell et al. (1987) shifted the whole speech spectrum of PWS and reported a marked reduction in concurrent stutters. This reduction under FSF has been replicated using monologue, conversation and reading materials and for a range of frequency shifts usually up to an octave (Armson & Stuart, 1998; Hargrave et al., 1994; Kalinowski et al., 1993; Natke et al.,2001; Ritto et al., 2016; Stuart & Kalinowski, 2004). Fluency enhancement does not correlate with the magnitude of the shift and there is no particular shift that has maximum effect. For instance, Stuart et al. (1996) suggested that the entire spectrum had to be shifted by at least ¼ of an octave to induce fluency-enhancing effects in PWS but upward shifts of ¼ octave and above all led to similar fluency enhancements for PWS (Kalinowski et al., 1993; Hargrave et al., 1994; Stuart et al., 1996). Some studies report that groups of PWS only compensate to upward FSF perturbations (Bosshardt et al., 1997; Natke et al., 2001). However, downward shifts are known to reduce the likelihood of F0 compensations (Natke et al., 2001) and to promote fluency (Bauer et al. 2007; Natke et al., 2001). As with fluent speakers, it is not known why direction-specific effects occur and, additionally for PWS, whether these indicate differences in underlying neural pathology. Nevertheless, this review suggests that downward shifts are recommended for clinical use, assuming F0 compensations should be avoided, even though upward shifts are studied most often.

FSF improves speech fluency without adversely affecting other aspects of speech including intensity (Howell, 1990): FSF does not affect speech naturalness in PWS other than partial compensatory shifts in F0 (Natke et al., 2001); FSF does not slow speech (Howell, et al., 19877 Howell & Sackin, 2000; Natke et al., 2001).

There is no work that has studied individual susceptibility to the fluency-enhancing effects of FSF *a priori* (studies have looked at individual differences *post facto*). Although PWS differ in whether or not they respond to F0 perturbations, compensatory response to F0 perturbation does not predict fluency-enhancing responses to FSF (Natke et al., 2001). The fluency enhancement does, however, seem to relate to the implementation method with speech-change procedures proving most effective (Howell, 2004a). Although the fluency-enhancing effects of short-delay DAF have been reported to be "equal" (i.e. not significantly different) to that of whole-spectrum FSF, DSP implementation of FSF were used in the studies (Hargrave et al., 1994; Kalinowski et al., 1993; Stuart et al., 1996, 2004, 2006). As mentioned, these introduce delays because they use the FFT to shift the speech spectrum (Howell & Sackin, 2000). Thus, estimating an FSF effect separate from short-delay DAF is not possible in these studies (Howell & Sackin, 2000).

Clinical trials using FSF prostheses

The reasons FSF is commended for clinical work are that it has few side effects on intensity, speech rate and F0, but large effects on fluency. These findings led to clinical trials to establish whether enhanced fluency under FSF persists over time. Stuttering symptoms decrease by up to 80% in PWS under FSF (Armson & Stuart, 1998; Howell et al., 1987; Howell 1990; Kalinowski et al., 1993; Natke et al., 2001). Consequently, prostheses that employ FSF have appeared including SpeechEasy© (Janus Development Group Inc.), Casa Futura Technologies, VoiceAmp, National Association for Speech Fluency, A.S. General Limited, Digital Recordings and Kay Elemetrics. There are important differences in the way FSF is implemented in these prostheses and as compared to laboratory set-ups. Prostheses that are worn have limited processing power. Consequently, prostheses often have significant additional delays between the speech input and when the perturbed output is returned to the speaker. Unlike laboratory implementations, SpeechEasy© loses harmonic information (Stuart et al., 2003). For example, if a harmonic complex of 500, 1,000 and 2,000 Hz (first, second and fourth harmonics of 500 Hz) received a 400 Hz shift, components would be at 900, 1,400 and 2,400 Hz. The latter components are not harmonically-related which may affect perceived pitch of the complex. Delays and distortions to harmonics are important when considering the efficacy of prostheses.

FSF prostheses improve fluency in PWS and provide an effective treatment for stuttering (Armson et al., 2006; Kalinowski et al., 1993; Stuart et al., 2003, 2004). However, the effect size is not as large as laboratory results would suggest whether comparisons are made with the sampling or DSP methods. Thus, Armson et al. (2006) documented the effect sizes for the SpeechEasy© device in different speaking tasks both in and out of their laboratory. Reductions in laboratory conditions were about 49% for conversations, 36% for monologues and 74% for readings (Armson et al., 2006). When the SpeechEasy© was used outside the laboratory, no reduction was apparent either in "Situation of Daily Living" (SDL) or at follow-up (O'Donnell et al., 2008). Rate of stuttering even increased for some participants when the device was used for 16 weeks.

Gallop and Runyan (2012) reported similar findings over a longer time-period (59 months). Reductions in stuttering for the whole group did not occur but some individuals showed appreciable reductions after 59months of use (others showed increased stuttering rate). Extended use also changed the stuttering frequency from before the prosthesis was used, even when the prosthesis was not used frequently by individuals. The reasons for these individual differences are not clear. Assuming, as argued with fluent speakers, that changes to speech control are mediated by neural changes, participants may have either adapted to maintain the fluency-inducing effect or to ignore the perturbation and continue speech as they did before baseline. The findings highlight that brains respond to long-term perturbation in different ways. Intermittent presentation of FSF could prevent extinction of responses (PREE described earlier). Consistent with this, although most applications have applied FSF throughout speech, it has been focused on syllables onsets and this "pulsed" form of FSF provides the same level of fluency enhancement as continuous FSF (Howell et al., 1987). Implementation of pulsed FSF in prostheses would require increased processing power which may explain why continuous presentation is used exclusively in current devices.

Despite prostheses providing a low-cost alternative to conventional treatments intended to reduce stuttering, the long-term effects remain unclear and may even be detrimental to certain individuals. Theoretically-motivated ways of reducing adaptation remain to be explored (Howell, 2004b). Furthermore, from a conventional perspective, there is no consensus about what factors could predict whether an individual will respond positively or negatively, although, some research has suggested that PWS with a mild stutter are more likely to be affected detrimentally (Gallop & Runyan, 2012; O'Donnell et al., 2008). Nevertheless, FSF provides researchers and clinicians with a technique to induce fluency, at least temporarily, in most PWS.

It is interesting to consider how a speaker adjusts to these perturbations over a long period of time from a neuroplasticity perspective. As detailed, the extended use of AFB-prostheses generally results in a diminished fluency-enhancing effect (O'Donnell et al., 2008). Findings from all studies on PWS that observed effects over extended time-periods report highly variable response (Gallop & Runyan, 2012; O'Donnell et al., 2008; Ritto et al., 2016). Note that neither the longitudinal studies (Gallop & Runyan, 2012; O'Donnell et al., 2008) nor the randomized control trial (RCT) of Ritto et al., (2016) included a non-treatment control group of PWS for comparison. However, from research on formant manipulations detailed above, the brain adapts and recodes speech processes in response to manipulated feedback signals (Purcell & Munhall, 2006a). Although this research is restricted to formant manipulations, it is possible that extended use of whole-spectrum FSF causes an adaptive response from the brain. Unfortunately, no research to date has examined the neurophysiological effects of extended presentation of FSF to assess this point. Further research needs to elucidate whether neuroplastic changes to protracted AFB: (1) occur and (2) whether the changes aid long-term fluency versus whether they lead to dependency on the prosthesis.

In sum, due to technological constraints, prostheses induce fluency improvement in PWS but not to the extent reported in lab studies. Nonetheless, the improvements are significant and are at least as good as current behavioral therapies at a group level (Ritto et al., 2016). As discussed, responses to the prostheses vary markedly in different contexts (Armson et al., 2006) and the outcomes after long-term use are not clear. Again, it must be stressed that prostheses: (1) include delays (both long-delay and short-delay) in conjunction with FSF adding a further factor that makes responses variable; and (2) perturb entire utterances which is not necessary and possibly disadvantageous insofar as it resulted in several users criticizing the accompanying noise (Pollard et al., 2009).

F0 perturbation

Scanning evidence suggests that PWS have a deficit in sensorimotor integration (Tourville & Guenther, 2011; Watkins et al., 2008). This has been tested in tasks where responses to F0 perturbations have been examined. Consistent with the proposed deficit, PWS show a variable and diminished compensatory response to the instantaneous F0 perturbation compared to fluent speakers (Sares et al., 2018).

PWS show similar responses to fluent speakers when magnitude of spectral perturbation to F0 or speech intensity are varied, but responses are reduced (amplitude) and delayed (phase) for PWS (Loucks et al., 2012). The deficient responses indicate an inability for PWS to appropriately account for perceived errors both in strength and timing of corrective response, compared to fluent speakers. Bauer et al. (2007) reported that the abnormal responses in both amplitude and phase in PWS did not apply when the magnitude of the shift was 600 cents. It is unclear why PWS, compared to fluent speakers, are no less able to respond to F0 perturbations when the magnitude of the perturbation is relatively large but unable to respond adequately to smaller perturbations (100cents in Loucks et al., 2012). Unlike FSF, F0 perturbations have no reported clinical benefit and do not promote fluent speech.

Formant perturbation

As noted previously, F1 and F2 perturbations provide information about how an individual integrates, compensates and adapts their articulator movements. PWS show similar responses to fluent speakers in: (1) adaptation where, after formants are incrementally shifted over utterances, PWS reconfigure articulatory actions to restore the perceived (afferent) speech to match more closely to the intended speech (efferent) output (Daliri et al.,2018); and (2) immediate compensation where PWS compensate for unexpected F1 and F2 perturbations by adjusting their articulators by reducing or increasing formant values (Cai et al., 2012, 2014).

There are, however, some subtle differences between PWS and fluent speakers: Unlike response to F0 where PWS showed lagged response times to F0 perturbation (Loucks et al., 2012), PWS took a similar time (150 ms) to fluent speakers to adjust to formant perturbation (Cai et al., 2012). The magnitude of compensation was significantly reduced compared to fluent speakers (Cai et al., 2014). These findings suggest a deficit in ability to integrate spectral, but not temporal, formant information. Furthermore, the differences noted between PWS and fluent controls only apply to adult PWS since children's responses were not distinguishable from their fluent peers (Daliri et al., 2018). This suggests that adults acquire this deficit.

There is no evidence whether formant perturbations influence vocal intensity. PWS may have a similar response to the one they have to FSF (intensity reduces slightly, Howell, 1990). Also, although there is no research about whether formant perturbation affects speech rate, it seems likely that it would have a similar effect to FSF and F0 shifts (no slowing of speech rate).

Although formant manipulation permits better probing of what aspects of speech are deficient in PWS, there are no known clinical benefits in using such forms of altered feedback as yet. Nevertheless, since whole-spectrum shifts (which includes the formants) improve speech fluency, formant manipulations may help reveal the as-yet unknown mechanisms driving this fluency enhancement.

Vibrotactile feedback

Several parts of the body vibrate during articulation and provide sensory information about speech activity. As with altered *auditory* feedback, vibration can be altered to investigate how this form of afferent input affects speakers. Vibration during articulation possibly only carries information about F0 (Howell & Powell, 1984). Nevertheless, there are several features of vibrotactile feedback (VTF) that make it interesting. VTF: (1) operates over different neural pathways to AFB (Cheadle et al., 2018); (2) does not interfere with auditory information[3]; and (3) induces corresponding fluency changes to AFB (Cheadle et al., 2018; Kuniszyk-Jozkowiak et al., 1996; Snyder et al., 2009; Waddell et al., 2012).

Vibratory information is sensed by two types of mechanoreceptors in the skin which code for the intensity and frequency of the vibration: Meissner's and Pacinian corpuscles (see Figure 32.1). Meissner's corpuscles code for 20–70 Hz vibrations and their resonant frequency is 30 Hz (Iggo, 1986). Pacinian corpuscles code for 100–400 Hz vibrations and have a resonant frequency of 250 Hz (Griffin, 1990; Siegel & Sapru, 2006). Vibratory stimulation at different frequencies, therefore, activates different mechanoreceptors. Vibratory information ascends to the primary somatosensory cortex via two main pathways: (1.) the main sensory trigeminal cranial nerve (CN), transducing stimulation to the facial and scalp areas including the vocal system and (2) the posterior column-medial lemniscal (non-CN) pathways, carrying all stimulatory information presented to everything caudal to the cranium (Juliano & Mclaughlin, 1999). In particular, vibrotactile stimulation at the facial and cranial tissues will ascend through the CN-pathway whilst stimulation at all parts of the body otherwise ascend through the non-CN pathway. The CN-pathway also transmits vibratory information through the brainstem at the level of the mid-pons, the trigeminal lemniscus and the thalamus. The non-CN pathway transmits to the medulla, thalamus and primary somatosensory cortex. Note that both pathways meet at the thalamus and, unlike AFB, neither carries information to the cerebellum (Hendelman, 2015; Juliano & Mclaughlin, 1999).

Vibrotactile feedback Figure

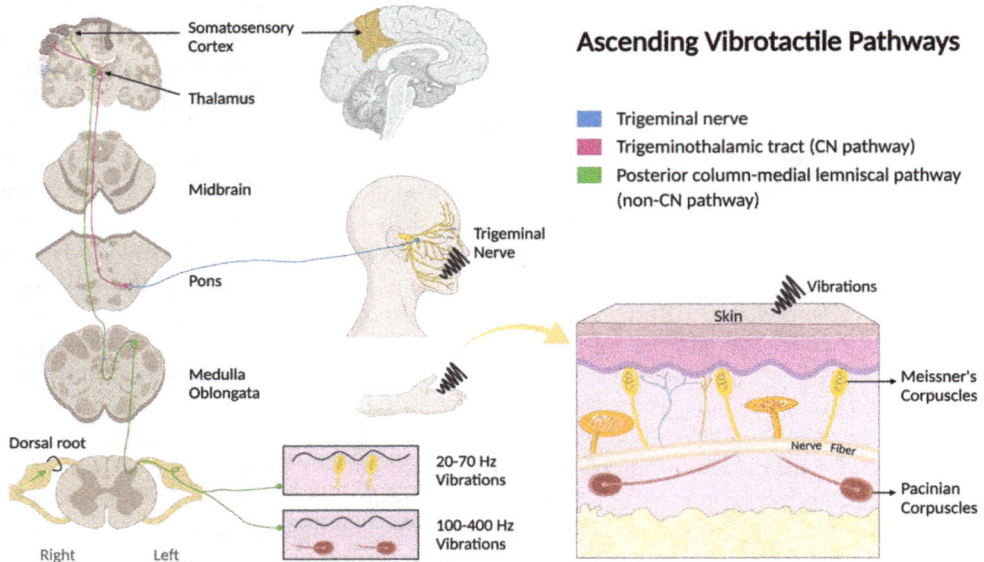

Figure 32.1 Detailing the vibrotactile pathway from sensation at skin level to the primary sensory cortex. The figure illustrates the two pathways: 1.) The main sensory trigeminal cranial nerve (CN) which emanates from the facial nerves (top-left) and posterior column-medial lemniscal (non-CN) pathways (Juliano & Mclaughlin, 1999). The CN pathway also transmits vibratory information through the brainstem at the level of the mid-pons, the trigeminal lemniscus and the thalamus. The non-CN pathway transmits to the medulla, thalamus and primary somatosensory cortex. Note, although the illustration joins the pathways at the mid pons the information is shared only at the thalamus and above. Unlike AFB, neither carries information to the cerebellum (Juliano & Mclaughlin, 1999; Hendelman, 2005).

Fluent speakers

Work on VTF with fluent speakers has mainly been conducted on perception rather than production. Thus, Fucci et al. (1985, 1991) compared effects of VTF on fluent speakers (and PWS) in perceptual work. They investigated individual sensitivity to vibrotactile stimulation at 250 Hz (activated the Pacinian corpuscles), delivered to the hand and the tongue. The experimenter controlled a master attenuator and participants had their own attenuator to modulate the intensity of stimulation. Intensity was gradually increased to the threshold of sensation for the participant. The experimenter then modulated the intensity of stimulation and the participants had to follow this modulation by adjusting their own attenuator. In effect, they estimated how the participant judged that the experimenter had changed intensity. Fluent speakers had more accurate representations of somatosensory information emanating from the tongue, not the hand, compared to PWS. PWS integrated somatosensory information from the arm as well as fluent speakers (Fucci et al., 1985). This suggests that VTF should have little or no effect on speech in fluent speakers, possibly due to a fully functional somatosensory feedback system. Further work using VTF with fluent speakers is required to verify this.

With respect to production studies, VTF has not usually included a fluent control group (Cheadle et al., 2018; Kuniszyk-Jozkowiak et al., 1996, 1997; Snyder et al., 2009; Waddell et al., 2012). Kuniszyk-Józkowiak and Adamczyk (1989) is the only study on the effects of VTF on fluent speakers and results were reported as comparisons with PWS. This is discussed in the following section.

People who stutter

Fucci et al.'s (1985, 1991) investigations tested whether PWS have poor sensorimotor integration for vibratory information similar to that claimed for auditory stimulation (Cai et al., 2014; Loucks, Chon & Han, 2012). Their perceptual studies, discussed in the previous section, provides evidence that fluent speakers have more accurate somatosensory representations about the articulators relative to PWS.

Research has considered how VTF affects fluency of PWS and how this varies when VTF is perturbed. VTF improves fluency (Cheadle et al., 2018; Kuniszyk-Jozkowiaket al., 1996; Snyder et al., 2009; Waddell et al., 2012).

The intensity of VTF affects speech production in PWS, however the effect shows a quadratic relationship with intensity: Low (0.5–1 m/s^2) and high (2.5–3 m/s^2) amplitudes of vibration induce greater reductions in stuttering than mid-range (1–2.5 m/s^2) amplitudes (Cheadle et al., 2018). Placement of the vibrator, and therefore the neural pathway stimulated, did not influence stuttering frequency during VTF (Cheadle et al., 2018). This contrasts with the perceptual work that found vibration applied to the articulators had different effects than when vibration was applied to the hand for PWS compared to fluent speakers (Fucci et al., 1985).

Kuniszyk-Józkowiak and Adamczyk (1989) included PWS and compared their results with a control group. Concurrent and delayed VTF were compared for stimulation delivered separately to the left and right middle fingers at 230 Hz with 0.5 mm maximum amplitude of oscillation. There were no differences in speech rate in response to VTF between fluent speakers and PWS rather, speech rate slowed for all participants when stimulation was delayed. The rate-slowing effect is at odds with Cheadle et al. (2018) who found that, PWS did not change their speech rate in response to VTF whether the stimulation was concurrent or delayed. However, procedural differences may account for this discrepancy, Cheadle et al. stimulated at a lower peak frequency (~100 Hz) whereas, Kuniszyk-Józkowiak and Adamczyk (1989) used a high resonant frequency (230 Hz). Hence, there are two possible accounts for the difference:

1. Compared to Cheadle et al., Kuniszyk-Józkowiak and Adamczyk stimulated at a higher resonant frequency than would activate Pacinian corpuscles. Thus they may have been more successful than Cheadle et al. at perturbing speech when VTF was delayed and this led to a reduction in speech rate.
2. High frequency VTF stimulation (Kuniszyk-Józkowiak & Adamczyk, 1989) can result in audible noise. The noise arising from the delayed VTF would act like DAF when delayed and would slow speech (Howell et al., 1992).

As mentioned, the neural pathway for VTF differs from the auditory pathway until the post-thalamic pathways. Consequently, VTF does not pass through the cerebellum and therefore VTF cannot affect timekeeping processes in the lateral cerebellum reasoned to be implicated in fluent speech control (Howell, 2011). This may explain why DAF has greater effects on stuttering reduction (up to 85% according to Lincoln et al., 2006)) compared to VTF (maximum of 80%). Furthermore, Cheadle et al.'s (2018) recent study on VTF with PWS found effect size to be 21.82% across all conditions. Finally, the way the effect size varies as a function of intensity, frequency of vibration, frequency of use, timing of vibration and inter-individual differences are not fully understood. This point is underlined by the lack of such information on other patient groups and fluent speakers.

Although early research showed that delaying VTF further reduced dysfluency (Kuniszyk-Jozkowiak et al., 1996), this was not replicated by Cheadle et al. (2018). Hence, the role this parameter could play in clinical applications using VTF is unclear. No research has looked at whether auditory parameters of speech such as F0 and formant frequencies change with respect to VTF for PWS.

Conclusion

Speech production can be modulated by altering sensory feedback. With respect to PWS, all procedures that have been reviewed promote fluency. The principles and parameters of each sensory feedback manipulation have been outlined and areas where future work is needed have been indicated. Clearly the effects of altered sensory feedback are diverse and vary by technique, whether individuals are fluent or not (PWS) and between individuals within each fluency group.

Looking at fluency-enhancing effects in PWS, the techniques lend themselves, and have been implemented, as prostheses. As the fluency-enhancing effects depend on the prosthesis being active, there should not necessarily be any carry-over of fluency enhancement. However, the alterations induced by long-term use of the devices may lead to neuroplastic changes that change speech permanently (Purcell & Munhall, 2006a). Present implementations of techniques to alter sensory feedback in prostheses are not optimized to counteract adaptation and to achieve effects at low dosages. We have suggested prosthetic procedures may need to be modified so that they are only active for a percentage of utterances on parts of the utterance (Hochman & Erev, 2013; Reed & Howell, 2000)) at points where problems are being experienced (Howell, El-Yaniv, & Powell, 1987).

Notes

1 Speech error here includes medial vowel elongations. If medial elongations are not considered to be an error then the estimated effect of DAF would be less.
2 Note, Frequency Shifted Feedback or FSF refers to the shifting of the whole spectrum, not specific manipulations like F1 perturbation.
3 Note, VTF can generate auditory signals if presented at a too high a frequency and intensity. Low resonant frequencies of ~100 Hz are unlikely to generate an auditory signal. However, 230–250 Hz are often used in the literature as this allows maximal stimulation of Pacinian corpuscles (Griffin, 1990; Siegel & Sapru, 2006) and stimulating at this high frequency may provide some undesired noise and therefore masking.

References

Antipova, E. A., Purdy, S. C., Blakeley, M., & Williams, S. (2008). Effects of altered auditory feedback (AAF) on stuttering frequency during monologue speech production. *Journal of Fluency Disorders*, *33*(4), 274–290. https://doi.org/10.1016/j.jfludis.2008.09.002

Armson, J., Kiefte, M., Mason, J., & De Croos, D. (2006). The effect of SpeechEasy on stuttering frequency in laboratory conditions. *Journal of Fluency Disorders*, *31*(2), 137–152. https://doi.org/10.1016/j.jfludis.2006.04.004

Armson, J., & Stuart, A. (1998). Effect of extended exposure to frequency-altered feedback on stuttering during reading and monologue. *Journal of Speech, Language, and Hearing Research*, *41*(3), 479–490. https://doi.org/10.1044/jslhr.4103.479

Atkinson-Clement, C., Sadat, J., & Pinto, S. (2015). Behavioral treatments for speech in Parkinson's disease: meta-analyses and review of the literature. *Neurodegenerative Disease Management, 5*(3), 233–248. https://doi.org/10.2217/nmt.15.16

Basi, M., Farazi, M., & Bakhshi, E. (2016). Evaluation of Effects of Gradual Increase Length and Complexity of Utterance (GILCU) treatment method on the reduction of dysfluency in school-aged children with stuttering. *Iranian Rehabilitation Journal, 14*(1), 59–62. https://doi.org/10.15412/J.IRJ.08140109

Bauer, J. J. (2004). *Task dependent modulation of voice F0 responses elicited by perturbations in pitch of auditory feedback during English speech and sustained vowels*, PhD dissertation, Northwestern University.

Bauer, J. J., Hubbard Seery, C., LaBonte, R., & Ruhnke, L. (2007). Voice F0 responses elicited by perturbations in pitch of auditory feedback in individuals that stutter and controls. *The Journal of the Acoustical Society of America, 121*(5), 3201–3201. https://doi.org/10.1121/1.4782465

Bauer, J. J., & Larson, C. R. (2003). Audio-vocal responses to repetitive pitch-shift stimulation during a sustained vocalization: Improvements in methodology for the pitch-shifting technique. *The Journal of the Acoustical Society of America, 114*(2), 1048–1054. https://doi.org/10.1121/1.1592161

Bauer, J. J., Mittal, J., Larson, C. R., & Hain, T. C. (2006). Vocal responses to unanticipated perturbations in voice loudness feedback: An automatic mechanism for stabilizing voice amplitude. *The Journal of the Acoustical Society of America, 119*(4), 2363–2371. https://doi.org/10.1121/1.2173513

Black, J. W. (1951). The effect of delayed side-tone upon vocal rate and intensity. *Journal of Speech and Hearing Disorders, 16*(1), 56–60. https://doi.org/10.1044/jshd.1601.56

Bosshardt, H. G., Sappok, C., Knipschild, M., & Hölscher, C. (1997). Spontaneous imitation of fundamental frequency and speech rate by nonstutterers and stutterers. *Journal of Psycholinguistic Research, 26*(4), 425–448. https://doi.org/10.1023/A:1025030120016

Bothe, A. K., Davidow, J. H., Bramlett, R. E., & Ingham, R. J. (2006). Stuttering treatment research 1970–2005: I. Systematic review incorporating trial quality assessment of behavioral, cognitive, and related approaches. *American Journal of Speech-Language Pathology, 15*, 321–341. https://doi.org/10.1044/1058-0360(2006/031)

Burnett, T. A., Freedland, M. B., Larson, C. R., & Hain, T. C. (1998). Voice F0 responses to manipulations in pitch feedback. *The Journal of the Acoustical Society of America, 103*(6), 3153–3161. https://doi.org/10.1121/1.423073

Burnett, T. A., & Larson, C. R. (2002). Early pitch-shift response is active in both steady and dynamic voice pitch control. *The Journal of the Acoustical Society of America, 112*(3), 1058–1063. https://doi.org/10.1121/1.1487844

Cai, S., Beal, D. S., Ghosh, S. S., Guenther, F. H., & Perkell, J. S. (2014). Impaired timing adjustments in response to time-varying auditory perturbation during connected speech production in persons who stutter. *Brain and Language, 129*(1), 24–29. https://doi.org/10.1016/j.bandl.2014.01.002

Cai, S., Beal, D. S., Ghosh, S. S., Tiede, M. K., Guenther, F. H., & Perkell, J. S. (2012). Weak responses to auditory feedback perturbation during articulation in persons who stutter: Evidence for abnormal auditory-motor transformation. *PLoS ONE, 7*(7), 1–13. https://doi.org/10.1371/journal.pone.0041830

Cai, S., Ghosh, S. S., Guenther, F. H., & Perkell, J. S. (2011). Focal manipulations of formant trajectories reveal a role of auditory feedback in the online control of both within-syllable and between-syllable speech timing. *Journal of Neuroscience, 31*(45), 16483–16490. https://doi.org/10.1523/JNEUROSCI.3653-11.2011

Cheadle, O., Sorger, C., & Howell, P. (2018). Identification of neural structures involved in stuttering using vibrotactile feedback. *Brain and Language, 180–182*(May), 50–61. https://doi.org/10.1016/j.bandl.2018.03.002

Chen, S. H., Liu, H., Xu, Y., & Larson, C. R. (2007). Voice F0 responses to pitch-shifted voice feedback during English speech. *The Journal of the Acoustical Society of America, 121*(2), 1157–1163. https://doi.org/10.1121/1.2404624

Costello-Ingham, J. C. (1993). Current status of stuttering and behavior modification—I: Recent trends in the application of behavior modification in children and adults. *Journal of Fluency Disorders, 18*(1), 27–55.

Daliri, A., Wieland, E. A., Cai, S., Guenther, F. H., & Chang, S. E. (2018). Auditory-motor adaptation is reduced in adults who stutter but not in children who stutter. *Developmental Science, 21*(2), 1–11. https://doi.org/10.1111/desc.12521

Donath, T. M., Natke, U., & Kalveram, K. T. (2002). Effects of frequency-shifted auditory feedback on voice F0 contours in syllables. *The Journal of the Acoustical Society of America, 111*(1), 357–366. https://doi.org/10.1121/1.1424870

Elman, J. L. (1981). Effects of frequency-shifted feedback on the pitch of vocal productions. *Journal of the Acoustical Society of America, 70*(1), 45–50. https://doi.org/10.1121/1.386580

Fairbanks, G. (1955). Selective vocal effects of delayed auditory feedback. *The Journal of Speech and Hearing Disorders, 20*(4), 333–346. https://doi.org/10.1044/jshd.2004.333

Fucci, D., Petrosino, L., Gorman, P., & Harris, D. (1985). Vibrotactile magnitude production scaling: A method for studying sensory-perceptual responses of stutterers and fluent speakers. *Journal of Fluency Disorders, 10*(1), 69–75. https://doi.org/10.1016/0094-730X(85)90007-5

Fucci, D., Petrosino, L., Schuster, S., & Belch, M. (1991). Lingual vibrotactile threshold shift differences between stutterers and normal speakers during magnitude-estimation scaling. *Perceptual and motor skills, 73*(1), 55–62. https://doi.org/10.2466%2Fpms.1991.73.1.55

Gallop, R. F., & Runyan, C. M. (2012). Long-term effectiveness of the SpeechEasy fluency-enhancement device. *Journal of Fluency Disorders, 37*(4), 334–343. https://doi.org/10.1016/j.jfludis.2012.07.001

Geetha, Y. V., Sangeetha, M., Sundararaju, H., Sahana, V., Akshatha, V., & Antonye, L. (2017). Effects of altered auditory and oro-sensory feedback on speech naturalness in persons with and without stuttering. *Journal of the All India Institute of Speech & Hearing, 36*, 12–19..

Goldiamond, I. (1965) Stuttering and fluency as manipulatable operant response classes. In: L. Krasner, L. Ullman (Eds., pp. 106–156). *Research in behavior modificaton*. Holt, Rhinehart and Winston

Griffin, J. W. (1990). Basic pathologic processes in the nervous system. *Toxicologic Pathology, 18*(1 II), 83–88. https://doi.org/10.1177/019262339001800113

Hain, T. C., Burnett, T. A., Kiran, S., Larson, C. R., Singh, S., & Kenney, M. K. (2000). Instructing subjects to make a voluntary response reveals the presence of two components to the audio-vocal reflex. *Experimental Brain Research, 130*(2), 133–141. https://doi.org/10.1007/s002219900237

Hargrave, S., Kalinowski, J., Stuart, A., Armson, J., & Jones, K. (1994). Effect of frequency-altered feedback on stuttering frequency at normal and fast speech rates. *Journal of Speech and Hearing Research, 37*(6), 1313–1319. https://doi.org/10.1044/jshr.3706.1313

Heinks-Maldonado, T. H., & Houde, J. F. (2005). Compensatory responses to brief perturbations of speech amplitude. *Acoustic Research Letters Online, 6*(3), 131–137. https://doi.org/10.1121/1.1931747

Hendelman, W. (2015). *Atlas of functional neuroanatomy*. London: CRC press.

Hochman, G., & Erev, I. (2013). The partial-reinforcement extinction effect and the contingent-sampling hypothesis. *Psychonomic Bulletin and Review, 20*(6), 1336–1342. https://doi.org/10.3758/s13423-013-0432-1

Houde, J. F., & Jordan, M. I. (1998). Sensorimotor adaptation in speech production. *Science, 279*(5354), 1213–1216. https://doi.org/10.1126/science.279.5354.1213

Houde, J. F., & Jordan, M. I. (2002). Sensorimotor adaptation of speech I: Compensation and adaptation. *Journal of Speech, Language, and Hearing Research, 45*(2), 295–310. https://doi.org/10.1044/1092-4388(2002/023)

Howell, P. (1990). Changes in voice level caused by several forms of altered feedback in fluent speakers and stutterers. *Language and Speech, 33*(4), 325–338. https://doi.org/10.1177%2F002383099003300402

Howell, P. (2004a). Assessment of some contemporary theories of stuttering that apply to spontaneous speech. *Contemporary Issues in Communication Science and Disorders, 31*(Spring), 123–140. https://doi.org/10.1044/cicsd_31_s_123

Howell, P. (2004b). Assessment of some contemporary theories of stuttering that apply to spontaneous speech. *Contemporary Issues in Communication Science and Disorders, 31*(Spring), 123–140. http://www.speech.psychol.ucl.ac.uk/PAPERS/PDF/Howell1.pdf

Howell, P. (2011). Listen to the lessons of The King's Speech: A film that shows King George VI struggling with a stammer could raise awareness and change treatments. *Nature, 470*(7332), 7–8. https://doi.org/10.1038/470007a

Howell, P., & Archer, A. (1984). Susceptibility to the effects of delayed auditory feedback. *Perception & Psychophysics, 36*(3), 296–302. https://doi.org/10.3758/BF03206371

Howell, P., El-Yaniv, N., & Powell, D. J. (1987). Factors affecting fluency in stutterers when speaking under altered auditory feedback. In *Speech motor dynamics in stuttering* (pp. 361–369). Vienna: Springer.

Howell, P., & Powell, D. J. (1984). Hearing your voice through bone and air: Implications for explanations of stuttering behavior from studies of normal speakers. *Journal of Fluency Disorders, 9*(4), 247–263. https://doi.org/10.1016/0094-730X(84)90019-6

Howell, P., & Powell, D. J. (1987). Delayed auditory feedback with delayed sounds varying in duration. *Perception & Psychophysics*, *42*(2), 166–172. https://doi.org/10.3758/BF03210505

Howell, P., & Sackin, S. (2000). Speech rate manipulation and its effects on fluency reversal in children who stutter. *Journal of Developmental and Physical Disabilities*, *12*, 291–315.

Howell, P., & Sackin, S. (2002). Timing interference to speech in altered listening conditions. *The Journal of the Acoustical Society of America*, *111*(6), 2842–2852.

Howell, P., Sackin, S., & Glenn, K. (1997a). Development of a two-stage procedure for the automatic recognition of dysfluencies in the speech of children who stutter: I. Psychometric procedures appropriate for selection of training material for lexical dysfluency classifiers. *Journal of Speech, Language and Hearing Research*, *40*, 1073–1084.

Howell, P., Sackin, S., & Glenn, K. (1997b). Development of a two-stage procedure for the automatic recognition of dysfluencies in the speech of children who stutter: II. ANN recognition of repetitions and prolongations with supplied word segment markers *Journal of Speech, Language and Hearing Research*, *40*, 1085–1096.

Howell, P., Wingfield, T., & Johnson, M. (1988). "Characteristics of the speech of stutterers during normal and altered auditory feedback" *In Proceedings Speech 88*, edited by W. A. Ainswoth and J. N. Holmes. Institute of Acoustics, Edinburgh, Vol. 3, pp. 1069–1076.

Howell, P., Young, K., & Sackin, S. (1992). Acoustical changes to speech in noisy and echoey environments. *Speech processing in adverse conditions*. 223-226. Retrieved from: https://www.isca-speech.org/archive_open/spac/spac_223.html

Iggo, A. (1986). Sensory receptors in the skin of mammals and their sensory function. *Pain*, *26*(1), 121. https://doi.org/10.1016/0304-3959(86)90184-3

Jones, J. A., & Munhall, K. G. (2002). The role of auditory feeback during phonation: Studies of Mandarin tone production. *Journal of Phonetics*, *30*(3), 303–320. https://doi.org/10.1006/jpho.2001.0160

Jones, J. A., & Munhall, K. G. (2000). Perceptual calibration of F0 production: Evidence from feedback perturbation. *The Journal of the Acoustical Society of America*, *108*(3), 1246. https://doi.org/10.1121/1.1288414

Juliano, S. L., & Mclaughlin, D. F. (1999). Somatic senses 2: Discriminative touch. *Neuroscience for rehabilitation*(2nd ed., pp. 111–130). Washington DC: Lippincott Williams & Wilkins.

Kalinowski, J., Armson, J., Stuart, A., & Gracco, V. L. (1993). Effects of alterations in auditory feedback and speech rate on stuttering frequency. *Language and Speech*, *36*(1), 1–16. https://doi.org/10.1177%2F002383099303600101

Kalinowski, J., Stuart, A., Sark, S., & Armson, J. (1996). Stuttering amelioration at various auditory feedback delays and speech rates. *International Journal of Language and Communication Disorders*, *31*(3), 259–269. https://doi.org/10.3109/13682829609033157

Kalveram, K. Th. Neurobiology of speaking and stuttering. In: Bosshardt, HG.; Yaruss, JS.; Peters, HFM., editors. Fluency Disorders: Theory, Research, Treatment and Self-help. *Proceedings of the Third World Congress of Fluency Disorders;* Nijmegen: Nijmegen University Press; 2001. p. 59–65.

Kalveram, K. T., & Jäncke, L. (1989). Vowel duration and voice onset time for stressed and nonstressed syllables in stutterers under delayed auditory feedback condition. *Folia Phoniatrica*, *41*(1), 30–42.

Kuniszyk-Józkowiak, W., & Adamczyk, B. (1989). Effect of tactile echo and tactile reverberation on the speech fluency of stutterers. *International Journal of Rehabilitation Research*, *12*(3), 312–317. Retrieved from http://ovidsp.ovid.com/ovidweb.cgi?T=JS&PAGE=reference&D=ovfta&NEWS=N&AN=00004356-198909000-00009.

Kuniszyk-Jóźkowiak, W., Smołka, E., & Adamczyk, B. (1996). Effect of acoustical, visual and tactile echo on speech fluency of stutterers. *Folia phoniatrica et Logopaedica*, *48*(4), 193–200. https://doi.org/10.1159/000266408

Kuniszyk-Jóźkowiak, W., Smołka, E., & Adamczyk, B. (1997). Effect of acoustical, visual and tactile reverberation on speech fluency of stutterers. *Folia Phoniatrica et Logopaedica*, *49*(1), 26–34. https://doi.org/10.1159/000266434

Lametti, D. R., Nasir, S. M., & Ostry, D. J. (2012). Sensory preference in speech production revealed by simultaneous alteration of auditory and somatosensory feedback. *Journal of Neuroscience*, *32*(27), 9351–9358. https://doi.org/10.1523/JNEUROSCI.0404-12.2012

Lane, H., & Tranel, B. (1971). The Lombard sign and the role of hearing in speech. *Journal of Speech and Hearing Research*, *14*(4), 677–709. https://doi.org/10.1044/jshr.1404.677

Larson, C. R., Sun, J., & Hain, T. C. (2007). Effects of simultaneous perturbations of voice pitch and loudness feedback on voice F0 and amplitude control. *The Journal of the Acoustical Society of America, 121*(5), 2862–2872. https://doi.org/10.1121/1.2715657

Lee, B. S. (1950). Effects of delayed speech feedback. *Journal of the Acoustical Society of America, 22*(6), 824–826. https://doi.org/10.1121/1.1906696

Lincoln, M., Packman, A., & Onslow, M. (2006). Altered auditory feedback and the treatment of stuttering: A review. *Journal of Fluency Disorders, 31*(2), 71–89. https://doi.org/10.1016/j.jfludis.2006.04.001

Liu, H., & Larson, C. R. (2007). Effects of perturbation magnitude and voice F0 level on the pitch-shift reflex. *The Journal of the Acoustical Society of America, 122*(6), 3671–3677. https://doi.org/10.1121/1.2800254

Lotzmann, G. (1961). On the use of varied delay times in stammerers. *Folia Phoniatrica, 13*, 276–310.

Loucks, T., Chon, H., & Han, W. (2012). Audiovocal integration in adults who stutter. *International Journal of Language and Communication Disorders, 47*(4), 451–456. https://doi.org/10.1111/j.1460-6984.2011.00111.x

Macleod, J., Kalinowski, J., Stuart, A., & Armson, J. (1995). Effect of single and combined altered auditory feedback on stuttering frequency at two speech rates. *Journal of Communication Disorders, 28*(3), 217–228. https://doi.org/10.1016/0021-9924(94)00010-W

Max, L., Guenther, F. H., Gracco, V. L., Ghosh, S. S., & Wallace, M. E. (2004). Unstable or insufficiently activated internal models and feedback-biased motor control as sources of dysfluency: A theoretical model of stuttering. *Contemporary Issues in Communication Science and Disorders, 31*(Spring), 105–122. https://doi.org/10.1044/cicsd_31_s_105

Natke, U., Donath, T. M., & Kalveram, K. T. (2003). Control of voice fundamental frequency in speaking versus singing. *The Journal of the Acoustical Society of America, 113*(3), 1587–1593. https://doi.org/10.1121/1.1543928

Natke, U., Grosser, J., & Kalveram, K. T. (2001). Fluency, fundamental frequency, and speech rate under frequency-shifted auditory feedback in stuttering and nonstuttering persons. *Journal of Fluency Disorders, 26*(3), 227–241. https://doi.org/10.1016/S0094-730X(01)00099-7

Natke, U., & Kalveram, K. T. (2001). Effects of frequency-shifted auditory feedback on fundamental frequency of long stressed and unstressed syllables. *Journal of Speech, Language, and Hearing Research, 44*(3), 577–584. https://doi.org/10.1044/1092-4388(2001/045)

Nessel, E. (1958). Die verzögerte Sprachrückkopplung (Lee-Effekt) bei Stotterern. *Folia Phoniatrica et Logopaedica, 10*(4), 199–204.

Novak, A. (1978). The influence of delayed auditory feedback in stutterers. *Folia Phoniatrica, 30*, 278–285.

O'Donnell, J. J., Armson, J., & Kiefte, M. (2008). The effectiveness of SpeechEasy during situations of daily living. *Journal of Fluency Disorders, 33*(2), 99–119. https://doi.org/10.1016/j.jfludis.2008.02.001

Pollard, R., Ellis, J. B., Finan, D., & Ramig, P. R. (2009). Effects of the SpeechEasy on objective and perceived aspects of stuttering: A 6-month, phase i clinical trial in naturalistic environments. *Journal of Speech, Language, and Hearing Research, 52*(2), 516–533. https://doi.org/10.1044/1092-4388(2008/07-0204)

Purcell, D. W., & Munhall, K. G. (2006a). Adaptive control of vowel formant frequency: Evidence from real-time formant manipulation. *The Journal of the Acoustical Society of America, 120*(2), 966–977. https://doi.org/10.1121/1.2217714

Purcell, D. W., & Munhall, K. G. (2006b). Compensation following real-time manipulation of formants in isolated vowels. *The Journal of the Acoustical Society of America, 119*(4), 2288–2297. https://doi.org/10.1121/1.2173514

Reed, P., & Howell, P. (2000). Suggestions for improving the long-term effects of treatments for stuttering: A review and synthesis of frequency-shifted feedback and operant techniques. *European Journal of Behavior Analysis, 1*(2), 89–106. https://doi.org/10.1080/15021149.2000.11434158

Ritto, A. P., Juste, F. S., Stuart, A., Kalinowski, J., & de Andrade, C. R. F. (2016). Randomized clinical trial: The use of SpeechEasy® in stuttering treatment. *International Journal of Language and Communication Disorders, 51*(6), 769–774. https://doi.org/10.1111/1460-6984.12237

Rosen, S., & Howell, P. (2011). *Signals and systems for speech and hearing* (Vol. 29). Leiden, the Netherlands: Brill.

Ryan, B. (1974). *Programmed therapy for stuttering in children and adults*. Springfield, IL: Charles C Thomas Publisher.

Sares, A. G., Deroche, M. L. D., Shiller, D. M., & Gracco, V. L. (2018). Timing variability of sensorimotor integration during vocalization in individuals who stutter. *Scientific Reports, 8*(1), 1–10. https://doi.org/10.1038/s41598-018-34517-1

Siegel, A., & Sapru, H. N. (2006). *Essential neuroscience*. Philadelphia, PA: Lippincott Williams & Wilkins.

Sivasankar, M., Bauer, J. J., Babu, T., & Larson, C. R. (2005). Voice responses to changes in pitch of voice or tone auditory feedback. *The Journal of the Acoustical Society of America*, *117*(2), 850–857. https://doi.org/10.1121/1.1849933

Soderberg, G. A. (1969). Delayed auditory feedback and the speech of stutterers: A review of studies. *Journal of Speech and Hearing Disorders*, *34*(1), 20–29.

Sparks, G., Grant, D. E., Millay, K., Walker-Batson, D., & Hynan, L. S. (2002). The effect of fast speech rate on stuttering frequency during delayed auditory feedback. *Journal of Fluency Disorders*, *27*(3), 187–201. https://doi.org/10.1016/S0094-730X(02)00128-6

Stuart, A., & Kalinowski, J. (2004). The perception of speech naturalness of post-therapeutic and altered auditory feedback speech of adults with mild and severe stuttering. *Folia Phoniatrica et Logopaedica*, *56*(6), 347–357. https://doi.org/10.1159/000081082

Stuart, A., Kalinowski, J., Armson, J., Stenstrom, R., & Jones, K. (1996). Fluency effect of frequency alterations of plus/minus one-Half and one-quarter octave shifts in auditory feedback of people who stutter. *Journal of Speech, Language, and Hearing Research*, *39*(2), 396–401. https://doi.org/10.1044/jshr.3902.396

Stuart, A., Kalinowski, J., Rastatter, M. P., Saltuklaroglu, T., & Dayalu, V. (2004). Investigations of the impact of altered auditory feedback in-the-ear devices on the speech of people who stutter: Initial fitting and 4-month follow-up. *International Journal of Language and Communication Disorders*, *39*(1), 93–113. https://doi.org/10.1080/13682820310001616976

Stuart, A., Kalinowski, J., Saltuklaroglu, T., & Guntupalli, V. (2006). Investigations of the impact of altered auditory feedback in-the-ear devices on the speech of people who stutter: One-year follow-up. *Disability and Rehabilitation*, *28*(12), 757–765. https://doi.org/10.1080/09638280500386635

Stuart, A., Xia, S., Jiang, Y., Jiang, T., Kalinowski, J., & Rastatter, M. P. (2003). Self-contained in-the-ear device to deliver altered auditory feedback: Applications for stuttering. *Annals of Biomedical Engineering*, *31*(2), 233–237. https://doi.org/10.1114/1.1541014

Snyder, G. J., Waddell, D., Blanchet, P., & Ivy, L. J. (2009). Effects of digital vibrotactile speech feedback on overt stuttering frequency. *Perceptual and Motor Skills*, *108*(1), 271–280.

Tourville, J. A., & Guenther, F. H. (2011). The DIVA model: A neural theory of speech acquisition and production. *Language and Cognitive Processes*, *26*(7), 952–981. https://dx.doi.org/10.1080/2F01690960903498424

Van Borsel, J., Reunes, G., & Van Den Bergh, N. (2003). Delayed auditory feedback in the treatment of stuttering: Clients as consumers. *International Journal of Language and Communication Disorders*, *38*(2), 119–129. https://doi.org/10.1080/1368282021000042902

Villacorta, V. M., Perkell, J. S., & Guenther, F. H. (2007). Sensorimotor adaptation to feedback perturbations of vowel acoustics and its relation to perception. *The Journal of the Acoustical Society of America*, *122*(4), 2306–2319. https://doi.org/10.1121/1.2773966

Waddell, D. E., Goggans, P. M., & Snyder, G. J. (2012). Novel tactile feedback to reduce overt stuttering. *NeuroReport*, *23*(12), 727–730. https://doi.org/10.1097/WNR.0b013e328356b108

Watkins, K. E., Smith, S. M., Davis, S., & Howell, P. (2008). Structural and functional abnormalities of the motor system in developmental stuttering. *Brain : A Journal of Neurology*, *131*(Pt 1), 50–59. https://doi.org/10.1093/brain/awm241

Weidig, T. (2005). The statistical fluctuation in the natural recovery rate between control and treatment group dilutes their results. Rapid response to "Randomised controlled trial of the Lidcombe programme of early stuttering intervention" by Jones, Onslow, Packman, Williams, Ormond, Schwarz & Gebski (2005). *British Medical Journal* [Announcement posted on the World Wide Web]. 27-11-2009, from: http://bmj.bmjjournals.com/cgi/eletters/331/7518/659#115238

33

DICHOTIC LISTENING

Mária Gósy and Ruth Huntley Bahr

Introduction

Hemispheric asymmetry is one of the fundamental principles of neuronal organization (Hugdahl & Westerhausen, 2010). Dichotic listening (DL) is one way to evaluate hemispheric asymmetry. The term dichotic listening refers to a broad variety of experimental paradigms that assess hemispheric differences in auditory processing (Westerhausen, 2019).

Interpretation of DL results provides insight into the functional specificity of cerebral organization as an overall phenomenon, without regard to native language. The classical DL method is that two auditory stimuli are presented simultaneously to the subject's right and left ears, and he/she has to report the stimuli (syllables, words, etc.) that are heard after each trial. Responses are then calculated and compared across ears. The results depict hemispheric superiority. Most individuals demonstrate a right ear advantage (REA) for language functions because the right-ear has priority over the left-ear in accessing the left-hemisphere language processor (Yund et al., 1999). A large number of papers using various methods (such as PET, fMRI, MEG, electrophysiological measurements, etc.) along with the DL technique have confirmed the anatomical basis of REA (e.g. Bethmann et al., 2007; Brancucci et al., 2005; Hakvoort et al., 2016; Hugdahl et al., 2000; Penna et al., 2007).

Brief historical overview

In 1954, Broadbent conducted the first experiment using DL. His research question focused on the role of auditory localization in the maintenance of attention and memory span of air traffic controllers as they simultaneously received information about multiple flights. He reported that when two different digits were presented to the right and left ear of his participants simultaneously, they could accurately recognize more words heard in their right ear. The REA is a consequence of the anatomy of the auditory projections from the cochlear nucleus to the primary auditory cortex, which demonstrates a left hemisphere superiority for the processing of language and speech. Broadbent surmised that spatially separated sounds might pass through the perceptual mechanism successively, rather than simultaneously, based on the findings that the sound in one ear produces a response that occurs before the other ear perceives the signal (Broadbent, 1954).

A few years later, Doreen Kimura developed the present-day version of the DL technique while studying hemispheric function in normal individuals and patients with brain lesions (Kimura, 1961a, 1961b). Following Broadbent's procedure, she used digits in her dichotic tests and obtained an REA with her participants. She interpreted this finding as the crossed auditory pathways seemed to be stronger or more numerous than the uncrossed ones and that the left temporal lobe played a more important part than the right in the perception of spoken material. Kimura's findings received support from several studies that followed (e.g. Bryden, 1967; Bryden, 1970; Satz, 1968; Studdert-Kennedy et al., 1970).

The methodology used in Kimura's classical DL paradigm has been modified over time in terms of preparation and nature of speech material, the test procedures used, the instructions the participants received and with changes in technology. Early investigators prepared their stimuli using natural speech with a two-channel tape, modified to permit the length of leader tape passing between two playback heads to be varied (until the onsets of the two syllables coincided). Synthesized speech stimuli became available in the 1970s (see Studdert-Kennedy et al., 1972).

Description of the DL technique

In a typical DL experiment, the subject is presented with pairs of various types of speech or speech-like stimuli via headphones. One stimulus is presented to the right ear, while the other one is presented simultaneously to the left ear (see Figure 33.1). The timing and intensity of the stimuli are carefully manipulated to ensure that the test stimuli are similar in duration and their inputs and outputs are appropriately synchronized.

Development of a DL test consists of decisions on the nature of the stimuli, the number of the pairs and the trials in the test (single or multiple stimulus-pair presentations per trial) according to the goal and the participants in the experiments.

Stimulus material

The stimuli used in DL tests can be categorized by their relationships to authentic language (i.e. sound sequences, real words, strings of words), stimulus length (number of segments and syllables utilized), whether the stimuli were natural or synthesized and if stimuli were selected

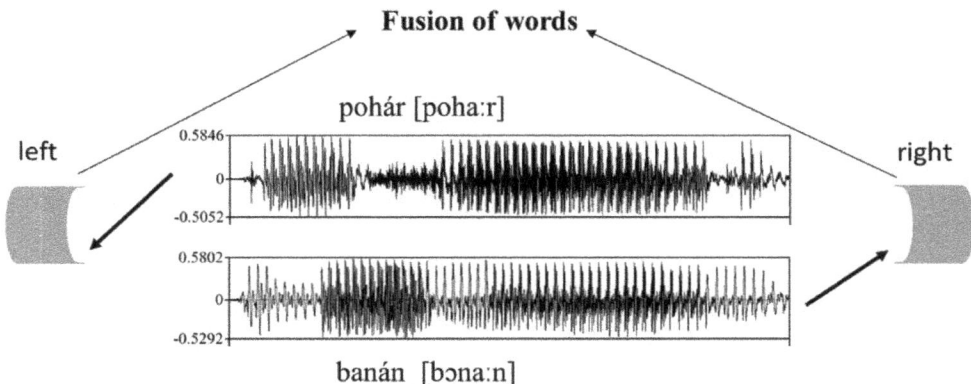

Figure 33.1 Schematic display of the DL technique using Hungarian disyllabic words indicated by oscillograms (*pohár* "cup" played to the left ear and *banán* "banana" played to the right ear simultaneously).

for their perceptual difficulty. The first DL tests used digits that differed in list length. Digits have several advantages, which include relative frequency of the words, ease of perception, easy access to the mental lexicon, limited possible sequences from 1 to 10 and neighborhood density of the words.

Other DL tests contain CV-syllables that frequently differ only in the initial consonants. These stimuli are often stop consonants and are placed in pairs that differ in voicing (e.g. *ba/pa*) and/or in place of articulation (e.g. *ba/da*). The vowel is either the same (frequently an [a]), but other vowels have also been used (e.g. Hugdahl et al., 2009; Westerhausen et al., 2018). The syllable stimuli can be CV or CVC, and rarely VCV (e.g. *bap*, *dab*, *deb* vs. *aga*, *aka*). Longer sound sequences (or pseudo words), monosyllabic (rhyming) words (*gage* and *cage* or *Preis* "price" and *Kreis* "circle") and mono- and disyllabic words (mostly nouns, e.g. *way* vs. *day* and *airplane* vs. *wetpaint*) have been used (Fernandes et al., 2006; Meyers et al., 2002; McCulloch et al., 2017). Word pairs selected for a DL test should have similar spectral and temporal properties or differ by one or two phonemes for the stimuli to perceptually fuse. The frequency of phonemes, syllables and words differ by their occurrence in spontaneous speech, which has an influence on stimulus identification.

Many types of stimulus materials are thought to be appropriate for the assessment of hemispheric asymmetry, but according to Westerhausen (2019), they assess different stages of speech processing. Various speech units (syllables, words, etc.) also are processed differentially during speech perception. According to Moncrieff (2011), words involve the highest verbal workload for dichotic testing. There are some DL tests that use sentences. In one case, six meaningless strings of meaningful words were created (e.g. *go change your car color is red*) and the participants were asked to identify them from a closed set of six possible responses (Noffsinger et al., 1994). Even arithmetic problems phrased as true/false statements were used in a dichotic experiment with young adults (Mildner, 2001). Finally, the Dichotic Sentence Identification (DSI) test uses 30 pairs of sentences presented dichotically in order to analyze binaural separation in the case of hearing impairment (Auditec, Inc.). Normative data for the DSI are available for adults (Jerger, 2019).

Preparation of stimuli

In case of natural speech, speakers are asked to produce the stimuli in a neutral voice, without intonational variation. The two paired stimuli should be synchronously presented to the left and right audio channel. In practice, each pair of stimuli is displayed on a computer screen and synchronized for simultaneous onset and offset between the right and left channels. Average root mean square (RMS) amplitude should be equalized for each stimulus. The sound level of the stimuli should be set at a comfortable hearing intensity between 70 and 80 dB(A) with the same mean intensity in the two ears. The inter-stimulus interval is kept constant at 4,000 ms, in general. Currently, no systematic analysis is available about the possible effects on DL results depending whether female or male voices are used.

Procedure

To be included in a DL experiment, the participants must have good hearing (i.e. below 20 dB across all tested frequencies in each ear) and no inter-aural acuity differences between ears. If the participants do not have equal hearing ability in both ears, the DL procedure should balance the hearing level differences between ears. DL experiments have even been conducted with hearing-impaired subjects (see Wesarg at al., 2015).

DL experiments involve two basic techniques: (1) a non-forced condition (NF) and (2) a forced condition (e.g. Hugdahl & Westerhausen, 2010). During the NF condition (also known as free-report or a free recall condition), the subject is asked to report what he or she heard irrespective of ear. The free recall method requires lower cognitive demands of participants, making it a simpler task. During the forced condition, the participant is instructed to report the stimuli from a particular ear. There are two subtypes of the forced condition: the forced-right (FR) and the forced-left (FL) conditions (Hugdahl & Andersson, 1986). The forced condition is harder as it requires greater attentional resources than the free recall condition.

Stimuli for a DL test are presented using headphones. The participants are asked to repeat what they hear after each trial (i.e. a verbal response format). The participant's response is the repetition of either one stimulus on each trial or as many stimuli the subject is able to recall. The other response format is manual (checking off stimuli on a prepared sheet of paper; using keyboards, a mouse click, touch screen or an external response button box). Participants' responses are either recorded directly on to a computer or written down by the experimenter. The greater the number of trials in a test increases its reliability. Most experimenters use 90 to 120 trials depending upon stimulus material and participant age (Hiscock et al., 2000). It seems that DL tests with single-pair trials are better for laterality estimates since those types of tasks simplify the cognitive processing involved.

More recently, Westerhausen and Samuelsen (2020) decided to develop a DL task that reduced the influence of cognitive factors on participant performance. Their assessment device utilized stop consonant-vowel (CV) stimuli that are matched by voicing. These voicing pairs were alternated to avoid priming effects. Free recall was used to reduce the cognitive effects associated with attention. Participants heard single trials and were asked to provide a single response. Finally, there were only 120 trials, presented in both directions (right-left and left-right) with equal frequency, and binaural trials (i.e. both stimuli were the same) were included. Test-retest reliability results were strong, indicating that these modifications resulted in a DL test that focused on stimulus-driven factors with the fewest trials while also reducing participant variability. More testing is needed to validate this procedure.

Scoring

Correctly recalled stimuli are scored for the right and left ear independently. The data of the correctly recalled stimuli can be used to calculate ear advantage by subtracting the score for the left ear from the score for the right ear, yielding a positive number for a REA, a negative number for a left-ear-advantage (LEA) and zero for no ear advantage (NEA). Ear advantages also can be calculated by subtracting the score for the nondominant ear (the lower score) from the score for the dominant ear (see Moncrieff, 2011).

The laterality index (LI) is a measure of the relative difference between the ear scores, demonstrating the magnitude of lateralized processing (Fernandes & Smith, 2000; Hakvoort et al., 2016; Studdert-Kennedy & Shankweiler, 1970, etc.). A DL LI is calculated using the following formula: [(right ear score) − (left ear score)]/[right ear score + left ear score)] * 100 (Hugdahl et al., 2003a). In this formula, "right ear" or "left ear" refers to the number of stimuli heard and recalled correctly from that ear. LI can also be calculated using the natural logarithm of the ratio between right and left ear responses. In both calculations, a negative LI shows right-hemisphere dominance, while a positive LI shows dominance of the left hemisphere. The determination of ear advantage is then used in future statistical treatment of the data.

DL paradigm and cognitive functions

In addition to assessing language laterality, the DL technique taps into a broad spectrum of cognitive functions, including memory, attention, speech perception, etc. The relationship between memory and performance in a dichotic listening task was introduced in the late 1960s and has since been confirmed (e.g. Bentin et al., 1995; Murray & Hitchcock,1969; Penner et al., 2009). REA has been shown to be relatively robust in free recall DL tasks, but it might be influenced by attentional processes (Asbjørnsen, & Hugdahl, 1995; Bryden et al. 1983; Haakvoort et al., 2016; Hiscock and Kinsbourne 2011). In 1971, Bryden published a DL experiment where the participants were instructed to attend to the digit stimuli arriving at one ear and to indicate either the attended or unattended stimuli (Bryden, 1971). Poorer performance was noted with stimuli from the unattended ear. These "biased attenders" demonstrated an asymmetry in the forced responses between ears (Bryden et al., 1983, p. 246). This meant that they allowed stimuli from the dominant ear to frequently intrude into their responses from the nondominant ear.

In 1986, Hugdahl and Andersson used DL for studying the interaction between attention and speech laterality. They used the "forced-attention" paradigm when comparing the responses of children ages 8–9 years with young adults. A significant REA was obtained for all groups during the free recall condition. During the forced-attention conditions, adults' scores differed from those of children depending upon condition. During the FR condition, significantly more correct responses were obtained from the right compared to the left ear in both groups. However, in the FL condition, significantly more correct responses from the left ear were obtained only in the adult group. The investigators related this to attentional factors influencing the DL performance differently between children and adults.

Handedness and its connection with laterality was well known prior to the use of the DL technique (McManus, 2009). Considerations of handedness and DL performance started in the early 1960s (e.g. Curry, 1967; Zurif & Bryden, 1969; Briggs & Nebers, 1976) and has been studied for years (Brunswick & Rippon, 1994; Foundas et al., 2006; Hugdahl, 1988; Obrzut et al., 1997). In a large-scale study of over 1,800 participants – children (5–9 years), adolescents (10–15 years), young adults (16–49 years) and adults older than 50 years – REA was found in all groups. However, handedness did not seem to be an influencing factor and no sex differences were noted (Hirnstein et al.,2014). Another large-scale study of subjects (from age 10 to older adults) showed that neither handedness, nor gender influenced ear advantage in children and older adults (Hirnstein et al., 2013). A study by Mildner and her colleagues (2005) focused on the effects of handedness and gender on ear advantage with adult Croatian speakers in their first language and in their L2 (English). Data revealed significant relationships between handedness and ear advantage in Croatian, but not in English. There was a significant effect of gender on ear advantage in responses to English stimuli (where males showed a lower REA than females), but not for Croatian stimuli.

DL paradigm and speech perception

The DL technique was used to study "dichotic fusion" in relation to speech perception as early as the 1950s. Initially, Broadbent (1955) presented the higher-frequency components of sounds (high-pass filtered at 2,000 Hz with an attenuation of 18 dB/octave) in one ear while the lower-frequency components of another sound (low-pass filtered at 450 Hz with an attenuation of 18 dB/octave) were presented to the other ear. This procedure resulted in some perceptual fusion. Hence, the majority of the participants heard a single sound as a result of the fusion of the different stimuli from the two ears. This phenomenon was further investigated by Broadbent and Ladefoged (1957) who employed two-formant synthetic syllables (and various fundamental frequencies) in a DL experiment. The first formant was presented in one ear while the second formant was presented in the other ear. The fusion occurred when these two formants were presented to different ears at the same fundamental frequency. Differing fundamental frequencies prevented fusion. Their findings highlighted the role of multiple cues in speech perception.

Similarly, intensity modifications were added to the synthetic speech stimuli presented to separate ears (Rand, 1974) and when consonants were masked by vowels (Repp, 1975) in DL experiments. Cutting (1976) studied factors that could influence the strength of perceptual fusion. He determined that variation in the relative onset time of two stimuli, relative intensity and relative fundamental frequency affected perceptual fusion. Six fusions (sound localization, psychoacoustic fusion, spectral fusion, spectral/temporal fusion, phonetic feature fusion and phonological fusion) were analyzed by means of the DL paradigm. Results confirmed the arrangement of the six fusions in a hierarchy for speech perception: first perceptual integration influences sound localization and psychoacoustic fusion. Perceptual disruption and recombination characterize the other four types of fusion.

Studdert-Kennedy and Shankweiler (1970) focused on vowel and consonant perception in American English CVC syllables. They observed (i) a significant REA for initial stop consonants, (ii) a significant, though reduced, REA for final stop consonants, (iii) a non-significant REA for six medial vowels and (iv) significant and independent REAs for the articulatory features of voicing and place in initial stop consonants (p. 592). Based on these findings, the authors suggested that differences in REA between stops and vowels may be due to differences in the susceptibility of these segments to information loss during transmission.

Speech perception was examined using the DL method in order to highlight the distinction between auditory and phonetic processes (Studdert-Kennedy et al., 1972). These authors used various synthesized CV syllables where the Cs were stops and the V was either a [u] or an [i] vowel. Their results revealed that there was a distinction between auditory and phonetic processes in speech since the common properties at the two levels affected ear advantage differently. Phonetic features influenced the subjects' performance, but not their ear advantage. Auditory similarities or contrasts, however, had an effect on ear advantage, but not on overall performance.

Voicing perception was analyzed using a DL method in Australian children (Arciuli, 2011) who demonstrated a developmental trajectory, where long VOTs gradually dominated over short VOTs. In a cross-language study using a free-report DL paradigm (Westerhausen et al., 2018), Norwegian and Estonian subjects were tested on their sensitivity to a voicing contrast. Norwegian native speakers were found to be more sensitive to the voicing of the initial stop consonants than the Estonian speakers (whose language has only unvoiced initial stops).

The development of cognitive control of speech perception across the life span in 2,988 subjects was examined in a forced-attention CV DL paradigm by Westerhausen et al. (2015). Their results confirmed an increase in performance level throughout childhood, with the highest performance noted in young adults followed by a continuous decline into old age.

DL paradigm and language laterality

The DL method is useful in the determination of language lateralization for speakers of various languages. REA is seen in the majority of older children and adults, while a LEA is seen in about 10–20% of the population (De Andrade et al., 2015; Hugdahl et al., 2001; Jerger & Martin, 2004; McCulloch et al., 2017; Obrzut et al., 1986; Roup et al., 2006). However, the magnitude of ear advantage varies across experiments, participants and the methods used. Nevertheless, the similarity of findings noted across languages supports the nature of auditory processing. Specifically, the auditory input to the contralateral hemisphere is supposed to be more strongly represented in the left hemisphere of the brain in right-handers. The rationale proposed for this phenomenon is that auditory information sent along the ipsilateral pathways is suppressed or blocked by the contralateral stimuli. In turn, information that reaches the ipsilateral right hemisphere has to be transferred crossing the corpus callosum to the left hemisphere language processing areas (e.g. Davidson & Hugdahl, 1996). Therefore, similar laterality effects should exist across languages.

Most of the laterality studies that used the DL technique have tested relatively small groups of participants and the majority of them utilized English speakers. A smartphone application (*i-Dichotic*) has been developed and used to increase both the number of the participants and the variety of languages (Bless et al., 2015) used in DL experiments. This application uses CV syllables (/ba/, /da/, /ga/, /ta/, /ka/ and /pa/) spoken by native speakers of (British) English, Norwegian, German and Estonian. Participants are asked to download the app and self-administer the DL test. This procedure resulted in the testing of 4,408 subjects (mean age: 33 years) representing 64 native languages. Findings confirmed that left-hemispheric language dominance is in fact a general phenomenon and that the phoneme inventory and acoustic properties of the language influenced the magnitude of ear advantage.

DL paradigm and the development of language laterality

Hemispheric asymmetry is one of the fundamental principles of neuronal organization that develops during language acquisition. The DL paradigm has been used to study the development of language laterality in children and adolescents. These results have confirmed an REA in these young subjects with various first languages and also showed an increase of correct responses with age (Gósy & Krepsz, 2018; Hirnstein et al., 2013; Hiscock & Decter, 1988; Hugdahl et al., 2001; Jerger & Martin, 2004; Kershner & Chyczij, 1992; Lebel & Beaulieu, 2009; Moncrieff & Musiek, 2002; Moncrieff & Wilson, 2009, Moncrieff, 2011; Norrelgen et al., 2012; etc.).

Nevertheless, results reporting age and gender effects on the development of laterality in children have been varied. In a longitudinal study, Harper and Kraft (1994) observed no significant change in REA in children between 3;4 to 3;8 years. However, significant increases were found between 4 and 7;6 years. Kimura's results with children (Kimura, 1963, 1967) revealed a REA for both boys and girls at the age of 6. Five-year-old girls showed a significant right-ear effect, but the 5-year-old boys did not. Kimura concluded that boys seemed to lag behind girls in the development of dichotic speech perception with no further explanation. Similarly, Hynd and Obrzut (1977) studied 2nd-, 4th- and 6th-grade children using the DL method and noted a significant REA irrespective of age or gender. Moncrieff (2011) studied children between five and twelve years of age using a DL paradigm with monosyllabic words and digits. Her data showed an REA for nearly 60% of the 5- to 7-year-olds tested, over 75% of 8- to 10-year-olds and roughly 70% of 11- to 12-year-old participants. In contrast, almost 30% of the youngest participants, over 20% of the 8- to 10- year-olds and slightly more than 25% of the oldest group exhibited an LEA.

REA prevalence was shown to be greater among females and lower among males (Moncrieff, 2011). She concluded that gender has a decisive effect on ear advantage in a DL task. In an early study, results of 9-, 13- and 17-year-old subjects revealed that older participants repeated the DL stimuli better than younger ones (Piazza et al., 1985). In another experiment, 11-year-olds showed correct recall of 88% of words administered to their right ear, while 82% of the words presented to the left ear were accurate (Moncrieff & Musiek, 2002). In conclusion, findings with schoolchildren confirmed left-hemisphere dominance and no change in dominance was documented after the age of 6, with girls demonstrating a stronger LEA than boys (Asbjørnsen & Helland, 2006; Bryden, 1970; Moncrieff, 2011; Obrzut & Mahoney, 2011; Rosenberg, 2011).

DL paradigm and clinical populations

From the beginning, experimenters have applied the DL technique to clinical populations. DL testing can be used to identify difficulties in language processing, specifically related to laterality, but also the influences of attention, arousal and higher cortical functioning (Hugdahl, 2, 62–84. 2000). In his review of DL experiments, Hugdahl identified how stimulus-driven tasks, i.e. digits, CV syllables, words, etc., influenced the degree of laterality results in different ways than instruction-driven laterality tasks, i.e. selective attention versus free report. Given the noted limitations of DL tasks in evaluating language processing, a brief review of the findings by age and clinical population is provided. Results related to the use of DL in assessment and treatment will be described.

Language processing in adults

DL has been used to identify cerebral dysfunction in adults. Studies in patients with traumatic brain injury and aphasia (Hugdahl, 2003; Meyers et al, 2002; Nascimento et al., 2014; Richardson et al., 1994; Roberts et al., 1990) have shown that dichotic word listening tests can differentiate between the degrees of traumatic brain injury, mild, moderate and severe, based on the duration of unconsciousness and differences in language processing associated with left and right hemisphere damage. Hugdahl (2003) compared patients with left and right frontal lobe damage on the standard CV syllables DL test to evaluate the effects of site of lesion on speech perception. An REA was found with the right lesioned patients, while no ear advantage was noted with the left lesioned patients. However, during the forced-right attention condition, a significant REA was found in both groups. The authors suggested that the left frontal lobe patients had impairments of both stimulus processing and attentional modulation, while the right frontal lobe patients only experienced deficits in attentional modulation.

Continued research demonstrated that DL tasks could identify differences in language processing associated with a disruption in subcortical pathways, as in cerebral malaria patients and those with Parkinson's Disease (Richardson et al., 1994). The results of these studies (and others like them) demonstrated that the use of DL procedures can supplement other neuropsychological testing by demonstrating the impact of neurological injury on language processing. There is even evidence that treatment utilizing a variety of DL tasks can result in positive changes in auditory processing, resulting in the improved comprehension of complex commands in patients with acquired brain injuries (Richardson et al., 1994; Purdy & McCullagh, 2019;).

DL also has been used in the study of language processing in adults who stutter (Robb et al., 2013). Using both directed and undirected attention tasks, adults who stutter demonstrated a weaker REA than adults who do not stutter. The latter finding suggested a stronger right hemisphere involvement in speech processing. However, no difference was noted between these groups in the directed attention condition. Nevertheless, these results should be interpreted with caution due to the small sample size.

Other clinical research has considered the utility of DL tests to identify language processing differences in patients with emotional and behavioral difficulties. Bruder and colleagues (1996) studied changes in DL asymmetries after fluoxetine treatment for patients with depression. They noted that greater left than right hemisphere activation was associated with better treatment outcomes. In other words, a greater REA for dichotic words and less LEA for complex tones was noted in patients that positively responded to the drug therapy. A major weakness with this study was the absence of a no-treatment group. However, more recent research has substantiated these findings at two different test sites (Bruder et al., 2017; Kishon et al., 2015). These researchers concluded that patients with a REA were better at activating the cognitive processes essential for treatment success.

Language processing in children

In children, deficits in DL have been associated primarily with language and reading difficulties (e.g. Moncrieff, 2010). Many of the studies that addressed language difficulties focused on the use of central auditory processing (CAP) tests. Children with autism spectrum disorders demonstrated a wide range of performance on CAP tests, from scores within the typically developing range to those indicating significant difficulties in language processing (Kozou et al., 2018; Richardson et al., 1994). However, these same students were able to improve their language processing skills with auditory training.

Other researchers have shown that boys with disruptive behavior disorders (i.e. attention-deficit; Pine et al., 1997) exhibited a lower REA, which was indicative of poorer verbal processing ability. These boys also had lower test scores in reading and language comprehension. Such findings support the notion that attention plays a critical role in language development.

Many DL studies have focused on students with dyslexia. Typically, these researchers reported a reduced or no REA on DL tests with poor readers and dyslexic children (Asbjørnsen & Helland, 2006; Gósy et al., 2018; Hakvoort et al., 2016; Heiervang et al., 2000; Moncrieff & Musiek,). Likewise, no REA was found when testing adolescents and adults with dyslexia (Hugdahl et al., 1995). These researchers reasoned that a left temporal lobe processing dysfunction identified in childhood persisted into adulthood. However, Brunswick and Rippon (1994) found no difference in the performances of the children with dyslexia and controls on their DL task. Yet, they noted significantly greater N100 amplitudes in the left temporal region during a DL test in students without dyslexia while students with dyslexia displayed approximately equivalent levels of N100 amplitude bilaterally. Other studies have revealed an increased occurrence of LEA and no ear advantage (NEA) in some groups with dyslexia (see Helland et al., 2008). In this case, a significant correlation was found between activity in the planum temporale and dichotic listening asymmetry in children with dyslexia, supporting a positive relationship between brain structure and function in this clinical population (Hugdahl et al.,2003b). Researchers reasoned that the differing results among the studies on students with dyslexia are related to poor phonological processing skills. DL tasks might not sufficiently test these subtle differences in auditory processing disorders or be sensitive to subtypes of dyslexia (e.g. Cohen et al., 1992; Hakvoort et al., 2016; Helland et al., 2018; Lamm & Epstein, 1994). In addition, attention seems to play a decisive role in the performance of DL tasks with individuals with reading difficulties. No attentional shifts were observed during a DL test in the students with reading disabilities as opposed to those in the control group (Asbjørnsen & Bryden, 1998). Hence, the poor performance of the children with learning disabilities was related to their selective attention deficit (Obrzut & Mahoney, 2011).

DL use with disorders of central auditory processing and hearing

DL tasks are an essential component of CAP test batteries. CAP Deficits reflect difficulties with speech processing and selective attention, which is related to difficulties in auditory comprehension. In older adults, DL testing can be divided into three patterns when tested with the Dichotic Sentence Identification (DSI) task in both the divided and directed attention modes (Jerger & Martin, 2004). The first pattern occurred in 19% of the study population and revealed normal scores in both conditions. Pattern II (58% of the participants) evidenced an abnormal DSI score in one ear (usually the left) in the divided attention mode, but no difference in the directed attention condition. Central auditory dysfunction characterized Pattern III (23% of the elders). In this case, the participants had abnormal scores in one ear in both testing modes.

DL tasks are also useful in hearing assessment. Elders (ages between 61 and 80 years) who had bilateral hearing loss but chose to use one hearing aid at 6 months post-bilateral hearing aid fitting were assessed with a DL task (Martins et al., 2017). Results revealed that the participants preferred use of the hearing aid in their dominant ear because this reduced the auditory competition they experienced when two hearing aids were used. On the other hand, in a group of children who received bilateral cochlear implantation, DL testing did not reveal an ear advantage using a German DL task that incorporated trisyllabic words that could be broken down into two words. Their results did not support the hypothesis that bilateral implantation would result in an REA. While other auditory tests demonstrated improvement in speech perception for these children with cochlear implants, DL tests were not helpful in predicting improvements in speech perception (see also Koopmann et al., 2020).

A recent study has considered the utility of DL tasks in a training protocol for children with auditory processing disorder (Delphi & Abdollahi, 2018). Twelve children (ages 8–9 years) participated into two different training tasks: Differential Interaural Intensity Difference (DIID) and Dichotic Offset Training (DOT). Improvements in auditory processing were noted in both training conditions; however, DOT required more training sessions. The authors reported that DIID training specifically targets the poorer ear and helps it improve to the level of the better ear. While both tasks were effective, the researchers suggested that DIID might be a more effective procedure for improving DL.

Conclusion

Six decades of research on DL have described its role in determining cerebral dominance, illustrating aspects of speech perception and demonstrating similarities/differences attributable to age, gender and language disabilities. This work has expanded from experimental designs to clinical applications. Recent research has focused on establishing best practices in the design of DL experiments (Westerhausen & Samuelsen, 2020) and understanding the role of native language on DL (Bless et al., 2015), as well as bilingualism (Westerhausen et al., 2018). DL has proven to be a useful task in determining the role of laterality, attention and other cognitive factors in language processing.

References

Arciuli, J. (2011). Manipulation of voice onset time during dichotic listening. *Brain and Cognition, 76*, 233–238.

Asbjørnsen, A., & Hugdahl, K. (1995). Attentional effects in dichotic listening. *Brain and Language, 49*, 189–201.

Asbjørnsen, A., & Helland, T. (2006). Dichotic listening performance predicts language comprehension. *Laterality, 11*(3), 251–262.

Asbjørnsen, A., & Bryden, M. P. (1998). Auditory attentional shifts in reading-disabled students: quantification of attentional effectiveness by the Attentional Shift Index. *Neuropsychologia, 36*(2), 143–148.

Bentin, S., Kutas, M., & Hillyard, S. A. (1995). Semantic processing and memory for attended and unattended words in dichotic listening: Behavioral and Electrophysiological evidence. *Journal of Experimental Psychology: Human Perception and Performance, 21*(1), 54–67.

Bethmann, A., Tempelmann, C., De Bleser, R., Scheich, H., & Brechmann, A. (2007). Determining language laterality by fMRI and dichotic listening. *Brain Research, 1133*(1), 145–157.

Bless, J. J., Westerhausen, R., von Koss Torkildsen, J., Gudmundsen, M., Kompus, K., & Hugdahl, K. (2015). Laterality across languages: Results from a global dichotic listening study using a smartphone application. *Laterality, 20*(4), 434–452.

Brancucci, A., Babiloni, C., Vecchio, F., Galderisi, S., Mucci, A., Tecchio, F., ... & Rossini, P. M. (2005). Decrease of functional coupling between left and right auditory cortices during dichotic listening: An electroencephalography study. *Neuroscience, 136*(1), 323–332.

Briggs, G., & Nebers, R. D. (1976). The effects of handedness, family history and sex on the performance of a dichotic listening task. *Neuropsychologia, 14*(1), 129–133.

Broadbent, D. E. (1954). The role of auditory localization in attention and memory span. *Journal of Experimental Psychology, 47*(3), 191–196. doi:10.1037/h0054182

Broadbent, D. E. (1955). A note on binaural fusion. *Quarterly Journal of Experimental Psychology, 7*(1), 46–47. doi:10.1080/17470215508416672

Broadbent, D. E., & Ladefoged, P. (1957). On the fusion of sounds reaching different sense organs. *Journal of Acoustical Society of America, 29*, 708–710. doi:10.1121/1.1909019

Bruder, G. E., Otto, M. W., McGrath, P. J., Stewart, J. W., Fava, M., Rosenbaum, J. F., & Quitkin, F. M. (1996). Dichotic listening before and after fluoxetine treatment for major depression: relations of laterality to therapeutic response. *Neuropsychopharmacology, 15*(2), 171–179. doi:10.1016/0893-133X(95)00180-L

Bruder, G. E., Haggerty, A., & Siegle, G. J. (2017). A quick behavioral dichotic word test is prognostic for clinical response to cognitive therapy for depression: A replication study. *Psychiatry Research, 248*, 13–19. doi:10.1016/j.psychres.2016.12.011.

Brunswick, N., & Rippon, G. (1994). Auditory event-related potentials, dichotic listening performance and handedness as indices of lateralisation in dyslexic and normal readers. *International Journal of Psychophysiology, 18*(3), 265–275. doi:10.1016/0167-8760(94)90012-4

Bryden, M. P. (1967). An evaluation of some models of dichotic listening. *Acta Oto-Laryngology, 63*, 595–604.

Bryden, M. P. (1970). Laterality effects in dichotic listening: Relations with handedness and reading ability in children. *Neuropsychologia, 8*(4), 443–450.

Bryden, M. P. (1971) Attentional strategies *and* short-term memory *in* dichotic listening. *Cognitive Psychology, 2*(1), 99–116. doi:10.1016/0010-0285(71)90004-1

Bryden, M.P., Munhall, K., & Allard, F. (1983). Attentional biases and the right-ear effect in dichotic listening. *Brain and Language, 18*(2), 236–248. doi:10.1016/0093-934X(83)90018-4

Cohen, M., Hynd, G.W., & Hugdahl, K. (1992). Dichotic listening performance in subtypes of developmental dyslexia and a left temporal lobe brain tumor contrast group. *Brain and Language, 42*(2), 187–202. doi:10.1016/0093-934X(92)90124-W

Curry, F. K. W. (1967). A comparison of left-handed and right-handed subjects on verbal and nonverbal dichotic listening tasks. *Cortex, 3*, 343–352.

Cutting, J. E. (1976). Auditory and linguistic processes in speech perception: Inferences from six fusions in dichotic listening. *Psychological Review, 83*(2), 114–140. doi:10.1037/0033-295X.83.2.114

Davidson, R.J., & Hugdahl, K. (1996). Brain asymmetry in brain electrical activity predict dichotic listening performance. *Neuropsychology, 10*(2), 241–246. doi:10.1037/0894-4105.10.2.241

De Andrade, A. N., Gil, D., & Iorio, M. C. (2015). Benchmarks for the dichotic sentence identification test in Brazilian Portuguese for ear and age. *Brazilian Journal of Otorhinolaryngology, 81*(5), 459–465.

Delphi, M., & Abdollahi, F. Z. (2018). Dichotic training in children with auditory processing disorder. *International Journal of Pediatric Otorhinolaryngology, 110*, 114–117.

Fernandes, M. A., & Smith, M. L. (2000). Comparing the fused dichotic words test and the intracarotid amobarbital procedure in children with epilepsy. *Neuropsychologia, 38*(9), 1216–1228. doi:10.1016/s0028-3932(00)00035-x

Fernandes, M. A., Smith, M., Logan, W., Crawley, A., & McAndrews, M. (2006). Comparing language lateralization determined by dichotic listening and fMRI activation in frontal and temporal lobes in children with epilepsy. *Brain and Language*, *96*(1), 106–114. doi:10.1016/j.bandl.2005.06.006

Foundas, A. L., Corey, D. M., Hurley, M. M., & Heilman, K. M. (2006). Verbal dichotic listening in right and left-handed adults: Laterality effects of directed attention. *Cortex*, *42*(1), 79–86. doi:10.1016/s0010-9452(08)70324-1

Gósy, M. & Krepsz, V. (2018). Dichotic word recognition across ages. *Govor*, *35*, 3–26. doi.org/10.22210/govor.2018.35.01

Gósy, M., Huntley Bahr, R., Gyarmathy, D., & Beke, A. (2018). Dichotic listening and sentence repetition performance in children with reading difficulties. *Clinical Linguistics and Phonetics*, *32*(9), 115–133. doi.org/10.1080/02699206.2018.1431807

Hakvoort, B., Leij van der, A., Setten van, E., Maurits, N., Maassen, B., & Zuijen van, T. (2016). Dichotic listening as an index of lateralization of speech perception in familial risk children with and without dyslexia. *Brain and Cognition*, *109*, 75–83. doi:10.1016/j.bandc.2016.09.004

Harper, L.V., & Kraft, R. H. (1994). Longitudinal change of ear advantage for receptive language function in 2 1/2- to 9-year-old children. *Perceptual and Motor Skills*, *79*(3), 1091–1092.

Heiervang, E., Hugdahl, K., Steinmetz, H., Smievoll, A. I., Stevenson, J., Lund, A., Ersland, L., & Lundervold, A. (2000). Planum temporale, planum parietale and dichotic listening in dyslexia. *Neuropsychologia*, *38*(13), 1704–1713. doi:10.1016/S0028-3932(00)00085-3

Helland, T., Asbjørnsen A.E., Hushovd A.E., & Hugdahl, K. (2008). Dichotic listening and school performance in dyslexia. *Dyslexia*, *14*(1), 42–53. doi:10.1002/dys.343

Helland, T., Morken, F., Bless, J. J., Valderhaug, H. V., Eiken, M., Helland, W. A., & Torkildsen, J. V. (2018). Auditive training effects from a dichotic listening app in children with dyslexia. *Dyslexia*, *24*, 336–356.

Hirnstein, M., Westerhausen, R., Korsnes, M. S., & Hugdahl, K. (2013). Sex differences in language asymmetry are agedependent and small: A largescale, consonant–vowel dichotic listening study with behavioral and fMRI data. *Cortex*, *49*(7), 1910–1921. doi:10.1016/j.cortex.2012.08.002

Hirnstein, M., Hugdahl, K., & Hausmann, M. (2014). How brain asymmetry relates to performance – a large-scale dichotic listening study. *Frontiers in Psychology*, *4*, 146–155. doi:10.3389/fpsyg.2013.00997

Hiscock, M., & Decter, M. H. (1988). Dichotic listening in children. In Hugdahl, K. (Ed.), *Handbook of dichotic listening: Theory, methods and research* (pp. 431–473). Oxford, England: John Wiley & Sons.

Hiscock, M., Cole, L. C., Benthall, J. G., Carlson, V. L., & Ricketts, J. M. (2000). Toward solving the inferential problem in laterality research: Effects of increased reliability on the validity of the dichotic listening right-ear advantage. *Journal of the International Neuropsychological Society*, *6*(5), 539–547.

Hiscock, M., & Kinsbourne, M. (2011). Attention and the right-ear advantage: What is the connection? *Brain and Cognition*, *76*(2), 263–275. doi:10.1016/j.bandc

Hugdahl, K. (Ed). (1988). *Handbook of dichotic listening: Theory, methods, and research*. Chichester, UK: John Wiley and Sons. doi.org/10.1002/acp.2350040307

Hugdahl, K. (2000). What can be learned about brain function from dichotic listening. *Revista Española di Neuropsicologia*, *2*, 62–84.

Hugdahl, K. (Ed.) (2003). *Experimental methods in neuropsychology*. Boston, Dordrecht, New York, London: Kluwer Academic Publishers. doi:10.1007/978-1-4615-1163-2

Hugdahl, K., & Andersson, L. (1986). The "forced-attention paradigm" in dichotic listening to CV-syllables: A comparison between adults and children. *Cortex*, *22*(3), 417–432. doi:10.1016/S0010-9452(86)80005-3

Hugdahl, K., Helland, T., Færevåg, M. K., Lyssand, E. T., & Asbjørnsen, A. (1995). Absence of ear advantage on the consonant–vowel dichotic listening test in adolescent and adult dyslexics: specific auditory phonetic dysfunction. *Journal of Clinical and Experimental Neuropsychology*, *17*(6), 833–840.

Hugdahl, K., Law, I., Kyllingsbaek, S., Bronnick, K., Gade, A., & Paulson, O. B. (2000). Effects of attention on dichotic listening: A 15O-PET study. *Human Brain Mapping*, *10*(2), 87–97.

Hugdahl, K., Carlsson, G., & Eichele, T. (2001). Age effects in dichotic listening to consonant-vowel syllables: Interactions with attention. *Developmental Neuropsychology*, *20*(1), 445–457. doi:10.1207/S15326942DN2001_8

Hugdahl, K., Bodner, T., Weiss, E., & Benke, T. (2003a). Dichotic listening performance and frontal lobe function. *Brain Research. Cognitive Brain Research, 16*(1), 58–65. doi: 10.1016/s0926-6410(02)00210-0

Hugdahl, K., Heiervang, E., Ersland, L., Lundervold, A., Steinmetz, H., & Smievoll, A. I. (2003b). Significant relation between MR measures of planum temporale area and dichotic processing of syllables in dyslexic children. *Neuropsychologia, 41*(6), 666–675. doi: 10.1016/s0028-3932(02)00224-5

Hugdahl, K., Westerhausen, R., Alho, K., Medvedev, S., Laine, M., & Hämäläinen, H. (2009). Attention and cognitive control: Unfolding the dichotic listening story. *Scandinavian Journal of Psychology, 50*(1), 11–22. doi.org/10.1111/j.1467-9450.2008.00676.x

Hugdahl, K., & Westerhausen, R. (2010). *The two halves of the brain*. Cambridge, MA: MIT Press. doi. org/10.7551/mitpress/9780262014137.001.0001

Hynd, G. W., & Obrzut, J. E. (1977). Effects of grade level and sex on the magnitude of the dichotic ear advantage. *Neuropsychologia, 15*(4-5), 689–692. doi:10.1016/0028-3932(77)90074-4

Jerger, J. (2019). Dichotic listening in elderly, hearing-impaired persons: An exercise in pattern recognition. *Hearing Review, 26*(3), 18–22.

Jerger, J., & Martin, J. (2004). Hemispheric asymmetry of the right ear advantage in dichotic listening. *Hearing Research, 198*, 125–136. doi:10.1016/j.heares.2004.07.019

Kershner, J., & Chyczij, M. (1992). Lateral preference in six to nine-year-old children: Relationships to language lateralization and cognitive ability. *Learning and Individual Differences, 4*(4), 347–367. doi.org/10.1016/1041-6080(92)90019-B

Kimura, D. (1961a). Some effects of temporal-lobe damage on auditory perception. *Canadian Journal of Psychology, 15*, 156–165.

Kimura, D. (1961b). Cerebral dominance and the perception of verbal stimuli. *Canadian Journal of Psychology, 15*, 166–171.

Kimura, D. (1963). Speech lateralization in young children as determined by an auditory test. *Journal of Comparative and Physiological Psychology, 56*(5), 899–902.

Kimura, D. (1967). Functional asymmetry of the brain in dichotic listening. *Cortex, 3*, 163–168.

Kishon, R., Abraham, K., Alschuler, D. M., Keilp, J. G., Stewart, J. W., McGrath, P. J., & Bruder, G. E. (2015). Lateralization for speech predicts therapeutic response to cognitive behavioral therapy for depression. *Psychiatry Research, 228*(3), 606–611. doi:10.1016/j.psychres.2015.04.054

Koopmann, M., Lesinski-Schiedat, A., & Illg, A. (2020). Speech perception, dichotic listening, and ear advantage in simultaneous bilateral cochlear implanted children. *Otology & Neurotology, 41*(2), e208–e215.

Kozou, H., Azouz, H. G., Abdou, R. M., & Shaltout, A. (2018). Evaluation and remediation of central auditory processing disorders in children with autism spectrum disorders. *International Journal of Pediatric Otorhinolaryngology, 104*, 36–42. doi:10.1016/j.ijporl.2017.10.039

Lamm, O., & Epstein, R. 1994. Dichotic listening performance under high and low lexical workload in subtypes of developmental dyslexia. *Neuropsychologia, 32*(7), 757–785. doi.org/10.1006/jecp.1996.2359

Lebel, C., & Beaulieu, C. (2009). Lateralization of the arcuate fasciculus from childhood to adulthood and its relation to cognitive abilities in children. *Human Brain Mapping, 30*(11), 3563–3573. doi:10.1002/hbm.20779

Martins, J., Ribas, A., & Moretti, C. (2017). Dichotic listening in the elderly: Interference in the adaptation of binaural prosthesis. *Innovation in Aging, 1*, S1, 588. 10.1093/geroni/igx004.2064

McCulloch, K., Lachner Bass, N., Dia, l H., Hiscock, M., & Jansen, B. (2017). Interaction of attention and acoustic factors in dichotic listening for fused words. *Laterality, 22*(4), 473–494. doi:10.1080/1357650X.2016.1219361

McManus, I. (2009). The history and geography of human handedness. In Sommer, I. E. C. & Kahn, R. S. (Eds.), *Language lateralization and psychosis*. (pp. 37–57). Cambridge: Cambridge University Press. doi:10.1016/j.bandc.2008.02.107

Mildner, V. (2001). Some quick arithmetic. *Brain and Cognition, 46*(1-2), 205–209.

Mildner, V., Stanković, D., & Petković, M. (2005). The relationship between active hand and ear advantage in the native and foreign language. *Brain and Cognition, 57*, 158–161. doi:10.1016/j.bandc.2004.08.036

Moncrieff, D. W. (2010). Hemispheric asymmetry in pediatric development disorders: autism, attention deficit/hyperactivity disorder, and dyslexia. In Hugdahl, K. & Westerhausen, R. (Eds.), *The two halves of the brain*. (pp. 561–601). Cambridge, MA: The MIT Press. doi.org/10.7551/mitpress/9780262014137.001.0001

Moncrieff, D. W. (2011). Dichotic listening in children: Age-related changes in direction and magnitude of ear advantage. *Brain and Cognition, 76*, 316–322. doi:10.1016/j.bandc.2011.03.013

Moncrieff, D. W., & Musiek, F. E. (2002). Intra-aural asymmetries revealed by dichotic listening tests in normal and dyslexic children. *Journal of the American Academy of Audiology, 13*, 428–437.

Moncrieff, D. W., & Wilson, R. H. (2009). Recognition of randomly presented one-, two-, and three-pair dichotic digits by children and young adults. *Journal of the American Academy of Audiology, 20*, 58–70. doi:10.3766/jaaa.20.1.6

Murray, D. J., & Hitchcock, C. H. (1969). Attention and storage in dichotic listening. *Journal of Experimental Psychology, 81*(1), 164–169.

Meyers, J. E., Roberts, R. J., Bayless, J. D., Volkert, K., & Evitts, P. E. (2002). Dichotic listening: Expanded norms and clinical application. *Archives of Clinical Neuropsychology, 17*(1), 79–90.

Nascimento, M. D. S. R. D., Muniz, L. F., & Costa, M. L. G. D. (2014). Auditory processing and aphasia: A systematic review. *Revista CEFAC, 16*, 634–642. doi.org/10.1590/1982-021620144912

Noffsinger, D., Martinez, Ch. D., & Wilson, R. H. (1994). Dichotic listening to speech: Background and preliminary data for digits, sentences, and nonsense syllables. *American Academic Audiology, 5*, 248–254.

Norrelgen, F., Lilja, A., Ingvar, M., Gisselgård, J. and Fransson, P. (2012). Language lateralization in children aged 10 to 11 years: A combined fMRI and dichotic listening study. *PLoS One, 7*(12): e51872. doi:10.1371/journal.pone.0051872

Obrzut, J., Boliek, C., & Obrzut, A. (1986). The effect of stimulus type and directed attention on dichotic listening with children. *Journal of Experimental Child Psychology, 41*, 198–209. doi. org/10.1016/0022-0965(86)90058-5

Obrzut, J., Boliek, C., & Bryden, M. (1997). Dichotic listening, handedness, and reading ability: A meta-analysis. *Developmental Neuropsychology, 13*, 97–110. doi.org/10.1080/87565649709540670

Obrzut, J. E., & Mahoney, E. B. (2011). Use of the dichotic listening technique with learning disabilities. *Brain and Cognition, 76*, 323–331. doi:10.1016/j.bandc.2011.02.012

Penna, S. D., Brancucci, A., Babiloni, C., Franciotti, R., Pizzella, V., Rossi, D., Torquati, K., Rossini, P. M., & Romani, G. L. (2007). Lateralization of dichotic speech stimuli is based on specific auditory pathway interactions: Neuromagnetic evidence. *Cerebral Cortex, 17*(10), 2303–2311. doi:10.1093/cercor/bhl139

Penner, I. K., Schläfli, K., Opwis, K., & Hugdahl, K. (2009). The role of working memory in dichotic-listening studies of auditory laterality. *Journal of Clinical Experimental Neuropsychology, 31*(8), 959–966. doi:10.1080/13803390902766895

Piazza, M., Gordon, D. P., & Lehman, R. (1985). Reading ability and the development of lateralization of speech. *Language Sciences, 7*(1), 73–84.

Pine, D. S., Bruder, G. E., Wasserman, G. A., Miller, L. S., Musabegovic, A., & Watson, J. B. (1997). Verbal dichotic listening in boys at risk for behavior disorders. *Child and Adolescent Psychiatry, 36*(10), 1465–1473. doi.org/10.1097/00004583-199710000-00030

Purdy, M., & McCullagh, J. (2019). Dichotic listening training following neurological injury in adults: A pilot study. *Hearing, Balance and Communication, 18(1), 16–28*. doi:10.1080/21695717.2019.1692591

Rand, T. (1974). Dichotic release from masking for speech. *Journal of the Acoustical Society of America, 55*(3), 678–680.

Repp, B. H. (1975). Dichotic forward and backward "masking" between CV syllables. *Journal of the Acoustical Society of America, 57*, 483–496.

Richardson, E. D., Springer, J. A., Varney N. R., Struchen, M. A., & Roberts, R. J. (1994) Dichotic listening in the clinic: New neuropsychological applications. *The Clinical Neuropsychologist, 8*(4), 416–428. doi:10.1080/13854049408402044

Roberts, R. J., Varney, N. R., Paulsen, J. S., & Richardson, E. D. (1990). Dichotic listening and complex partial seizures. *Journal of Clinical and Experimental Neuropsychology, 12*(4), 448–458. doi. org/10.1080/01688639008400992

Robb, M. P., Lynn, W. L., & O'Beirne, G. A. (2013). An exploration of dichotic listening among adults who stutter. *Clinical Linguistics & Phonetics, 27*(9), 681–693. doi.org/10.3109/02699206.2013.791881

Roup, C. M., Wiley, T. L., & Wilson, R. H. (2006). Dichotic word recognition in young and older adults. *Journal of the American Academy of Audiology, 17*(4), 230–240. doi: 10.3766/jaaa.17.4.2

Rosenberg, G. G. (2011). Development of local child norms for the dichotic digits test. *Journal of Educational Audiology, 17*, 6–10.

Satz, P. (1968). Laterality effects in dichotic listening. *Nature, 218,* 277–278. doi.org/10.1038/218277a0

Studdert-Kennedy, M., & Shankweiler, D. (1970). Hemispheric specialization for speech perception. *Journal of the Acoustical Society of America, 48,* 579–594.

Studdert-Kennedy, M., Shankweiler, D. & Pisoni, D. (1972). Auditory and phonetic processes in speech perception: Evidence from a dichotic study. *Cognitive Psychology, 3*(3), 455–466.

Wesarg, T., Richter, N., Hessel, H. Günther, S. Arndt, S. Aschednforff, A. Laszig, R., & Hassepass, F. (2015). Binaural integration of periodically alternating speech following cochlear implantation in subjects with profound sensorineural unilateral hearing loss. *Audiology, Neurology 20,* Suppl. 1, 73–78. doi:10.1159/000380752

Westerhausen, R. (2019): A primer on dichotic listening as a paradigm for the assessment of hemispheric asymmetry, laterality: Asymmetries of body. *Brain and Cognition, 24*(6), 1–32. doi:10.1080/1357 650X.2019.1598426

Westerhausen, R., Bless, J. J., Passow, S., Kompus, K., & Hugdahl, K. (2015). Cognitive control of speech perception across the lifespan: A large-scale cross-sectional dichotic listening study. *Developmental Psychology, 51*(6), 806–815. doi.org/10.1037/dev0000014

Westerhausen, R., Põldver, N., Naar, R., Radziun, D., Kaarep, M. S., Kreegipuu, K.,… & Kompus, K. (2018). Effect of voicing on perceptual auditory laterality in Estonian and Norwegian native speakers. *Applied Psycholinguistics, 39*(2), 259–273. doi.org/10.1017/S014271641700017

Westerhausen, R., & Samuelsen, F. (2020). An optimal dichotic-listening paradigm for the assessment of hemispheric dominance for speech processing. Preprint at Psyarciv.com.

Yund, W. E., Uno, A., & Woods, D. L. (1999). Preattentive control of serial auditory processing in dichotic listening. *Brain and Language, 66*(3), 358–376. doi:10.1006/brln.1998.2034

Zurif, E. B., & Bryden, M. P. (1969). Familial handedness and left-right differences in auditory and visual perception. *Neuropsychologia, 7*(2), 179–187. doi.org/10.1016/0028-3932(69)90015-3

34
PERCEPTUAL PHONETIC EXPERIMENTATION
Grant McGuire

Introduction

The goal of this chapter is to provide a brief overview of the common methods for gathering speech perception data. The field of speech perception is very broad and encompasses everything from psycho-acoustic investigations of basic hearing abilities to the exploration of learning and memory. Despite this broadness, the methods employed are fairly uniform and easily adaptable to many different research goals. Here they are grouped into three general categories, *discrimination, identification* and *scaling*. Though certainly not the only way to classify such experiments, they are unified broadly by the type of data generated and common analytical techniques. Following these descriptions is a more general discussion of experimental considerations for gathering speech perception data. This chapter complements Chapter 4, "Perceptual phonetics for the speech clinician," and the techniques discussed in Chapter 10, "Analyzing phonetic data with generalized additive mixed models" are broadly applicable to analyzing data produced in speech perception experiments. Due to space concerns, this chapter does not discuss experiment designs for infants and pre-verbal children which can be quite divergent from the designs and considerations reported here.

Basic experimental designs

Discrimination

A discrimination experiment measures subjects' ability to differentiate stimuli and frequently involve multiple stimulus presentations on a single trial. These designs excel at exploring the architecture of perceptual space and how it is affected by differences among subject populations or changes due to learning or exposure. As defined here, all discrimination experiments involve correct and incorrect responses from subjects, meaning that these designs all have similar analyses of percent correct data in common, including the use of sensitivity measures, such as d'.

Same – Different (AX)

The *same – different* design is quite common in speech research due to its simplicity. In this design two stimuli are presented in each trial, separated by a specified amount of time, the interstimulus interval ISI. The stimuli are paired such that on any given trial they are either the same or different in some way and the subject's task is to identify which type of trial was presented. For example, if there are two stimuli, *A* and *B*, then there are two possible *different* pairs, <AB> <BA>, and two *same* pairs, <AA> <BB>. Generally, the number of same pairs presented to the subject matches the number of different pairs, though if discrimination is difficult then the number of same pairs may be reduced. This is due to the assumption that subjects expect an even number of same and different pairs and this assumption should be met or else the subjects will be alarmed and change strategies. This could be addressed in instructions by explicitly telling the subjects that there's an even number of same and different pairs. It could also be argued that accuracy feedback would have the same effect. The most common measures from this design include accuracy (proportion correct, or a sensitivity measure such as *d'*) and reaction time. Note that the order of the pairs, often ignored for simplification or due to lack of statistical power, can be a consistent effect (see Best et al., 2001, Francis and Ciocca, 2003).

This design is very simple to explain to subjects. However, it has a further "ease of explanation" advantage: the differences and similarities of the stimuli do not need to be described to the subject. That is, subjects only need decide that two sounds are different in some way and do not need to consciously identify or be told the difference or know a particular label (i.e. compare to the labeling examples below). Moreover, because subjects obligatorily make decisions based only on the second stimulus, reaction times derived from this paradigm are easy to measure and generally reliable.

There are a few concerns to be noted when using the *Same – Different* design. The first is that it can encourage bias toward responding same when the task is difficult, i.e. the number of erroneous "same" responses becomes greater than the number of erroneous "different" responses. This can cause deeper problems when different pairs do not have similar perceptual distances; where the bias to respond "same" varies by pair rather than being comparable across all pairs. Another complication is that for many experiments only the *different* trials are of interest the "same" stimuli are thrown out as uninterpretable or uninteresting, removing as many as half the trials.

Many researchers employ variants of the *same – different* design to tap into different modes of perception. In a *speeded* design, subjects are directed to base their decision on a highly detailed short-term memory trace of each stimulus. The theory underlying this is that there are two modes of perception, an *auditory mode* consisting of a highly detailed but quickly decaying trace memory, and a *phonetic mode*, consisting of a more abstracted or categorical representation of the sound in question (Pisoni, 1973). Under such an analysis, the auditory mode has been seen as being analogous to a non-speech mode of perception and used to compare raw perceptual distance independent of language specific effects (see e.g. Johnson & Babel, 2007). In order to get this effect it is necessary for the task to have a low memory load, usually by making subjects respond very quickly, at least less than 800 ms and preferably below 500 ms (Fox, 1984; Pisoni & Tash, 1974). This is accomplished in two ways. First, the ISI must be sufficiently short, less than 500 ms, with 100 ms being a common duration. Note that an ISI of 0 is actually too short and results in slower RTs (Pisoni, 1973). Second, the subjects need to be encouraged to respond quickly, typically by giving them an RT goal (such as < 500 ms), frequent feedback as to their RTs (usually every trial) and a cut-off time when the RT is too long (e.g. 1500 ms).

Additionally, RTs, because they tend to be more constrained on their upper bound by the task, usually show less variability than in other designs. Moreover, it is possible to get two measures of performance, RT and accuracy. The speed of the task also allows many trials in a reasonable amount of time. Unfortunately, data may be lost due to the difficulty of the task as subjects are encouraged to choose speed over accuracy and the incorrect responses must be thrown out for reaction time analyses. Moreover, different subjects or different groups may choose to respond more accurately or more quickly, independently of each other, complicating statistical analyses. For this reason, accuracy feedback is often given in addition to RT feedback and subjects are given a target for both.

ABX (AXB, XAB, matching-to-sample)

In an ABX discrimination design three stimuli are presented in a series and the listener compares which stimulus, the *A* or the *B,* is the same or most similar to the *X* stimulus. This is also called *matching-to-sample* as the subject's task is to "match" the *X* stimulus to the sample, *A* or *B*. Other variations have the sample stimuli flanking the target (e.g. Harnsberger, 1998), or less commonly, following (XAB). There are consequently two ISIs, nearly always the same.

The unique advantage of this task is that listeners are comparing a stimulus to two possibilities and thus know on each trial that either *A* or *B* must be the correct answer. This reduces the bias problems inherent in AX discrimination as "same" is not an option. The cost of this advantage is that recency effects due to memory become a greater consideration. This usually means a bias toward the *B* token as it is more current in memory. This effect can be accommodated by strict balancing of *AB* ordering and treating it as a factor in analyses. This also means that this design does not have a speeded analogue (except for possibly very short stimuli). This is due to both sample stimuli necessarily being stored in memory and the assumed decay in detail of these memories, theoretically making the *A* stimulus more abstracted than the *B* one.

Two Alternative Forced Choice (2AFC)

In some linguistic phonetics traditions, the term *two alternative forced choice* is used for the number of response options a listener has, such as a *same-different* experiment. In this tradition a *three alternative* experiment would have three possible choices for the listener to make, and so on. In psychology it is more commonly used to refer to an experiment where two stimuli are presented and the listener is forced to choose between the two. Having two distinct meanings for this term is unfortunate and quite confusing, yet any experimenter working in speech should be aware of the different uses. This chapter will cleave to the latter meaning of the term as is common in psychology.

Essentially, in this design two stimuli are presented on each trial and subjects are asked to discern their order. Instructions usually take the form of, "Which stimulus came first, A or B?" This design is considered highly valuable as it minimizes bias and can be used for stimuli that are very similar. Because subjects hear two stimuli on each trial and know that each order is possible, subjects should assume that either order is equally possible.

This task only works well for binary choices and more choices require different blocks. For example, if there are three different categories (ABC) that a researcher wants listeners to compare, it would require three blocks of stimuli, *AB, AC, BC*. Another consideration is that it requires some sort of explicit label to determine the order. This can make instructions difficult, if not impossible to relate to subjects, or requires some sort of subject training.

4-Interval Forced Choice (4IAX)

This design is considered analytically identical to 2AFC (Macmillan & Creelman, 2005) and consists of a presentation of four sounds and only a binary choice for the subject. This task has two subtle alternatives in design and subject explanation. In one, subjects are instructed to determine whether the second or third sound is different from the other three. Possible stimulus presentations are limited to <ABAA>, <AABA>, <BABB> and <BBAB>. This is a very specific version of the *oddity* design (see below) and usually has identical ISIs across all intervals. The first and last stimuli are called "flankers" or "flanking stimuli." The other version of this design is explicitly related to *same – different* discrimination such that two pairs are presented, one a *same* pair and the other *different*. This is usually paired with a somewhat longer medial ISI compared to the first and third ones to more explicitly separate the stimuli into pairs for the subjects. It can be designed identically to the previous description (with slightly different instructions) or further complicated such that <AB AA>, <BA AA> pairs are allowed (though this may only complicate the analysis and is probably not recommended). For both types the subject is really being tasked with deciding the order of given stimuli, just as with 2AFC, so the analysis for *d'* is considered identical.

This design is another way to remove the bias problems that can occur with AX discrimination. Because both *same* and *different* options are available on each trial, subjects shouldn't be biased toward *same* (both are present on each trial and therefore equally likely). This also means that very difficult discrimination tasks can be performed without assumed bias and pairs differing in similarity should not differ in bias.

The primary drawback to this design is that RTs are difficult to measure. Although theoretically subjects could make a decision upon hearing the second stimulus, it is possible and even likely that subjects will wait until the third or even fourth stimulus for reassurance. More worryingly, subjects could differ dramatically on what decision point they chose, or even differ by pair contrasted, or vary unpredictably trial by trial. Practically, their decision point is unpredictable and RTs are likely to be highly variable and unusable, except for the grossest distinctions.

Category change (oddball)

This design was created to be an adult analogue to a common infant perception task in which the infant hears a stream of syllables and responds by looking (in interest) when the stream changes in some detectable way. In the adult version, the stream of syllables is presented and the subject presses a button when they hear the change. The measure in this task is whether a change is detected or not, making it essentially a kind of Yes-No task (see below) where stimuli designed for infant research can be used. Versions of the design are used in brain imaging tasks where continuous stimulus presentation is important (e.g. fMRI, NIRS, etc.).

Identification tasks

In identification tasks subjects are presented one or more sounds and asked to give them an explicit label. This usually requires a category label, although some designs avoid this, essentially making them the same as the discrimination experiments previously described.

Labeling (identification, forced choice identification)

In the very popular labeling task only a single stimulus is presented in each trial and the subject must apply a label to that stimulus, either from a closed set (e.g. two buttons labeled *s* or *sh*) or some open set (e.g. "write what you hear"). This design is generally used to assess categorical knowledge; ambiguous or continuous stimuli are often categorized in this way.

This design is simple and straightforward with generally simple analyses. It can be explained quickly with little likelihood of error. When the response set is small, many trials can be performed in fairly short period with little stress on the participant. The primary drawback to this design is that labels are required, imposing a categorical decision on the subject and all the ramifications that come with that fact.

Yes – No

This design subtype of identification experiment, and indeed the simplest kind, is one in which a stimulus is compared against one other stimulus and only one is presented per trial. This can take the form of asking the subject whether or not a stimulus was present or whether the stimulus was *x* with *not-x* implied. The classic example of this design is the Békésy hearing test, where a tone at a certain frequency and decibel level is presented and the subject responds whether they heard it or not. Though simple, this design is not as limited as it may seem and offers several options. For example, if there are two categories, <x y>, they can be compared as *x* ~ not *x* and *y* ~ not *y*. This potentially gives analytically a different result from an experiment where the task on each trial is to choose *x* or *y* (Macmillan & Creelman, 2005). Additionally, multiple categories can be compared by blocking, such as *x~y, y~z, x~z*.

This design is very simple to explain to subjects, "Did you hear *x* or not?" Proportion correct and RTs are common measures and are easy to calculate and generally reliable. However, this design quickly becomes unwieldy the more comparisons that are made. Also, there are no direct comparisons of stimuli in each trial so like difficult contrasts can be at a disadvantage.

Oddity

In this design multiple stimuli are presented, one is different from the rest and the subject determines which is the unique or odd one. It's often limited to three (also known as the *triangular* design) or four stimulus presentations on each trial. Note that 4IAX is a special case of a four interval oddity design. Guenther et al. (1999) offers an interesting example where oddity was used to train subjects. The difficulty of the task was increased over the course of the training by increasing the number of intervals from two (2AFC) to three (triangular) and finally to four.

Generally this style of experiment is easy to explain to subjects and no explicit label is necessary beyond order. Subjects must hold in memory the number of stimuli that have passed before the oddball, and possibly listen to them all for a difficult contrast, meaning that reaction times are unpredictable and recency effects are notable.

Scaling

Scaling experiments ask the participant to evaluate the stimuli on some sort of visual or numerical scale. Also called *rating,* scaling designs consist of subjective evaluations of a given dimension of a stimulus or stimulus pair, often using discrete points on a specified numerical scale (also known as a Likert-type scale). For example, subjects may rate the *word-likeness* of a nonce word on a scale of 1 to 5 or the *similarity* of pairs of sounds on a scale from 1 to 10. Because subjects may vary on the way they use a scale, it is common to transform the data into a standardized unit, such as a z-score.

The primary concern with such an experiment is that defined points along a continuum will bias participants to expecting evenly spaced stimuli in a continuum with discrete points along the way. A way of avoiding these possible biases is the Visual Analogue Scale. In this design the listener is presented a single line with only the endpoints labeled and otherwise unmarked and is instructed to identify a point anywhere along the line corresponding to their rating of the stimulus. While offering more detail and avoiding biasing, response consistency can be a problem; a hybrid model is a possible solution (Matějka et al., 2016).

A variant on scaling where there are no absolute endpoints is called *magnitude estimation* (Moskowitz, 1977). Here subjects decide the relative distance of given stimuli using ratios. Typically this takes the form of the presentation of a referent, called the modulus, and subsequent stimulus presentations where subjects judge the similarity to the modulus in terms of relative values. Numbers may be assigned such that the modulus is given a defined value and subjects label subsequent stimuli with numbers demonstrating similarity to the modulus. In general magnitude estimation data is considered more accurate than scaling data at the expense of being more challenging to explain the methodology to subjects and making accurate RT collection more difficult (or impossible).

These types of experiments provide very reflective, offline and conscious decisions and categorizations from participants and are often considered meta-judgments. When possible, response time data can be used to provide some data on the difficulty of the decision.

Elaborations on the basic designs

Many experiments use multiple designs to either acquire different kinds of data, have the difficulty of the task vary or use multiple designs to train subjects at some perceptual task. Having the same participants perform multiple experiments allows for statistical analyses to be within subject, rather than across subject, which makes most analyses easier and more reliable.

Multiple designs in one experiment

It is often desirable to acquire different kinds of data from the same subjects and different designs are better for different data. Care must be taken as earlier tasks may affect following tasks. Typically, less categorical tasks precede more categorical tasks, or they are balanced so that an equal number of subjects participate in each possible order. In the latter case, experiment order can be added as an additional factor in a statistical analysis. Famously, a categorical perception effect is shown by using a discrimination task and an identification task, where the expected outcome is for discrimination to be easiest across a categorical boundary and identification to be the most difficult across the boundary (Repp, 1984).

Adaptive testing (threshold measurement, staircase designs)

An adaptive design is one in which the difficulty or ease of the task is changed based upon the previous trial or trials with the goal of finding the threshold of detection or performance at a specific level (e.g. 75% accuracy). These designs are appropriate to stimuli that are in some sort of continuum such that stimulus comparisons can be made easier or harder by changing the *step size*, which is the distance between the stimuli (increasing step size makes the task easier by increasing the perceptual distance). These can be categorical data that have been made into a continuum (/pa/ to /ba/) or something inherently continuous such as loudness. Note that the aforementioned hearing test is an adaptive design to find the threshold of hearing for a tone at a given frequency and dB level. The task in such an experiment is usually some version of discrimination or Yes-No. Although an adaptive experiment may be done for its own sake (like the hearing test), it is more common as a first step in constructing stimuli that must fall into steps and those steps must be of an equal perceptual distance at a certain performance level.

The goals of adaptive test designs are efficiency and accuracy, i.e. the best adaptive test finds the given threshold accurately in the fewest number of trials. Efficiency is important as these tasks can be quite frustrating for subjects: they get more difficult as they go along and the subject may be performing near chance for a considerable number of trials. If a subject "gives up" or "fusses out" (to use the infant research terminology) they will perform poorly and the threshold will be inaccurate.

There are three basic components to an adaptive design that can all interact: performance level, the stepping rule and the termination rule.

The performance level is the actual threshold desired as the outcome of the experiment, e.g. a step size where discrimination is at 75%, or as in the hearing test, 50% accuracy (chance in a yes-no task). A performance level just above chance is appropriately called the just-noticeable-difference, or JND.

Generally if the stimuli are going to be used in another experiment, some higher level of performance is desired (or necessary). The stepping rule is the algorithm for determining when and how much to change the step size. While various algorithms have been proposed, the Kaernbach (1991) transformed up-down method is the most common. The simplest version is the *staircase* procedure where a correct answer results in a one-step increase in difficulty and an incorrect results in a one-step decrease in difficulty. This results in only the JND and no higher performance levels can be determined. To do that a *transformed* method is necessary where a single incorrect response results in a larger step change than an incorrect preceded by one or more correct answers.

Finally, the experiment requires a stopping rule, or the algorithm determining the end of the *run*. Commonly the run is ended using a set number of trials or a set number of *reversals*. A reversal is switch from increasing step size to decreasing step sizes or vice versa. This means that a steady increase or decrease in step size does not contribute to the stopping of the experiment, only a switch in movement. This method is considered a more efficient and accurate way of determining the desired threshold, though less predictable in the length of the experiment. The actual threshold is determined by either the step size at termination or an average across all or some sample of the trials.

Training experiments

In a training experiment the explicit goal is to get subjects to perform better at some task, usually with the goal of assessing how perceptual space has changed as a result of this (see Logan & Pruitt, 1995 for an overview), though sometimes training is necessary to perform adequately in some further task. They also have, in addition to the training task itself, some sort of testing paradigm. Because such experiments may be highly resource intensive (e.g. weeks of training for just one subject), extreme care should be taken in their design.

Training tasks vary considerably and many of the designs explained above can be used for training, with differing goals. Broadly, discrimination training is used to heighten subjects' sensitivity to differences in stimuli while identification training is used to encourage categorization and minimization of differences within a category. Multiple training tasks can be included to increase subject performance or make their learning well-rounded. Training can be used as goal in and of itself (e.g. how does perception change due to learning) or as an elaborate form of practice so that subjects can perform in some other task that is the primary experiment. Some experiments include a control group that receives no training and is only tested. The length of training can be fixed for all subjects regardless of performance (e.g. 3 sessions, 150 trials, etc.) or can be fixed to some criterion (e.g. >80% correct, 50 trials correct in a row, etc.).

For most training experiments a pre-test is administered to assess initial performance followed by training, which is followed by a test identical to the first called a post-test. In some experiments only a post-test is administered and performance across different groups with different training conditions is assessed. This minimizes the number of tests that must be administered, but means that within-subject changes in perception can't be observed directly, but must be inferred across groups. An option available in longer training experiments is to administer multiple tests at intervals during training. Any number of possible designs can be used in testing, the best being determined by the goals of the experiment. Multiple types of testing are usually desirable, when possible. Occasionally, pre-tests are used to determine a subject's suitability for further training, where subjects who either perform too poorly for training to be effective (floor effect) or too well for a training effect to be apparent (ceiling effect) are noted and rejected.

Many training experiments have tasks that are difficult enough to require multiple sessions of training. This can be over several consecutive days, several weeks or even months. The number of training sessions may be the same for all subjects or may be concluded when a certain criterion is reached (in which the number of sessions may vary). In situations with multiple sessions, testing may be done in an entirely different session from training. Also, to assess the long-term effects of training, testing may be repeated at some later interval with no intervening training.

General considerations

The data from perceptual experiments can vary, but special commentary is needed for response or reaction times. This measure is the speed of response, usually timed from the presentation of the stimulus, less commonly from some other point during presentation, and the timing of responses provides data on the difficulty of the decision. The faster a participant responds, the easier the decision is considered to be. Due to the rapid nature of such responses, special equipment is necessary. Keyboards, mouses and other peripheral devices should be assumed to have inadequate timing resolution unless shown otherwise. Usually only specially made "button boxes" and high speed keyboards are appropriate. RTs are often highly variable and the required motor response adds further variability (some researchers control for handedness, for example).

The start of the RT timing is crucial to accurate interpretation of results and when designing an experiment the subject's hypothesized time-course of decision making must be incorporated (i.e. at what point can a subject make an accurate decision relative to when timing began). Because collected RTs have a lower-bound, they are often skewed right and require a transformation (usually log) in order to be normally distributed. Only reaction times to correct answers are analyzed, meaning a considerable loss of data for very difficult tasks. An option for assessing a participant's reaction to a stimulus is to ask the participant to repeat the stimulus as quickly as possible. This is called *shadowing* and the time from the stimulus onset to the initiation of the participant's shadow production is measured.

Another, more sophisticated way of collecting response times is to use eye tracking, examining when and how long a participant's eyes look to a visual stimulus that is paired with or prompted by some auditory stimulus. It has two primary advantages compared to button pressing. First, the eyes have a much shorter time-course in reacting to stimuli than manual button pressing, reducing noise when assessing processing time. Second, the eyes scanning the visual field allow the researcher to directly observe which alternatives a subject considered before making a decision, rather than inferring such knowledge from comparing reaction times on different trials/blocks. A typical design involves subjects *fixating* on the center of a display screen. A sound is presented which the subject is instructed to identify on the screen (usually manually), and several (usually two to four) objects are presented on the screen. The subject's gaze is followed as they scan the possible objects until they "fixate" on the correct object. The two measures usually derived from such experiments are saccades and fixations. Saccades are the eye movements and fixations are locations of the pauses. Together they are referred to as the scanpath.

General to all experiments is controlling the flow of the stimuli. Blocks, subsets of stimuli, can be used simply to provide breaks for subjects or may be used for more sophisticated means. In a given block of trials, a subject may see only a subset of stimuli; for example one block may have a subject discriminate fricatives while in a second block they discriminate stops. In such an experiment the goal of blocking is to create a limited set of contrasts for the subject and presumably change their expectations. This only works if the subject can quickly identify what is possible, so the ratio of contrasts to trials should be low. One example of the use of blocks in this way is the Garner Paradigm (Garner, 1974, see also Kingston and Macmillan, 1995).

Breaks are frequently employed to increase subject performance by reducing stress. There are no hard rules on how many or how frequently they should be inserted, though the difficulty of the task should be a consideration. They may be strictly timed or the subject can advance the experiment on their own. If the experiment procedure is separated into blocks it is common to include breaks between them, otherwise they may be included at specified time intervals. Another option is to give subjects an escape button or key to pause the experiment at their discretion.

During an experiment, feedback alerts the subject to their performance. It can be used to give subjects a target to reach or expected performance level to hold. It often has the added benefit of increasing, or at least holding, a subject's attention in a tedious task and may be necessary for adequate performance. Feedback is given after every trial or at the end of a block of trials and often include summarized data. Typical feedback includes accuracy, response time and the labels assigned by the subject.

To ensure subjects understand the task and can perform adequately, a block of practice trials can be added at the beginning of the experiment. This block is usually brief (e.g. as few as four trials) and is either a random selection from the larger experimental set or a carefully selected group of trials that exemplify the expected performance demands placed on the subject (e.g. only the easiest and/or most difficult trials). Another option is to give accuracy feedback during practice even if no feedback is given in the main experiment. Of course, any practice may bias the subject and should be included with care.

Indeed, biasing participants before the experiment is to be avoided, unless it is an explicit part of the design (Goldinger & Azuma, 2003, Hay & Drager, 2010). Written instructions are usually given to subjects before the experiment with minimal verbal input. Ideally, instructions give just enough information for the subject to perform the task correctly without extraneous information that might introduce bias. One way this may be accomplished is to mislead the subject as to the experiment's purpose. IRB's require significant deception to be revealed upon completion of the experiment and the subject again be asked for consent to use their data.

After the conclusion of an experiment it is common to give a questionnaire to the subject asking questions about the experiment itself. The goals of such questionnaires are usually to find out the strategies used by the subject to complete the experiment, their impressions of the stimuli (naturalness, for example) or to alert the experimenter concerning any abnormalities. Though not often reported as data, they are useful when interpreting the data and designing subsequent experiments.

Stimulus considerations

Just as crucial to the successful answer to a research question as the design of an experiment is the construction of the stimuli used in it. The types of stimuli used in speech perception can be broadly grouped into three types: natural, synthetic and hybrid.

A common experimental consideration is avoiding subjects performing too well (ceiling effect) or too poorly (floor effect) to properly analyze differences in performance. There are several solutions to this problem. One is simply to adapt the experimental design to the stimuli. As noted above, tasks that reduce memory load allow listeners to make finer distinctions among stimuli that are otherwise difficult for listeners to distinguish.

A common way to make stimuli vary in their perceptual difficulty is to embed them in different levels of noise. This is done at a specific signal-noise-ratio determined to make the task sufficiently hard. A classic example of this technique is Miller and Nicely (1955). Individual stimuli may be embedded in white or pink noise or played over a continuous stream of noise. Sometimes "cocktail party" noise is used–this consists of many unintelligible voices talking at a low level. Special concern should be taken when constructing such stimuli (Simpson & Cooke, 2005).

Naturally-produced stimuli

Natural stimuli are produced by a talker and are not modified further other than by minor adjustments, such as trimming silence or overall amplitude normalization. Because they are produced by an actual talker, they should most accurately represent sounds "in the wild," though at the expense of precise control of the stimulus parameters.

Usually such stimuli are recorded in a sound attenuated booth or at least a very quiet room using the best recording equipment available. In some cases the stimuli may have been recorded for some other purpose such as building a corpus and the recording conditions are out of the researcher's control. The producer of the stimuli is usually called a *talker*. Talkers are chosen for their ability to reliably reproduce the linguistic categories needed for the experiment in a controlled and consistent manner. They may speak the same language as the listeners in the experiment or may speak another language in the case of a cross-linguistic perceptual experiment. When more controlled stimuli are necessary, or when a speaker of a language natively having all the relevant contrasts cannot be found, a phonetically trained talker may be used. In such cases the productions can be checked for naturalness by a speaker of languages that have those contrasts. Often several talkers are used to increase the variety of stimuli or to explore the role of individual variability.

When recorded for express purposes of an experiment, the talker's instructions are crucial. For example the subject may be asked to produce very careful speech or very natural, conversational speech (possibly difficult given the context unless some deception is involved). A subject may also be given much more explicit instructions, such as "use the same vowel as in *hood*," or a phonetically trained talker may be asked to produce very specific stimuli, such as syllables with only unreleased stops or a variety of "exotic" sounds. In all cases, however, care should be taken to ensure that productions are consistent, including intonational contours. List intonation is usually acceptable, but the falling tone at the end of a list should be avoided by either repeating the final stimulus in a list (and discarding it) or adding filler stimuli at the end that are not to be used. An alternative strategy is to put the target tokens in a syntactic frame such as, "Please say X again." A good, if more time consuming, strategy is to ensure the stimuli are representative of natural categories by recording many examples, making relevant acoustic measurements and then selecting tokens that match most closely to previously reported values and rejecting anomalous ones.

Synthetic stimuli

Synthetic stimuli are constructed from scratch usually using either acoustic or perceptual models of speech. Various programs are available for these purposes with varying levels of control or user friendliness. Such stimuli are used when very tight control of specific aspects of the stimuli is necessary, such as when investigating the value of specific perceptual cues. A concern with such stimuli is their ability to represent natural categories. Different programs and manipulations result in stimuli that are more or less natural, so care should be taken in choosing a construction method.

By far the most widely used program for stimulus construction is the Klatt cascade/parallel synthesizer (Klatt, 1980, Klatt & Klatt, 1990). Users specify various parameters for source and filter characteristics and build stimuli based on how these parameters change over time. Various more or less user-friendly interfaces have been developed over the years (e.g. McMurray et al., 2008). The freely available Praat acoustic analysis software (Boersma & Weenink, 2020) offers a simple but useful source-filter synthesizer along with reasonable instructions. Often a naturally produced token is used as a model to create a token from scratch; the parameters measured in the model token are used to make the synthetic token and only certain parameters are further manipulated.

Some synthesis programs use models of articulator and vocal tract characteristics to produce an acoustic output. Such models are useful when production aspects are important to the research question at hand or when the stimuli must be producible by a human vocal tract. Examples include the Haskins CASY model (Iskarous et al., 2003) and ArtiSynth (Lloyd et al., 2012) designed at the University of British Columbia.

Hybrid stimuli

Hybrid stimuli attempt to combine these two methods to produce very naturalistic but controlled stimuli and are sometimes known as "modified naturally produced" stimuli. For such stimuli naturally produced tokens are resynthesized in various ways to change very specific aspects of the signal (changing intonational contours, vowel quality, vocal tract length etc.). The resulting naturalness is dependent on the nature and number of modifications made. Generally, if at least one stimulus is resynthesized for an experiment, all should be resynthesized as the process does produce noticeable changes. The most common programs used for resynthesis are Praat (Boersma & Weenink, 2020) and Matlab (MATLAB, 2010).

References

Best, C.T., McRoberts, G.W., & Goodell, E. (2001). Discrimination of non-native consonant contrasts varying in perceptual assimilation to the listener's native phonological system. *Journal of the Acoustical Society of America. 109*(2), 775–794.

Boersma, P. & Weenink, D. (2020). Praat: doing phonetics by computer [Computer program]. Version 5.1.43, retrieved August 4, 2010 from http://www.praat.org/

Fox, R.A. (1984). Effect of lexical status on phonetic categorization. *Journal of Experimental Psychology: Human perception and performance, 10*(4), 526–540.

Francis, A.L. & Ciocca, V. (2003). Stimulus presentation order and the perception of lexical tones in Cantonese. *Journal of the Acoustical Society of America, 114*(3), 1611–1621

Garner, W.R. (1974). *The processing of information and structure.* Hillsdale, NJ: Erlbaum,

Goldinger, S. D., & Azuma, T. (2003). Puzzle-solving science: The quixotic quest for units in speech perception. *Journal of Phonetics, 31*(3–4), 305–320.

Guenther, F.H., Husain, F.T., Cohen, M.A. & Shinn-Cunningham B.G. (1999). Effects of categorization and discrimination training on auditory perceptual space. *Journal of the Acoustical Society of America, 106*(5), 2900–2912.

Harnsberger, J. D. (1998). The perception of place of articulation in three coronal nasal contrasts. *The Journal of the Acoustical Society of America, 103*(5), 3092–3093.

Hay, J. & Drager, K. (2010). Stuffed toys and speech perception. *Linguistics, 48*(4), 865–892.

Iskarous, K., Goldstein, L., Whalen, D. H., Tiede, M. & Rubin, P. (2003). CASY: The Haskins configurable articulatory synthesizer. In *International Congress of Phonetic Sciences*, Barcelona, Spain (pp. 185–188).

Johnson, K., & Babel, M. (2007). Perception of fricatives by Dutch and English speakers. *UC Berkeley PhonLab Annual Report, 3*(3), 302–325.

Kaernbach, C. (1991). Simple adaptive testing with the weighted up-down method, *Perception & Psychophysics 49*, 227–229.

Kingston, J. & Macmillan, N.A. (1995). Integrality of nasalization and F1 in vowels in isolation and before oral and nasal consonants: A detection-theoretic application of the Garner paradigm, *The Journal of the Acoustical Society of America, 97*, 1261–1285.

Klatt, D. H. (1980). Software for a cascade/parallel formant synthesizer. *Journal of the Acoustical Society of America, 67*, 971–995.

Klatt, D. H., & Klatt, L. C. (1990). Analysis, synthesis, and perception of voice quality variations among female and male talkers. *Journal of the Acoustical Society of America, 87*, 820–857.

Lloyd, J.E., Stavness, I. & Fels, S. (2012). ArtiSynth: A fast interactive biomechanical modeling toolkit combining multibody and finite element simulation. In *Soft tissue biomechanical modeling for computer assisted surgery* (pp. 355–394). Springer, Berlin, Heidelberg.

Logan, J.S. & Pruitt, J.S. (1995). Methodological considerations in training listeners to perceive nonnative phonemes. In W. Strange (Ed.), *Speech perception and linguistic experience: Theoretical and methodological issues in cross-language speech research* (pp. 351–377). Timonium, MD: York Press.

Macmillan, N.A. & Creelman, C.D. (2005). *Detection theory: A user's guide* (2nd ed.). Mahwah, NJ: Erlbaum.

Matějka, P., Glembek, O., Novotný, O., Plchot, O., Grézl, F., Burget, L., & Cernocký, J. H. (2016, March). Analysis of DNN approaches to speaker identification. In *2016 IEEE international conference on acoustics, speech and signal processing (ICASSP)* (pp. 5100–5104). IEEE.

MATLAB. (2010). *version 7.10.0 (R2010a)*. Natick, Massachusetts: The MathWorks Inc.

McMurray, B., Clayards, M. A., Tanenhaus, M. K., & Aslin, R. N. (2008). Tracking the time course of phonetic cue integration during spoken word recognition. *Psychonomic bulletin & review, 15*(6), 1064–1071.

Miller, G.A. & Nicely P. E. (1955). An analysis of perceptual confusions among some English consonants. *Journal of the Acoustical Society of America, 27*(2): 338–352.

Moskowitz, H.R. (1977). Magnitude estimation: Notes on what, how, when, and why to use it. *Journal of Food Quality, 1*(3), 195–227.

Pisoni, D.B. (1973). Auditory and phonetic memory codes in the discrimination of consonants and vowels. *Perception and Psychophysics, 13*, 253–260.

Pisoni, D.B. & Tash, J. (1974). Reaction times to comparisons within and across phonetic categories. *Perception and Psychophysics, 15*, 285–290.

Repp, B.H. (1984). Categorical perception: Issues, methods, findings. In *Speech and language (Vol. 10*, pp. 243–335). Elsevier.

Simpson, S.A. & Cooke, M. (2005). Consonant identification in N-talker babble is a nonmonotonic function of N. *The Journal of the Acoustical Society of America, 118*(5), 2775–2778.

Speech recognition and speech synthesis

35

AUTOMATIC SPEECH RECOGNITION IN THE ASSESSMENT OF CHILD SPEECH

Loridana Buttigieg, Helen Grech, Simon G. Fabri,
James Attard, and Philip Farrugia

Introduction

Speech sound disorders (SSD) is an umbrella term referring to any difficulty or combination of difficulties with perception, motor production or phonological representation of speech sounds and speech segments (ASHA, 2020). SSD can be organic or functional in nature (ASHA, 2020): functional SSD refer to idiopathic disorders while organic SSD have a known cause, often reflecting anatomical, physiological or neurological deficits.

Speech language pathologists (SLPs) are trained to make use of phonetic transcription to record and evaluate their clients' speech production abilities (McLeod & Verdon 2017; Ray, 2014). The International Phonetic Alphabet (IPA) (International Phonetic Association, revised to 2005) is used to transcribe the clients' speech in terms of the place and manner of articulation. It is critically important that SLPs who assess and treat SSD and researchers who study children's speech production, make accurate judgments and measures of children's speech (Munson, Schellinger & Carlson, 2012).

Since manual phonetic transcriptions have been reported to be time-consuming, costly and prone to error (Cucchiarini & Strik, 2003), automatic procedures have the potential to offer a quicker, cheaper and more accurate alternative (Van Bael, Boves, van den Heuvel & Strik, 2007). In fact, researchers have been investigating ways of automating the process of phonetic transcriptions, for example by utilizing speech recognition algorithms and automatic speech recognition (ASR) systems (Cucchiarini & Strik, 2003). ASR refers to the process by which a machine recognizes and acts upon an individual's spoken utterance (Young & Mihailidis, 2010). An ASR system typically consists of a microphone, computer, speech recognition software and some type of audio, visual or action output (Young & Mihailidis, 2010). The automatic conversion of speech to text is one of the most popular ASR applications (Young & Mihailidis, 2010). ASR systems require algorithms to analyse pauses between syllables, relative syllable stress between strong and weak syllables and phonemic accuracy devices which recognize the child's speech as correct or incorrect.

ASR of adults' speech has improved significantly lately, yet less progress has been made in recognizing the speech of young children (Shivakumar, Potamianos, Lee & Narayanan, 2014; Yeung & Alwan, 2018). In fact, ASR for children is still a poorly understood area (Benzeghiba et al., 2007; Yeung & Alwan, 2018), particularly because children's speech is highly variable. Children's voices and speech differ through development and across age groups (Gong et al. (2016). Additionally, both the pronunciation and rate of speech of children differ immensely from those of adults (Gong et al., 2016; Knowles et al., 2015). It has been shown that children younger than 10 exhibit more variations in vowel durations and larger suprasegmental features (Benzeghiba et al., 2007). Consequently, many existing speech recognition algorithms based on adults may not transfer well to children (Gerosa, Giuliani & Brugnara, 2007). The high variability in the typical children's speech suggests that differentiating children with impairments from those who are typically developing is a much more challenging task (Gong et al., 2016).

ASR data collected in the Maltese context

ASR technology for Maltese remains under-resourced (Gatt, 2018). A group of Maltese researchers are currently involved in a project called "Maltese Automatic Speech Recognition" (MASRI). As part of this project, researchers are creating speech corpora for the Maltese language and investigating different data augmentation techniques (MASRI, 2020). This, however, is meant to be used by the general public and not for clinical purposes. Another group of Maltese researchers, who worked on the "SPEECHIE" project, have investigated the use of an ASR system with both monolingual and bilingual typically developing Maltese children and others receiving speech and language therapy services in Malta (SPEECHIE, 2020). The objective of the SPEECHIE project was to design an assessment and therapeutic smart device, named "Olly Speaks," in the form of a toy that will support young children with speech and language impairment to be better communicators (SPEECHIE, 2020). A robust ASR system needed to be designed for "Olly Speaks" in order to recognize the words produced by young children and to detect any varieties from the adult target form, mainly substitutions, insertions and deletions of phonemes (i.e. for automatic phonetic transcription – APT) (Attard, 2018).

Currently, the Maltese and English Speech Assessment (MESA) (Grech, Dodd, & Franklin, 2011) is the only standardized manual assessment available for clinicians working in Malta to assess and review the speech of monolingual and bilingual Maltese children presenting with SSD. The SR system that was designed included words from the MESA, whereby a clinician administered the assessment specifically to validate the constructed ASR system for Maltese bilingual children. This comprised a total of 37 different phonemes, including the "SIL" phoneme (representing the silence before and after a word), and a total of 43 English words and 42 Maltese words. The system used a Hidden Markov Model (HMM) to recognize children's speech (Attard, 2018). A number of possible pronunciation errors for each word were identified and the list of combinations increased the number of words from a total of 85 to 463 words.

ASR systems require multiple recordings in order to train acoustic models and HMM parameters (Venkatagiri, 2002). Although Maltese phonemes can be associated with those of other languages, the pronunciation is quite unique, given the local bilingual context. Hence, using a corpus from another language was not possible as it does not serve as a good acoustic model representation. A speech corpus was therefore created by recording Maltese children producing vocabulary from the MESA assessment. In this study, due to logistical and time-constraint reasons, the speech corpus that could be practically collected for the purpose of training and testing of the ASR system was limited to a relatively short recording time of 1 hour 22 minutes in total. The ASR system designed by Attard (2018) was installed on an android application for the purpose of data collection. This system was coded as an Android application and implemented in an embedded device incorporating a touch-sensitive screen (see Figure 35.1). Since the ultimate aim was to amalgamate the system to "Olly Speaks",

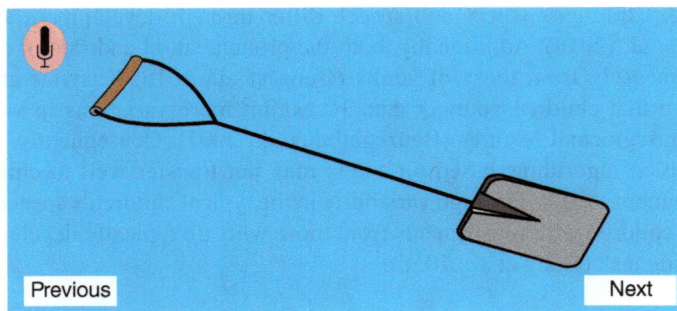

Figure 35.1 Android application used to train the ASR system.

the system was designed on the basis of isolated word recognition following picture naming (one word per picture) by the child.

A study was carried out (Buttigieg, 2019) to evaluate the ASR system that was designed explicitly to capture picture naming of children during the administration of the MESA. The aim of this study was to compare the automatic derived transcriptions to the phonetic transcriptions derived from a human expert (i.e. a qualified SLP). For this purpose, the administrator transcribed the speech production of the young participants during the testing procedure, whilst the software was simultaneously analyzing their performance and generating APT. The ultimate research question that was addressed by this study was meant to answer how accurate the novel Maltese-English ASR system is in comparison to the human expert. More specifically, the researchers needed to check the sensitivity and specificity of the ASR system during the initial assessment as well as whether the system proved to be more specific and sensitive following algorithm improvements.

For this study, a group of typically-developing (TD) children and another group of children with SSD were recruited (27 children in total). Their age ranged between 2;0 and 8;0 years old (developmental age) and they were Maltese and/or English speaking children residing in Malta. The participants were reported by the parents not to have significant neurodevelopmental disorder, cognitive difficulties or problems with hearing acuity. More than half of the sample population (52%) had a diagnosis of SSD and thus formed part of the clinical group, whilst 48% of the sample population did not have a diagnosis of SSD and did not receive speech therapy services. These were therefore part of the TD group. Out of the 27 children that were recruited, 19 children (70%) were reported to use Maltese only at home. Only 4% of the sample (i.e. one participant) was reported to use English only at home. The rest of the participants (26%) were reported to speak both Maltese and English at home. The majority of the children (89%) were reported to have Maltese as their primary language, whilst only 11% of the children were primarily English speaking.

All participants were assessed by a SLP using the designed android application. Participants of the study were shown (1) 42 pictures from the MESA sub-test of articulation, (2) 42 pictures from the MESA sub-test of phonology and (3) 17 pictures from the consistency sub-test of the MESA, on the android application. Children were prompted to label the images displayed on the screen, using either Maltese or English. As the child produced the word, the administrator pressed the "record" button and the child's responses were recorded. Their responses were automatically recognized by the system and a manual phonetic transcription of their responses was completed by the administrator of the test. Twenty-two participants (79% of the original sample population) went through the procedure again on another occasion. Children's responses for each word were recorded and the administrator transcribed each word using the IPA format. The android application recognized the speech characteristics of the individual recordings and converted speech to text. Following the initial assessment, the engineer who designed the system included the words that were not part of the possible errors combinations and that were produced by children during the initial assessment, in the corpus of the SR system.

The recognized words of both the initial sessions and the reassessment sessions were organized in a list. These phonetic transcriptions were compared to those written by the administrator. In order to determine the accuracy of the ASR system, the results of each transcribed word were categorized in four types: (1) true positive (TP), (2) true negative (TN), (3) false positive (FP) and (4) false negative (FN). Those words that were recognized as being mispronounced by both the ASR system and the administrator were marked as TP. The words that were recognized as being pronounced correctly by both the ASR system and the administrator were categorized as TN. Those words that were recognized as being mispronounced by the ASR system and pronounced correctly by the administrator were considered as FP. Finally, those words that were recognized as being produced correctly by the ASR system and mispronounced by the administrator were categorized as FN. This was required to generate the sensitivity and specificity of the ASR system. Sensitivity refers to the ability of the test to identify correctly those who have a particular condition, in this case SD, whilst specificity refers to the ability of the test to identify correctly those who do not have the condition (Lalkhen & McCluskey, 2008). For the purpose of this study, sensitivity reflected the ability of the ASR system to detect mispronounced words when the child produced the word differently from the adult target word and specificity reflected the ASR's ability to detect words which were produced correctly by the child. The accuracy levels of the ASR system during the initial assessment were compared to those of the second assessment in order to determine any improvements (T1 referring to the initial assessment and T2 to re-assessment).

Those words that were marked as TP in both the initial and the reassessment session were qualitatively investigated to determine the accuracy of the ASR system at the phonemic level and not merely at the word level.

Accuracy of the ASR system in T1 and T2

In order to determine the accuracy of the Maltese ASR system, the phonetic transcriptions of the SLP (i.e. the current gold standard method) were compared to the transcriptions generated by the ASR system. Word utterances covered 2038 words in T1 and 1539 words in T2. The APT was compared to the manual transcriptions and then categorized as TP, FP, TN and FN to investigate the accuracy of the ASR system. The sensitivity of the ASR system was obtained for both T1 and T2 to determine the system's ability to detect mispronounced words. This was generated using the TP/(TP+FN) formula. The generated sensitivity of the ASR system was 0.631 during T1 and 0.712 during T2. The specificity of the system was also generated to understand the system's ability to recognize words that were produced correctly. The specificity was generated through the TN/(TN+FP) formula. The value of accuracy was also generated to determine the proportion of true positive results (including the true positives and the true negatives) in the selected population (Zhu, Zeng & Wang, 2010). Accuracy was calculated using the (TN + TP)/(TN+TP+FN+FP) formula. The value of accuracy obtained during T1 was 0.650 and 0.698 was obtained in T2. The receiver operation characteristics (ROC) curve was obtained by calculating the sensitivity and specificity of the ASR system and plotting sensitivity against 1-specificity (Akobeng, 2007). The ROC analysis indicated that the ASR system had poor accuracy during the initial assessment (see Table 35.1). Similar to the findings of the current result, Attard (2018)

Table 35.1 Area under the curve: Initial assessment

			95% Confidence interval	
Area	*Std. error*	*P-value*	*Lower bound*	*Upper bound*
0.642	0.016	0.000	0.612	0.673

Note: Null hypothesis: true area = 0.5

Table 35.2 Area under the curve: Reassessment

			95% Confidence interval	
Area	*Std. error*	*P-value*	*Lower bound*	*Upper bound*
0.703	0.017	0.000	0.669	0.737

Note: Null hypothesis: true area = 0.5

found that the accuracy of the same Maltese-English ASR system tested during this study is relatively poor and cannot yet be considered as an accurate system for speech recognition. Yet, Attard (2018) emphasized that despite not having good levels of accuracy, this system can be used to provide basic feedback. This study also exhibited that in spite of not being accurate as the human expert, the accuracy of the ASR system is a better detector of speech error productions than what is attributed to chance. Other researchers, such as Benzeghiba et al. (2007) and Gong et al. (2016) proved that automated SR for young children is still a poorly understood area, particularly because their speech varies immensely from one another.

As shown in Table 35.1 and Table 35.2, the area under the curve for the initial assessment was 0.642 and for the second assessment 0.703 ($p < 0.05$). This suggests a slight increase of 0.061, and whilst the initial assessment was classified as having poor accuracy, the reassessment was classified as having fair accuracy in detecting correct and incorrect production of words.

Likewise, the specificity, sensitivity and accuracy level improved slightly from the initial assessment to the reassessment, with an increase of 0.081 for sensitivity, 0.041 for specificity and 0.048 for the level of accuracy. These scores suggest that although the SLP cannot yet be replaced by the ASR system and the accuracy needs to be further improved, the slight improvement from T1 to T2 indicates that in spite of not obtaining high accuracies the system has the potential to be further improved following additional training of the corpus and the gathering of more recordings. This finding also conforms to the findings of Attard (2018) who found that the average accuracy improved from one session to another, indicating that having more recordings would lead to better acoustic models. The participants of this study and those of Attard (2018) were identical, since both researchers were working concurrently on the same project. Such an agreement in findings could therefore be predicted. The findings of this study also conform to the findings of Dudy, Bedrick, Asgari, and Kain (2018) who found that the accuracy of the ASR system improved significantly through specific models aimed to improve system performance. Yet, Dudy et al. (2018) stated that further training is required to improve the performance of the system and to approach the performance of the human expert, which findings are similar to those of the current study. Contrastively, Maier et al. (2009) showed that significant correlations between the automatic analysis and the analysis of the human expert was found for the system which was tested on adults who had their larynx removed due to cancer and on children with a cleft lip and palate. The correlations were found to be comparable to the human inter-rater.

Such findings differ from findings of the current study. It should however be noted that Maier et al.'s reported system was tested on a much larger sample size than what was included for the system of this study and a variety of dialects were included. Also, it took a span of 6 years for data to be collected in the latter study. These differences amongst the 2 studies explain the variation in the outcomes of both studies.

Qualitative investigation and phonetic analysis of APT

For the system to be highly accurate and useful, it should not only recognize words as being mispronounced but also transcribe the words accurately at the phonemic level, allowing the SLP to identify any particular speech sound errors and to explore the child's phonetic and phonemic repertoire and his/her phonological errors. For this reason, the APT of the words classified as TP were analyzed in further detail. This was done to determine whether the words that were correctly identified by the ASR system as being mispronounced, were correctly transcribed at a phonemic level.

Out of the 251 TP results of the initial assessment, 118 words were automatically transcribed and identical to the administrator's manual phonetic transcription. The other 133 words were transcribed differently by the ASR system. This indicates that approximately half of the words that were categorized as being true positives (i.e. 47.01%) were recognized and transcribed accurately by the ASR system. The other approximate half (i.e. 52.99%), although identified as being mispronounced, were not transcribed accurately by the ASR system and at times these were different from those produced by the child and hence transcribed by the SLP. Similar results were obtained in T2. Out of the 200 TP results of T2, 97 words (48.5% of the words) were transcribed accurately so that the ASR system was in agreement with the manual transcriptions. Yet, the other 51.5% of the words (i.e.103 words of 200), although recognized as being mispronounced by the ASR system, were transcribed differently from the manual transcriptions provided by the administrator. These results suggest that the system is not yet highly accurate at the phonetic level. The APT varied from the manual phonetic transcription in three main ways: (1) at a phonemic level, (2) syllabic level and (3) word level. The inaccuracies of the system's APT of mispronounced words could be clustered into six main groups. These are: (1) insertion/addition of a phoneme, (2) insertion/addition of a syllable, (3) substitution of a phoneme, (4) omission of a phoneme and (5) omission of a syllable. Table 35.3 demonstrates an example of each type and the total number of occurrences in both the initial assessment (T1) and the reassessment (T2) sessions.

Table 35.3 The types of ASR inaccuracies

ASR inaccuracies	Manual transcription	ASR transcription	Total in T1	Total in T2
Insertion of a phoneme *e.g. addition of /l/*	dʒɛ	dʒɛl:	26	16
Insertion of a syllable *e.g. addition of /ɪn/*	kantau	ɪnkantaʊ	3	1
Substitution of a phoneme *e.g. k→g*	sɪnkɪ	sɪngɪ	105	88
Omission of a phoneme *e.g. omission of /l/*	rafjʊl	ravjʊ	23	22
Omission of a syllable *e.g. omission of /an/*	anʔbuta	ʔbʊta	2	2
A complete different word *e.g. 'banju' (in English, 'bath') → 'balloon'*	banju	bɛjʊn	22	18

This finding confirms the affirmation that the ASR system cannot yet replace the gold standard method (i.e. the traditional SLP's role). Duenser et al. (2016) reported that most of the existing ASR systems focus on the word or sentence level and not much on the phonemic level. Similarly to the system investigated in this study, the ASR system of Duenser et al. (2016) aimed to focus at the phonemic level. In their study, Duenser et al. (2016) found that through the use of adequate models, phoneme classification for disordered speech is possible even though it is not highly accurate. The current study exhibited that the Maltese-English speech recognition (SR) system detected phonemic errors accurately for approximately half of the mispronounced words that were recognized as being produced incorrectly by the system. Yet, errors at the phonemic level were not detected correctly by the SR system for the other half. This also suggests that despite having a low accuracy rate, recognition at the phonemic level can be further improved if more recordings are collected and hence if the overall accuracy of the system is improved.

Other studies, such as that of Meyer, Wächter, Brand, and Kollmeier, (2007), found that when comparing the performance of an ASR to a human speech recognition (HSR), HSR led to better accuracies than the ASR system under equivalent conditions. This study also found that the performance of the human expert's recognition was superior to that of the ASR system during both T1 and T2.

Conclusion

This study was the first of its kind in Malta and its findings have set the path for a new era in the provision of speech and language therapy in Malta. Based on the results outlined above, the Maltese ASR system is less accurate than the human expert is, and accuracy at the phone level is particularly low. Hence, more efforts to improve the Maltese-English ASR system are required and more recordings need to be collected to train the ASR system more extensively. Despite this, results have shown that the system has the potential to be developed even further in order to assist SLPs in the assessment of young children and the generation of APT within the clinical context. Furthermore, in the future, the ASR system may also be amalgamated with therapy games, in which it provides feedback to the young clients, serving to be more interesting for the child. This therefore shows the importance of further improving the system and its word and phonemic error rates.

Acknowledgements

This work was supported by the Malta Council for Science and Technology (MCST), through the FUSION Technology Development Programme 2016 (R&I-2015-042-T). The authors would like to thank all the volunteers for participating in this study. Special thanks go to Ing. Emanuel Balzan who developed the device Olly Speaks to which it is planned to link the on-line MESA.

References

Akobeng, A. K. (2007). Understanding diagnostic tests 3: receiver operating characteristic curves. *Acta paediatrica*, *96*(5), 644–647.

American Speech-Language-Hearing Association (ASHA). (2020). Speech sound disorders: articulation and phonology. Practice Portal. nd. Accessed April, 2020 from: https://www.asha.org/PRPSpecificTopic.aspx?folderid=8589935321&section=Roles_and_Responsibilities

Attard, J. (2018). A speech recognition system for SPEECHIE: A device supporting children with language impairment. Unpublished master's dissertation. University of Malta, Malta.

Benzeghiba, M., De Mori, R., Deroo, O., Dupont, S., Erbes, T., Jouvet, D., ... & Rose, R. (2007). Automatic speech recognition and speech variability: A review. *Speech Communication, 49*(10–11), 763–786.

Buttigieg, L. (2019). *Facilitating the assessment and analysis of child's speech in the Maltese context,* Master's Dissertation, University of Malta.

Cucchiarini, C. & Strik, H. (2003). Automatic phonetic transcription: An overview. In *Proceedings of ICPHS* (pp. 347–350).

Duenser, A., Ward, L., Stefani, A., Smith, D., Freyne, J., Morgan, A. & Dodd, B. (2016). Feasibility of technology enabled speech disorder screening. *Studies in Health Technology and Informatics, 227,* 21–27.

Dudy, S., Bedrick, S., Asgari, M. & Kain, A. (2018). Automatic analysis of pronunciations for children with speech sound disorders. *Computer Speech & Language, 50,* 62–84.

Gatt, A. (2018). Maltese Speech Recognition. *The Malta Business Weekly.* Retrieved April, 2020 from https://www.pressreader.com/malta/the-malta-business-weekly/20180628/281719795321176

Gerosa, M., Giuliani, D. & Brugnara, F. (2007). Acoustic variability and automatic recognition of children's speech. *Speech Communication, 49*(10–11), 847–860.

Gong, J.J., Gong, M., Levy-Lambert, D., Green, J. R., Hogan, T. P. & Guttag, J. V. (2016, October). Towards an automated screening tool for developmental speech and language impairments. In *INTERSPEECH* (pp. 112–116).

Grech, H., Dodd, B. & Franklin, S. (2011). *Maltese-English speech assessment (MESA). Msida, Malta: University of Malta.*

International Phonetic Association. (2005). The International Phonetic Alphabet (Revised to 2005). *Retrieved* 1 January, 2011.

Knowles, T., Clayards, M., Sonderegger, M., Wagner, M., Nadig, A. & Onishi, K. H. (November, 2015). Automatic forced alignment on child speech: Directions for improvement. In *Proceedings of Meetings on Acoustics 170ASA* (Vol. 25, No. 1, p. 060001). Acoustical Society of America.

Lalkhen, A. G. & McCluskey, A. (2008). Clinical tests: Sensitivity and specificity. *Continuing Education in Anaesthesia Critical Care & Pain, 8*(6), 221–223.

Maier, A., Haderlein, T., Eysholdt, U., Rosanowski, F., Batliner, A., Schuster, M. & Nöth, E. (2009). PEAKS–A system for the automatic evaluation of voice and speech disorders. *Speech Communication, 51*(5), 425–437.

MASRI (2020). Maltese Automatic Speech Recognition. Retrieved April, 2020 from https://www.um.edu.mt/projects/masri/

McLeod, S. & Verdon, S. (2017). Tutorial: Speech assessment for multilingual children who do not speak the same language(s) as the speech-language pathologist. *American Journal of Speech-Language Pathology,* 1–18.

Meyer, B. T., Wächter, M., Brand, T. & Kollmeier, B. (2007). Phoneme confusions in human and automatic speech recognition. Presented at *Eighth Annual Conference of the International Speech Communication Association.* Antwerp, Belgium, August 27–31, 2007.

Munson, B., Schellinger, S. K. & Carlson, K. U. (2012). Measuring speech-sound learning using visual analog scaling. *Perspectives on Language Learning and Education, 19*(1), 19–30.

Ray, A. (2014). Phonetic transcription for speech language pathologists: A Practice Manual. Retrieved from http://www.linguaakshara.org/yahoo_site_admin/assets/docs/PTSLP_MANUAL_for_Lingua_Akshara.6363003.pdf

Shivakumar, P. G., Potamianos, A., Lee, S. & Narayanan, S. (September, 2014). Improving speech recognition for children using acoustic adaptation and pronunciation modeling. In *WOCCI* (pp. 15–19).

SPEECHIE (2020). Speaking.Loud.And.Clear. Retrieved April, 2020, from https://www.um.edu.mt/projects/speechie/

Van Bael, C., Boves, L., Van Den Heuvel, H. & Strik, H. (2007). Automatic phonetic transcription of large speech corpora. *Computer Speech & Language, 21*(4), 652–668.

Venkatagiri, H. S. (2002). Speech recognition technology applications in communication disorders. *American Journal of Speech-Language Pathology, 11*(4), 323–332.

Yeung, G., & Alwan, A. (September, 2018). On the Difficulties of Automatic Speech Recognition for Kindergarten-Aged Children. In *INTERSPEECH* (pp. 1661–1665).

Young, V. & Mihailidis, A. (2010). Difficulties in automatic speech recognition of dysarthric speakers and implications for speech-based applications used by the elderly: A literature review. *Assistive Technology, 22*(2), 99–112.

36

CLINICAL APPLICATIONS
OF SPEECH SYNTHESIS

Martine Smith and John Costello

Introduction

Roughly 0.5% of the population have such difficulties producing speech that is intelligible to others that they require some way of augmenting or replacing their natural speech (Creer, Enderby, Judge, & John, 2016). This group includes children with developmental conditions such as cerebral palsy, who may never produce speech that can be understood even by their parents; it also includes young people and adults who lose the ability to speak, sometimes abruptly (e.g. post brain injury) and sometimes gradually due to neurodegenerative illnesses such as Motor Neurone Disease (MND)/Amyotrophic Lateral Sclerosis (ALS). For all these individuals, synthetic speech offers a potential opportunity to participate as a speaker in social interactions, to gain or regain a voice and to represent themselves as individuals in their speech community. Over recent years, synthetic speech has found its way into routine technologies, including navigation systems, gaming platforms, utility company service supports and a host of other industries. It is easy to assume that replacing natural speech with synthetic speech should be straightforward, but such an assumption underestimates the complexity of the contribution that natural spoken voice makes to communication, as well as the role it plays in identity formation and social participation.

The production of human speech is both complex and rapid. The speaker must decide what to say, how to say it and modulate that *how* in order to achieve a specific communicative goal. Each speaker generates a unique and personal voice, and each message uttered carries features specific to that moment of production. Although the linguistic content of the message spoken is represented by the articulated form spoken, the communicative intent of that message is carried in other acoustic features of the speech signal, as well as through aspects of nonverbal communication. The same sounds or words uttered with different intonation, pacing or stress can convey quite different intents. Given the complexity of these multiple layers of activity, replicating these processes using technology has presented many challenges.

Individuals with severe impairments often need to augment their speech using a broad range of strategies and tools, all of which come under the umbrella term of augmentative and alternative communication (AAC). Within these tools, devices that produce synthetic speech (variously termed Voice Output Communication Aids, VOCAs, or Speech Generating Devices, SGDs) can play an important role. The rest of this chapter considers current clinical applications of speech synthesis, recognizing that high-tech communication devices represent only one component of rich multi-modal communication systems for individuals who use AAC. We start with some key concepts and a very brief review of how speech synthesis has evolved over the past decades.

Terminology and the historical context

Digitized speech is a recorded sample of natural speech that is transformed into a digitized format. Once recorded, content can be stored, replayed, segmented and reconfigured. If high quality recording equipment is used, digitized speech can be almost indistinguishable acoustically from natural speech. On the other hand, what can be replayed (i.e. "spoken") is restricted to the content that has been recorded, making unplanned, spontaneous comments impossible. Synthetic speech, by contrast, is computer-generated, using algorithms. Although some very early "speech machines" produced at the end of the eighteenth century could produce single phonemes, the VODER presented by Homer Dudley in 1939 is often regarded as the first synthesizer capable of producing continuous human speech electronically (Delić et al., 2019). Speech sounds were generated using a special keyboard, essentially the basis of what is known as a text-to-speech (TTS) procedure, now ubiquitous in speech synthesis. The advantage of a TTS system is that, unlike with digitized speech, there are no constraints on what can be generated in text and therefore what can be "spoken." However, a disadvantage is that text is composed of distinct units—letters and words with discrete boundaries, unlike the fluid acoustic wave form of continuous speech. As a consequence, early speech synthesizers sounded very robotic and unnatural. Much of the early work in speech synthesis focused on achieving a more human-sounding speech output. The emergence of Dennis Klatt's DECTalk synthesizer in 1976 heralded a new era of speech technologies. DECTalk was pioneering in that it incorporated sentence-level phonology into the algorithms used to generate speech (e.g. Klatt, 1987), thereby capturing some of the features of coarticulation so fundamental in speech production and it offered a range of different voices (male, female and child versions; see https://acousticstoday.org/klatts-speech-synthesis-d/ for some recorded examples of these early voices). From the outset, Klatt was interested in the application of this technology to support those with disabilities. The most widely-used DECTalk voice, *Perfect Paul*, based on Klatt's own voice, became best known as the voice of Stephen Hawking, the renowned theoretical physicist who died in 2018.

Since the emergence of DECTalk, both the technology underpinning speech synthesis as well as the applications in which it is now embedded have changed fundamentally. Boundaries between assistive and mainstream technology have blurred. The divisions between pre-recorded digitized speech and text-to-speech synthesis have shifted. Most modern speech synthesizers are based on extensive recorded samples of natural speech. The range of synthetic voices available has expanded greatly through advances in capturing and reconfiguring natural voice data (Pullin & Hennig, 2015). Ironically, the increasingly natural-sounding synthetic voices have led to new concerns about involuntary voice capture, ethics and cyber security (Bendel, 2019; Delić et al., 2019). Despite such concerns, these advances have brought significant benefits to people with severe speech impairments.

Clinical considerations: Speech synthesis for communication

Synthetic speech and intelligibility

Clearly for any speech synthesis to be useful for functional communication, it must be intelligible to interaction partners. Historically, synthetic speech has been found to be consistently less intelligible than natural speech (Giannouli & Banou, 2019), but over recent decades there has been considerable progress in enhancing the quality of the acoustic signal. Manipulating speech rate, fundamental frequency variation and the overall duration of the acoustic wave (i.e. single words versus sentences) can all impact perceived intelligibility (Alamsaputra, Kohnert, Munson, & Reichle, 2006; Vojtech, Noordzij, Cler, & Stepp, 2019). However, intelligibility is not just a function of the speech signal: signal-independent variables, such as background noise, context and the "ear of the listener" (Beukelman & Mirenda, 2013) are equally important. Among native speakers of English, variables such as linguistic redundancy within the message generated, visual display of key words, contextual information and practice or familiarity with synthesized speech have all been found to enhance performance on intelligibility tasks (e.g. Alamsaputra et al., 2006; Koul & Clapsaddle, 2006). The language competence of the listener (particularly receptive vocabulary) is another important signal-independent variable. Young children, those with additional disabilities, and non-native speakers all perform less well on tasks involving synthetic speech (Alamsaputra et al., 2006; Drager & Reichle, 2001; Drager, Clark-Serpentine, Johnson, & Roeser, 2006). These groups are also more impacted by background noise, the complexity of the intelligibility task and extraneous distractions. These differences are not insignificant. Young children acquiring language using SGDs may abstract less information from the acoustic signal of synthetic speech than adults, making it more difficult for them to determine if the message generated matches the intended target and providing them with less rich phonological and phonetic information. They may also be more vulnerable to the impact of background noise in a busy classroom when they are using their SGDs. This difference may partly explain the inconsistent findings on the benefits of providing speech output in supporting literacy skills and in enhancing graphic symbol acquisition (Koul & Schlosser, 2004; Schlosser & Blischak, 2004). The low-paid status of many caring roles means that personal assistants employed to support people who rely on AAC are often migrant workers, for whom the intelligibility of synthetic speech may exacerbate other communication barriers related to linguistic competence.

Prosody and naturalness in synthetic speech

Even if synthesized speech is intelligible, inferring what others really *mean* by what they say involves more than decoding the words that have been uttered. Communicative intent is largely expressed through vocal tone, volume, intonation and stress. Natural voice can convey a speaker's personal state, regardless of the words spoken (think of the multiple meanings of "*I'm fine*"), and can even reveal information on health status (Podesva & Callier, 2015). Capturing these features using synthetic speech is particularly challenging in spontaneous utterances, constructed in-the-moment, in response to a specific communicative situation. Prosody allows speech to be intelligible, but also to sound natural. Without access to intonation or stress, individuals who rely on SGDs cannot easily express irony, humor, sarcasm, frustration or sadness. For natural speakers, calling someone's name in a particular tone of voice simultaneously attracts attention and gives an indication as to whether simply responding "*I'm here*" is sufficient or whether urgent assistance is needed (see also Pullin & Hennig, 2015). Without access to prosodic cues, these distinctions must be expressed through words, requiring far greater effort of the speaker – but also of the listener, who must interpret what has been said. Most work on incorporating prosody into synthetic speech involves generating algorithms based on linguistic rules or inferences about phrase structure from a source text, or through voice conversion, where linguistic content is mapped onto target spectral and prosodic features of a given natural voice (Vojtech, Noordzij, Cler, & Stepp, 2019). However, such systems work optimally when there is adequate grammatical information available, unlike the output of many individuals who use aided communication (e.g. von Tetzchner, 2018). While it may be possible to develop an interface that allows a user to directly control prosody, explicitly manipulating prosody may come at a cost of user effort, in what is already an exceptionally effortful communication process.

Speech naturalness allows listeners to focus on the meaning of the message, but also impacts on the extent to which they are willing to engage with a speaker. In general, listeners have been found to prefer listening to natural speech over synthesized speech, but if natural speech is dysarthric (as is the case for many people who rely on SGDs), they may switch preference to synthesized speech (Stern, Chobany, Patel, & Tressler, 2014). Such preferences are complicated by factors such as the listener's familiarity with the speaker, the nature of the interaction and even simply knowing that the speaker has a disability. Listeners are predisposed to make judgements about a speaker based on vocal characteristics and so vocal quality is important not only for communication but also for social identity.

Clinical considerations: Voice, identity, and speech synthesis

Each individual's voice represents their unique acoustic fingerprint (Costello, 2000) and a core part of their identity (Nathanson, 2017). That aspect of identity is important to self, but is also important in building and maintaining social connections (McGettigan, 2015). Familiar voices have a unique impact on listeners who have a personal relationship with that speaker (Sidtis & Kreiman, 2012), capable of instantly evoking a whole range of emotions. Hearing a familiar voice can impact stress levels (as measured by levels of hydrocortisol) in much the same way as being in the physical presence of that person (Seltzer, Prososki, Ziegler, & Pollak, 2012).

Children who have never had the ability to produce natural speech themselves risk missing out on this core aspect of identity formation – hearing their own personal voice – as well as experiencing the changes in the acoustic properties of that voice as a tangible marker of aging. Adults who lose the ability to produce intelligible speech face a potential associated loss of identity, while their loved ones face the risk of losing this critical dimension of that person, and with it the loss of personal connection over distance. These distinctions between developmental and acquired conditions create particular sets of expectations of what a synthetic voice might offer and enable, as well as impacting the willingness of individuals to accept a voice that is not their "own."

The role of personal voice in identity raises a number of questions for individuals who rely on synthetic speech. Can a synthetic voice become "personal"? If so, what are the implications if that synthetic voice is used by others, becomes obsolete or is no longer available due to technological developments? In the 80s and early 90s, the choice of synthetic voices available for communication aids was extremely limited. Many individuals with speech impairments opted to use the same voice, regardless of their age or gender. This preference often resulted in unusual interactions where several speakers (male and female) sounded exactly the same. In one day center familiar to the first author, a blind service user became adept at identifying speakers by the pacing of speech output and the sound of switch activations unique to that speaker. Despite the fact that they were not unique owners of a particular synthetic voice, some individuals (including Stephen Hawking) became attached to that voice, perceiving it as part of their identity, and rejecting offers to upgrade to more advanced, natural voices.

For those who can use natural speech, changes in voice quality and range are most rapid and pronounced in childhood, remaining relatively stable across early and middle adulthood, with very gradual, even imperceptible change in older age (Stathopoulos, Huber, & Sussman, 2011). This pattern is in marked contrast to the step-wise changes in synthetic speech that have characterized the past decades and the abrupt and often unplanned transitions in voice that are often associated with upgrading or replacing SGDs. Individuals may start out using a child voice and in adolescence face explicit choices about transitions to a new voice that is unfamiliar to those in their environment, who may not "recognize" their voice. Furthermore, despite technical advances, available voice types continue to largely reflect gender norms with US or British standardized accents for English-language synthesizers. Alan Martin, a long-time user of an SGD commented, "Although I now have an English male voice, I sound more like a BBC news reader than the 'Scouser' that is the real ME" (Martin & Newell, 2013, p. 99) (see https://www.youtube.com/watch?v=xsqInns6LXQ where Lee Ridley comments on the familiarity of his voice because of the listeners' experience of automated train timetable announcements). The aspiration of capturing the unique nuances of individual voices so that individuals can express their identity is still a work in progress.

Voice banking, message banking, and double dipping

Two innovations in speech technology have brought the holy grail of truly personalized voices closer: voice banking and message banking. Voice banking involves using a large number of high-quality digital recordings of an individual's speech and segmenting those recordings to generate a unique phonetic database. These phonetic segments can then be combined in novel sequences to create synthetic utterances with personalized synthesized voice that can be accessed through text-to-speech (Bunnell & Pennington, 2010; Pullin, Treviranus, Patel, & Higginbotham, 2017). To complete this process, individuals register with a voice banking service and using a computer with internet connection, record in a quiet environment with a high-quality microphone. Up to 1600 phrases may be needed to establish a sufficiently large data set to create a personal voice. More recently, some voice banking services have applied Deep Neural Network (DNN) technology to this process; for example, Acapela® allows for a personalized voice to be created with only 50 recordings. VocalID™ (www.vocalid.com) was an early innovator in creating unique synthesized voices by combining the residual vocalization of an individual potential user and the recordings of a matched-speech donor from an extensive database (VocalID's Human Voicebank™; www.vocalid.com). This database was generated by volunteer donations of over 20,000 speakers representing a diversity of age, gender, cultures and geography (Patel & Threats, 2016; Pullin et al., 2017). More recent initiatives include SpeakUnique (www.speakunique.co.uk) where users can opt to bank their own voice, even if it is mildly dysarthric, or generate a bespoke voice, based on voices from an existing database or donors they nominate themselves.

Despite significant reductions in the quantity of recordings now required to create a bespoke personalized voice, individuals already experiencing speech deterioration may still find the demands of recording challenging, and there can be significant cost implications with some service providers. Voice banking is an important development in recognizing the unique and specific role of personal voice in maintaining identity; however, apart from cost and the physical demands of recording, even high-quality bespoke voices lack the facility to generate the intonation and prosody that characterizes natural speech and that reflects an individual's way of speaking.

In Message banking™ (Costello, 2000) the goal is not to generate a phonetically balanced recorded sample of speech to re-construct, but rather to capture recordings of phrases, sayings and utterances that reflect the identity and personality of the speaker. Because the emphasis is on messages rather than on words, aspects such as intonation, phrasing and emotional content are key. There are no specific constraints on the quantity of messages needed, as the focus is not on deconstructing and reconstructing the messages. Each recorded message is stored in a specific location on a speech-generating device (SGD). Message banking is a collaborative process involving individuals at risk of losing their speech, their loved ones and their clinician. The goal is to capture that person's unique ways of speaking, their individual turns of phrase, so they can utter important messages in their own unique way (for demonstrations, see https://tinyurl.com/messagebankingprocessvideos).

Typically, individuals who use Message banking™ combine their use of these recorded messages with conventional TTS-based synthetic speech output. Double dipping™, a recent innovation pioneered by the Augmentative Communication Program at Boston Children's Hospital in collaboration with a range of partners, uses recorded messages that were completed through message banking as the script for creating a synthetic voice. The option of using one effort for both purposes (i.e. "double dipping") eliminates the need to choose which process to complete or whether to expend additional energy to complete each process separately. Successful Double dipping™ ideally requires 750 or more banked messages of sufficient quality as a database source. As one example, using their My-Own-Voice™, Acapela® uses audio files of an individual's banked messages from MyMessagebanking.com to create a personalized synthetic voice that can be fully integrated into Windows-based or iOS-based communication technology. Dozens of high-quality, synthetic voices have been created in multiple languages using 750 or more recordings from banked messages (for an Italian example, see https://youtu.be/umGQZmvRSH8).

Conclusion

There have been remarkable advances in the intelligibility and naturalness of synthetic speech since the first SGDs were introduced. Voice banking and message banking represent complementary approaches with a common purpose, that of ensuring that individuals can continue to use their own unique voice, even if vocal quality has changed due to disease progression. Both approaches recognize the importance of voice as a marker of identity and social connection, as well as a channel for communication. The next phases of innovation in speech synthesis must address the crucial role of prosody in supporting effective communication, using interfaces that are intuitive. When synthetic speech can naturally age with a user, effectively conveys emotion and communicative intent, and is uniquely configured for each individual user, all without any additional effort on the part of the user, then it will truly be approaching the power of natural speech.

References

Alamsaputra, D. M., Kohnert, K. J., Munson, B., & Reichle, J. (2006). Synthesized speech intelligibility among native speakers and non-native speakers of English. *Augmentative and Alternative Communication, 22*(4), 258–268.

Bendel, O. (2019). The synthesization of human voices. *AI & Society, 34,* 83–89. doi:10.1007/s00146-017-0748-x

Beukelman, D. R., & Mirenda, P. (2013). *Augmentative and Alternative Communication: Supporting children and adults with complex communication needs* (4th ed.). Baltimore MD: Brookes Publishing.

Bunnell, H., & Pennington, C. (2010). Advances in computer speech synthesis and implications for assistive technology. In J. Mullennix & S. Stern (Eds.), *Computer synthesized speech technologies: Tools for aiding impairment* (pp. 71–91). Hershey, PA: IGI Global.

Costello, J. (2000). AAC intervention in the intensive care unit: The Children's Hospital Boston model. *Augmentative and Alternative Communication, 16,* 137–153.

Creer, S., Enderby, P., Judge, S., & John, A. (2016). Prevalence of people who could benefit from augmentative and alternative communication (AAC) in the UK: Determining the need. *International Journal of Language and Communication Disorders, 51,* 639–653. doi:10.1111/1460-6984.12235

Delić, V., Peric, Z., Sećujski, M., Jakovljevic, N., Nikolić, N. J., Mišković, D., … Delić, T. (2019). Speech technology progress based on new machine learning paradigm. *Computational Intelligence and Neuroscience* (Article ID 4368036), 1–19. doi:10.1155/2019/4368036

Drager, K., & Reichle, J. (2001). Effects of age and divided attention on listeners' comprehension of synthesized speech. *Augmentative and Alternative Communication, 17*(2), 109–119.

Drager, K., Clark-Serpentine, E. A., Johnson, K. E., & Roeser, J. L. (2006). Accuracy of repetition of digitized and synthesized speech for young children in background noise. *American Journal of Speech Language Pathology, 15*(2), 155–164. doi:15/2/155 [pii]10.1044/1058-0360(2006/015)

Giannouli, V., & Banou, M. (2019). The intelligibility and comprehension of synthetic versus natural speech in dyslexic students. *Disability and Rehabilitation: Assistive Technology.* doi:10.1080/174 83107.2019.1629111

Klatt, D. (1987). Review of Text-to-Speech conversion for English. *Journal of the Acoustical Society of America, 82*(3), 737–793.

Koul, R., & Clapsaddle, K. (2006). Effects of repeated listening experiences on the perception of synthetic speech by individuals with mild-moderate intellectual disabilities. *Augmentative and Alternative Communication, 22*(2), 112–122. doi:10.1080/07434610500389116

Koul, R., & Schlosser, R. (2004.). Effects of synthetic speech output on the learning of graphic symbols of varied iconicity. *Disability and Rehabilitation, 26*(21/22), 1278–1285.

Martin, A. J., & Newell, C. (2013). Living through a computer voice: A personal account. *Logopedics Phoniatrics Vocology, 38*(3), 96–104. doi:10.3109/14015439.2013.809145

McGettigan, C. (2015). The social life of voices: Studying the neural bases for the expression and perception of the self and others during spoken communication. *Frontiers in Human Neuroscience, 9*, 1–4. doi:10.3389/fnhum.2015.00129

Nathanson, E. (2017). Native voice, self-concept and the moral case for personalized voice technology. *Disability and Rehabilitation, 39*(1), 73–81. doi:10.3109/09638288.2016.1139193

Patel, R., & Threats, T. (2016). One's voice: A central component of personal factors in augmentative and alternative communication. *Perspectives of the ASHA Special Interest Groups, SIG 12*, 94–98. doi:10.1044/persp1.SIG12.94

Podesva, R., & Callier, P. (2015). Voice quality and identity. *Annual Review of Applied Linguistics, 35*, 173–194.

Pullin, G., & Hennig, S. (2015). 17 ways to say 'Yes': Toward nuanced tone of voice in AAC and speech technology. *Augmentative and Alternative Communication, 31*(2), 170–180. doi:10.3109/0743461 8.2015.1037930

Pullin, G., Treviranus, J., Patel, R., & Higginbotham, J. (2017). Designing interaction, voice, and inclusion in AAC research. *Augmentative and Alternative Communication, 33*(3), 139–148. doi:10.1080/07 434618.2017.1342690

Schlosser, R., & Blischak, D. (2004). Effects of speech and print feedback on spelling by children with autism. *Journal of Speech, Language and Hearing Research, 47*(4), 848–862.

Seltzer, L., Prososki, A., Ziegler, T., & Pollak, S. (2012). Instant messages vs speech: Why we still need to hear each other. *Evolution and Human Behavior, 33*, 42–45. doi:10.1016/j.evolhumbehav.2011.05.004

Sidtis, D., & Kreiman, J. (2012). In the beginning was the familiar voice: Personally familiar voices in evolutionary and contemporary biology of communication. *Integrative Psychological and Behavioral Science, 46*, 146–159.

Stathopoulos, E., Huber, J. E., & Sussman, J. E. (2011). Changes in acoustic characteristics of the voice across the lifespan: measures from individuals 4-93 years of age. *Journal of Speech Language Hearing Research, 54*(4), 1011–1021. doi:10.1044/1092-4388

Stern, S., Chobany, C., Patel, D., & Tressler, J. (2014). Listeners' preference for computer-synthesized speech over natural speech of people with disabilities. *Rehabilitation Psychology, 59*(3), 289–297. doi:10.1037/a0036663

Vojtech, J., Noordzij, J., Cler, G., & Stepp, C. (2019). The effects of modulating fundamental frequency and speech rate on the intelligibility, communication efficiency and perceived naturalness of synthetic speech. *American Journal of Speech-Language Pathology, 28*, 875–886. doi:10.1044/2019_AJSLP-MSC18-18-0052

von Tetzchner, S. (2018). Introduction to the special issue on aided language processes, development, and use: An international perspective. *Augmentative and Alternative Communication, 34*(1), 1–15. doi: 10.1080/07434618.2017.1422020

AUTHOR INDEX

McGettigan, C., 519
McGurk, H., 387–8
McLean, A.E., 257
McLeod, S., 96, 179, 230, 237, 342, 344, 352, 508
McManus, I., 484
McMicken, B., 381–2
McMurray, B., 47, 505
McNeil, M.R., 258
McNutt, J., 102
McWilliams, B., 84
Mefferd, A.S., 436
Mehta, D.D., 292, 294, 299, 302
Ménard, L., 407
Mendelsohn, A.H., 302
Merletti, R., 253
Messaoud-Galusi, S., 47
Meyer, B.T., 514
Meyer, J., 50–1
Meyers, J.E., 482, 487
Miceli, G., 29
Michi, K., 352
Milberg, W., 47
Mildner, V., 421, 482, 484
Miller, G.A., 504
Miller, J.D., 79
Millgård, M., 62
Milner, B., 421
Minifie, F.D., 248
Mirman, D., 47
Mohd Ibrahim, H., 326
Moll, K.L., 323, 332
Moncrieff, D.W., 482–3, 486–8
Monsen, R., 201
Moore, C.A., 258, 378
Moore, P., 282, 292
Moritani, T., 249
Morris, R.J., 21, 71
Morrison, M.D., 295
Mortensen, M., 300
Moskowitz, H.R., 500
Moulonget, A., 248
Moya-Galé, G., 258
Mra, Z., 330
Müller, N., 68, 75, 173, 175, 203, 421
Mundt, J.C., 218
Munhall, K.G., 362, 387–8, 467
Munson, B., 147, 508
Murakami, K., 48
Murdoch, B.E., 369
Murray, D.J., 484
Musiek, F., 32

Nabelek, A.K., 459
Nacci, A., 316
Nakagawa, H., 158
Nakano, K.K., 258
Narayanan, S.S., 342, 344, 375, 378

Nascimento, M.D.S.R.D., 487
Nathanson, E., 519
Natke, U., 465, 467–9
Nawka, T., 297–8, 300
Nayak, K.S., 378
Nearey, T.M., 93
Neger, T., 419
Neilson, P.D., 259
Nellis, J.L., 326, 331
Nelson, T.L., 176, 178
Nemec, R.E., 258
Nespoulous, J.L., 435
Nessel, E., 463
Neto Henriques, R., 362–5, 367
Netsell, R., 258
Neumeyer, V., 425, 436
Newby, H.A., 27
Ng, I., 377
Nguyen, N., 362
Nguyen, V.T., 326
Ni, X.G., 300
Nicolaides, K., 160, 348–9, 425, 436
Nijland, L., 45
Nittrouer, S., 428
Nixon, J.S., 137
Noffs, G., 225
Noffsinger, D., 482
Noiray, A., 401
Noordzij, J.P., 297
Nooteboom, S.G., 48
Norrelgen, F., 486
Norris, D., 47
Novak, A., 463
Nycz, J., 425
Nyquist, H., 223

O'Connor, J.D., 60, 172
O'Donnell, J.J., 469–70
Obrzut, J., 484–5, 487–8
O'Dwyer, N.J., 253–4
Ohala, J.J., 418
Ohde, R.N., 429
Öhman, S., 248
Okalidou, A., 326
Oliveira, G., 224
Oller, D.K., 144–5
Olson, K.S., 160
Oostdijk, N.H.J., 142, 146–7
Orlikoff, R.F., 311

Padareva-Ilieva, G., 434
Palethorpe, S., 421
Palmer, P.M., 254
Pantano, K., 282
Pantelemidou, V., 201–2
Papakyritsis, I., 108
Park, M., 326

SUBJECT INDEX

AAC, *see* augmentative and alternative communication
absolute (knowledge), 181
acceleration, 395
accent, 77
accredited, 175
acoustic analysis, 421–425, 431–33, 435–37
  dynamic analysis, 425, 431, 436
  spectrogram, 17–21, 24
  target analysis, 425
  types of acoustic analysis, 17–19
acoustic phonetics, 16–26, 27–8
acquisition/development, 77–8, 81–6, 229–30
active nasal air emission, 265, 278
African American English, 89, 94–96
aglossia, 381–2
airstream mechanisms, 5–7, 153
  glottalic, 7
  non-pulmonic, 153
  pulmonic, 6–7, 153
  velaric, 7
  see also non-pulmonic egressive sounds
alphabet, 153
  Greek, 153
  Latin, 153
  See also International Phonetic Alphabet
altered sensory feedback, 461
  clinical trials using sensory feedback prostheses 464–5, 468, 470–1, 474
  delayed auditory feedback, 462–65
  frequency shifted feedback, 465–71
  neuroplasticity, 470
  partial resistance to extinction effect, 464
  prostheses, 463–5, 468–70, 474
  somatosensory feedback, 461, 466, 471–3
  vibrotactile feedback, 471–4
Alzheimer's disease, 435

American English, 89, 91–97
analogue to digital conversion, 223
anatomy and physiology of the auditory system, 28–33
  acoustic reflex (AR), 32
  auditory cortex, 480
  cochlea, 30–1
  cerebral cortex, 32
  internal auditory system (IAS), 32
  organ of Corti, 30
  ossicular chain, 29–31
  otoacoustic emission (OAE), 31
  peripheral auditory system (PAS), 29–31
  tinnitus, 32–3
  tinnitus tones, 33
  tonotopy, 31
aphasia, 38, 44, 46–7, 58, 68, 91, 434–5, 487
  paraphasias, 68
aphonia, 516
  see also dysphonia
Appearance Models, 392
apraxia of speech, 18, 20, 56, 68–9, 257–63, 381–4, 407, 425, 430, 432, 434–5
  childhood apraxia of speech (CAS), 45, 70, 407, 411
approximant-r, 101–2, 105–6
  apical-r, 101–2
  bunched-r, 102
articulation, 3–15, 155
  alveolar ridge, hard palate and velum, 10
  double articulation, 12, 155
  estimation, 393
  impossible, 155
  lips and teeth, 10
  overview of, 3–5
  pharynx and glottis, 11
  secondary, 83–4, 159

tongue, 11
voiced and voiceless, 9
See also manner of articulation, place of articulation
articulator, 155
active, 155
passive, 155
articulatory phonetics, 3–15, 27
Articulograph, 358–71
AG500, 358, 359, 360, 369, 371
AG501, 358, 359, 360, 362, 369, 371
Artificial Neural Network, 392–3
assessment, 230, 237
assimilation, 41
attention, 480, 483–5, 487–9
audiogram, 445
configuration, 453, 455
interpretation, 446, 447, 451, 453
audiology, 27
medical: pediatrics, gerontology, neurology, 27
non-medical: physics, psychology, education, 27
audiometry, 34
pure tone audiometry, 444, 447–8, 455, 459
speech audiometry, 447, 455–9
auditory judgement, 156
auditory phonetics, 27
auditory-visual speech, 387–9
interference, 387
augmentative and alternative communication, 516–8

baseline competencies, 176
benchmark, 176–77, 179, 183
bilingual, 77–8, 82–5, 89–91, 96–7
biofeedback 256–62, 399, 407
biomarker
speech as, 225
botulinum toxin 256, 262–3
brackets, square, 153
breathy voice, *see* phonation

categorical perception, 45–7
group differences in, 46
in clinical research, 46–7
child speech disorders, 69–70
articulation disorders, 70
phonological disorders, 70–1
CHILDES, 228–230
see also speech corpus / corpora
cleft palate, 9, 46, 62, 65–6, 84, 102, 199–201, 264, 274, 277, 279, 315, 326, 332, 341, 346, 350–2, 376, 381–3, 407, 427, 430
clinical, 77–8, 82, 84, 86
clinical assessment, 89–93, 95–97
coarticulation, 40–44, 425, 428
anticipatory, 41
carry-over, 41
compensation for, 44
C-to-V, 425, 428

factors affecting, 42
in clinical research, 44
resistance, 42
second formant transitions, 433
V-to-C, 425, 434
window model, 43
competency/proficiency-based standards, 175
consonant articulation, 20–21, 78–84, 153
VOT (voice onset time), 20–21
oral stops, 20–21
consonant manner of articulation, 12–13
affricate, 12–13
approximant, 13
obstruent, 13
plosive, 12–13
sonorant, 13
tap/flap, 13
constructively aligned, 181, 183
cranio-facial anomalies, *see* cleft palate
creaky voice, *see* phonation
crosslinguistic, 77–86

data, *see* speech data
database, 228–30, 244
declarative knowledge, 180
deep learning, 179–81, 393
delayed auditory feedback, *see* altered sensory feedback
dementia, 435, 451
diacritic, 157, 159–60
dialect, 77–9, 82, 85–6, 89, 91–4
dichotic listening, 480–9
Stimuli for Dichotic Listening Tasks, 481–485
difference curve/surface, 126–7, 134–5
differential diagnosis, 177
digital signal processing, 418
FFT, 421, 427
PCA, 421
power spectra, 421, 427
dysarthria, 18, 21, 60, 62, 69–70, 108–11, 196
258–9, 261–2, 384, 411, 428, 434
ataxic, 20, 69–70
dyskinesia, 70
flaccid, 69
hyperkinetic, 69
hypokinetic, 69
mixed, 69
spastic, 69–70
dyslexia, 488
dysphonia, 315–6, 319
see also aphonia

ear, 29
EGG, *see* electroglottography
electrode 250–6, 259–62
intramuscular 250–1, 254–6,
monopolar 252–3
surface 251–4, 256, 260–3

For Product Safety Concerns and Information please contact our EU
representative GPSR@taylorandfrancis.com
Taylor & Francis Verlag GmbH, Kaufingerstraße 24, 80331 München, Germany

www.ingramcontent.com/pod-product-compliance
Lightning Source LLC
Chambersburg PA
CBHW072006230326
41598CB00082B/6790

* 9 7 8 0 3 6 7 3 3 6 2 8 8 *